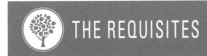

THE REQUISITES

NUCLEAR MEDICINE AND MOLECULAR IMAGING

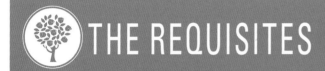

THE REQUISITES

NUCLEAR MEDICINE AND MOLECULAR IMAGING

5th EDITION

JANIS P. O'MALLEY, MD, FACR

Professor of Radiology
University of Alabama at Birmingham
Division of Molecular Imaging & Therapeutics
Birmingham, Alabama

HARVEY A. ZIESSMAN, MD

Professor of Radiology
Division of Nuclear Medicine and Molecular Imaging
The Johns Hopkins University
Baltimore, Maryland

Series Editor

JAMES H. THRALL, MD

Radiologist-in-Chief Emeritus
Massachusetts General Hospital
Distinguished Juan M. Taveras Professor of
  Radiology
Harvard Medical School
Boston, Massachusetts

ELSEVIER

Elsevier
1600 John F. Kennedy Blvd.
Ste 1800
Philadelphia, PA 19103-2899

NUCLEAR MEDICINE AND MOLECULAR IMAGING:
THE REQUISITES, 5th EDITION

ISBN: 978-0-323-530378

Library of Congress Control Number: 2019941296

Senior Content Strategist: Kayla Wolfe
Content Development Specialist: Ann R. Anderson
Publishing Services Manager: Shereen Jameel
Project Manager: Radhika Sivalingam
Designer: Brian Salisbury

Printed in India

Last digit is the print number: 9 8 7 6 5

CONTRIBUTOR

Frederic H. Fahey, DSc
Director of Nuclear Medicine/PET Physics, Department of Radiology,
    Boston Children's Hospital, Boston; Professor, Department of
    Radiology, Harvard Medical School, Boston, Massachusetts
Chapter 1: Radioactivity and Radionuclides;
Chapter 2: Radiation Detection and Ancillary Instrumentation;
Chapter 3: Single-Photon Emission Tomography, Positron Emission
Computed Tomography, and Hybrid Imaging

FOREWORD

Nuclear Medicine and Molecular Imaging: The Requisites is a new title for this well-received text now appearing its fifth edition. The change in title reflects the remarkable advances in tracer-based medical imaging that have taken place over the last two decades. These advances have clearly extended the diagnostic utility and value of nuclear medicine and molecular imaging in clinical patient care.

Predictably much of the fifth edition of *Nuclear Medicine and Molecular Imaging: The Requisites* is focused on new molecular imaging methods and the latest advances in their clinical application including positron emission tomography (PET), SPECT/CT, PET/CT and PET/MRI hybrid imaging. The intense interest in hybrid imaging provides clear recognition of the increased value now placed on functional and molecular information in disease diagnosis.

Although retitled, *Nuclear Medicine and Molecular Imaging: The Requisites* continues to follow the format of the first four editions. The basic science chapters are designed to present important principles of physics, instrumentation, and nuclear pharmacy in the context of how they help shape clinical practice. The physics content of the fifth edition has been expanded and integrated to reflect current technology. Topics on regulatory issues, radiation safety and quality control have been added as well as material on the "non-interpretive" aspects of nuclear medicine and molecular imaging practice.

The clinical chapters continue to follow a logical progression from basic principles of tracer distribution and localization to practical clinical applications. Knowledge of how radiopharmaceuticals localize temporally and spatially in normal and diseased tissues is the best deductive tool available for analyzing images. The best use of new tracers such as Ga-68 DOTA, the F-18 amyloid agents and F-18 PMSA agents requires this kind of knowledge of the underlying mechanisms of disease and therewith tracer localization.

Adding new tracers and new SPECT, PET, PET/CT, and PET/MRI applications to the nuclear medicine armamentarium has injected new, unprecedented, vitality into the specialty.

Readers of *Nuclear Medicine and Molecular Imaging: The Requisites* will feel this vitality almost palpably as they work their way through the book. In particular, PET and PET/CT have become cornerstones in cancer diagnosis and management with PET/MRI becoming more important in both cancer diagnosis and neurological studies.

The Requisites in Radiology titles have now become old friends to generations of radiologists. The original intent of the series was to provide the resident or fellow with a text that might be reasonably read within several days at the beginning of each subspecialty rotation and perhaps reread several times during subsequent rotations or during board preparation. The series is not intended to be exhaustive but rather to provide the basic conceptual, factual, and interpretive material required for clinical practice. After more than 30 years of experience with the series, it is now clear that the books are also sought out by practicing imaging specialists for the efficiency of their presentation format and the quality of their material. With more people reaching the point of requiring re-certification, the Requisites books are again proving helpful.

The first four editions of *Nuclear Medicine and Molecular Imaging: The Requisites* were well received in the radiology and nuclear medicine community. For the retitled fifth edition, Dr. Janis M. O'Malley and Dr. Harvey A. Ziessman have again done a terrific job in putting together this substantially updated edition. Congratulations to them. I expect that this fifth edition will be deemed to be even more outstanding than its predecessors.

We hope that *Nuclear Medicine and Molecular Imaging: The Requisites* will serve residents in radiology as a concise and useful introduction to the subject and will also serve as a very manageable text for review by fellows and practicing nuclear medicine specialists and radiologists.

James H. Thrall, MD
Radiologist-in-Chief Emeritus, Massachusetts General Hospital
Distinguished Juan M. Taveras Professor of Radiology, Harvard
Medical School, Boston, Massachusetts

PREFACE TO THE 5TH EDITION OF THE REQUISITES, NUCLEAR MEDICINE

This is the 5th edition of *Nuclear Medicine: The Requisites*. However, we are now titled *Nuclear Medicine and Molecular Imaging: The Requisites*. We are deeply indebted to Dr. James H. Thrall for developing the concept of the Requisite series and his involvement as a coauthor of *Nuclear Medicine: The Requisites* for the first four editions, in 1995, 2001, 2006, and 2014. Since the last edition, there have been many exciting changes in the field, particularly concerning new PET agents and therapy techniques. The 5th edition builds on the success of the prior editions, providing a concise, easy to read review that is suitable not only for radiology and nuclear medicine residents and fellows preparing for their service rotations or board exams but also serves a useful tool for those in practice at all levels of expertise, particularly when targeting knowledge gaps during maintenance of board certification reviews.

All chapters have been significantly updated and contain numerous stunning new images. The first section of the book is again devoted to technical matters: basic principles and concepts of radiation production, instrumentation and detection, radiopharmaceuticals and quality control, radiation safety, and regulatory matters. New topics have been introduced including PET/MR, and important facts the Authorized Users of radiopharmaceuticals are highlighted. The second section of the book is focused on clinical imaging and therapy, emphasizing physiological mechanisms and pharmacokinetics. Because of the rapid progress in oncology, particularly in the areas of prostate cancer and neuroendocrine tumor imaging and treatment, these section have been extensively updated with important details on the use of newly approved imaging and therapy agents highlighted. The popular chapter, "Pearls, Pitfalls, and Frequently Asked Questions," again provides an excellent concluding summary. Protocols and key facts are again organized in many boxes and tables for easy identification.

Over the years, it has been an honor to help guide and train the most incredibly gifted physicians and introduce them to the incredible field of nuclear medicine. Our students have also taught us a lot along the way, and their feedback has been essential as we continue to strive to improve as educators. In addition, hearing from colleagues around the globe how the text has helped them or their trainees has been another wonderful way to continue developing new material. Hopefully, our experiences are reflected here and provide a foundation for another successful text.

ACKNOWLEDGEMENTS

We would like to thank those who have contributed to the preparation of this book. Selected images were provided by: Suzanne Lapi, PhD; Kirk Fry, MD, PhD; Jonathon McConathy, MD, PhD; Steven P Rowe, MD, Bital Savir Baruch MD, Corina M Millo, MD; Khun Visith Keu, MD; Lauren L Radford, PhD; Mark Muzi, PhD; Les Foto; Farrokh Dehdashti, MD; and Hong-gang Liu. Hong-gang Liu also produced some of graphics in animated images. Suzy Lapi and Jon McConathy helped with editing the chapters on brain imaging and Molecular Imaging.

We would also like to thank our spouses and family for all their support during our work on each of these editions.

Janis O'Malley thanks her mom, Lanis Petrik.

CONTENTS

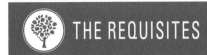

THE REQUISITES

NUCLEAR MEDICINE AND MOLECULAR IMAGING

Radioactivity and Radionuclides

In nuclear medicine, radiopharmaceuticals given to the patient emit the radiation used to create images or perform therapy. In order to understand how these agents perform and what safety considerations are involved in their use, it is necessary to be familiar with some basic aspects of the physics behind radioactive decay. This chapter discusses radioactive molecules, different types of radioactive decay, and how these emissions interact with matter.

ATOMIC STRUCTURE OF MATTER

Electronic Structure of the Nucleus

All matter is made up of atoms, which in turn are made up of protons, electrons, and neutrons. Positively charged protons and uncharged neutrons have a similar mass and are known as nucleons because they are located in the nucleus. Although much less massive, electrons orbiting the nucleus possess an opposite negative charge equal in magnitude to that of the protons (Table 1.1). Some properties of atomic particles are listed, along with important constant values, in Table 1.2.

The attraction of the opposite charges keeping the electron in orbit around the nucleus is known as an electrostatic force (or coulombic force; the coulomb is the unit for electric charge). On the other hand, there is also a repulsive, electrostatic force in the nucleus from the like-charged protons pushing apart. The nucleus is held together by the attractive *strong nuclear force* each nucleon exerts on the other nucleons. Although more powerful than electrical forces, these strong forces act only over extremely short distances. The actual atomic mass is less than the sum of the masses of all its nucleons. This difference in mass, or mass deficit, is manifest in the nuclear binding energy holding the nucleus together (as related by the equation $E = mc^2$).

Elements are organized in the periodic table of the elements (see Appendix 2). All atoms of the same element have the same number of protons. The proton number is also referred to as the *atomic number* or Z. Thus, all carbon atoms have 6 protons, all oxygen atoms have 8 protons, and all iodine atoms have 53 protons—that is, they have Z numbers of 6, 8, and 53, respectively. Atoms of a particular element can, however, have a varying number of neutrons (referred to as the *neutron number, N*). For example, in addition to their 8 protons, some oxygen atoms have 8 neutrons, and others have 7 or 10 neutrons. The total number of nucleons (Z plus N) is known as the *atomic mass* or *atomic number, A*. Therefore, in the oxygen example, A would be 15, 16, and 18 for atoms that have 8 protons plus 7, 8, or 10 neutrons, respectively.

Unlike an element, which is characterized only by its number of protons (Z), a *nuclide* is a nuclear entity characterized by a certain nuclear composition of protons and neutrons as well as a certain energy level. Shorthand notation has been agreed on to describe the makeup of specific nuclides:

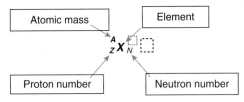

To illustrate this, consider the element iodine, which has 53 protons (Z = 53). If one particular nuclide of the element iodine has 78 neutrons (N = 78), the atomic mass (A) of 53 + 78 equals 131. It can be written as:

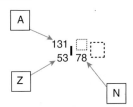

Because the atomic number can be inferred by the element's symbol, and N = A − Z, this can be shortened:

$${}^{131}_{53}I_{78} \Longrightarrow {}^{131}I_{78} \Longrightarrow {}^{131}I$$

This can also be written as I-131 or iodine-131. The term *isotope* describes nuclides of the same element, that is, nuclides

TABLE 1.1	Properties of Atomic Particles			
Particle	Charge	Mass (amu or u)[a]	Mass (MeV)[b]	Mass (kg)
Proton	+1	1.0073	938.21	1.673×10^{-27}
Neutron	0	1.0087	939.51	1.675×10^{-27}
Electron	−1	0.000549	0.511	9.11×10^{-31}

[a]One amu = 1.661×10^{-27} kg or 1/12 atomic mass carbon (1 nucleon from carbon-12 atom).
[b]Energy as related by $E = mc^2$.

TABLE 1.2	Summary of Physical Constants
Unit of charge	1 amp·sec
Coulomb (C)	6.24×10^{18} electrons
Electron volt (eV)	1.602×10^{-19} J
Charge of 1 electron	-1.6×10^{-19} C
Charge of 1 proton	$+1.6 \times 10^{-19}$ C
Planck's constant (h)	6.63×10^{-34} m²·kg/s
Avogadro's number	6.02×10^{23} molecules/g·mole
Calorie (cal)	4.2 Joules
Speed of light in a vacuum	3.0×10^{8} m/sec
Angstrom (Å)	10^{-10} m

BOX 1.1	Important Terms Related to Atomic Matter
Nucleon	components of the atomic nucleus: protons and neutrons
Atomic number	Number of protons, or Z
Neutron number	Number of neutrons, or N
Atomic mass	Sum of the nucleons—protons and neutrons (Z + N)—or atomic number or A
Elements	Atoms with the same number of protons (Z)
Nuclides	Nuclear entity comprised of a particular number of protons (Z) and neutrons (N) as well as energy state of the nucleus
Radionuclides	Unstable nuclides: isotopes emitting radiation attempting to reach stability
Isotopes	Atoms with the same number of protons: P for proton, **P** for isoto**p**e.
Isotones	Atoms with the same number of neutrons: **N** for isoto**n**e
Isobars	Atoms with the same atomic number A: **A** for isob**a**r
Isomer	Nuclide with same Z and N (so same A) but a different energy level

M for metastable; **M** for iso**m**er.

with the same number of protons (Z) but potentially differing atomic numbers. *Radioisotopes* are isotopes that undergo radioactive decay. For example, some common isotopes of iodine are as follows:

$$^{131}_{53}I_{78}, \,^{125}_{53}I_{72}, \,^{124}_{53}I_{71}, \,^{123}_{53}I_{70}$$

In medicine, different isotopes have varying properties, such as the types of radiation they emit and how long they remain radioactive, which can determine their usefulness. For example, the beta and high-energy gamma emitter ^{131}I (I-131) is used for treating thyroid cancer and performing thyroid uptake measurements; ^{125}I (I-125), a low-energy gamma and x-ray emitter, is used in biological assays and prostate cancer brachytherapy; ^{124}I (I-124), a positron emitter, can image thyroid cancer with a positron emission tomography (PET) scanner; and ^{123}I, a moderate-energy gamma emitter, is very commonly used to image benign thyroid diseases and thyroid cancers as well as to calculate thyroid activity (radioactive iodine uptake).

In addition to isotopes, other special terms include *isotones*, nuclides with the same number of neutrons (e.g., $^{14}_{8}O$, $^{13}_{7}N$, $^{12}_{6}C$ where N = 6); and *isobars*, those with similar atomic mass numbers (e.g., ^{14}O, ^{14}N, ^{14}C). Nuclides that have the same Z and N numbers (and, therefore, A) but differ in their energy states are called *isomers*. A well-known example of an isomer in nuclear medicine is technetium-99 (Tc-99) and its metastable state technetium-99m (Tc-99m). Several key terms to know concerning atomic structure are listed in Box 1.1.

Structure of the Orbital Electrons

Our understanding of the atom has evolved, but it is still useful to picture the classic Bohr atom (Fig. 1.1) with electrons arranging themselves into discrete orbital shells (Table 1.3). The innermost shell is referred to as the *K shell*, and subsequent shells are referred to as *L, M, N, O,* and beyond. Each shell holds only a set maximum number of electrons, given by $2n^2$, where *n* is the shell number). Based on this, for example, the K shell (*n* = 1) contains 2 electrons, and the L shell (*n* = 2) has 8.

Because electrons are bound by the electrical forces, energy is required to remove an electron from an atom. This orbital *binding energy* (BE) is characteristic for each particular atom, depending on its Z number, as well as which shell is involved (i.e., it is harder to remove an inner-shell electron than an outer-shell electron; Fig. 1.2).

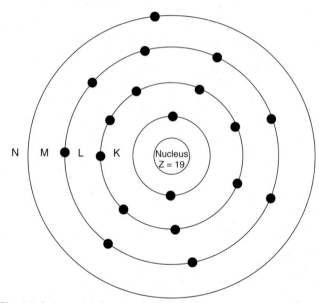

Fig. 1.1 Bohr model diagram of the potassium atom. Potassium has an atomic (Z) number of 19; that is, it has 19 protons in the nucleus and 19 orbital electrons.

ELECTROMAGNETIC RADIATION

Electromagnetic (EM) radiations, such as visible light, have long been known to have a duality to their nature: behaving in some situations as a wave and in others as a particle, or *photon*. The EM spectrum (Fig. 1.3) varies in wavelength and frequency, from low-energy radio waves up to high-energy x-rays and gamma (γ) rays as used in medical imaging and therapy.

The unit of energy typically used in atomic and nuclear physics is the electron volt (eV), which is the amount of energy an electron garners when crossing an electronic potential difference of 1 volt. One eV is equivalent to 1.6×10^{-9} joules. EM radiations travel at the speed of light (*c*) with the known relationship:

$$c = v\lambda$$

TABLE 1.3   Terms Used to Describe Electrons

Term	Comment
Electron	Basic elementary particle
Orbital electron	Electron in one of the shells or orbits in an atom
Valence electron	Electron in the outermost shell of an atom; responsible for chemical characteristics and reactivity
Auger electron	Electron ejected from an atomic orbit by energy released during an electron transition
Conversion electron	Electron ejected from an atomic orbit because of internal conversion phenomenon as energy is given off by an unstable nucleus
Photoelectron	Electron ejected from an atomic orbit as a consequence of an interaction with a photon (photoelectric interaction) and complete absorption of the photon's energy
Compton electron	Electron ejected from orbit after absorbing a portion of a photon's energy during Compton scatter

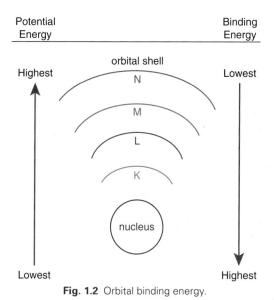

Fig. 1.2 Orbital binding energy.

where v is frequency, λ is the wavelength, and $c = 3 \times 10^8$ m/s.

The photon energy (E) is related to the frequency of the EM wave by

$$E = hv$$

where h is Planck's constant (6.626×10^{-34} J/s)

Relating these equations, $v = \dfrac{c}{\lambda}$ so $E = \dfrac{hc}{\lambda}$, thus:

$$E \,(keV) = \frac{12.4}{\left(\mathring{A}\right)} \text{ with the } \lambda \text{ measured in angstroms } \left(\mathring{A}\right).$$

Visible light has energy slightly less than 1 eV, whereas x-rays and gamma rays have energies in the range of several thousand eV (or keV) to tens of millions eV (MeV).

X-rays and gamma-ray photons do not differ in their energy levels but in their origin. X-rays are generated from interactions outside the nucleus, whereas gamma rays are generated by transitions within the nucleus. Once created, nothing distinguishes an x-ray from a gamma ray (e.g., A 100-keV x-ray is absolutely identical and indistinguishable from a 100-keV gamma ray).

Production of X-Rays

X-rays are produced in two ways: (1) as a result of the transition of atomic electrons from one orbit to another and (2) from the deacceleration of passing charged particles as they interact with other charged particles, usually as a result of columbic electrical interactions.

Characteristic X-Rays

In the first instance, excited electrons may be removed from their atomic orbit or elevated to a higher-energy orbit. An electron from an outer orbit can drop down to fill the vacancy, and the excess energy, the difference in the binding energy of the shells, can be emitted as an x-ray photon, a fluorescent x-ray (Fig. 1.4A). This is also known as a *characteristic x-ray* because it is specific to not only each element but also to the orbital shell from which it originated. Consider the case of fluorescent or characteristic x-rays from electronic transitions within an iodine atom with the following binding

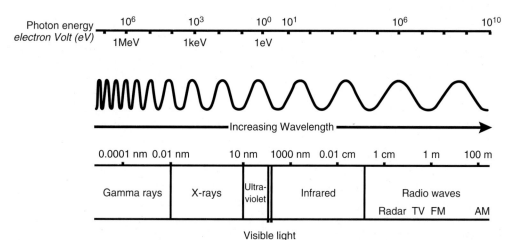

Fig. 1.3 Electromagnetic energy spectrum. Photon energies (eV) and wavelengths of x-rays and gamma ultraviolet, visible light, infrared, and radio waves.

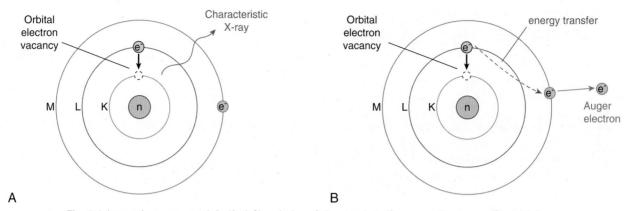

Fig. 1.4 Interactions may result in (A, *left*) emission of characteristic (fluorescent) x-rays or (B, *right*) Auger electrons.

energies: K = 35, L = 5, and M = 1 keV. Thus, the energy of the fluorescent x-rays resulting from the transition of electrons from the L to the K shell (referred to as *Kα fluorescent x-rays*) is 30 keV (35 − 5 keV) and that from the transition from the M to the K shell (referred to as *Kβ x-rays*) is 34 keV (35 − 1 keV).

Auger Electrons

There is an alternative outcome to characteristic x-ray emission, where the transition can cause an outer-shell electron to be ejected. This electron is called an Auger (pronounced *oh-zhey*) electron (see Fig. 1.4B). The kinetic energy (KE) of the resultant Auger electron is determined by the binding energy of the orbits involved:

$$KE_{Auger} = BE_{Inner} - BE_{Outer} - BE_{Auger}$$

Using the example of the iodine atom binding energies again for the transitions shown in Fig. 1.4B, the calculation would then be:

$$KE_{Auger} = BE_K shell - BE_L shell - BE_{M\ shell}$$
$$= 35 keV - 5 keV - 1 keV = 29 keV$$

The probability of an Auger electron being emitted is greater in lower Z elements and from outer shells where the binding energy is lower. X-ray fluorescence, on the other hand, is the more likely outcome when binding energy is higher, such as in higher Z elements and from inner-shell electrons.

Particle Deceleration and Bremsstrahlung X-Rays

X-rays can also be produced as a charged particle deaccelerates as it passes an atom. In nuclear medicine, this commonly involves electrons or beta particles passing through soft tissue. In this case, the negatively charged particle is slowed as it interacts with the positively charged nucleus it is passing, causing it to slow. The energy it loses is emitted as radiation referred to as *bremsstrahlung* (from the German for "braking") radiation. The magnitude of the bremsstrahlung production increases linearly with the kinetic energy of the incident electron and the Z number of the target material. Thus, bremsstrahlung x-ray production is more likely to occur at higher energies and with high-Z targets. As a result, radiographic systems can generate x-rays by directing an energetic electron beam into a tungsten (Z = 74) target. On the other hand, the intensity of the bremsstrahlung radiation is relatively low when beta particles pass through soft tissue.

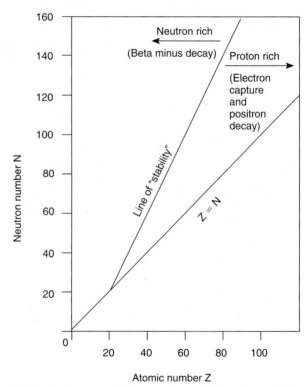

Fig. 1.5 Graph of neutrons (N) versus protons (P) for various nuclides. For elements with a low atomic number, the two are roughly equal (Z = N). With increasing atomic number, the relative number of neutrons increases. Stable nuclear species tend to occur along the "curve of stability."

RADIOACTIVITY AND RADIOACTIVE DECAY

The protons and neutrons can only exist in the nucleus in a limited number of combinations. The remaining unstable atoms may transform to a lower-energy stable state through *radioactive decay* (or *disintegration*), with the excess energy resulting in either particulate emissions or electromagnetic radiation. The initial nuclide, or radionuclide, is known as the *parent*, and the resultant one after radioactive decay is known as the *daughter*. Although the daughter nucleus created from a radioactive decay has a lower energy than the parent nucleus, it may not be stable, and thus subsequent radioactive decays may result.

Fig. 1.5 shows a plot of the stable nuclides as a function of the Z number on the *x*-axis and the N number on the *y*-axis. At

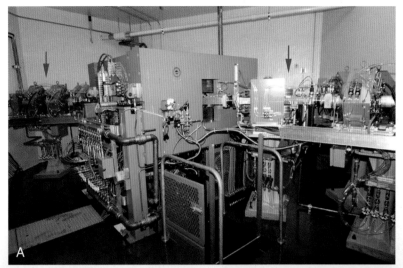

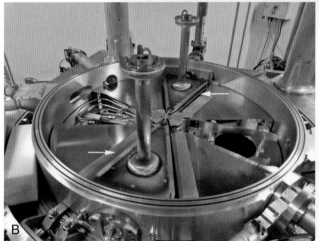

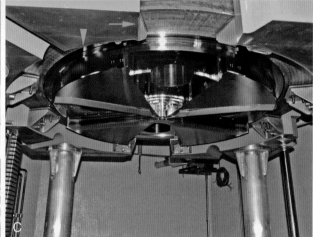

Fig. 1.6 "Proton-rich" radionuclides that decay by positron emission can be made in a cyclotron or particle accelerator. (A) Varying in size and appearance, cyclotrons may be self-shielded or housed in a thick cement vault (as shown) to reduce radiation exposure. Beam lines *(arrow)* extending from the central unit direct high-speed charged particles to bombard desired targets. (B) The bottom of the cyclotron contains the accelerating electrodes *(short arrows)*. (C) Electromagnetic fields created by a large magnet *(arrowhead)* in the upper portion of the cyclotron constrain the particles to circular orbits. (Photos courtesy of Anthony F. Zagar, University of Alabama at Birmingham.)

low Z numbers, stable elements tend to have equal numbers of protons and neutrons (e.g., carbon-12, nitrogen-14, and oxygen-16) and lie along or near the Z = N line. However, as the nucleus becomes larger, the repulsive force of the nuclear protons grows, and more neutrons are necessary in the stable nucleus to provide additional attractive nuclear force. Other factors also contribute to the stability and instability of the nucleus. For example, nuclides with even numbers of protons and neutrons tend to be more stable than those with odd Z and N configurations.

Unstable nuclides fall to either the right or the left of the curve of stability, with those to the right considered *proton rich* and those to the left *neutron rich.* As unstable radionuclides decay to entities that are closer to the curve of stability, proton-rich radionuclides tend to decay in a manner that will reduce the Z number and increase the N number, and neutron-rich radionuclides tend to decay in a way that decreases the N number and increases the Z number.

Proton-rich radionuclides can be created by bombarding a certain target material with high-energy protons that can overcome nuclear forces. Typically, a particle accelerator such as a cyclotron is used, increasing kinetic energy by accelerating charged particles to high speeds in a spiral path using alternating high-frequency voltage and electromagnetic fields (Fig. 1.6). Conversely, in artificial production of neutron-rich radionuclides, one typically must use a nuclear reactor to bombard a target with a neutron flux (Fig. 1.7).

Modes of Radioactive Decay

A *decay scheme* is a way to illustrate the transition from parent to daughter nuclides. In a decay scheme, higher energy levels are toward the top of the figure, and higher Z numbers are to the right of the figure. Transitions that lead to a reduction in energy are represented by an arrow pointing down. If it also results in a daughter nuclide with a change in the Z number, the arrow will point to the left with a decrease in the Z number and to the right if Z is increased.

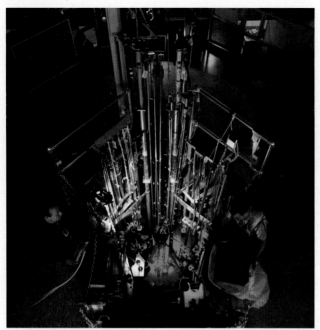

Fig. 1.7 Fission and neutron capture radionuclide production in a nuclear reactor. Samples can be lowered into the reactor as shown, with water acting as shielding against neutrons. The blue glow is caused by the emission of electrons from the radioactive products; when charged particles move faster than the speed of light in a medium such as water, the emitted radiation is called Cherenkov radiation. (Courtesy of the University of Missouri Research Reactor Center.)

Alpha Decay

An unstable heavy atom may decay to a nuclide closer to the curve of stability by emitting an alpha particle (α) consisting of 2 protons and 2 neutrons (essentially an ionized helium atom):

$$^A_Z X \rightarrow\ ^{A-4}_{Z-2} Y + \alpha =\ ^{A-4}_{Z-2} Y_{jo9} +\ ^4_2 He$$

The daughter nucleus may not be stable, and thus the emission of an alpha particle often will lead to the emission of a series of radiations until the nucleus is stable. The decay scheme for the decay of radium-226 (Ra-226) to radon-222 (Rn-222) is shown in Fig. 1.8.

Beta-Minus Decay

Neutron-rich radionuclides tend to stabilize by decreasing the number of neutrons through a radioactive-decay process referred to as *beta-minus* (β^-), also known as negatron or beta decay. Factors such as weak forces between nucleons transfer energy, transforming a neutron into a proton (N – 1 and Z + 1). This is an isobaric transition with no change to the atomic mass (A). An example of the beta-minus decay scheme for I-131 is shown in Fig. 1.9. Excess energy is emitted from the nucleus as an antineutrino and a negative *beta particle* (or *negatron*). This process can be written as follows:

$$^A_Z X_N =\ ^A_{Z+1} Y_{N-1} + \beta^- + \bar{v}\ _{\text{antineutrino}}$$

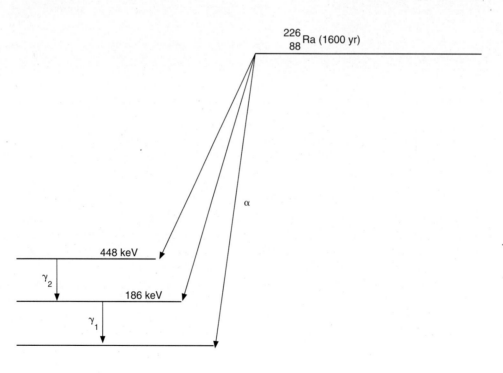

Fig. 1.8 Alpha decay. The emission of an alpha particle (2 protons and 2 neutrons) results in the atomic number (Z) decreasing by 2 and the atomic mass (Z + N) decreasing by 4. Decay of radium-226 to the daughter Rn-222 shows the arrow pointed down, indicating a decrease in energy, and to the left because of the decrease in Z.

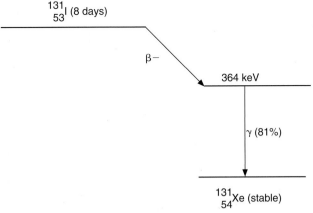

Fig. 1.9 Beta minus (β^-) decay scheme for iodine-131 to the daughter Xe-133. β^- decay (negatron emission) results in the daughter with one more proton in the nucleus (Z + 1), so the arrow points to the right. Because a neutron is lost (N − 1), this is an isobaric transition with the atomic mass unchanged.

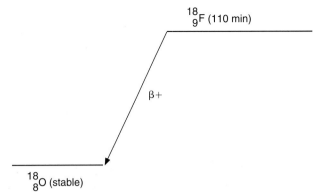

Fig. 1.10 Positron (β^+) decay results in a loss of 1 proton (Z − 1) in proton-rich radionuclides. Because 1 neutron is gained, the atomic mass of the daughter is unchanged, another example of isobaric transition. F-18 decay by positron emission results in the daughter product, O-18. The arrow points down and to the left, indicating the decrease in Z.

The antineutrino is very difficult to measure because it has virtually no mass or charge associated with it, only energy. The negative beta particle is indistinguishable from an electron with the same mass and electric charge, differing only in that the beta particle is emitted from the nucleus and the electron orbits the nucleus. In addition to the Mo-99 used to make Tc-99m, several β^--emitting radionuclides play an important role in nuclear medicine for therapy applications: I-131, phosphorus-32 (P-32), yttrium-90 (Y-90), and lutetium-177 (Lu-177).

Beta-Plus (Positron) Decay

Unstable proton-rich radionuclides can reduce Z and increase N numbers through either *beta-plus decay* or *electron capture*. In beta-plus decay, the parent nucleus emits a positively charged beta particle, a *positron* (β^+). The resulting daughter nucleus has one fewer proton and one more neutron than the parent, an *isobaric transition*:

$$^A_Z X_N = ^A_{Z-1} Y_{N+1} + \beta^+ + \bar{v}_{neutrino}$$
$$(\text{average } \beta^+ \text{ kinetic energy: } E_{\beta^+} \approx E_{max}/3)$$

The positron has the same mass as a beta-minus particle or electron, with a charge of the same magnitude but the opposite. In fact, the positron is the *antiparticle* of the electron; if they are brought into close contact, they will be annihilated and transformed into two 511-keV photons, traveling at 180 degrees in opposite directions. This annihilation process is the basis of PET imaging. The 511-keV value derives from the energy equivalence of the mass of the beta particle, similar to the rest mass of an electron (using $E = mc^2$ as previously discussed).

For positron decay to occur, the transition energy must be in excess of a 1022-keV threshold (twice 511 keV) to overcome the production of the positron and addition of an orbital electron to maintain electric neutrality. These radionuclides are typically produced using a cyclotron. Some positron-emitting radionuclides of interest include fluorine-18 (F-18; Fig. 1.10), nitrogen-13 (N-13), carbon-11 (C-11), gallium-68 (Ga-68), and rubidium-82 (Rb-82).

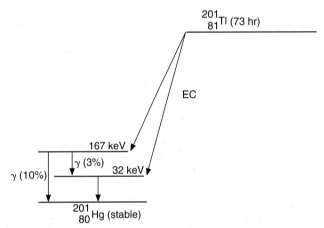

Fig. 1.11 Electron capture is an alternate transition that can occur to reduce the proton number and does not require that an energy threshold be met. Tl-201 decays by electron capture, with the daughter (Hg-201) containing one fewer proton (Z − 1) than the parent.

Electron Capture. An alternative to beta-plus decay for proton-rich radionuclides is electron capture (EC). In this process, an inner-shell, orbital electron is absorbed into the nucleus, leading to the reduction of Z and increase of N by 1. However, no energy threshold exists for EC to occur. In cases in which the transition energy is less than the 1022-keV threshold, EC is the only possible decay process, but either process is possible when the energy is greater than 1022 keV. For F-18, positron decay occurs 97% of the time, and EC occurs 3% of the time. The capture of an orbital electron leads to an inner-shell vacancy, which in turn leads to the emission of fluorescent x-rays or Auger electrons. Radionuclides that decay through EC exclusively include thallium-201 (Tl-201; Fig. 1.11), gallium-67 (Ga-67), and indium-111 (In-111). These are all produced in a cyclotron.

Isomeric Transition. In some cases, an excited radionuclide decays from one energy level to another while retaining the same Z and N numbers. This is referred to as an *isomeric transition* because the nuclide decays from one isomer (energy level) to another. This transition may result in the emission of a gamma ray, the energy of which is determined by the energy

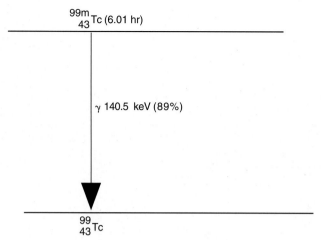

Fig. 1.12 Isomeric transitions involve a change in the energy state of a radionuclide, such as Tc-99m to Tc-99.

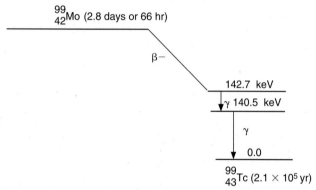

Fig. 1.13 Decay scheme of Mo-99. Beta-minus emission to Tc-99m, followed by isomeric transition to Tc-99.

difference of the initial and eventual energy levels. In some cases, an alternate process called *internal conversion* can occur, resulting in the emission of an orbital electron, a *conversion electron*. The kinetic energy is calculated as the difference in the two energy levels minus the electron's binding energy.

Perhaps the most important isomeric transition for nuclear medicine involves technetium. The term *metastable* (i.e., almost stable) is used if the daughter nucleus remains in the excited state for a considerable amount of time (>1 microsecond, which is long by nuclear standards). Mo-99 decays to an excited, or metastable, Tc-99m that in turn transitions to Tc-99 (Figs. 1.12 and 1.13). Tc-99m has a 6-hour half-life. Tc-99m is so commonly used because of its reasonable half-life, as well as its gamma-ray energy (140 keV) and lack of beta- or alpha-particle emissions. Another example of isomeric transition is seen in the decay scheme of I-131 (see Fig. 1.9). Xenon-131 (Xe-131), formed from the beta-minus decay of I-131, is in an excited state and immediately decays by isomeric transition with the emission of a 364-keV gamma ray.

Radioactive Decay Calculations

Atoms in a sample containing a certain number (N) of radioactive atoms will not all decay at the same time but with a *mean time* (T_m) that is characteristic of a particular radionuclide. The

reciprocal of T_m, the fraction of the radioactive atoms that decay per unit time, is referred to as the *decay constant, λ*:

$$\lambda = \frac{1}{T_m}$$

Thus, the number of atoms (dN) that decay in a short time interval (*dt*) is given by:

$$dN = \lambda dt$$

Integrating this equation over time leads to:

$$N = N_0 e^{-\lambda t}$$

where N_0 is the initial number of radioactive atoms, and N is the number remaining after some time, *t*.

This equation describes exponential decay in which a certain fraction of the material is lost in a set period. This fraction is referred to as the *decay fraction*, DF:

$$DF = e^{-\lambda t}$$

Thus, the number of radioactive atoms remaining, N, is also given by:

$$N = N_0 \times DF$$

Also, N_d is the number of atoms that have decayed in time, *t*, and can be calculated with:

$$N_d = N_0 \times (1 - DF)$$

The time necessary for half of the material to decay is defined as the *half-life ($T_{1/2}$)*. The half-life is related to the mean life and the decay constant by the following equations:

$$T_{1/2} = \ln(2)T_m = \frac{0.693}{\lambda}$$

Alternatively, one can determine the decay constant from the half-life by:

$$\lambda = \frac{0.693}{T_{1/2}}$$

One can also express the radioactive decay equation using the half-life:

$$N = N_0 e^{\frac{-0.693t}{T1/2}}$$

If a sample contains 10,000 radioactive atoms at a particular point in time, one half-life later, there will be 5000 atoms; another half-life later, there will be 2500 atoms; and so on. This process of a certain fraction of the material decaying in a certain time is representative of exponential decay (Fig. 1.14A). When graphed using a log scale on the y-axis (semilog plot), the result is a straight line with the negative slope equal in magnitude to the decay constant (Fig. 1.14B).

The amount of *activity* (A) is the number of nuclear transformations—decays or disintegrations—per unit time. The activity is characterized by the number of radioactive atoms in the sample, N, divided by the mean time to radioactive decay, T_m:

$$A = N/T_m$$

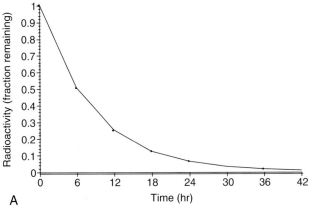
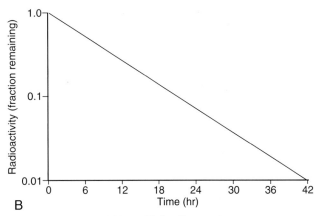

Fig. 1.14 Decay plot for Tc-99m. (A) Standard graph showing the exponential loss. (B) Semilog graph.

Activity is thus the product of the decay constant and the number of radioactive atoms:

$$A = \lambda N$$

Conversely, if the amount of activity of a particular radionuclide is known, the number of radioactive atoms can be calculated:

$$N = A/\lambda$$

Because the activity is directly related to the number of radioactive atoms, all of the equations for radioactive decay apply to activity, as well as the number of atoms:

$$A = A_0 e^{-\lambda t}$$

And

$$A = A_0 e^{-(0.693t)/(T1/2)}$$

The units associated with activity are the *becquerel* (1 Bq = 1 disintegration per second) and the *curie* (1 Ci = 3.7 × 10^{10} disintegrations per second; Box 1.2). Their relationship is as follows:

$$1\ \text{mCi} = 37\ \text{MBq, and } 1\ \text{MBq} = 27\ \mu\text{Ci}$$

Example 1. The radiopharmacy is preparing a dose of an I-123–labeled agent (13-hour half-life) for the clinic. If 10 mCi is to be administered at 1 PM, how much activity should be placed in the syringe at 7 AM?

$$A = A_0 e^{-(0.693t)/(T1/2)}$$

Thus

$$10\text{mCi} = A_0 e^{(-0.693)(6\ hr)/(13\ hr)}$$

$$A_0 = 10\text{mCi}/e^{(-6.693)(6\ hr)/(13\ hr)} = 10\text{mCi}/0.726 = 13.8\text{mCi}$$

Example 2. The staff at the nuclear medicine clinic is testing their equipment with a cobalt-57 source (270-day half-life) that was calibrated to contain 200 MBq on January 1 of this year. How much activity remains on September 1 (243 days)?

BOX 1.2 Conversion of International System and Conventional Units of Radioactivity

Mathematical
c (centi-) 10^{-2}
m (milli-) 10^{-3}
k (kilo-) 10^{3}
μ (micro-) 10^{-6}
M (mega-) 10^{6}
n (nano-) 10^{-9}
G (giga-) 10^{9}
p (pico-) 10^{-12}
T (tera-) 10^{12}

Conventional Unit
1 curie (Ci) = 3.7 × 10^{10} disintegrations per second (dps)

SI Unit
1 becquerel (Bq) = 1 dps

Curies → Becquerels
1 Ci = 3.7 × 1010 dps = 37 GBq
1 mCi = 3.7 × 107 dps = 37 MBq
1μCi = 3.7 × 104 dps = 37 KBq

Becquerels → Curies
1 Bq = 1 dps = 2.7 × 10^{-11} Ci = 27 pCi
1 MBq = 106 dps = 2.7 × 10^{-5} Ci = 0.027 mCi
1 GBq = 109 dps = 27 mCi
  Probability of radiative losses directly proportional to Z of target and energy incident particle.

$$A = A_0 e^{-(0.693t)/(T1/2)}$$

Thus

$$A = 200 e^{\frac{-0.693 \times 243\ days}{270\ days}} = 200\ \text{MBq} \times 0.536 = 107\ MBq$$

INTERACTIONS BETWEEN RADIATION AND MATTER

Charged-Particle Interactions With Matter

A charged particle may transfer energy in different ways. First, it can be attracted and slowed by the opposite charge of the nucleus or orbiting electrons in target material atoms. The resulting kinetic energy loss is released as radiation *(radiative losses)*. Bremsstrahlung radiation occurring with a β^- emitter is one example of this type of interaction. The energy of radiative losses is directly proportional to the Z number of the target as well as to the incident particle's energy.

Charged particles can also directly transfer energy to the atom's orbital electrons, resulting in electron excitations and ionizations. While excited, electrons can temporarily move to a shell farther from the nucleus. As de-excitation occurs, transferred energy leads to the emission of Auger electrons or electromagnetic radiation. This radiation can have a wide range of energies, including visible or ultraviolet radiation for outer-shell transitions and fluorescent x-rays for the inner-shell transitions.

When the energy from charged-particle interactions produces ionized electrons and atoms in tissues, the majority of the ionized electrons are low energy. However, some interactions result in high-energy electrons, referred to as *delta rays,* which in turn can also cause excitation and ionization. In the energies of practical interest in nuclear medicine, nearly all of the energy from a charged-particle interaction (greater than 99%) is expended in excitation and ionization (or *collisional losses*) compared with radiative losses.

The rate at which a material causes a charged particle to lose energy (per unit length of the matter) is referred to as its *stopping power.* A related quantity is *linear energy transfer (LET),* which is the amount of energy deposited locally (i.e., not lost to energetic electrons, delta rays, or radiative loss) per unit length. The stopping power and LET values depend on the type of radiation, its energy, and the density of the material through which it travels. Radiation with a higher LET value has been shown to cause more damage to cells. Alpha particles have a higher LET than beta particles or electrons.

Although densely ionizing, alpha particles deposit their energy over a very short distance, a small fraction of a millimeter in soft tissues. Also, although they are easily stopped by the skin, these high-energy particles cause substantial cell death when internalized, making them both extremely dangerous if accidentally ingested as well as highly effective in therapeutic applications (e.g., Ra-223 in prostate cancer).

Comparatively, β^- particles travel for much longer distances, ranging from several millimeters to several centimeters depending on their initial energy. They can be stopped by material such as a thin sheet of aluminum or a few millimeters of soft tissue.

The β^- kinetic energy is variable because it shares energy with the antineutrino produced during the decay event. The maximum kinetic energy of the beta particle (E_{max}) is defined by the difference in the energy levels of the parent and daughter nuclide. However, it is the average kinetic energy that is used when calculating the impact of the β^- on cells and tissues, estimated as 1/3 of E_{max} ($E_\beta \approx E_{max}/3$), similar to the calculation previously described for positrons.

Photon Interactions in Matter

High-energy photons (gamma rays, x-rays, bremsstrahlung radiation, and annihilation radiation) can also transfer energy to the electrons, nuclei, or atoms as a whole that they encounter. Unlike charged particles, which directly create ionized atoms, the high-energy photons act indirectly, transferring their energy to charged particles, specifically electrons, which in turn create most of the excitations and ionizations that occur in the matter. Thus they are considered secondary ionizing radiations.

At low energy levels (a few keV), photons are scattered in a manner that does not deposit energy, referred to as *Rayleigh scattering.* Photons with energy in excess of several MeV can result in *pair production* of a negatron and a positron (effectively a negative and positive electron). However, in energy ranges most common in nuclear medicine (from several tens of keV to approximately 1 MeV), the two most prominent modes of photon interaction are the *photoelectric effect* and *Compton scattering.* Factors involved in the various types of interaction are outlined in Table 1.4.

Photoelectric Effect

The photoelectric effect (Fig. 1.15) occurs when a photon transfers all of its energy to an orbital electron, causing it to be ejected from the atom and creating an electron-shell vacancy. The kinetic energy of the liberated *photoelectron* equals the incident photon's energy minus the binding energy of the electron's initial orbital shell. As the shell vacancy is filled by electrons from outer shells, fluorescent x-rays and Auger electrons are also emitted. Paradoxically, the probability of photoelectric interactions is highest for tightly bound orbiting electrons (i.e., those in the inner shells of high Z elements). These electrons are most likely the ones in the innermost orbital shell where the binding energy is just under the photon's energy. In addition, the chance of this interaction dramatically decreases as incident photon energy increases. The probability of the photoelectric interaction (or P_{PE}) is given by:

$$P_{PE} \, \alpha \, Z^3/E^3$$

where Z = atomic number, and E = incident photon kinetic energy.

TABLE 1.4 Photon Interactions in Matter

Interaction	Occurrence	Effect of Target Material Z	Incident Photon E Range (E_0)	Target	Resulting Particle Emissions	Secondary Photon Emissions
Compton	Predominant in soft tissues at diagnostic E range	Nearly independent of Z Depends on e^- density (therefore on target density) Hydrous > anhydrous material	Mid E range ($\approx$26 keV–30 MeV)	Outer-shell e^-	Recoil e^-	Scattered photon Degrades image
Photoelectric effect	Predominates in shielding and detector crystals/PMT	High-Z materials	Low-E photon Z^3/E^3	Innermost-shell e^- possible	Photoelectrons Auger e^-	Characteristic x-ray
e^- cascade produces						
Characteristic x-ray		$\uparrow$ with $\uparrow$ Z-detector material, shielding		$\uparrow$ when weakly bound valence (e.g., PMT photocathode materials)		
Auger e^-		$\uparrow$ in soft tissues		e^- binding E less a factor in tissue		
Pair production	Not typically seen in energies used in medicine		1.02-MeV minimum but actually >>1.02 MeV (not present at diagnostic E ranges)	Usually nucleus, sometimes orbital e^-	β^+ and β^- (or e^+ and e^-)	Annihilation photons (from β^+) Two 5110 keV at 180 degrees

E, Energy; *Z*, atomic number (number of protons); *PMT*, photomultiplier tube; *e^-*, electron; *β^+*, positron (or a positive electron); *β^-*, negatron (same as negative electron or beta-minus particle).

In soft tissues (low Z), the photoelectric effect is much less common than Compton scatter. It is, however, more prevalent in the high-Z materials used for shielding (e.g., lead) or for photon detection (sodium iodide crystals). Photoelectric effect interactions can also occur in the gamma camera's photomultiplier tubes, which contain high-Z materials, such as cesium.

Compton Scatter

The incident photon does not disappear in Compton scatter. Rather, it transfers a portion of its energy to an orbital electron (a Compton electron), which is then ejected from the atom. The photon is deflected or scattered, at an angle θ from its original path (Fig. 1.16). The electron and scattered photon may go on to ionize or excite other atoms.

The sum of the kinetic energies of the scattered photon and the Compton electron will equal the initial photon's energy. With lower-energy incident photons, more energy is transferred to the electron, and there is greater backscatter of the resulting photon (i.e., the angle between the incident and scattered photons tends to be wider), with even 180 degrees of backscatter occurring. Higher-energy incident photons lose less energy to the electron, and deflection is less significant (i.e., the scatter angle is narrower), such that both the scattered photon and electron tend to travel in a more forward direction.

Whereas the photoelectric effect is important at lower energies and more likely involves inner-shell electrons in high-Z materials, Compton scatter predominates in soft tissues in the moderate-energy ranges of gamma-ray and x-ray photons in nuclear medicine imaging and tends to involve outer-shell electrons. Because the energy of the incident photon is much greater than the shell's binding energy, the collision occurs as if involving a free electron. Compton interactions tend to depend on electron density but are relatively independent of the Z number or incident photon energy. Because electron density is fairly consistent among the atoms in soft tissues, the probability increases with increasing material density rather than its Z number. Electron density is higher when hydrogen atoms are present, so tissues with high water content are more affected than anhydrous tissues.

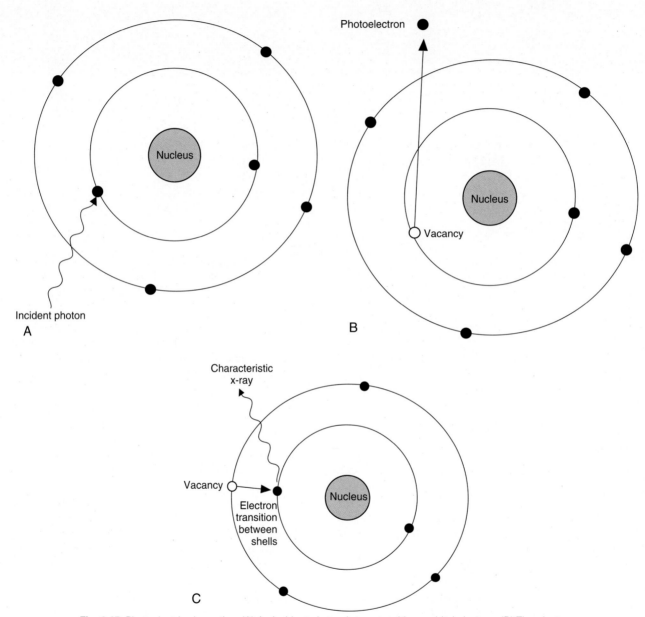

Fig. 1.15 Photoelectric absorption. (A) An incident photon interacts with an orbital electron. (B) The electron is ejected from its shell, creating a vacancy. The electron is either ejected from the atom or moved to a shell further from the nucleus. (C) The orbital vacancy is filled by the transition of an electron from a more distant shell. Consequently, a characteristic x-ray is given off.

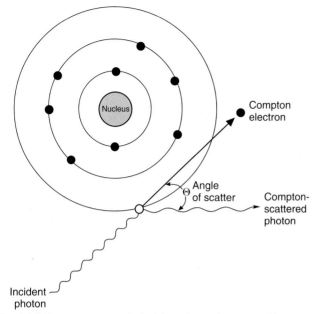

Fig. 1.16 Compton scatter. An incident photon interacts with an outer or loosely bound electron, giving up a portion of its energy to the electron and undergoing a change in direction at a lower kinetic energy level.

SUGGESTED READING

Chandra R, Rahmin A. *Nuclear Medicine Physics: The Basics*. 8th ed. Philadelphia: Williams & Wilkins; 2012.

Cherry SR, Sorenson JA, Phelps ME. *Physics in Nuclear Medicine*. 4th ed. Philadelphia: WB Saunders; 2012.

Eckerman KF, Endo A. *MIRD: Radionuclide Data and Decay Schemes*. 2nd ed. Reston, VA: Society of Nuclear Medicine; 2008.

Loevinger R, Budinger TF, Watson EE. *MIRD Primer for Absorbed Dose Calculations*. Reston, VA: Society of Nuclear Medicine; 1988.

Powsner RA, Powsner ER. *Essentials of Nuclear Medicine Physics*. 3rd ed. West Sussex, UK: Wiley-Blackwell; 2013.

Saha GP. *Physics and Radiobiology of Nuclear Medicine*. 4th ed. New York: Springer; 2013.

2

Radiation Detection & Ancillary Instrumentation

Janis M. O'Malley, Harvey Ziessman, Frederic Fahey

The passage of radiation, such as x-rays and gamma rays, through a given material leads to ionizations and excitations that can be used to quantify the amount of energy deposited. This property allows measurement of the level of intensity of a radiation beam or small amounts of radionuclides, including from within the patient. The appropriate choice of detection approach depends on the purpose. In some cases, the efficient detection of minute amounts of the radionuclide is essential, whereas in other cases the accurate determination of the energy or location of the radiation deposited is most important. A variety of approaches to radiation detection are used, including those that allow for in vivo imaging of radiopharmaceuticals.

RADIATION DETECTION

Consider the model of a basic radiation detector, as shown in Fig. 2.1. The detector acts as a transducer that converts radiation energy to electronic charge. Applying a voltage across the detector yields a measurable electronic current. Radiation detectors typically operate in either of two modes, *current mode* or *pulse mode*. Detectors that operate in current mode measure the average current generated within the detector over some characteristic integration time. This average current is typically proportional to the exposure rate to which the detector is subjected or the amount of radioactivity within the range of the detector. In pulse mode, each individual detection is processed with respect to the peak current (or pulse height) for that event. This pulse height is proportional to the energy deposited in the detection event. The histogram of pulse heights is referred to as the *pulse-height spectrum*. It is also referred to as the *energy spectrum* because it plots a histogram of the energy deposited within the detector.

Certain properties of radiation detectors characterize their operation. Some are applicable to all detectors, whereas others are used for detectors that operate in pulse mode. These characterizations are not only useful for describing the operation but can also give insight into the benefits and limitations of the particular detector.

The detection efficiency depends on several factors, including the intrinsic and extrinsic efficiency of the detector. The *intrinsic efficiency* is defined as the fraction of the incident radiation particles that interact with the detector. It depends on the type and energy of the radiation and the material and thickness of the detector. For photons, the intrinsic efficiency, D_I, is given to first order by:

$$D_I = (1 - e^{-\mu x})$$

where μ is the linear attenuation coefficient for the material of interest at the incident photon energy, and x is the thickness of the detector. Thus the intrinsic efficiency can be improved by using a thicker detector or choosing a photon energy and detector material that optimizes the value of μ.

The *extrinsic efficiency* is the fraction of photons or particles emitted from the source that strike the detector. It depends on the size and shape of the detector and the distance of the source from the detector. If the detector is a considerable distance from the source (i.e., a distance that is >5 times the size of the detector), the extrinsic efficiency, D_E, is given by:

$$D_E = A/\left(4\pi d^2\right)$$

where A is the area of the detector, and d is the distance from the source to the detector. This equation defines the *inverse square law*. For example, if the source-to-detector distance is doubled, the intensity of the radiation beam is reduced by a factor of 4. The total detection efficiency is the product of the intrinsic and extrinsic efficiencies:

$$D_T = D_I \times D_E$$

In pulse mode, the pulse height is proportional to the energy deposited within the detector. However, the uncertainty in the energy estimation, referred to as the *energy resolution*, depends on the type of detector used and the energy of the incident radiation. For a photon radiation source of a particular energy, the feature associated with that energy is referred to as the *photopeak*, as shown in Fig. 2.2. The width of the photopeak, as characterized by the full width at half of its maximum (FWHM) value normalized by the photon energy represented as a percentage, is used as a measure of the energy resolution of the detector.

When the detector is subjected to a radiation beam of low intensity, the count rate is proportional to the beam intensity. However, the amount of time it takes for the detector to process an event limits the maximum possible count rate. Two models describe the count rate limitations: *nonparalyzable* and *paralyzable*. In the nonparalyzable model, each event takes a certain

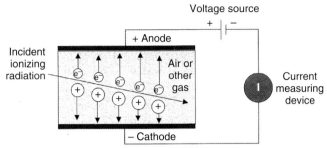

Fig. 2.1 Block diagram of basic detector. The radiation detector basically acts as a transducer, converting radiation energy deposited into an electrical signal. In general, a voltage has to be supplied to collect the signal, and a current or voltage measuring device is used to measure the signal. In some instances, the average current over a characteristic integration time is measured, which is referred to as *current mode.* In other cases, the voltage pulse of each detection event is analyzed, referred to as *pulse mode.* (From Cherry, Sorenson JA, Phelps ME. *Physics in Nuclear Medicine.* 3rd ed. Philadelphia: WB Saunders; 2003.)

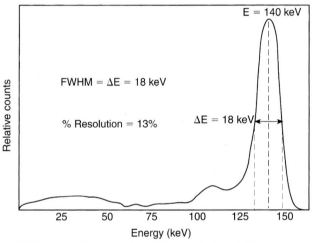

Fig. 2.2 Spectrum for technetium-99m (Tc-99m) in air. The energy resolution is characterized by the width of the photopeak (the full width at half maximum [FWHM]) normalized by the photon energy. For the particular detector system illustrated, the FWHM is 18 keV. The energy resolution of the detector system for Tc-99m is 13% (100 × 18/140).

amount of time to process, referred to as the *dead time,* which defines the maximum count rate at which the detector will saturate. For example, if the dead time is 4 μs, the count rate will saturate at 250,000 counts per second. With the paralyzable model, the detector count rate not only saturates but can "paralyze"—that is, lose counts at very high count rates. Gamma cameras, for example, are paralyzable systems.

The three basic types of radiation detectors used in nuclear medicine are *gas detectors, scintillators,* and *semiconductors.* These three operate on different principles and are typically used for different purposes.

Gas detectors are used every day in nuclear medicine for assaying the amount of radiopharmaceutical to be administered and to survey packages and work areas for contamination. However, because of the low density of gas detectors, even when the gas is under pressure, the sensitivity of gas detectors is not high enough to be used for clinical counting and imaging applications.

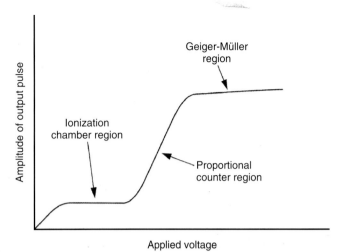

Fig. 2.3 Amplitude of gas detector output signal as a function of applied voltage. This graph shows the relationship between the magnitude of the output signal from the gas detector (related to the amount of ionized charge collected) as a function of the voltage applied across the detector. There is no signal with no voltage applied. As the voltage is increased, the detector signal starts to increase until the *saturation voltage* is reached, the start of the plateau defining the *ionization chamber region,* where all of the initially liberated charge is collected. Further increasing the voltage leads to the *proportional counter region,* at which the liberated electrons attain sufficient energy to lead to further ionization within the gas. Finally, the *Geiger-Müller region* is reached, at which each detection yields a terminal event of similar magnitude (i.e., a "click"). (From Cherry, Sorenson JA, Phelps ME. *Physics in Nuclear Medicine.* 3rd ed. Philadelphia: WB Saunders; 2003.)

A gas radiation detector is filled with a volume of gas that acts as the sensitive material of the detector. In some cases it is air, and in others it is an inert gas such as argon or xenon, depending on the particular detector. Electrodes are located at either end of the sensitive volume. The detector circuit also contains a variable voltage supply and a current detector. As radiation passes through the sensitive volume, it causes ionization in the gas. If a voltage is applied across the volume, the resulting ions (electrons and positive ions) will start to drift, causing a measurable current in the circuit. The current will last until all of the charge that was liberated in the event is collected at the electrodes. The resulting current entity is referred to as a *pulse* and is associated with a particular detection event. If only the average current is measured, this device operates in *current* mode. If the individual events are analyzed, the device is operating in *pulse* mode.

Fig. 2.3 shows the relationship between the charge collected in the gas detector and the voltage applied across the gas volume. With no voltage, no electric field exists within the volume to cause the ions liberated in a detection event to drift, and thus no current is present and no charge is collected. As the voltage is increased, the ions start to drift, and a current results. However, the electric field may not be sufficient to keep the electrons and positive ions from recombining, and thus not all of the originally liberated ions are collected. This portion of Fig. 2.3 is referred to as the *recombination region.* As voltage is increased, the level is reached at which the strength of the electric field is sufficient for the collection of all of the liberated ions (no recombination). This level is referred to as the *saturation voltage,* and the resulting plateau in Fig. 2.3 is the *ionization chamber* region. When operating in this region, the amount of charge collected is proportional to the amount of ionization caused in the detector and thereby to the energy deposited within the detector. Ionization detectors or chambers typically operate in current mode and are the detectors of choice for determining the radiation beam intensity level at a particular location. They can directly measure this intensity level in either exposure in roentgens (R) or air kerma in rad. Dose calibrators and the ionization meters used to monitor the output of an x-ray device or the exposure level from a patient who has received a radiopharmaceutical are examples of ionization (or *ion*) chambers used in nuclear medicine.

If the voltage is increased further, the drifting electrons within the device can attain sufficient energy to cause further ionizations, leading to a cascade event. This can cause substantially more ionization than with an ionization chamber. The total ionization is proportional to the amount of ionization initially liberated; therefore these devices are referred to as *proportional counters* or *chambers*. Proportional counters, which usually operate in pulse mode, are not typically used in nuclear medicine. If the voltage is increased further, the drifting electrons attain the ability to cause a level of excitations and ionizations within the gas. The excitations can lead to the emission of ultraviolet radiation, which also can generate ionizations and further excitations. This leads to a terminal event in which the level of ionization starts to shield the initial event, and the level of ionization finally stops. This is referred to as the *Geiger-Müller process*. In the Geiger-Müller device, every event leads to the same magnitude of response, irrespective of the energy or the type of incident radiation. Thus the Geiger-Müller meter does not directly measure exposure, although it can be calibrated in a selected energy range to milliroentgens per hour (mR/hr). However, the estimate of exposure rate in other energy ranges may not be accurate. The Geiger-Müller survey meter is excellent at detecting small levels of radioactive contamination and thus is often used to survey radiopharmaceutical packages that are delivered and work areas within the nuclear medicine clinic at the end of the day.

SCINTILLATION DETECTORS

Some crystalline materials emit a large number of light photons upon the absorption of ionizing radiation. This process is referred to as *scintillation,* and these materials are referred to as *scintillators*. As radiation interacts within the scintillator, a large number of excitations and ionizations occur. On de-excitation, the number of light photons emitted is directly proportional to the amount of energy deposited within the scintillator. In some cases, a small impurity may be added to the crystal to enhance the emission of light and minimize the absorption of light within the crystal. Several essential properties of scintillating materials can be characterized, including density, effective Z number (number of atomic protons per atom), amount of light emitted per unit energy, and response time. The density and effective Z number are determining factors in the detection

efficiency because they affect the linear attenuation coefficient of the scintillation material. The amount of emitted light affects both energy and, in the gamma camera, spatial resolution. Resolution is determined by the statistical variation of the collected light photons, which depends on the number of emitted photons. Finally, the response time affects the temporal resolution of the scintillator. The most common scintillation crystalline material used in nuclear medicine is thallium-doped sodium iodide (NaI) with lutetium oxyorthsilicate (LSO) or lutetium yttrium oxyorthosilicate (LYSO) most commonly used in positron emission tomography (PET).

Once the light is emitted in a scintillation detector, it must be collected and converted to an electrical signal. The most commonly used device for this purpose is the *photomultiplier tube* (PMT). Light photons from the scintillator enter through the photomultiplier entrance window and strike the *photocathode,* a certain fraction of which (approximately 20%) will lead to the emission of photoelectrons moving toward the first dynode. For each electron reaching the first dynode, approximately a million electrons will eventually reach the anode of the photomultiplier tube. Thus the photomultiplier tube provides high gain and low noise amplification at a reasonable cost. Other solid-state light-detection approaches are now being introduced into nuclear medicine devices. In *avalanche photodiodes* (APDs), the impinging light photons lead to the liberation of electrons that are then drifted in the photodiode, yielding an electron avalanche. The gain of the APD is not as high as with the PMT (several hundred compared with about a million), but the detection efficiency is substantially higher (approximately 80%). A second solid-state approach is the *silicon photomultiplier tube (SiPMT)*. This device consists of hundreds of very small APD channels that operate like small Geiger-Müller detectors—that is, each detection is a terminal event. The signal from the SiPMT is the number of channels that respond to a particular detection event in the scintillator. SiPMTs have moderate detection efficiency (approximately 50%) and operate at low voltages. One further advantage of APDs and SiPMTs compared with PMTs is that they can operate within a magnetic field. Thus the development of positron emission tomography/magnetic resonance (PET/MR) scanners has involved the use of either APDs or SiPMTs.

Solid-state technology is used to detect the light from a scintillation detector and also can be used to directly detect gamma rays. The detection of radiation within a *semiconductor detector* leads to a large number of electrons liberated, resulting in high energy resolution. The energy resolution of the lithium-drifted germanium (GeLi) semiconductor detector has approximately 1% energy resolution compared with the 10% energy resolution associated with a sodium iodide scintillation detector. However, thermal energy can lead to a measurable current in some semiconductor detectors such as GeLi, even in the absence of radiation, and thus these semiconductor detectors must be operated at cryogenic temperatures. On the other hand, semiconductor detectors such as cadmium telluride (CdTe) or cadmium zinc telluride (CZT) can operate at room temperature. CdTe and CZT do not have the excellent energy resolution of GeLi, but at approximately 5%, it is still significantly better than that of sodium iodide.

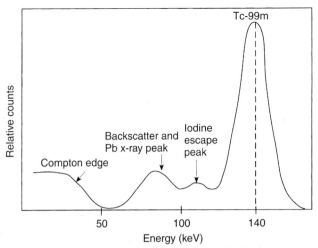

Fig. 2.4 Energy spectrum for technetium-99m (Tc-99m) in air for a gamma scintillation camera with the collimator in place. Note the iodine escape peak at approximately 112 keV. The 180-degree backscatter peak at 90 keV merges with the characteristic x-ray peaks for lead (Pb). The Compton edge is at 50 keV.

The pulse height spectrum corresponding to the detection of the 140-keV gamma rays from technetium-99m (Tc-99m) is illustrated in Fig. 2.4. The photopeak corresponds to events where the entire energy of the incident photon is absorbed within the detector. These are the events of primary interest in most counting experiments, and thus the *good* events are within an energy acceptance window about the photopeak. Other events correspond to photons scattered within the detector material and depositing energy, which can range from very low energy from a very-small-angle scatter to a maximum 180-degree scatter (in the spectrum referred to as the *Compton edge*). Events below the Compton edge correspond to these scattered events. In some cases, photons can undergo multiple scatters and possibly result in events between the Compton edge and the photopeak. Photons scattered within the patient and then detected may also result in events in this energy region. Finally, the pulse-height spectrum will be blurred depending on the energy resolution of the detector. Thus in Fig. 2.4, the photopeak has approximately a 10% spread because of the energy resolution associated with NaI, rather than the narrow spike that might be expected from the emission of a monoenergetic gamma ray.

ANCILLARY NUCLEAR MEDICINE EQUIPMENT

Besides the imaging equipment in the nuclear medicine clinic, other additional ancillary equipment may be necessary from either a medical or regulatory point of view or to otherwise enhance the operation of the clinic. This equipment will be reviewed, including the quality. control required for proper operation.

As previously discussed, the two basic radiation meters commonly used in the nuclear medicine clinic are the Geiger-Müller (GM) meter and the ionization chamber. Both are gas detectors, although they operate differently. With the GM meter, all detections lead to a terminal event of the same magnitude—a "click." The device is excellent for detecting small amounts of

contamination. It is routinely used to determine whether there is contamination on packages of radiopharmaceutical that are delivered to the clinic and to test working surfaces and the hands and feet of workers for contamination. GM meters often are equipped with a test source of cesium-137, with a very small amount of radioactivity, that is affixed to the side of the meter. On calibration, the probe is placed against the source, and the resulting exposure rate is recorded. The probe is tested daily using the source to ensure that the meter's reading is the same at the time calibration. The GM meter should be calibrated on an annual basis.

The ionization chamber meter (ion chamber) operates in current mode and assesses the amount of ionization within an internal volume of gas (often air) and thus can directly measure exposure or air kerma rate. The ion chamber is used to evaluate the exposure rate at various locations within the clinic. For example, it could be used to measure the exposure rate in an uncontrolled area adjacent to the radiopharmaceutical hot laboratory. The ion chamber is also used to evaluate the exposure rate at a distance from a patient who has received radionuclide therapy (e.g., iodine-131 for thyroid cancer) to determine that the patient can be released without exposing the general public to unacceptable radiation levels. The ion chamber also should be annually calibrated.

The dose calibrator is an ionization chamber used to assay the amount of activity in vials and syringes. This includes the assay of individual doses before administration to patients, as required by regulation. The dose calibrator operates over a very wide range of activities, from tens of microcuries to a curie (hundreds of Bq to tens of GBq). The device is also equipped with variable settings for each radionuclide to be measured, with typically about 10 buttons for ready selection of the radionuclides commonly used in the clinic. In addition, buttons are available for user-defined radionuclide selection. Others can be selected by entering the appropriate code for that radionuclide into the system.

The dose calibrator is used to assay the activity administered to the patient, and thus a comprehensive quality control program is necessary. Regulations specify dose calibrator quality control program must meet the manufacturer's recommendations or national standards. Typically, the program comprises four basic quality control tests: geometry, accuracy, linearity, and constancy.

The geometry protocol tests that the dose calibrator provides the same reading for the same amount of activity irrespective of the volume or orientation of the sample. A reading of a certain amount of activity in a 0.5-mL volume is obtained. The volume is then increased by augmenting the sample with amounts of nonradioactive water or saline and taking additional readings. The subsequent readings should not vary from the original readings by more than 10%. The geometry test is performed during acceptance testing and after a major repair or move of the equipment to another location.

For accuracy, calibrated sources (typically cobalt-57 and ^{137}Cs) are assayed; the resultant reading cannot vary by more than 10% from the calibrated activity decay corrected to the day of the test. The accuracy test should be performed during acceptance testing, annually thereafter, and after a major repair or move.

The linearity protocol tests that the dose calibrator operates appropriately over the wide activity range to which it is applied. The device is tested from 10 μCi (370 kBq) to a level higher than that routinely used in the clinic and perhaps as high as 1 Ci (37 GBq). The activity readings are varied by starting with a sample of the radioactivity of Tc-99m at the highest value to be tested (e.g., tens of gigabequerels). The activity readings are then varied by either allowing the source to radioactively decay over several days or using a set of lead shields of varying thicknesses until a reading close to 370 kBq is obtained. Each reading should not vary by more than 10% from the line drawn through the calculated activity values. The linearity test should be performed during acceptance testing, quarterly thereafter, and after a major repair or move.

The constancy protocol tests the reproducibility of the readings compared with a decay-corrected estimate for a reference reading obtained from the dose calibrator on a particular day. Today's constancy reading cannot vary from the decay-corrected reference reading by more than 10%. The constancy test varies from accuracy in that it evaluates the precision of the readings from day to day rather than accuracy. The constancy test should be performed on every day that the device is used to assay a dose to be administered to a patient.

There are two nonimaging scintillator devices, the well counter, and the thyroid probe that are routinely used in the nuclear medicine clinic. The well counter is used for both radiation protection and clinical protocols. The thyroid probe can provide clinical studies with a fraction of the equipment costs and space requirements of the use of nuclear imaging equipment. However, these devices also require comprehensive quality control programs.

The well counter consists of an NaI crystal with a hole in it, allowing for test tubes, and other samples can be placed within the device for counting. The samples to be placed in the counter is practically surrounded by the detector, with a geometrical efficiency in excess of 90%. Thus the well counter can measure very small amounts of radioactivity, on the order of a kilobecquerel. The well counter should not be confused with the dose calibrator, which is a gas-filled ionization chamber that can measure activities up to 37 GBq. It is used to test packages of radiopharmaceuticals to ensure that no radioactivity has been spilled on the outside of the package or leaked from the inside. The device also can be used to measure removable activity from working surfaces where radioactivity has been handled or from sealed sources such as calibration sources to ensure that the radioactivity is not leaking out.

The well counter can also be used for the assay of biological samples for radioactivity for a variety of clinical evaluations. For example, after the administration of Tc-99m diethylenetriamepentaacetic acid (DTPA), blood samples can be counted at several time points (e.g., at 1, 2, and 3 hours) to estimate the patient's glomerular filtration rate (GFR). The amount of radioactivity in a 0.2-mL blood sample will be very small, and thus the well counter is the appropriate instrument for these measurements. By making these measurements and the measurements of standards of known activity concentration (kilobecquerel per milliliter), the patient's GFR can be estimated.

The thyroid probe consists of an NaI crystal on a stand with the associated counting electronics. The patient is administered a small amount of radioactive iodine. The probe is placed at a certain distance from the thyroid, and a count is obtained. In addition, a count is acquired of a known standard at the same distance. The thyroid uptake of iodine can be estimated from these measurements.

The quality control program for both the well counter and the thyroid probe includes the energy calibration, the energy resolution, the sensitivity, and the chi-square test. For the energy calibration, the energy window is set for the calibration source of a particular radionuclide—for example, the 662-keV peak of Cs-137. The amplifier gain is varied until the maximum count is found that corresponds with the alignment of the window with the 662-keV energy peak. In addition, the counts in a series of narrow energy windows across the peak can be measured to estimate the energy resolution. A standard window can be set, and the counts of a known calibration source can be counted and normalized by the number of nuclear transformations to estimate the sensitivity in counts per transformation (or counts per second per becquerel). Finally, the chi-square test evaluates the operation of the counter by comparing the uncertainty of the count to that expected from the Poisson distribution.

THE PATIENT AS A RADIOACTIVE SOURCE

In nuclear medicine, the patient is administered a radiopharmaceutical that distributes according to a specific physiological or functional pathway. The patient is then imaged using external radiation detectors to determine the in vivo distribution and dynamics of the radiopharmaceutical through which the patient's physiology can be inferred, providing this essential information to the patient's doctor to aid in diagnosis, prognosis, staging, and treatment. The equipment used to acquire these data will be described in the sections ahead. Single-photon emission computed tomography (SPECT) and PET are described in the next chapter. However, before examining how the instrumentation operates, it is instructive to understand the nature of the signal itself—that is, the radiation being emitted from within the patient.

The radiopharmaceutical is administered to the patient most commonly by intravenous injection but also in some cases through other injection routes, such as intraarterial, intraperitoneal, or subdermal. In other cases, the radiopharmaceutical may be introduced through the gastrointestinal tract or through the breathing of a radioactive gas or aerosol. After administration, the path and rate of uptake depend on the particular radiopharmaceutical, the route of administration, and the patient's individual physiology. However, the characteristics and parameters associated with the radiopharmaceutical in vivo distribution and dynamics are of considerable clinical importance. In some cases, the enhanced uptake of the radiopharmaceutical in certain tissues (e.g., the uptake of fluorodeoxyglucose [FDG] in tumors) may be of most clinical importance, whereas in other cases it may be the lack of uptake (e.g., the absence of Tc-99m sestamibi in infarcted myocardium). In the first case, this would be referred to as a *hot-spot* imaging task, and in the latter would be a *cold-spot* task. In other situations, it may be the rate of uptake *(wash in)* or clearance *(wash out)* that may be considered the essential characteristic of the study. In a Tc-99m mercapto-acetyltriglycine (MAG3) renal study, fast wash in may indicate a well-perfused kidney, and delayed clearance may indicate renal obstruction. In the Tc-99m DTPA counting protocol described previously, a slow clearance of the radiopharmaceutical from the blood would indicate a reduced GFR. In some cases, the ability to discern uptake in a particular structure that is adjacent to other nonspecific uptake may require the ability to spatially resolve the two structures, whereas other tasks may not require such specific resolution. The choice of instrumentation, acquisition protocol, and data-processing approach fundamentally depend on the clinical task at hand.

To characterize the rate, location, and magnitude of radiopharmaceutical uptake within the patient, the emitted radiation must be detected, in most cases, by detectors external to the patient's body. Some instruments are specially designed for internal use—for example, interoperative radiopharmaceutical imaging—but in most the cases, the imaging device is located outside the body while detecting radiation internally. This requirement limits the useful emitted radiations for nuclear medicine imaging to energetic photons—that is, gamma rays and x-rays. The amount of overlying tissue between the internally distributed radiopharmaceutical and the radiation detector may vary from several centimeters to as much as 20 to 30 cm. Alpha and beta particles will not be of use in most cases because their ranges in tissue are limited to a few millimeters, and thus they will not exit the body and cannot be measured by external radiation detectors. Even x-rays and gamma rays must have energies in excess of 50 keV to penetrate 10 cm of tissue. On the other hand, once the radiation exits the patient, it is best that the radiation not be so energetic as to be difficult to detect with reasonable-size detectors. Thus the radiation types optimal for most nuclear medicine imaging applications are x-rays and gamma rays in the 50- to 600-keV energy range, depending on the equipment and collimation being used.

Consider a situation in which a radiopharmaceutical labeled with Tc-99m leads to a point source at some depth within the patient's body. The 140-keV gamma rays will be emitted isotropically from the point source. Therefore it would be advantageous to place the radiation detector close to the source or to place several detectors around the source to collect as many of the emitted photons as possible. In fact, acquiring data from several angles may allow the source to be better localized. Those emitted photons that exit the body without interaction and are subsequently detected will yield the highest quality spatial information. Conversely, those photons that scatter within the patient compromise spatial information. Photons that undergo very-small-angle scatter will perhaps not be of much consequence, but those that undergo scatter at larger angles will not be of much use. Noting that the Compton-scattered photons have less energy than the incident photons, and that small-angle scatter leads to less energy loss than large-angle scatter, energy discrimination (i.e.,

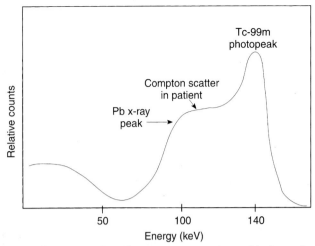

Fig. 2.5 Energy spectrum from a gamma camera with the technetium-99m (Tc-99m) activity in the patient. Note the loss of definition of the lower edge of the Tc-99m photopeak. This spectrum illustrates the difficulty of discriminating Compton-scattered photons within the patient using pulse-height analysis.

only allowing photons to be counted within a narrow energy window about the photopeak energy) will lead to the elimination of a significant number of scattered photons from the nuclear medicine image. In contrast to the case of a point source, a more challenging clinical case with regard to scatter may be the imaging of a cold-spot feature, such as an infarction in a myocardial perfusion scan or a renal scar in a Tc-99m DMSA scan. In these cases, scattered photons in the neighboring tissue may be displaced into the cold spot, leading to a loss in image contrast and an inability to properly discern the extent of the feature. It must also be kept in mind that in a true clinical case, the distribution of the radiopharmaceutical is unknown, and background levels in other tissues may compromise the situation. The pulse-height spectrum from a patient is shown in Fig. 2.5.

GAMMA CAMERAS

In the earliest days of nuclear medicine, counting devices similar to the thyroid probe described in the previous section were used to evaluate the amount of activity in a particular tissue. For example, probes could be used to evaluate the iodine uptake of the thyroid gland. However, it was not long before clinicians realized that it would be helpful to not only know the total uptake of the radiopharmaceutical within the tissue of interest but also to be able to discern the spatial distribution of the uptake within the tissue. In the early 1950s, Benedict Cassan attached a focused collimator to an NaI crystal and a mechanism for acquiring the counts from the patient at multiple locations in a raster fashion and plotting the spatial distribution of the counts. This device, the *rectilinear scanner*, provided nuclear medicine images of physiological function. As a result the term *scan*, as in a thyroid or bone scan, has remained in the nuclear medicine lexicon. However, these scans took a long time to acquire and did not allow for the acquisition of time-sequence or dynamic studies. Still, the rectilinear scanner continued to be used in nuclear medicine clinics through the late 1970s.

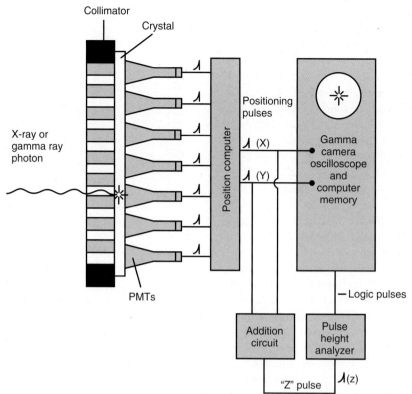

Fig. 2.6 Schematic of gamma scintillation camera. The diagram shows a photon reaching the NaI crystal through the collimator and undergoing photoelectric absorption. The photomultiplier tubes (PMTs) are optically coupled to the NaI crystal. The electrical outputs from the respective PMTs are further processed through positioning circuitry to calculate *(x, y)*-coordinates and through additional circuitry to calculate the deposited energy of the pulse. The energy signal passes through the pulse height analyzer. If the event is accepted, it is recorded spatially in the location determined by the *(x,y)*-positioning pulses.

In the mid-1950s, Hal Anger developed his first prototype of the *gamma camera,* which allowed a section of the body to be imaged without a raster scan, opening the door for the possibility of both dynamic and physiologically gated studies. Further developments of the technology took place over the next 10 years, and the first commercial gamma camera was introduced in the mid-1960s. With further advances that have improved and stabilized the operation of the instrument, along with the addition of tomographic capability, the gamma camera remains the most commonly used imaging device in the nuclear medicine clinic.

A block diagram of the gamma camera is shown in Fig. 2.6. Gamma rays emitted from within the patient pass through the holes of an absorptive collimator to reach the NaI crystal. On interaction of the gamma ray with the NaI scintillating crystal, thousands of light photons are emitted, a portion of which are collected by an array of PMTs. By taking weighted sums of the PMT signals within the associated computer, the two-dimensional (2D) *x*- and *y*-location and the total energy of the detection event deposited are estimated. If the energy deposited is within a prespecified energy window (e.g., within 10% of the photopeak energy), the event is accepted, and the location of the event recorded. In this manner, the gamma camera image is constructed on an event-by-event basis, and a single nuclear medicine image may consist of hundreds of thousands of such events. Each component of the gamma camera will be described.

The detection material of the gamma camera is typically a single, thin large-area NaI scintillation crystal. Some smaller cameras rely on a 2D matrix of smaller crystals, but most rely on a single large crystal. In the most common gamma camera designs, the NaI crystal is about 30 cm × 50 cm in area and 9.5 mm thick. Some cameras designed for imaging only photons with energies below 150 keV may have thinner crystals. Others used more commonly for higher-energy photons may be thicker, but the 9.5-mm thickness provides a reasonable compromise because it detects more than 85% of the photons with energies of 140 keV or lower and stops about 28% of the 364-keV gamma rays emitted by I-131. NaI is hygroscopic and thus damaged by water. It is hermetically sealed and has a transparent light guide on the side adjacent to the PMT array and aluminum on the side closer to the collimator. The NaI crystal is the most fragile component of the gamma camera, being susceptible to both physical and thermal shock. When the collimator is not in place, the bare NaI crystal must be treated with extreme care. In addition, the environment in the room must be controlled so that the air temperature is maintained at a reasonable level (18-24°C) and is not subject to wide variations over a short period.

The PMT array consists of about 60 to 100 photomultiplier tubes that are each about 5 cm in diameter. The PMTs are usually hexagonal and arranged in a hexagonal close-packed array to collect as many light photons as possible. Although PMTs are used in practically all gamma cameras, some small camera designs are using avalanche photodiodes to collect the scintillation light. The signal from each PMT is input into the gamma camera host computer. First, the sum of all of the PMT signals is used to estimate the energy deposited in the detection event. In addition, each PMT has a weight associated with its position in both the x- and y-direction. For example, the PMTs on the left side of the camera may have a low weight, and those on the right side of the camera would have a higher weight. For a particular detection event, if the weighted sum of the signal is low, the event would be on the left side, and if it were high, it would be on the right side of the camera. However, the weighted sum as described is dependent not only on the position of the event but also on the total amount of light collected, which is directly proportional to the energy deposited. Therefore the sum must be normalized by the energy estimate. This approach to determining the position of the detection event is often referred as *Anger logic,* in honor of the developer of the gamma camera, Hal Anger. This leads to an estimate of the detection event location to within 3 to 4 mm, which is referred to as the intrinsic spatial resolution of the camera.

However, distortions can occur in images with respect to both the energy and position estimates. Detection events directly over PMTs lead to the collection of slightly more light than the events between PMTs and therefore to a slightly higher pulse height. *Energy calibration* notes the shift in the pulse height spectrum as a function of position. Subsequently, an opposite shift is applied on an event-by-event basis, leading to improved energy resolution and greater energy stability. In addition, there is an inherent nonlinearity, with events being bunched over PMTs and spread out between PMTs. Analogous to energy calibration, *linearity calibration* determines the spatial shift from linearity as a function of position across the entire field of view. Again, these shifts in both energy and position are applied on an event-by-event basis, providing an image that is free of linear distortion. A very-high-count *uniformity calibration* map is acquired that characterizes the remaining nonuniformities inherent in the gamma camera acquisition process. These uniformity calibration maps are used to generate uniformity corrections that are applied during each acquisition.

COLLIMATORS

Although the NaI crystal, PMTs, and electronics can estimate the location of a detection event to within 3 to 4 mm, the directionality of the event is not known. Gamma rays from a point source could be detected anywhere across the field of view, and the counts detected at a particular location in the NaI crystal could have also originated from practically anywhere within the patient. Thus collimation is required to determine the directionality of the detected event. Because gamma rays cannot be easily focused, absorptive collimation must be used—that is, all photons *not* heading in the desired direction will be absorbed by the collimator, and those heading in the correct direction will be allowed to pass. Therefore absorptive collimation is inherently very insensitive because practically all of the emitted photons will be absorbed and only a very few will be accepted. In general, only 0.01% (i.e., 1 in 10,000) of the photons emitted from the patient will be accepted by the collimator and incorporated into the image.

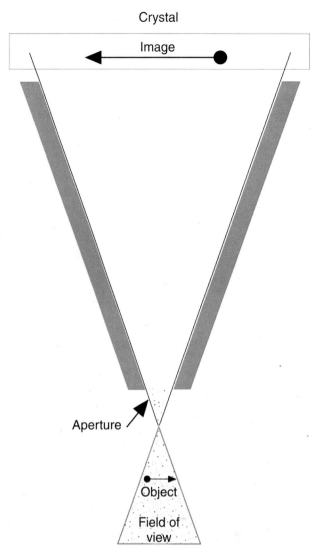

Fig. 2.7 Pinhole collimator. The image is inverted. The image is magnified if the distance from the aperture to the object is smaller than the distance from the aperture to the gamma camera crystal. Spatial resolution improves and sensitivity decreases as the aperture diameter decreases. The sensitivity also decreases with the source-to-aperture distance, according to the inverse square law. In general, the pinhole collimator provides the best spatial resolution and the lowest sensitivity of any collimator used in nuclear medicine.

The simplest is the *pinhole collimator* (Fig. 2.7). It consists of a single, small hole or aperture located a set distance (typically on the order of 20 cm) from the surface of the NaI crystal. Photons from one end of the source that pass through the aperture will be detected on the opposite side of the detector. In addition, objects that are closer to the aperture will be magnified compared with those farther away. If b is the distance from the aperture to the object and f is the distance from the aperture to the detector, the amount of magnification, M, is given by:

$$M = f/b$$

Magnification can be of significant value when imaging small objects using a camera with a large field of view. Magnification will minimize the effect of the intrinsic spatial resolution of the camera and thus enhance overall system resolution. The

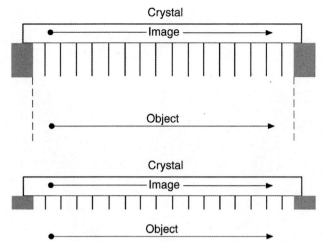

Fig. 2.8 Multihole, parallel-hole collimator. The collimator shown at the *top* has longer holes designed to provide higher resolution. However, it would also have a lower sensitivity than the collimator shown at the *bottom*. The septal thickness and thus energy rating are the same for both collimators.

collimator spatial resolution of the pinhole, R_{PH}, is determined by the diameter or the aperture, d (typically 4-6 mm) and the distances from both the object and the NaI crystal to the aperture.

$$R_{PH} = d \times (f + b)/f$$

It must be kept in mind that spatial resolution is typically characterized by the size of an imaged point source, and thus a large value corresponds to poor resolution, and a very small value indicates excellent spatial resolution. A system with 1-mm spatial resolution will lead to an image with greater acuity than one with 5-mm spatial resolution. For this reason, the term *high resolution* can be ambiguous because it may be unclear whether this system has very high resolution or a high R value (poor resolution). Based on the earlier formula, better spatial resolution is attained using a smaller aperture (small d value) with the source as close to the pinhole aperture as possible. In fact, all gamma camera collimators provide the best spatial resolution very close to the collimator, and spatial resolution will degrade as the object is moved farther from the collimator. The geometrical sensitivity of the pinhole collimator, G_{PH}, depends on the area of the pinhole (πd^2) compared with the squared distance of the source from the pinhole (b^2):

$$G_{PH} \approx 1/16 \, (d/b)^2$$

Thus the geometrical collimator sensitivity is highest with a large aperture diameter and drops off as the inverse square of the distance from the source to the aperture—that is, it follows the inverse square law. A larger aperture diameter leads to better geometrical sensitivity but poorer spatial resolution, whereas the converse is true for a smaller aperture diameter. As is true in some other instances in nuclear medicine imaging, a trade-off occurs between sensitivity and spatial resolution such that improvement in one area may cause degradation of another. The choice of whether to use high sensitivity or better resolution may depend on the clinical imaging task at hand, but often a compromise will lead to a reasonable value for both parameters. The pinhole collimator typically provides the best spatial resolution and the lowest sensitivity of all

of the collimators commonly used in nuclear medicine. It is often used when imaging small organs (e.g., the thyroid gland) with a gamma camera with a large field of view or in special cases when a very-high-resolution spot view image is required, such as when trying to discern which bone in the foot may be demonstrating increased radiopharmaceutical uptake on a bone scan.

The *multihole collimator* provides substantially better geometrical sensitivity compared with the pinhole collimator because the object is viewed through many small holes rather than through a single hole. The most commonly used multihole collimators consist of a very large number of parallel holes with absorptive septa between the holes to restrict the emitted gamma rays from traversing from one hole to a neighboring hole. The holes are typically hexagonal and arranged in a hexagonal, close-packed array (Fig. 2.8). A typical low-energy, parallel-hole collimator may have hole diameters and lengths of about 1 and 20 mm, respectively, and septal thicknesses between holes of about 0.1 mm. No magnification occurs with a parallel-hole collimator. The collimator spatial resolution depends on the diameter (d) and the length (a) of the collimator holes and the distance from the source to collimator (b):

$$R_P = (d/a)(a + b)$$

A parallel-hole collimator with either small or long holes will provide the best spatial resolution (Fig. 2.8, *top*). Similar to the pinhole collimator, the spatial resolution of the parallel-hole collimator is best at the surface of the collimator and degrades with distance from the collimator. The geometrical sensitivity of the parallel-hole collimator also depends on the thickness of the septa between the holes (t) in addition to the hole diameter and length:

$$G_P \approx 1/16 \, (d/a)^2 \, d/ \, (d + t)^2$$

The geometrical sensitivity will be the highest for a collimator with the thinnest interhole septa. On the other hand, the septa must be thick enough to minimize *septal penetration* when a photon enters one hole, traverses the septa, and enters the neighboring hole. The septa are typically designed to be as thin as possible while limiting the amount of septal penetration to less than 5% of photons striking the septa. As a result, collimators designed for higher energy photons (over 200 keV) will require thicker septa than those designed for lower energies. Converse to collimator spatial resolution, the best geometrical sensitivity is attained with a collimator with either large or short holes. Thus again, a trade-off exists between spatial resolution and geometrical sensitivity. Because the geometrical sensitivity is proportional to $(d/a)^2$ and the spatial resolution is proportional to (d/a), the geometrical sensitivity of the collimator is roughly proportional to the square of the spatial resolution:

$$G_P \propto R_P^2$$

Finally, it is notable that the geometrical sensitivity of a parallel-hole collimator does not depend on the distance between the source and the collimator. The sensitivity is the same at the surface as it is at a distance removed from the surface. This fact may be counterintuitive because it might be expected that the sensitivity would drop off with distance as it does with the pinhole collimator.

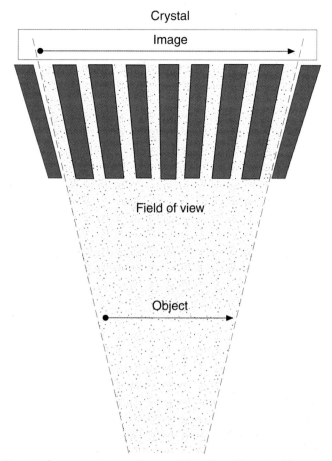

Fig. 2.9 Converging-hole collimator. With this collimator, objects are magnified, which tends to minimize the blurring effects of the intrinsic spatial resolution and thus provide higher system spatial resolution. In addition, the sensitivity increases with distance as the collimator's focal distance is approached, and thus it provides both improved spatial resolution and higher sensitivity, but with a decreased field of view.

In fact, the sensitivity of a single hole of the collimator does go down with distance, but the degrading spatial resolution leads to the irradiation of more holes, and these two facts cancel each other.

The *converging* multihole collimator provides both enhanced spatial resolution and improved sensitivity. With the converging collimator (Fig. 2.9), the direction of the holes is focused at a point some distance from the collimator surface. The distance from the collimator to the focal point is typically on the order of 50 cm and thus far beyond the boundaries of the patient. The focusing provides magnification similar to that with the pinhole collimator. As a result, the spatial resolution is typically slightly better than that with a parallel collimator but not as good as that with a pinhole collimator. In addition, the geometrical sensitivity of the converging collimator improves as the source approaches the focal point, and thus the sensitivity improves at distances farther from the collimator. On the other hand, the field of view is slightly reduced at greater distances because of the increased magnification. The converging collimator is used in applications similar to those with the pinhole collimator—that is, for imaging smaller objects using a camera with a large field of view and to achieve a magnified image with slightly improved spatial resolution.

The extrinsic or system spatial resolution (R_E) depends on both the intrinsic and collimator geometrical spatial resolution (R_I and R_C, respectively). To first order, the relationship between these is given by:

$$R_E = \sqrt{R_I^2 = R_C^2}$$

Based on this equation, the larger of the two values, the intrinsic or the collimator resolution, will dominate the system resolution. Except at distances very close to the collimator face, the collimator spatial resolution is substantially greater than the intrinsic resolution, and thus the collimator spatial resolution is, in general, the more important factor. In cases involving magnification, the intrinsic spatial resolution, R_I, is modified by magnification, thus minimizing the effect of intrinsic spatial resolution on system spatial resolution:

$$R_E = \sqrt{\left(\frac{R_I}{M}\right)^2 = R_C^2}$$

The system spatial resolution and the collimator geometrical sensitivity vary as a function of the distance from the radioactive source to the collimator (Fig. 2.10). The system spatial resolution of all of the collimators degrades with increasing distance from the collimator (see Fig. 2.10). The pinhole provides the best spatial resolution, followed by the converging collimator and two types of parallel-hole collimators, the high-resolution and general-purpose collimators. On the other hand, the pinhole collimator has the poorest geometrical sensitivity, which varies as the square of the distance (see Fig. 2.10). For the two parallel-hole collimators, the sensitivity does not vary with distance, and the sensitivity of the converging collimator improves with distance.

The standard gamma camera can be used for various studies; however, some other nuclear medicine imaging devices are designed for very specific clinical applications. These often use novel approaches to either gamma ray or light detection. In some instances, they use a semiconductor detector such as CZT. In other cases, they may use avalanche photodiode or silicon PMTs for light detection in conjunction with a scintillator. The most notable clinical planar imaging application for these types of devices is breast imaging. The compact size allows the device to stay close to the breast, resulting in high spatial resolution. In addition, the camera can be designed with limited dead space between the edge of the field of view and the patient, allowing imaging close to the chest wall. All of these characteristics result in improved imaging with this device relative to the standard gamma camera.

QUALITY CONTROL

To ensure proper operation of any medical device, including the gamma camera, it is essential that a comprehensive quality control program be applied. This involves acceptance testing of the device before its initial use and a program of routine tests and evaluations applied on a regular basis. It is essential that the performance be evaluated regularly to ensure that the images adequately demonstrate the in vivo distribution of the administered

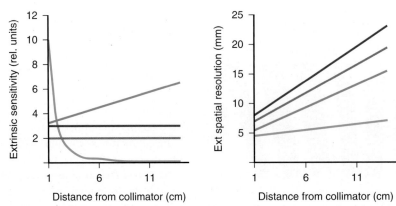

Fig. 2.10 System sensitivity *(left)* and spatial resolution *(right)* as a function of the source-to-collimator distance. The system spatial resolution of all collimators degrades (increases in value) with distance. The pinhole collimator *(blue)* provides the best spatial resolution (lowest value) but the lowest sensitivity, which varies according to the inverse square law. The converging collimator *(green)* provides very good spatial resolution with a sensitivity that increases with distance as the source approaches the focal distance of the collimator. The high-resolution parallel-hole collimator *(pink)* has good resolution and reasonable sensitivity. The general-purpose, parallel-hole collimator *(red)* has poorer spatial resolution than the high-resolution collimator but with a 50% increase in sensitivity. It is noted that the sensitivity of the two parallel-hole collimators does not vary with distance.

Fig. 2.11 Uniformity (flood) phantom image.

radiopharmaceutical and that any quantitation performed with the camera yields values that are as accurate and precise as possible.

Gamma camera quality control involves tests that are either quantitative or qualitative. For the quantitative tests, various parameters are used to measure the characteristics of the gamma camera system. Some of these parameters are evaluated intrinsically (i.e., without a collimator, to characterize the optics and electronics of the system) and other parameters extrinsically to include the collimator. If extrinsic tests are performed frequently (e.g., daily), they should be performed using the collimators most commonly used in the clinic. However, it may be best to perform the tests with all of the collimators used in the clinic at least annually. Certain parameters may be evaluated in different parts of the gamma camera's field of view. The *useful field of view* (UFOV) is the portion of the field of view the manufacturer has designated to be the proper extent for clinical imaging. Although the UFOV typically covers more than 95% of the total field of view, it may not extend to the very edge of the NaI crystal or collimator face. The *central field of view* (CFOV)

is the central 50% of the area of the UFOV. The U.S. National Electronic Manufacturers Association, a trade association of electronic manufacturers, has defined parameters for gamma camera manufacturers to use to characterize the performance of their equipment. Although some of these parameters may be difficult to assess in the clinic, they still provide the basis for many of the quantitative measures used in the gamma camera quality control program.

The *uniformity* (or *flood*) test evaluates the consistency of the response of the gamma camera to a uniform flux of radiation (Fig. 2.11). It should not be confused with the high-count uniformity calibration. The uniformity test can be applied either intrinsically or extrinsically. For the intrinsic test, the collimator is removed and exposed to the radiation from a point source of small activity (about .05 mCi (2 MBq) at a distance far enough to ensure uniform irradiation of the camera's field of view (at least 2 m). Extrinsic flood images are acquired with a large-area uniform source containing approximately 3 mCi to 10 mCi (111 to 370 MBq). This may consist of a thin water-filled source into which the radionuclide of choice (e.g., Tc-99m) is injected and thoroughly mixed. More commonly, a solid, sealed, large-area source of Co-57 (122-keV gamma ray, 270-day half-life) is used. For routine testing, 5 to 20 million counts are acquired and the images evaluated qualitatively for any notable nonuniformities. The daily flood should be acquired before administering the radiopharmaceutical to the first patient to ensure that the camera is working properly. Extrinsic floods for all collimators used with the camera may be acquired on an annual basis.

Gamma camera spatial resolution can be evaluated either intrinsically or extrinsically, qualitatively or quantitatively. In general, it may be evaluated quantitatively only during acceptance testing and perhaps during annual testing using very small point or line sources. The spatial resolution is characterized by the width of the image of the small source. Typical values for intrinsic spatial resolution range from 3 to 4 mm. Extrinsic values depend on the particular collimator being evaluated and the distance at which the test was performed, but for collimators commonly used in the clinic, the extrinsic spatial resolution at 10 cm ranges from about 8 to 12 mm. In the clinic, a qualitative assessment of extrinsic spatial resolution, typically a four-quadrant bar phantom (Fig. 2.12), is more commonly performed. Each quadrant of this phantom comprises alternating lead and spacing equal to the width of the bars of varying sizes (e.g., 2.0, 2.5, 3 0, and 3.5 mm). For extrinsic spatial resolution at the collimator surface, the phantom is placed on the collimator with the large-area uniformity source on top of it. The user reviews the resultant image and determines how many of the quadrants of the phantom can be discerned as separate bars. In general, the bars that can be discerned should be approximately 60% of the quantitative spatial resolution value. Thus, if the intrinsic spatial resolution is 3.5 mm, it should be possible to discern 2-mm bars of the four-quadrant bar phantom. The extrinsic spatial resolution at the surface of the most commonly used collimator in the clinic is qualitatively evaluated routinely on either a weekly or monthly basis. The number of quadrants that can be discerned should be compared with those determined during acceptance testing. The four-quadrant

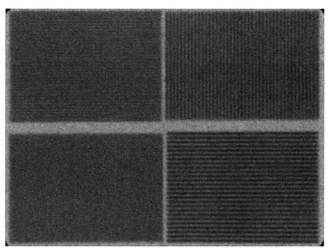

Fig. 2.12 Four-quadrant bar phantom image for spatial resolution.

bar phantom image can also be used to qualitatively test spatial linearity by evaluating the straightness of the bars in the image.

Other performance parameters or characteristics that can be tested include the sensitivity, energy resolution, count rate performance, and multiwindow registration. The sensitivity is most commonly evaluated extrinsically using a small-area source (e.g., 10 × 10 cm) of known activity (typically approximately 1.1 -3.2 mCi (40 - 120 MBq)` of Tc-99m) placed on the collimator being evaluated, counted for 1 minute and reported as the counts per minute per unit activity. For parallel-hole collimators, the distance of the source to the collimator is inconsequential because the sensitivity does not vary with distance. For the pinhole or focusing collimators, a standard distance such as 10 cm should be used. The sensitivity value will obviously depend on the collimator being evaluated, ranging from 5.0 to 8.5 cpm/kBq for typical high-resolution and general-purpose collimators. For the energy resolution, a pulse height (or energy) spectrum is acquired of a known radionuclide, typically Tc-99m, and the width of the photopeak is determined in a manner similar to that used for spatial resolution normalized by the gamma-ray energy. A typical gamma camera will have an energy resolution of 9% to 11% at 140 keV. As discussed previously, radiation detectors take a certain amount of time to process each event and, if events are registered too quickly, some may be lost as a result of dead time or count rate losses. The count rate performance can be evaluated by using two sources of reasonably high activity to calculate the dead time value in microseconds or by varying the exposure rate to which the camera is exposed and recording the observed count rate. For modern cameras, the maximum observable count rate is typically between 200,000 and 400,000 counts per second (cps). Finally, the multiwindow registration can be characterized. As previously discussed, the gamma camera position estimate obtained using Anger logic must be normalized by the energy deposited so that the position estimate does not vary as a function of photon energy. For this test, point sources of gallium-67, which emits photons of three different energies (90, 190, and 300 keV), are placed in several locations within the gamma camera field of view and the image location of each of the points sources

TABLE 2.1	Gamma Camera Quality Control Summary
Parameter	**Comment**
Daily	
Uniformity	Flood field; intrinsic (without collimator) or extrinsic (with collimator)
Window setting	Confirm energy window setting relative to photopeak for each radionuclide used with each patient
Weekly or Monthly	
Spatial resolution	Requires a "resolution" phantom such as the four-quadrant bar
Linearity check	Qualitative assessment of bar pattern linearity
Annually	
System uniformity	High count flood with each collimator
Multiwindow registration	For cameras with the capability of imaging multiple energy windows simultaneously
Count rate performance	Vary counts using decay or absorber method
Energy resolution	Easiest in cameras with built-in multichannel analyzers
System sensitivity	Count rate performance per unit of activity for each collimator

are evaluated to make sure that they do not vary depending on which photopeak was imaged.

These parameters should be evaluated and compared with manufacturer specifications during acceptance testing. It is highly recommended that these tests be performed by a qualified nuclear medicine physicist. After acceptance testing, quality control tests will be run at various frequencies (daily, weekly, monthly, quarterly, or annually), and the evaluation may be qualitative rather than quantitative in these cases. Table 2.1 summarizes the recommended frequency for each of the described tests. These recommendations are for the typical gamma camera, and the most

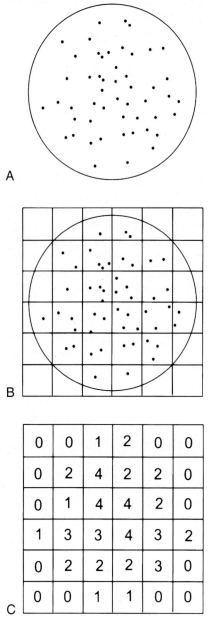

A

B

0	0	1	2	0	0
0	2	4	2	2	0
0	1	4	4	2	0
1	3	3	4	3	2
0	2	2	2	3	0
0	0	1	1	0	0

C

Fig. 2.13 Digital image. Consider a nuclear medicine image acquired in matrix mode using a 6 × 6 matrix. (A) The calculated positions based on Anger logic a number of events. (B) A 6 × 6 matrix superimposed onto these events demonstrates into which of the pixels of the matrix each event would fit. (C) The number of events (dots) in each pixel is recorded and assigned a particular shade of gray or another color to create the digital matrix.

appropriate quality control program for a specific gamma camera depends on manufacturer recommendations and the clinical use and stability of performance for that particular camera.

The x- and y-location of each accepted detection event is digitally stored within the acquisition host computer associated with the gamma camera. These data can be captured in two ways—matrix and list mode. In matrix mode, a specific matrix size (64 × 64, 128 × 128, 256 × 256, and so on) is predetermined depending on the assumed spatial resolution of the imaging task. For tasks that involve higher spatial resolution, a larger matrix would be required. The chosen matrix size is mapped to the field of view, and each estimated (x,y)-location is assigned to a particular picture element or *pixel* within the image matrix. The value of that pixel is then incremented by 1. In this manner, a 2D histogram of the event locations is generated, and at the end of the acquisition, the value in a particular pixel is the total number of events assigned to that pixel during the data acquisition process. An example with a 6 × 6 matrix is shown in Fig. 2.13. To display the image, the number of counts in a particular pixel is assigned a color or gray value according to a certain color scale lookup table on the computer monitor. An example might be that the pixel with the most counts is assigned the color white, pixels with no counts are assigned black, and all other pixels are assigned a shade of gray. Alternatively, the colors of the rainbow could be used, with violet indicating zero counts and red indicating the highest count. In addition, many other color tables could be used.

In many cases, more than one image is acquired during the imaging procedure. In some cases, a time-sequence of image frames, also known as a *dynamic study*, may be acquired. For example, a frame may be acquired every minute for 20 minutes. A multiphase study may be acquired, in which ten 30-second frames are followed by five 60-second frames, followed by five 120-second frames. In other instances, the data acquisition may be associated with a physiological gating signal such as the electrocardiogram (ECG) or a respiratory gate. In the cardiac example, counts from different parts of the heart cycle could be placed in different frames, resulting in frames from the end of diastole to the end of systole and back again. In matrix mode, these multiframe acquisitions would be obtained by establishing the desired number of the frames in the computer a priori. During the acquisition process, the appropriate pixel for each event would need to be determined, in addition to the appropriate frame within the heart cycle.

In list mode, the (x,y)-location of each event is stored using the highest level of digitization possible as a stream. In addition, timing and physiological gating marks may be stored periodically. For example, a timing mark may be stored every millisecond, as can the time of the R peak in the ECG (Fig. 2.14). After the acquisition is complete, the user can then select the desired matrix size and the temporal or physiological framing rate a posteriori. Based on these criteria, a postacquisition program is run to format the data as defined. The user could then decide to reformat the data to a different set of parameters. In this way, list mode acquisition is very flexible because it does not require the user to define the acquisition matrix and framing a priori. On the other hand, it typically requires more computer storage and running the formatting program to view the data. For these reasons, matrix mode is most commonly used.

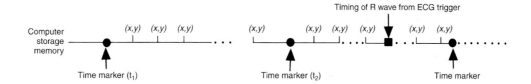

(x,y) = coordinates of each individual scintillation

Fig. 2.14 List-mode data acquisition. In *list mode*, the *(x,y)*-position of each detection event is determined at the highest available resolution and stored in sequence. In addition, time markers and physiological signals (such as the timing of the R wave from the electrocardiogram trigger) are periodically stored. Once the acquisition is completed, the desired matrix size, time sequence, and physiological gate framing can be selected, and a formatting program is run to provide the acquired data for viewing and analysis.

Each pixel in the planar nuclear medicine image can be considered its own detector, and thus the total counts in a pixel are governed by Poisson statistics similar to a well counter or a thyroid probe. Therefore the standard deviation of the pixel counts is simply estimated by the square root of the pixel counts. In addition, the sum of Poisson distributed values is also a Poisson distributed value. Therefore, if a region of interest is defined on a planar nuclear medicine image and the pixel values within that region are added, the result is also Poisson distributed. Nuclear medicine studies are often quantified by defining regions of interest (ROIs) over features of interest and subsequently comparing the counts. In some cases, the counts from different views of the patient can be combined to provide more accurate quantitation. For example, taking the geometrical mean (square root of the product of the counts) of similar regions from opposite, conjugate views such as the anterior and posterior views, can provide an estimate that, to first order, does not depend on the depth of the activity within the body. Theoretically, this approach works for point sources, but it also has been shown to work reasonably well for extended sources. The counts are determined from the ROIs drawn about each lung, right and left, on images acquired from both the anterior and posterior views of the patient. The geometrical mean of the counts in each lung is calculated, and the differential function of each lung is estimated by dividing the counts for that lung by the sum of counts for both lungs.

In a dynamic study, the region of interest counts in each frame can be plotted as a function of time. The resulting plot is referred to as the time–activity curve (TAC). In the case of relatively short-lived radionuclides, each value along the plot should be decay corrected to the beginning of the acquisition or the time of radiopharmaceutical administration. In the example of a Tc-99m MAG3 renal study, a TAC can be used to evaluate both renal perfusion and clearance of the agent.

Radiation detection and counting form the cornerstone of nuclear medicine. Detectors of all types—gas detectors, scintillators, and semiconductors—are used every day in the nuclear medicine clinic. Some are used for ancillary purposes that support the clinic, such as those used in the context of radiation protection. Others are used specifically to acquire biological data for a particular clinical purpose. Most notably, the gamma camera is used to obtain images of the in vivo distribution of the administered radiopharmaceutical from which the patient's physiology or function can be inferred to further define the patient's medical picture. A rigorous quality control program must be maintained for all equipment used in the nuclear medicine clinic to ensure the integrity of the data obtained from the patient. The quality control program for the gamma camera includes acceptance testing and tests that need to be performed on a routine basis. The nuclear medicine image acquired with the gamma camera provides a snapshot of the patient's in vivo radiopharmaceutical distribution from a certain view and at a particular point in time. These images can also be acquired as a dynamic (time-sequence) study or in conjunction with a physiological gate such as the ECG. ROIs can be drawn about specific features to provide regional quantitation or TACs of dynamic processes. Nuclear medicine instrumentation continues to evolve, including the development of devices designed for a specific clinical task, such as breast imaging. It is expected that this development will continue in the years ahead.

SUGGESTED READING

Chandra R, Rahmim A. *Nuclear Medicine Physics: The Basics.* 8th ed Philadelphia: Williams & Wilkins. 2018.

Cherry SR, Sorenson JA, Phelps ME. *Physics in Nuclear Medicine.* 4th ed. Philadelphia: WB Saunders. 2012.

International Atomic Energy Association. *Nuclear Medicine Physics: A Handbook for Teachers and Students.* Vienna, Austria: International Atomic Energy Agency. 2014.

International Atomic Energy Association. *Planning a Clinical PET Centre.* Vienna, Austria: International Atomic Energy Agency. 2010.

International Atomic Energy Association. *Quality Assurance for PET and PET-CT Systems.* Vienna, Austria: International Atomic Energy Agency. 2019.

International Atomic Energy Association. *Quality Assurance of SPECT Systems.* Vienna, Austria: International Atomic Energy Agency. 2009.

International Atomic Energy Association. *Quality Control Atlas for Scintillation Camera Systems.* Vienna, Austria: International Atomic Energy Agency. 2019.

National Electrical Manufacturers Association. *Performance Measurements of Positron Emission Tomographs.* Rosslyn, VA: National Electrical Manufacturers Association. 2018.

Powsner RA, Powsner ER. *Essentials of Nuclear Medicine Physics.* 3rd ed. Malden, MA: Blackwell Science. 2012.

3

Single-Photon Emission Computed Tomography, Positron Emission Tomography, and Hybrid Imaging

DATA ACQUISITION OF EMISSION TOMOGRAPHYN

Conventional or planar radionuclide imaging suffers a major limitation in the loss of object contrast as a result of background radioactivity. In the planar image, radioactivity underlying and overlying the object of interest is superimposed on that coming from the object. The fundamental goal of tomographic imaging systems is a more accurate portrayal of the three-dimensional (3D) distribution of radioactivity in the patient, with improved image contrast and definition of image detail. This is analogous to the way computed tomography (CT) provides better soft tissue contrast than planar radiography. The Greek *tomo* means "to cut"; tomography may be thought of as a means of "cutting" the body into discrete image planes. Tomographic techniques have been developed for both single-photon and positron imaging, referred to as single-photon emission computed tomography (SPECT) and positron emission tomography (PET), respectively.

Restricted or limited-angle tomography keeps the plane of interest in focus while blurring the out-of-plane data in much the same way as conventional x-ray tomography. Various restricted-angle systems have been investigated, including multi-pinhole collimator systems, pseudo-random, coded-aperture collimator systems, and various rotating slant-hole collimator systems. Although clinical use has been limited, resurgent interest has been shown for specific imaging applications, including those designed for cardiac and breast imaging.

Tomographic approaches that acquire data over 180 or 360 degrees provide a more complete reconstruction of the object and therefore are more widely used. Rotating gamma camera SPECT systems offer the ability to perform true transaxial tomography. PET uses a method called *annihilation coincidence detection* to acquire data over 360 degrees without the use of absorptive collimation. The most important characteristic of these approaches is that only data arising in the image plane of interest are used in the reconstruction of the tomographic image. This is an important characteristic leading to improved image contrast compared with methods using restricted-angle tomography. As will be discussed, the reconstruction of these data has historically been done with filtered back-projection. However, iterative techniques such as ordered subsets expectation maximization (OSEM) are increasingly used. This chapter reviews the current approaches to the acquisition and reconstruction of SPECT and PET, including the use of hybrid imaging such as PET/CT, PET/MR and SPECT/CT, and the quality control necessary to ensure high-quality clinical results.

All tomographic modalities used in diagnostic imaging, including SPECT, PET, CT, and magnetic resonance imaging (MRI), acquire raw data in the form of *projection data* at a variety of angles about the patient. Although SPECT and PET use different approaches to acquiring these data, the nature of the data is essentially the same. Image reconstruction involves the processing of these data to generate a series of cross-sectional images through the object of interest.

The geometries associated with the acquisition of SPECT and PET are illustrated in Fig. 3.1. In the simple SPECT example using a parallel-hole collimator, the data acquired at a particular location in the gamma camera crystal originated from a line passing through that point perpendicular to the surface of the sodium iodide (NaI) crystal face and is referred to in the figure as the *line of origin* (see Fig. 3.1, *left*). Thus the data at this point can be seen to represent the sum of counts that originated along this line, or *ray*, referred to as a *ray sum*. These ray-sum values across the patient are referred to as the projection data for this cross-sectional slice at this particular viewing angle. For PET, the ray sum represents the data collected along a particular line of response (LOR) connecting a pair of detectors involved in a coincidence detection event (see Fig. 3.1, *right*).

For a SPECT acquisition, the projection image acquired at each angle consists of the stack of projections for all slices within the camera field of view at that angle. Fig. 3.2, on the right, shows projections from a SPECT brain scan at five different viewing angles. For a particular slice (see Fig. 3.2, *dashed white line*), a row of the projection data for each angle can be stacked such that the displacement along the projection is on the *x*-axis and the viewing angle is on the *y*-axis (see Fig. 3.2, *right*). This plot is referred to as the *sinogram*, because the resulting plot of a point source resembles a sine-wave plot turned on its side. A more complicated object such as a brain scan can be perceived as many such sine waves overlaid on top of each other for each point within the object. The sinogram, represents the full set of projection data necessary to reconstruct a particular single slice. A separate slice is made in the sinogram for each cross-sectional slice through the object. The set of projection views and the set of

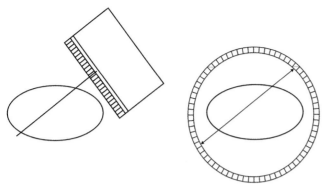

Fig. 3.1 Single-photon emission computed tomography (SPECT) and positron emission tomography (PET) acquisition geometries. For SPECT *(left)*, the gamma camera rotates about the patient, acquiring a projection image at each angle. Each projection image represents the projections of many slices acquired at that angle. For PET *(right)*, the patient is located within a ring of detectors. A positron annihilation event leads to two photons emitted in opposite directions. When two events are detected within a small timing acceptance window (5–12 ns), they are considered to be from the same event and are assumed to have originated along the line of response that connects the two detectors.

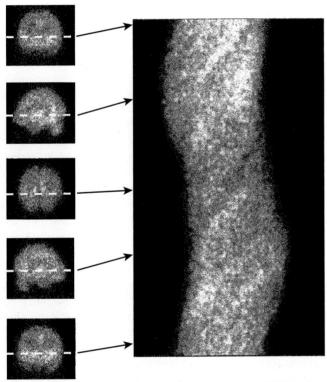

Fig. 3.2 Single-photon emission computed tomography (SPECT) projection images and sinograms. *Right,* projection images of a SPECT brain scan at five different viewing angles. For a particular slice (indicated by the *dashed white line*), the projection data can be stacked to form the sinogram *(left)*. (From Henkin RE. *Nuclear Medicine.* St. Louis: Mosby; 2006.)

sinograms are alternative means of displaying the projection data associated with a tomographic acquisition. Each projection view displays the projection data across all slices with a separate image for each angle, whereas the sinogram displays the projection data across all angles with a separate sinogram for each slice.

The geometry of PET acquisition (see Fig. 3.1, *right*) involves the data acquired along a particular LOR connecting two

detectors that may be involved in an annihilation coincidence detection event. These data thus represent the ray sum along this LOR. The data associated with a particular LOR are characterized in the sinogram by their distance from the center of the gantry (on the *x*-axis) and their angle of orientation (on the *y*-axis). In this manner, PET data acquisition directly into sinograms may be more straightforward than into projection views. In a PET detection event, the two detectors involved in the coincidence event are identified, and the LOR is recorded. The location in the sinogram corresponding to that particular LOR is localized, and its data are incremented. After the collection of many such events, the projection data are represented by a set of sinograms for each PET slice. However, these data also can be displayed as projection views similar to those acquired in SPECT studies. This simple example illustrates the acquisition of PET data in *2D mode,* in which each cross-sectional slice basically is acquired separately. Most current PET scanners acquire data only in *3D mode,* in which LORs cut across the parallel cross-section slices. The corresponding projection data will include oblique views or sinograms through the object. With time-of-flight PET (discussed later in this chapter), it is necessary to record not only the LOR but also the time difference between the two detections involved in the annihilation coincidence detection event, which will also be incorporated into the reconstruction of these data.

Tomographic data can be acquired in a dynamic or gated approach. For example, a PET study can be acquired as a time sequence of scans that might be simple or multiphase (e.g., ten 5-second frames, four 30-second frames, and five 60-second frames). In addition, the tomographic study can be acquired in association with a physiological gate such as the electrocardiogram (ECG) or a respiratory signal. For example, myocardial perfusion SPECT is acquired in conjunction with the ECG. In dynamic or gated tomographic acquisitions, a full set of projection data acquired at each time or gate point is to be reconstructed separately.

Tomographic Reconstruction

Images, like time signals, can be considered as either a spatial variation of the signal or a sum of signals of varying frequencies. It is intuitive to consider images as a spatial variation in the signal because some part of the image will be bright and other parts will be dark. In nuclear medicine, the bright and dark areas may correspond to regions of high and low radiopharmaceutical uptake, respectively. Conversely, it is not intuitive to consider an image to comprise signals of varying frequency, although this is in fact the case. On the other hand, we do naturally perceive audio signals in terms of frequencies. A choral performance comprises sopranos, altos, tenors, and basses, and the combination of these voices hopefully leads to a very pleasurable experience. On the other hand, we cannot perceive a presentation of the audio signal as a temporal variation of the signal and intuitively identify it as music. The music is fully described by either representation, and there may be cases in which either the temporal (i.e., real) or the frequency representation is the best approach for considering the audio data. The same is true for image data, except the variations are in space rather than time.

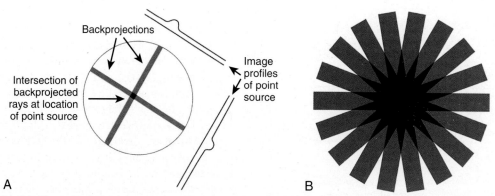

Fig. 3.3 Simple back-projection. (A) The counts in each position along the projection are back-projected across the reconstruction matrix because the algorithm has no knowledge as to the origin of the event. This process is referred to as *simple back-projection*. (B) Simple back-projection leads to streak artifacts that render all but the simplest objects discernable.

Image data may be best represented in either spatial (real) or frequency space. The mathematician Joseph Fourier noted in 1807 that any arbitrary signal can be generated by adding a large number of sine and cosine signals of varying frequencies and amplitudes. The plot of amplitude as a function of frequency is referred to as the *Fourier transform,* and it defines the components of the image at each frequency. The low frequencies provide the overall shape of the object, whereas the high frequencies help define the sharp edges and fine detail within the image. Audio signals can be manipulated by emphasizing certain frequencies (low or high); the same is true for images. Image noise is typically present in all frequencies; if the low frequencies are emphasized, the image may be less noisy but blurry, whereas emphasizing the high frequencies will accentuate both the edges of the objects and the noise. Such image manipulation is referred to as *filtering* because it allows certain spatial frequencies to be realized while removing others.

Since the initial development of CT 40 years ago, *filtered back-projection* has been the most common approach to reconstructing medical tomographic data, including SPECT, PET, and CT, although iterative techniques were introduced into the clinic for use with PET more than a decade ago. However, filtered back-projection is still used in SPECT and remains the most common method for CT. In back-projection, it is assumed that all of the data detected at a particular point along the projection originated from somewhere along the line emanating from this point. For SPECT using parallel-hole collimation, this would be the line of origin passing through the detection point and perpendicular to the NaI crystal surface. For PET, events would be assumed to have come from the LOR connecting the two detectors involved in the annihilation coincidence detection event. In general, back-projection makes no assumptions of where along the line the event occurred, and thus the counts are spread evenly along the line. In other words, the counts are *back-projected* along the line of origin or LOR. All of the counts from every location along every projection are *back-projected* across the reconstructed image (Fig. 3.3, *A*). The result is referred to as *simple back-projection;* it has substantial streak artifacts that, in all but the simplest objects, render the reconstructed image indiscernible (see Fig. 3.3, *B*). These streaks are

caused by uneven sampling of frequency space during the back-projection process, where low frequencies are sampled at a much higher rate than higher frequencies. To compensate for this, a filter, called the *ramp filter,* is applied during the reconstruction that increases linearly with frequency (Fig. 3.4). Applying back-projection in conjunction with such filtration is referred to as *filtered back-projection.* With a very large number of accurate, noiseless projections, filtered back-projection will yield an excellent, almost perfect reconstruction.

However, with true clinical data, the projections are noisy, and thus the ramp filter will tend to accentuate the high-frequency noise in the data. Therefore a *windowing filter* is applied, in addition to the ramp filter, to smoothly bring the filter back to zero at frequencies above the pertinent content in the study. Commonly used windowing functions include the Hamming and Butterworth filters (see Fig. 3.4). With these filters, a cutoff frequency is defined, which is the point at which they return to zero, with no higher frequencies being incorporated into the reconstructed image. Noting that low frequencies yield the overall shape and high frequencies yield the sharp edges and fine detail, the appearance of the resultant reconstructed image can be altered by varying the cutoff frequency. Selecting a cutoff frequency that is too low will yield a blurry reconstruction (Fig. 3.5, *A, far left*), and one that is too high will yield a noisy reconstruction (see Fig. 3.5, *C, second from the right*). However, an appropriate choice for cutoff frequency will provide an image that is a fair compromise between noise and detail (see Fig. 3.5, *B, second from left*). With an appropriate choice of cutoff frequency, filtered back-projection is a simple, fast, and robust approach to image reconstruction.

Iterative reconstruction provides an alternative to filtered back-projection that tends to be less noisy, tends to have fewer streak artifacts, and often allows for the incorporation of certain physical factors associated with the data acquisition into the reconstruction process, leading to a more accurate result. In iterative reconstruction, an initial guess as to the 3D object that could have led to the set of acquired projections is estimated. In addition, a model of the imaging process is assumed that may incorporate assumptions regarding photon attenuation and Compton scatter. It may also include other assumptions

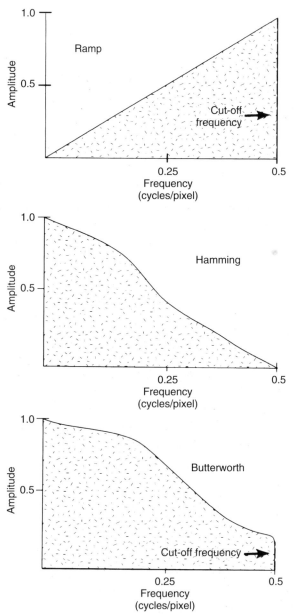

Fig. 3.4 Ramp, Hamming, and Butterworth filters. The ramp filter is a "high-pass" filter designed to reduce background activity and the star artifact. Hamming and Butterworth filters are "low-pass" filters designed to reduce high-frequency noise.

regarding the data-acquisition process, such as estimates of the device's spatial resolution that vary with position within the field of view; for example, the variation of collimator spatial resolution as a function of the distance between the object and the collimator can be incorporated into the reconstruction process.

Based on this model and the current estimate of the object, a new set of projections is simulated that is then compared with the real, acquired set. Variations between the two sets, parameterized by either the ratio or difference between pixel values, are then back-projected and added to the current estimate of the object to generate a new estimate (Fig. 3.6). These steps are repeated, or *iterated*, until an acceptable version of the object is reached. The goodness of the current estimate is typically based on statistical criteria such as the maximum likelihood. In other words, the process generates an estimate of the object that has the highest statistical likelihood to have led to the set of acquired projection data. A commonly used approach for the reconstruction of SPECT and PET data is the *maximum-likelihood expectation maximization* (MLEM) algorithm.

Iterative reconstruction often leads to a more accurate reconstruction of the data than that obtained through filtered back-projection. However, a large number of iterations, perhaps as many as 50, may be required to generate an acceptable estimation, and each iteration may take about the same time as a single filtered back-projection; thus the iterative approach may take 50 times longer to reconstruct. One approach to reducing the number of iterations is to organize the projection data into a series of ordered subsets of evenly spaced projections and update the current estimate of the object after each subset rather than after the complete set of projections. If the data are organized into 15 subsets, in general, the data can be reconstructed about 15 times faster while generating a result of similar image quality. A similar result can be produced with 15 ordered subsets and 3 iterations as would be obtained with 45 iterations using the complete set. The most common approach that uses ordered subsets in the clinic is referred to as OSEM. Fig. 3.5, *D (far right)* shows an OSEM reconstruction compared with a filtered back-projection of the same object. The use of faster algorithms such as OSEM and the development of faster computers have allowed iterative reconstruction of SPECT and PET data in 5 minutes or less, which is considered acceptable for clinical

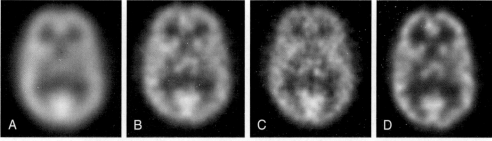

Fig. 3.5 Effect of different filtration on reconstruction. (A) Single-photon emission computed tomography (SPECT) study reconstructed with a cutoff frequency that is too smooth. The image is very blurry. (B) SPECT study reconstructed with an appropriate cutoff frequency, with a moderate noise level and sharpness. (C) SPECT study reconstructed with a cutoff frequency that is too sharp. The level of detail is good, but an excessive amount of image noise is present. (D) SPECT study acquired with iterative reconstruction ordered subsets expectation maximization (OSEM).

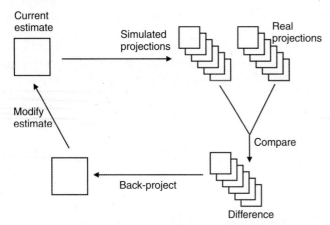

Fig. 3.6 Iterative reconstruction process. A set of simulated projections is generated from an initial guess of the object. This is compared with the real projection data, and the difference is back-projected and added to the initial guess. This process is iterated until the differences between the simulated and real projections are within an acceptable level.

work. With the development of even faster computers, iterative reconstruction may be routinely applied to the larger data sets associated with CT in the near future.

Attenuation Correction

A special problem of both SPECT and PET imaging is the attenuation of emissions in tissue. Photons emitted from deeper within the object are more likely to be absorbed in the overlying tissue than those emitted from the periphery. Therefore the signals from these tissues are *attenuated*. To obtain an image where the signal is not depth dependent, an *attenuation correction* must be performed to compensate for this effect. Good evidence indicates that studies that have not traditionally been attenuation corrected, such as myocardial perfusion imaging, benefit from proper attenuation correction. Two fundamentally different approaches are used for attenuation correction: analytic methods and those that incorporate transmission data into the process. Both are designed to create an image attenuation correction matrix, in which the value of each pixel represents the correction factor that should be applied to the acquired data. Some approaches are applied during reconstruction, whereas others are applied after reconstruction to the resultant images.

For portions of the body consisting almost entirely of soft tissue, an assumption of near-uniform attenuation can be made, and an analytic or mathematical approach such as the Chang algorithm can be used. The Chang algorithm is a postreconstruction approach. After the object is reconstructed, an outline of the body part is defined on the computer for each tomographic slice. From this outline, the depth, and therefore the appropriate correction factor, for each pixel location inside the outline can be computed. A correction matrix is generated, and a multiplicative correction is applied on a pixel-by-pixel basis. The linear attenuation coefficient for technetium-99m (Tc-99m) in soft tissue is 0.15/cm. This applies only to "good" geometry—that is, a point source with no scatter. Thus a value for Tc-99m of approximately 0.12/cm is often used to compensate for scatter. At a depth of 7 cm in a liver SPECT study, almost 60% of the corresponding activity is attenuated. The observed count value would have to be multiplied by a factor of 2.5 ($0.4 \times 2.5 = 1$) to

correct for attenuation. A similar analytic method has been developed for PET imaging, primarily of the brain.

The major limitation of the analytic approach occurs when multiple types of tissue, each with a different attenuation coefficient, are in the field of view. This can be particularly problematic for cardiac imaging, in which the soft tissues of the heart are surrounded by the air-containing lungs and the bony structures of the thorax. To correct for nonuniform attenuation, a transmission scanning approach is incorporated into the attenuation correction. In essence, a CT scan of the thorax is obtained using an x-ray tube. Older SPECT and PET systems also have used radionuclide sources for this purpose. The technique is similar to the use of CT, except radioactive sources incorporated into the scanner are used rather than an x-ray tube. The data are much noisier and require segmentation into the different tissue types before the attenuation map can be created. Manufacturers are moving away from the radioactive source methodology.

A hybrid SPECT-CT or PET-CT scanner is used to acquire a CT over the same axial range as the SPECT or PET scan. The CT scan is acquired with a tube voltage of 80 to 120 kVp, leading to an effective energy of about 40 to 60 keV. The range of the tube-current time product (milliamperes) is variable, depending on whether the CT scan is acquired for diagnostic purposes, for anatomical correlation, or for attenuation correction. Thus scans could be acquired with as little as 4 mA and as high as 400 mA. A lookup table is used to convert the Hounsfield units in the reconstructed CT scan to attenuation coefficients for the desired photon energy. The resulting attenuation map can then be applied as a postreconstruction correction or incorporated in the reconstruction process.

Display of Emission Tomographic Data

A particular advantage of gamma camera rotational SPECT is that a volume of image data is collected simultaneously. PET data may be acquired in several steps, but the resultant reconstructed data are also a volume. The pixel size for SPECT is the same in the three axes; for PET, the axial sampling might be slightly different from that in the transverse plane. However, in either case, once the transaxial tomographic volume is reconstructed, it easily can be resorted into other orthogonal planes. Thus the sagittal and coronal images can be directly generated from the reconstructed volume represented by the set of transaxial slices.

The data can be reformatted into planes oblique to the original transverse planes. This is particularly useful in cardiac imaging, in which the long axis of the heart does not coincide with any of the three major axes of the reconstructed data. It is desirable to reorient the data to obtain images that are perpendicular and parallel to the long axis of the left ventricle, which can be readily accomplished from the original volume data set. The computer operator defines the geometry of the long axis of the heart, and the data are reformatted to create cardiac long-axis and short-axis planes oblique to the transaxial slices (Fig. 3.7). The optimum angulation is highly variable across patients.

Another useful strategy is to view tomographic data as a sequence of planar images from different viewing angles in closed-loop cine. In the early days of SPECT imaging, this was accomplished by viewing the closed-loop cine of the raw projection data. This is still done in many cardiac imaging software

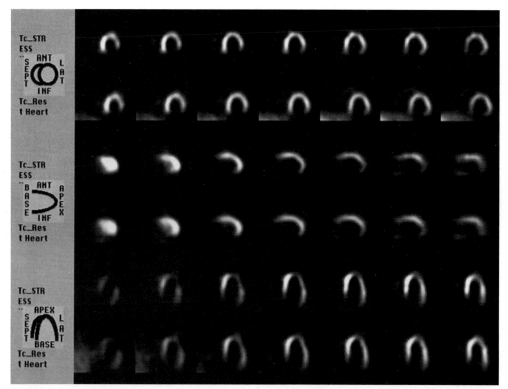

Fig. 3.7 Cardiac single-photon emission computed tomography (SPECT) images reformat data into multiple planes. The top two rows are short-axis views obtained perpendicular to the long axis of the left ventricle. The middle two rows are horizontal long-axis images, and the bottom two rows are vertical long-axis images. The patient has a large fixed perfusion defect involving the inferior wall of the left ventricle. The ability to reformat the data allows for more precise and accurate localization of abnormalities.

packages for quality control. However, these data tend to be noisy, making it difficult to view small variations in intensity. Currently, a common approach is to reproject the transaxial images to generate a series of planar images that have the benefit of greatly reduced noise. The reprojection method often used is the *maximum-intensity projection scan* (MIPS), created by reprojecting the hottest point along each particular ray for any given projection. These MIPS images emphasize areas of increased accumulation of radioactivity while providing an overall impression of the area of increased radioactivity in relation to the normal structures in individual tomographic slices. In some cases the MIPS images are distance weighted to make activity that is farther from the viewer appear less intense, thereby enhancing the 3D effect.

Single Photon Emission Computed Tomography

SPECT allows true 3D image acquisition, reconstruction, and display of the radiopharmaceuticals routinely used in conventional nuclear medicine. Over the past 30 years, SPECT has developed, particularly in the field of nuclear cardiology, to the point at which SPECT has become the standard imaging method. In SPECT, a series of projection images is acquired about the patient. In most cases, these projection images are acquired by rotating the imaging device about the object, but in other cases they may be acquired by viewing the object with multiple devices or through multiple pinhole apertures. These projection data are then reconstructed as described in the previous section, leading to the generation of a series of slices through the object.

The most common device used for SPECT is the rotating gamma camera, which consists of one or more gamma camera heads mounted onto a special rotating gantry. Nearly all gamma cameras marketed today incorporate SPECT capability. Early systems used a single gamma camera head, whereas modern systems more commonly have two detector heads. Dual-head systems that allow flexibility in configuration between the heads are very popular. For body imaging, the heads are typically arrayed parallel to each other; for cardiac imaging, they are often placed at right angles (Fig. 3.8). Some cameras are permanently configured in the 90-degree position for dedicated cardiac imaging. Multiple heads are desirable because they allow more data to be collected in a given period. Rotational SPECT is photon poor compared with x-ray CT, and thus SPECT imaging protocols commonly take 10 to 30 minutes for the acquisition of a data set. Therefore it is desirable to obtain as many counts as possible while completing the imaging within a reasonable time to limit the effects of patient motion and to minimize pharmacokinetic changes during the imaging time. Rotational SPECT has highlighted the need to improve every aspect of gamma camera system performance. Flood field nonuniformities are translated as major artifacts in tomographic images because they distort the data obtained from each view or projection. Desirable planar characteristics of a camera to be used for SPECT are an intrinsic spatial resolution of 3.5 mm (as estimated by the full width at half maximum [FWHM]), linearity distortion of 1 mm or less, and corrected integral uniformity within 3%. All contemporary

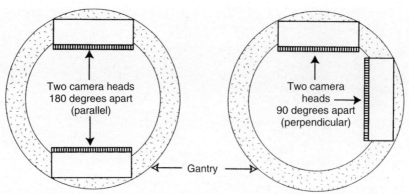

Fig. 3.8 Two configurations for a dual-detector single-photon emission computed tomography (SPECT) system.

rotational SPECT systems have online energy and uniformity correction, as described in Chapter 2.

Recently, dedicated SPECT systems have been developed for cardiac imaging only. These cameras may use Anger logic for event positioning; however, they are distinctly different in that they are not large, single-crystal detectors as are found in the traditional gamma camera, and many use solid-state detectors of cadmium zinc telluride (CZT) rather than NaI scintillating material. These detectors often use a pixelated design with detector elements of approximately 2 × 2 mm. Because of their multicrystal design, the scintillation-based systems often use either position-sensitive photomultiplier tubes or photodiodes for light detection. The systems that use CZT have higher intrinsic efficiency and enhanced energy resolution (6% at 140 keV compared with 9%-11% compared with NaI). This allows for the reduction of Compton scatter in the images and may also enhance the ability to perform dual-isotope acquisitions (e.g., Tc-99m and iodine-123). Finally, the detectors in these systems have physical design characteristics that improve sensitivity. For instance, multiple detectors or pinhole apertures may be viewing the heart simultaneously. These improvements in sensitivity can be used to shorten the acquisition time or lower the quantity of injected radioactivity and thereby lower the patient's radiation dose. Each system has different design characteristics, acquisition procedures, and quality control methods. Although these devices are promising, their use remains quite limited; therefore the rest of this section focuses on the rotating camera.

Box 3.1 summarizes factors that must be considered in performing SPECT with a rotating gamma camera. In addition to the calibrations described earlier and standard gamma camera quality control, careful attention to each of these factors will result in the high-quality SPECT images.

Although collimator selection is generally limited to those supplied by the manufacturer, the specific choice depends on the clinical imaging task at hand. For a given septal thickness and hole diameter, collimators with longer channels provide better resolution but at a cost of lower sensitivity. However, even though SPECT is relatively photon poor, collimator selection should favor high resolution over high sensitivity when possible because high-resolution collimators provide improved image quality compared with high-sensitivity or

---

BOX 3.1 Image-Acquisition Issues for Single-Photon Emission Computed Tomography

Collimator selection
Orbit
Matrix size
Angular increment: number of views
180- vs. 360-degree rotation
Time per view
Total examination time

---

general-purpose collimators, even with fewer counts. The use of multihead SPECT systems allows the operator to gain back some of the counts lost when using high-resolution collimators by longer acquisition at each step or projection angle.

In addition to the parallel-hole collimators routinely used for planar and SPECT imaging, there are special focused collimator options specifically designed for SPECT imaging of the brain and the heart. These typically are a type of converging collimator that permits more of the camera crystal to be used for radiation detection. These collimators cause magnification of the object and an increase in sensitivity proportional to the level of magnification. Thus given a parallel-hole collimator and a focused collimator with the same spatial resolution, the focused collimator will have an improvement in sensitivity compared with the parallel-hole collimator. The use of focused collimators results in a geometrical distortion that must be accounted for in the reconstruction.

The orbit selected (circular or noncircular) depends on the organ of interest (Fig. 3.9). Almost all systems today offer both circular and noncircular orbits. The ideal orbit keeps the detector as close to the object of interest as possible during the acquisition because the best resolution is at the face of the collimator for parallel-hole collimators. For imaging the trunk of the body, most cameras use a noncircular orbit for this reason. Both circular and noncircular orbits may be used for imaging the brain depending on whether the operator is able to position the detectors to clear the shoulders. When using special focused collimators, the orbit is often determined automatically by the system that keeps the organ of interest in the focused area.

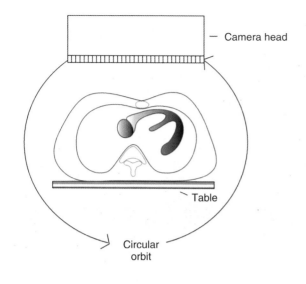

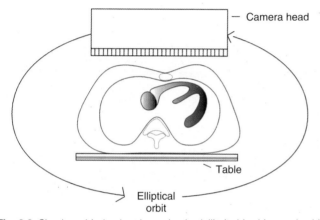

Fig. 3.9 Circular orbit *(top)* and noncircular (elliptical in this case) orbit *(bottom)*.

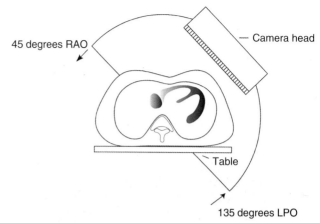

Fig. 3.10 The 180-degree arc frequently used for cardiac imaging from right anterior oblique (RAO; 45 degrees) to left posterior oblique (LPO; 135 degrees).

The choice of angular sampling and arc of acquisition depends on the clinical application and the collimator used. For body imaging applications, a full 360-degree acquisition arc is commonly used. Most SPECT data are acquired using a 128 × 128 image matrix with high-resolution collimators and Tc-99m radiopharmaceuticals. However, a 64 × 64 matrix may be used when the camera resolution is not as good or if the count density will be low because very little activity occurs in the patient at the time of imaging. Many SPECT/CT hybrid cameras in which a CT scan will be used for attenuation correction require that the emission data be acquired in a 128 × 128 matrix. If the 128 × 128 matrix is used, the angular sampling should be set to 3-degree increments. If the lower-resolution 64 × 64 matrix is used, the step size may be increased to 4- or 6-degree increments. These combinations of matrix size and angular sampling, along with the collimator selection, "balance" the resolution of the respective parameters. However, these parameters may be varied in some circumstances. For example, acquiring fewer steps may be acceptable for pediatric patients given their smaller size.

For cardiac imaging, a 180-degree acquisition arc is well accepted. Because the heart is located close to the anterior chest wall on the left side, the best data are obtained by imaging in a 180-degree arc that spans from the right anterior oblique to the left posterior oblique positions (Fig. 3.10). This acquisition paradigm is widely accepted in the clinical practice even when CT attenuation correction is applied to the data.

Another consideration is whether to use continuous or "step-and-shoot" data acquisition. Continuous acquisition has the advantage of not wasting time while the camera heads are moving from one angular position to the next. However, the data are blurred by the motion artifact of the moving camera head. The resulting trade-off between sensitivity and resolution favor step-and-shoot acquisition for most clinical applications. Exceptions are applications with rapidly changing tracer distribution and when the determination of overall tracer concentration is more important than spatial resolution.

In general, SPECT studies are count poor, and thus it is beneficial to acquire the studies for as long as possible. Within accepted limits for dosimetry and radiation exposure, a larger administered dosage may allow for more available counts. Although clinically accepted limits for administered radioactivity should never be exceeded, the radiation risk versus benefit must take into account the likelihood of obtaining a diagnostic-quality image. The goal of obtaining higher counting statistics is meaningless if the patient moves, causing data between the different angular sampling views to be misregistered. Most clinical protocols limit the total imaging time to 20 to 40 minutes. Correspondingly, the time per projection is usually 20 to 40 seconds, but as much as 60 seconds may be needed for particularly count-poor studies with gallium-67 and indium-111.

Even when restricting the total SPECT acquisition time to less than 30 minutes, patient motion may still be an issue. Some camera manufacturers provide motion-correction programs, but these work in only one dimension (vertical motion), not three dimensions. Patient compliance is improved by taking time during setup to position the patient comfortably. For scans of the head, the patient's arms can be in a natural position at the sides. For rotational SPECT studies of the heart, thorax, abdomen, or pelvis, the arms are typically raised out of the field of view so that they do not interfere with the path of photons toward the detector, which may increase the patient's

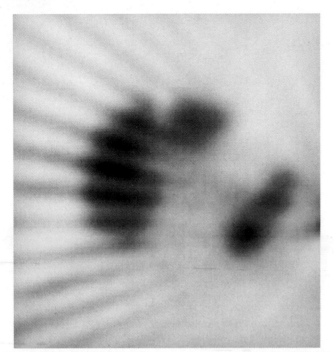

Fig. 3.11 Single-photon emission computed tomography (SPECT) artifact caused by injection-site activity in the field of view. Degraded SPECT image of the liver and spleen caused by including activity at the injection site in the imaging field of view. The starburst artifact is a result of back-projection of the hot-spot activity across the image. In this case the degree of activity in the injection site could not be accommodated in the reconstruction algorithm.

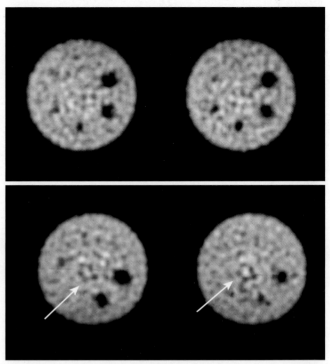

Fig. 3.12 Single-photon emission computed tomography (SPECT) ring artifacts. *Top,* SPECT phantom image with no ring artifact. *Bottom,* SPECT phantom image with significant ring artifacts (indicated by *arrows*) caused by inadequate uniformity calibration.

discomfort. In all applications, it is important to keep the injection site out of the field of view to prevent artifacts resulting from residual or infiltrated activity (Fig. 3.11). Compliance also can be improved by positioning the patient for maximum comfort by placing support under the knees to reduce strain on the lower back. If the patient's arms are over the head, additional support for the arms may be needed to alleviate shoulder pain.

Before a rotating SPECT camera is used, it must be properly calibrated. The calibrations necessary for proper operation are uniformity, center of rotation, and pixel size. For cameras that have more than one detector, the heads must be matched so that when each head is at the same projection angle—for example, directly above the patient—it will record events that occur in the same location within the object, at the same *(x, y)*-location in the acquired projection image. This is usually accomplished by imaging a set of sources at known locations and matching the pixel size and center of rotation for the two detectors. The head matching and pixel size adjustments may be performed by the field service engineer, with routine adjustments by the technologist. The technologist will usually perform the uniformity and center-of-rotation calibrations. Each manufacturer will specify how and with what frequency these calibrations should be performed. The most common frequency is to perform these calibrations on a monthly basis. However, some manufacturers may recommend longer frequencies of up to once per quarter.

All gamma cameras, regardless of how well tuned, will have residual nonuniformities. Minor variations in uniformity, not discernible in planar imaging, will result in significant *ring* or

bulls-eye artifacts in a SPECT study (Fig. 3.12, *arrows*). The usual 5- to 10-million-count uniformity image used for routine quality control is inadequate for uniformity calibration in SPECT imaging. For cameras with a large field of view and a 128 × 128 matrix, 100 to 200 million counts (roughly 10,000 counts per pixel) are required to achieve the desired pixel count that results in a relative standard deviation of 1%, which is necessary for artifact-free SPECT. Acquiring this number of counts requires a significant amount of time. The temptation to use very large amounts of radioactivity should be avoided because high count rates can also result in degraded performance of the gamma camera electronics and recording of spurious coincident events. Conservatively, the correction floods should be obtained at 20,000 to 30,000 counts per second. The uniformity calibration can be acquired either intrinsically using a point source or extrinsically with a flood source. The radioactivity in the flood source should have a uniformity of 1%. Although water-filled flood sources can be used for this calibration, they are difficult to mix and are subject to bulging. For this reason, sealed cobalt-57 sources are routinely used for acquiring the extrinsic uniformity calibration.

The center of rotation calibration matches the axis of rotation to the center of the image matrix. When viewing the rotational display of the raw SPECT data, it is the point about which the raw data rotates. Most importantly, it is the alignment point for the reconstruction. A common practice is to acquire the center of rotation correction on the same schedule as the uniformity correction. Many multiple-detector systems also use these data to match the heads. Each manufacturer has a very specific protocol for the center of rotation and multihead registration that

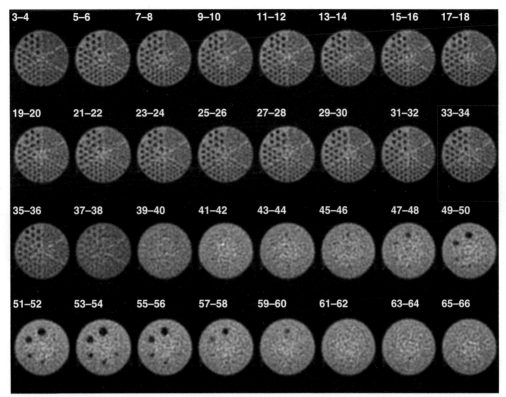

Fig. 3.13 Single-photon emission computed tomography (SPECT) quality control phantom. A series of slices from a phantom acquisition.

typically involves the acquisition of a series of images of a set of point or line sources of radioactivity.

As previously discussed, rotational SPECT requires maximum performance of the gamma camera. Performance that may be considered acceptable for planar imaging can render a SPECT study unreadable. In addition to the calibrations discussed earlier, all routine daily, weekly, and annual quality control procedures for gamma cameras should be performed. Particular attention should be paid to variations in uniformity because small variations in the field uniformity may result in significant artifacts.

A cylindrical tomographic phantom should be imaged periodically. An example of a phantom is shown in Fig. 3.13. Radioactivity can be added to this water-filled phantom to provide a uniform source that can be used to test for the presence of ring artifacts caused by inadequate uniformity calibration. In addition, other structures within the phantom can test SPECT system performance with respect to contrast and spatial resolution. In the example shown, solid Plexiglas rods of varying size and spacing and solid spheres of varying size are also imaged. These structures provide *cold* structures within the phantom—that is, areas of no activity. The phantom also may provide *hot* structures. It is customary to routinely acquire a SPECT study of such a phantom (e.g., quarterly) and compare the results to a reference study to determine whether a deterioration in SPECT performance has occurred.

An essential part of any imaging quality control program is the review of each patient's acquired data, and this is particularly true with SPECT. Excessive patient motion degrades the quality of SPECT scans because misregistration of the data in the different angular projections can lead to significant artifacts. Patient motion can be assessed in several ways. When the unprocessed projection images are viewed in a closed-loop cine, excessive patient motion is readily detected as a flicker or discontinuity in the display. Some laboratories use radioactive marker sources placed on the patient to further assess motion. Another approach is to view a sinogram of a slice in the study. The borders of the sinogram should be smooth, and interslice changes in intensity should be small. Any discontinuity may indicate patient motion (Fig. 3.14). Only up-and-down motion can be readily corrected. Discontinuities in the sinogram also may indicate an instrument malfunction. In addition to patient motion, the sinogram is useful for evaluation of head misregistration. A lateral shift at the point in the sinogram where the data from the first head ends and the second head begins can indicate a problem with the head registration. A tomographic acquisition of a point source can help determine whether these shifts are a result of head misregistration. Finally, the patient's reconstructed data should be carefully scrutinized for the presence of any irregularities or artifacts that may compromise the diagnostic quality of the study.

Positron Emission Tomography

PET, and particularly PET/CT, is a rapidly growing area of nuclear medicine. PET is made possible by the unique fate of positrons. When positrons undergo annihilation by combining with negatively charged electrons, two 511-keV photons are emitted in opposite directions, 180 degrees apart. In contrast to SPECT imaging, which detects single events, in PET imaging, two detector elements on opposite sides of the object are used to detect paired annihilation photons. If the photons are detected at the same time (or "in coincidence"), the event is assumed to have occurred along the line connecting the two

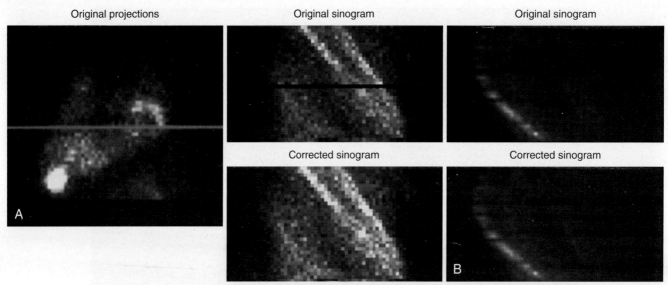

Original projections   Original sinogram   Original sinogram

Corrected sinogram   Corrected sinogram

Fig. 3.14 Patient quality control. (A) Sinogram from a myocardial perfusion study. The sinogram corresponds to the level of the cursor in the image on the *left*. Note the regular progression in the data across the projection profiles, indicating stability and lack of unwanted movement of the heart from one projection view to the next. (B) Sinogram illustrating multiple gaps in the sequential profile data. Compare these discontinuities with the regular progression of data in *A*. The discontinuities indicate unwanted motion of the object from one sampling position to the next.

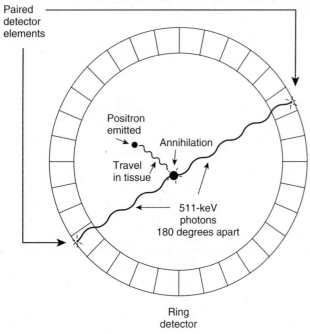

Paired detector elements

Positron emitted

Annihilation

Travel in tissue

511-keV photons 180 degrees apart

Ring detector

Fig. 3.15 Positron emission tomography (PET) ring detector. After emission, positrons travel a short distance in tissue before the annihilation event. The 511-keV protons are given off 180 degrees apart.

detectors involved (that is the line of response or LOR) (Fig. 3.15). Thus the direction of the photons can be determined without the use of absorptive collimation. This process is referred to as *annihilation coincidence detection* and is the hallmark of PET imaging.

Annihilation coincidence detection leads to at least a 100-fold increase in the sensitivity of PET relative to conventional nuclear medicine imaging and explains the higher image quality

compared with SPECT. The counts occurring between a single pair of detectors can be considered a ray, and projections can thereby be generated and reconstructed, just as in SPECT. Although both filtered back-projection and iterative approaches such as OSEM can be used to reconstruct the data, the latter is more common for PET because of the greatly improved image quality.

Instrumentation for PET has undergone several generations of development. Early systems had a single ring with multiple detectors and generated a single tomographic section at a time. Now, PET typically consists of many rings of multiple detectors that cover a 15- to 20-cm axial field of view. Each detector is typically paired with multiple other detectors on the opposite side of the detector ring. These detectors in coincidence are selected to encompass the field of view of the object or organ being imaged (Fig. 3.16). Multiple-ring systems allow a volume to be imaged simultaneously. Early systems typically had *septa* of absorptive material such as lead or tungsten inserted between the tomographic planes to reduce intraplane scatter and shield the detectors from crosstalk caused by activity outside of the plane of interest. These systems with interplane septa are referred to as *2D* systems because they limit the allowable coincidences to 2D transverse planes. Over time, the number of rings increased, and the ability to remove the septa to acquire data across planes (i.e., 3D mode) became common. The 3D design greatly increases the system sensitivity of the PET scanner and increases the number of Compton scattered and random events recorded. Most contemporary systems do not have septa between the planes and are referred to as *3D only systems*. This is made possible by improvements in scatter-correction algorithms and a reduction in the number of random coincidence events detected because of newer, faster detector materials.

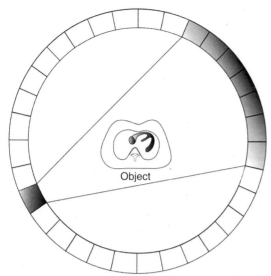

Fig. 3.16 Pairing of detectors. In the positron emission tomography (PET) tomograph, each detector is paired with multiple detectors on the opposite side of the ring to create an arc encompassing the object. This multiple-pairing strategy increases the sensitivity of the device.

When choosing the appropriate detector material for PET, the detection efficiency (related to the effective atomic number, Z, and mass density), resolution (spatial and energy, related to the number of scintillation light photons emitted per kiloelectron volt), and response time or decay time of the scintillator must be considered. The density and effective atomic number (Z) for NaI, the detector material commonly used in gamma cameras, are not optimal for the detection of the 511-keV photons in PET imaging. Bismuth germinate oxide (BGO) is approximately twice as dense as NaI and has an effective Z of 74, compared with the effective Z of 50 for NaI, leading to its use in PET for the past 30 years. However, its drawbacks include significantly lower light output per kiloelectron volt (i.e., lower energy resolution) and longer light decay time. This longer light decay time necessitated the use of coincidence timing windows of 10 to 12 nanoseconds (ns). New detector materials, such as lutetium oxyorthosilicate (LSO), lutetium-yttrium oxyorthosilicate (LYSO), and gadolinium oxyorthosilicate (GSO) combine high density with better timing resolution and superior light yield. Timing windows have been reduced to about 5 to 6 ns, which in turn reduces the number of random events by approximately 50%. It also provides the opportunity for time-of-flight PET. The better light output allows for better energy discrimination and thus a reduction in the number of scatter events acquired. For these reasons, state-of-the-art PET scanners are incorporating either LSO or LYSO as the detection material.

The spatial resolution of modern PET tomographs is excellent, primarily determined by the size of the detector modules. Resolution under clinical scanning conditions is superior in PET compared with SPECT. Resolution for clinical studies is in the 5- to 8-mm FWHM range with high-end contemporary PET scanners. Specialized devices designed for small animal imaging have a spatial resolution of about 1.5-mm.

The ultimate spatial resolution of PET is limited by two physical phenomena related to positrons and their annihilation. First, positrons are given off at different kinetic energies. Energetic positrons such as those emitted by oxygen-15, gallium-68, and rubidium-82 may travel several millimeters in tissue before undergoing annihilation (see Fig. 3.15). Thus the location of the annihilation event is some distance from the actual location of the radionuclide. This travel in tissue degrades the ability to truly localize the biodistribution of the radioactive agent in the patient and results in images with poorer resolution, particularly for radionuclides with higher positron kinetic energies, such as Ga-68 and Rb-82, compared with F-18. The second phenomenon limiting resolution is the noncollinearity of the annihilation photons. If the positron–electron pair is still moving at the time of annihilation, the result is a small deviation from true colinearity along a single ray (see Fig. 3.15), leading to a 1- to 2-mm spatial uncertainty in event localization. This leads to a limit of about 3-3.5 mm resolution in clinical whole-body PET scanners, irrespective of detector size.

Annihilation Coincidence Detection

Special circuitry in the PET tomograph allows the detection of two annihilation photons given off by a single positron annihilation event. The two events are considered to be from the same event if they are counted within a defined *coincidence timing window*. In current scanners, the coincidence window is on the order of 6 ns (although it may be as high as 12 ns in older, BGO-based scanners). Thus, when events are registered in paired detectors within 6 ns of each other, they are accepted as *true coincidence events* and recorded as occurring along the LOR that connects the two detectors. If a single recorded event is not matched by a paired event within the coincidence time window, the data are discarded. This approach effectively provides *electronic collimation* without the need for absorptive collimation. Therefore PET tomographs offer much higher sensitivity than gamma cameras. One complication in the coincidence approach occurs at higher count rates when two unrelated or random events are recorded within the coincidence timing window, leading to what is referred to as a *random coincidence*. Such random coincidences do not provide useful information with regard to localizing the radiopharmaceutical, thus, if no correction is applied, leading to a higher level of background signal that reduces the overall object contrast.

Data can be recorded in several ways, depending on whether the data are acquired in 2D or 3D format. PET data can be stored as sinograms (2D) or projections (3D). In either case, the counts in each pixel represent the coincidence events recorded along a particular LOR between a pair of detectors in coincidence. We know the coincidence event happened somewhere on the LOR but not specifically where along the LOR the event occurred. The sinogram or projection data are then reconstructed, most commonly using iterative reconstruction methods, although filtered back-projection may sometimes be used.

Time-of-flight PET uses the time difference in the arrival of the annihilation photons in the coincidence timing windows to estimate where on the LOR the event occurred. The estimated location of the event, Δd, is calculated from the time difference between the two events, Δt, using the formula: $\Delta d = (\Delta t \times c)/2$, where c is the speed of light. With the current detectors, such as LSO or LYSO, this methodology can be used to locate the annihilation event to within about 7 cm along the LOR, which can lead to a significant improvement in PET image quality, particularly in large patients. However, it has relatively little benefit when used for brain and pediatric imaging because of the smaller diameter of the object being imaged. Newer digitally based PET systems have been able to improve the temporal resolution leading to localization of the annihilation event to about 4 cm yielding a significant improvement in PET image quality.

PET Quality Control

A PET scanner has a very large number of detectors. A state-of-the-art scanner with 4-mm crystals and an 80-cm ring diameter can have as many as 32,000 crystals. As with any imaging system, variations occur in the response of the crystals to a uniform source of radiation. To correct for these variations, a high-count uniformity calibration is acquired, and a correction is applied. This correction is analogous to the uniformity correction applied to SPECT cameras. However, it differs in that the detectors are stationary, and therefore small variations in a given detector are not propagated over the complete 360 degrees of data. Thus whereas uniformity variations in SPECT will result in ring artifacts, this is not the case in PET. As a result, the uniformity correction for PET is done much less frequently, perhaps quarterly.

The PET scanner records detected annihilation coincidence events as counts or, more correctly, counts per second per pixel. It is preferred to have these data in units of microcurie or becquerels per milliliter. Therefore a calibration scan is performed to determine a conversion factor to convert counts to activity. This is accomplished by imaging a uniform phantom with a known concentration of activity (microcuries or becquerels per millimeter). The conversion factor is determined by calculating the ratio of activity concentration in the phantom to the counts per second per pixel in the image. This calibration factor is stored and later applied during image reconstruction so that the resultant image is reported in units of activity concentration. This conversion factor is crucial when activity quantitation is applied, such as in determining the standardized uptake value (SUV). The SUV is the ratio of the activity concentration in a pixel within the patient's PET study normalized by the administered activity and patient size (usually patient mass). If the radiopharmaceutical distributes uniformly within the patient, the SUV value will be 1. Inaccuracies in the count-to-activity calibration will result in inaccurate SUV values.

Each day, the detectors in a PET scanner are exposed to a uniform source of radioactivity to evaluate that each detector is working properly. Because of the large number of detectors, a small number of them may not be working. The data are presented to the user in a manner that allows an evaluation of which detectors are not working as expected. Each manufacturer has a different method, but the end result is a report that indicates whether the system is working properly. Systems that are identified as not working properly will need corrective action.

PET scans that are done for evaluation of different cancers are reconstructed, and the pixel values in some cases may be converted to SUVs. It is common for physicians to report changes in these values from one scan to the next as indicative of progression or regression of disease. It is important that the SUVs generated by the scanner are consistent from scan to scan. Drift in the electronics of the scanner can result in discordance between the calibration factor and patient data. One method of verifying the SUV is to image a uniform distribution of known radioactivity concentration. The phantom is imaged using clinical scan parameters. The amount of activity in the phantom and the mass of the phantom are entered into the acquisition data as if it were a patient. When these data are reconstructed, the average SUV in each reconstructed slice is determined. The resultant average SUV should be 1.0 ± 10%. Values outside this range would indicate that the scanner should be recalibrated. This test uses the methodology for calibrating the scanner as a check of the calibration. It has the advantage that, if necessary, the phantom is ready to be used for recalibration of the scanner.

Another method for evaluating the performance of PET scanners is to image a cylindrical, tomographic quality control phantom. These phantoms are similar to those used in SPECT, but they typically differ in that they often contain *hot* features in which the activity concentration is greater than that in the background for evaluating contrast (Fig. 3.17). They are usually imaged on a quarterly basis but could be imaged more frequently and combined with the quantitative accuracy value check. These phantoms typically allow for the evaluation of uniformity, resolution, contrast, and quantitative accuracy using one data acquisition. The hot features in the phantom are specified to have a certain target-to-background ratio (e.g., 2.5:1 or 4:1); the SUV of each is recorded. The targets may be spheres or cylinders of decreasing size. The resolution section typically consists of cold rods of decreasing size in a warm background, similar to those used in SPECT. The phantom is imaged using the clinical protocol. The SUV values in the hot features are compared with the expected value, and the sizes of the smallest rods and targets are recorded. The background is evaluated for an average SUV of 1.0 ± 10%. Because of the complexity in filling this phantom, it is typically used less frequently than the uniform phantom for checking the quantitative accuracy of the scanner.

Hybrid Imaging

Nuclear medicine images are excellent for looking at physiology, but they are organ specific and generally low resolution. Thus it is sometimes difficult to accurately localize features seen on the emission tomography scans. The introduction of hybrid PET-CT and SPECT-CT, allowing direct correlation of the functional information available from PET or SPECT with the anatomical information from CT, has greatly enhanced the clinical utility of these modalities. The addition of CT to both PET and SPECT has been very useful in anatomically defining both pathological and normal anatomy in the emission images. For PET, areas of increased uptake can be more easily correlated with a metastatic lymph node or a region of brown fat. The same is true for a variety of SPECT procedures, such as parathyroid imaging and bone SPECT for back pain.

The PET-CT places the CT scanner in front of the PET scanner. In the case of SPECT, the CT scanner is behind or parallel with the SPECT scanner. On either system, the CT scan may be acquired either before or after the emission study, although the

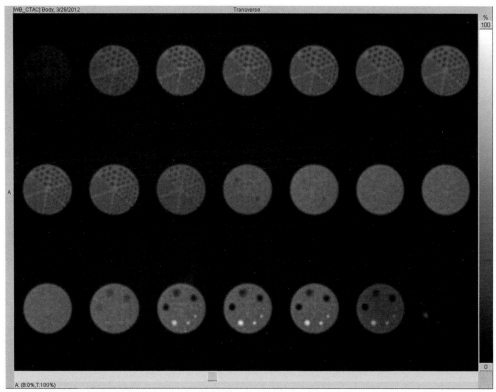

Fig. 3.17 Positron emission tomography (PET) quality control phantom. A series of slices from a phantom acquisition.

more common order is to acquire the CT first and then the emission study. The CT scan can then provide both the transmission scan for attenuation correction and anatomical correlation.

The CT scanner incorporated into these devices may be a state-of-the-art CT scanner, or in some cases, particularly with SPECT-CT, it may be a CT scanner of less capability but still adequate for the imaging task at hand. The quality control of the CT scanner is the same as that necessary for a clinical CT scanner and is therefore beyond the scope of this chapter. However, a test object should be imaged periodically that can be seen with both modalities to ensure alignment of the two devices.

When the CT is used for attenuation correction of the emission scan, artifacts can be introduced when misregistration exists between the emission and transmission data sets. The CT scan is acquired much more quickly than the emission studies. This can result in different breathing patterns between the two scans that can make registration of the data in the area of the diaphragm difficult. Therefore it is important to review both the attenuation-corrected images and the non–attenuation-corrected images in conjunction with the CT scan to evaluate misregistration. In cardiac imaging, misregistration of the heart can result in false-positive scans. This is true for both PET and SPECT.

In recent years, hybrid PET-MR scanners have been introduced by several vendors. In one case, the PET scanner is actually fitted within the MR device, and the two scans can be acquired simultaneously. In other cases, the PET and MR scanners are adjacent to each other and use a common bed that can service the two devices. Combined PET-MR acquisitions have the potential for interesting research applications; however, their clinical role is yet to be determined.

SUGGESTED READING

Chandra R, Rahmim A. *Nuclear Medicine Physics: The Basics*. 8th ed. Philadelphia: Williams & Wilkins. 2018.

Cherry SR, Sorenson JA, Phelps ME. 2012. *Physics in Nuclear Medicine*. 3rd ed. Philadelphia: WB Saunders.

International Atomic Energy Association. *Planning a Clinical PET Centre*. Vienna, Austria: International Atomic Energy Agency. 2010.

International Atomic Energy Association. *Quality Assurance for PET and PET/CT Systems*. Vienna, Austria: International Atomic Energy Agency. 2009.

International Atomic Energy Association. *Quality Assurance of SPECT Systems*. Vienna, Austria: International Atomic Energy Agency. 2009.

International Atomic Energy Association. *Quality Control Atlas for Scintillation Camera Systems*. Vienna, Austria: International Atomic Energy Agency. 2003.

National Electrical Manufacturers Association. *Performance Measurements of Positron Emission Tomographs*. Rosslyn, VA: National Electrical Manufacturers Association. 2018.

Powsner RA, Palmer MR, Powsner ER. *Essentials of Nuclear Medicine Physics*. 3rd ed. Hoboken NJ: Wiley Blackwell. 2013.

4

Radiopharmaceuticals

An unstable atom that undergoes radioactive decay in order to achieve stability is known as a radionuclide. The radiation these atoms emit can sometimes be used in medical imaging and therapy. Agents approved for such uses in humans that incorporate radioactive molecules are referred to as radiopharmaceuticals. Radiopharmaceuticals can portray physiology, biochemistry, or pathology in the body without causing any significant physiological effect. They are also referred to as "radiotracers" because they are given in subpharmacological doses that "trace" a particular physiological or pathological process in the body. This chapter presents general principles regarding clinically important radionuclides and radiopharmaceuticals, their production, radiolabeling, and quality assurance. Some terms related to radioactive imaging and therapy agents are defined in Box 4.1.

PRODUCTION OF RADIONUCLIDES

Naturally occurring radionuclides are often heavy, toxic elements (e.g., uranium, actinium, thorium, radium, and radon) with very long half-lives (>1000 years). Most of these radioactive elements have no role in nuclear medicine, and radionuclides for

---

BOX 4.1 Important Terms Concerning Radiopharmaceuticals and Their Properties

Radionuclide: Unstable isotope of an element that transitions to greater stability through radioactive decay.

Radiopharmaceutical: FDA-approved radioactive/radiolabeled agent (i.e., drug) for imaging or therapy.

Activity: The rate of decay; expressed as curies (3.7×10^{10} decays per second) or in metric units as becquerels (1 decay per second, 1 mCi = 37 MBq).

Half-life (or $T_{1/2}$): The time required for half the radioactive atoms in a sample to have decayed.

Equilibrium: Steady state or constant relationship that develops between a contained radioactive parent/daughter pair when the parent has a longer half-life than the daughter. Used for radionuclide production in a *generator.*

Carrier-free: Radiopharmaceutical free of contamination by other isotopes (stable or radioactive) of the same element. This is not to be confused with *carrier molecule.*

Carrier molecule: A chosen substance radiolabeled to allow evaluation or treatment of a particular physiologic parameter or cellular function, allowing or improving properties such as localization, accumulation, and/or background clearance.

Specific activity: The concentration of the radionuclide per unit volume or weight (i.e., in mCi/mg). High specific activity is optimal.

Radiative abundance: Also known as radiation yield; the likelihood that the decay of radioactive substance will result in desired emissions.

FDA, U.S. Food and Drug Administration.

---

clinical use are commonly produced artificially. Table 4.1 provides the physical properties of single-photon-emitting radionuclides used in medical imaging with a gamma camera. Dual-photon positron-emitting agents are listed in Table 4.2, and Table 4.3 notes several important radionuclides for therapy purposes. Appendix 2 contains a periodic table of the elements for reference.

Medical isotope production involves one of four methods: nuclear fission or neutron activation in a nuclear reactor, charged-particle bombardment in a particle accelerator (i.e., a cyclotron), or decay of a radioactive parent forming the desired agent in a radionuclide generator (Fig. 4.1). Production methods are outlined in Table 4.4. The various reactions involved in production can be annotated in equation form, noting the type of reaction, any particle involved in the transformation, as well as the initial isotope and final product, as presented in the examples listed in Box 4.2.

When a very heavy nuclide, such as uranium-235 (U-235), undergoes neutron bombardment in a reactor, a neutron can be captured. Rather than stabilizing through radioactive decay, this atom can undergo *nuclear fission,* a splitting of the atom. The process results in two smaller nuclides (e.g., those with masses ranging from 72 to 161, lying in the middle of the periodic table), along with a release of energy and multiple neutrons. Many of these are high-energy neutrons that can then cause further fission reactions, and this creates a chain reaction that can occur in a controlled fashion within the reactor. The daughters of the fission reaction include several radionuclides used in therapy or in imaging, such as molybdenum-99 (Mo-99), iodine-131 (I-131), xenon-133 (Xe-133), and cesium-137 (Cs-137). Radionuclides produced by this method are usually carrier-free.

In the process of neutron activation, a stable target material is exposed to thermal neutrons in the reactor, and neutron activation results if the target atom captures a neutron. The unstable atom that is formed in this scenario stabilizes by gamma-ray emission and/or β^- decay. In addition to the desired daughter product, contaminants are produced, including other isotopes of the same element. Because these isotopes will all have chemistries that are alike, it can be difficult separating the daughter. Therefore, the product is not carrier-free. The neutron-rich radionuclides produced almost always stabilize through β^- decay. Isotopes created by this method include P-32, Sr-89, and Sm-153. Mo-99 and I-131 can also be produced by this method, but unlike fission-produced material, these products are not carrier-free.

The third production method involves bombarding the target material with charged particles (protons, deuterons, alpha

TABLE 4.1 Physical Characteristics of Single-Photon Imaging Radionuclides for Clinical Use

Radionuclide	Principal Mode of Decay	Physical Half-Life	Principal Photon Energy in keV (% abundance)	Production Method
Mo-99	β^-	2.8 d	740 (12), 780 (4)	Reactor
Tc-99m	Isomeric transition	6 hr	140 (89)	Generator (Mo-99)
I-131	β^-	8 d	364 (81)	Reactor
I-123	EC	13.2 hr	159 (83)	Cyclotron
Ga-67	EC	78.3 hr	93 (37), 185 (20), 300 (17), 395 (5)	Cyclotron
Tl-201	EC	73.1 hr	69-83 (Hg x-rays), 135 (2.5), 167 (10)	Cyclotron
In-111	EC	2.8 d	171 (90), 245 (94)	Cyclotron
Xe-133	β^-	5.2 d	81 (37)	Reactor
Co-57	EC	272 d	122 (86)	Cyclotron
Cs-137	β^-	30.17 yrs	662	Reactor

β^-, beta minus; *EC,* electron capture

TABLE 4.2 Cyclotron-Produced Positron-Emitting Radionuclides: Physical Characteristics

Radionuclide	Physical Half-Life (min)	Positron Energy E_{max} (MeV)	E_{mean} (MeV)	Maximum Range in Soft Tissue (mm)	Mean Range in Soft Tissue (mm)
C-11	20.4 m	0.96	0.39	4.2	1.2
N-13	10 m	1.2	0.49	5.5	1.8
O-15[a]	2 m	1.73	0.73	8.4	3.0
F-18	110 m	0.63	0.25	2.4	0.6
Ga-68	67.8 m	1.90	0.84	10.3	2.9
Rb-82	1.3 m	3.38	1.56	8.6	5.9
Zr-89[a]	78.4 d	0.902	0.40	3.8	1.3
Cu-64[a]	12.7 hr	0.653	0.28	2.5	0.7

[a]Experimental applications
Conti M, Eriksson L. Physics of pure and non-pure positron emitters for PET: a review and discussion. *EJNMMI Phys.* 2016;3(1):8.

TABLE 4.3 Radionuclides Commonly Used for Therapeutic Applications

BETA MINUS EMITTERS							
Radionuclide	Half-Life	E_{max} (MeV)	E_{ave} (MeV)	Maximum Particle Range (mm)	Mean Particle Range (mm)	Gamma (γ) Photons Suitable for Imaging	Examples of Uses
Iodine-131 (I-131)	8.01 days	0.606	0.81	2.4	0.4	364 keV (81%)	Thyroid cancer, hyperthyroidism
Yttrium-90 (Y-90)	64.1	2.28	0.94	11.3	3.6	No γ; Bremsstrahlung radiation	CD20 Antibodies: lymphoma Microspheres: Colon cancer hepatic metastases Hepatocellular cancer
Lutetium-177 (Lu-177)	6.7 d	0.50	0.14	1.7	0.28	208 (11%)	Neuroendocrine tumor
Samarium-153 (Sm-153)	46.3 hr	0.81	0.22	3.1	0.7	103 (29%)	Bone metastases
Rhenium-186 (Re-186)	3.7 d	1.07	0.33	3.6	1.2	137 keV (9%)	Bone metastases
Strontium-89 (Sr-89)	50.5 days	1.496		8.0	2.4	910 (0.01%)	Bone metastases
Phosphorus-32 (P-32)	14.3 days	1.71	0.70	7.9	2.6	None	Bone metastases,[a] intraperitoneal ovarian cancer metastases, pleuroperitoneal fistulas

Continued

TABLE 4.3   Radionuclides Commonly Used for Therapeutic Applications—cont'd

			ALPHA EMITTERS		
Agent	Half-Life	Decay	Eα (MeV)	Principal Gamma (keV) and % Abundance	Uses
Radium-223 (Ra-223)	11.4 days	α multistep daughters also decay $\left(\frac{\alpha}{\beta^-}\right)$	5–7.5	82, 154, 270 (γ total 1.1%)	Prostate metastases
Actinium-225 (Ac-225)	10.0 days	α	5.9	99 (5.8%)	Experimental applications
Bismuth-213 (Bi-213)	45.6 min	α/β⁻	6.0	440 (27.3%)	Experimental applications
Lead-212 (Pb-212)	10.64 hours β⁻	Bi-212 daughter $\alpha/\beta\uparrow-$	6.1	238.6 (43.1%)	Experimental applications
Astatine-211 (At-211)	7.2 hr	α	6.0	500–900 keV (≤ 1%) 77–92 keV x-rays from Po-211	Experimental applications

^aSome applications are not approved by the U.S. Food and Drug Administration.

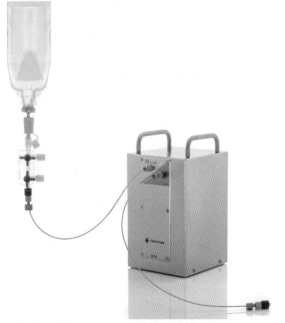

Fig. 4.1 Radionuclide generator. Given the short 68-minute half-life of Ga-68 and the lengthy process required to label agents like Ga-68 DOTATATE, on-site production is optimal. Commercially available generators make Ga-68 available to sites distant from a cyclotron. The germanium-68 parent is produced in a cyclotron and bonded to a borosilicate column through a titanium dioxide bed. The daughter Ga-68 can be eluted with sterile HCl. (GalliaPharm 68Ge/68Ga Generator, courtesy of Eckert & Ziegler Radiopharma GmbH, Berlin, Germany.)

particles) in a *cyclotron,* producing proton-rich radionuclides that will undergo positron decay (e.g., fluorine-18 [F-18]) or electron capture (e.g., iodine-123 [I-123], gallium-67 [Ga-67], thallium-201 [Tl-201], and indium-111 [In-111]). This production method produces radionuclides that are not only carrier-free but also usually contain fewer contaminants than agents produced in a reactor (which can contain other fission products).

Finally, medical isotopes can also be made in a *radionuclide generator,* consisting of a radioactive parent that decays to produce a radioactive daughter suitable for imaging. One key reason that generator systems have been so important to the field of nuclear medicine is their portability, allowing transport to locations far from a reactor or cyclotron, helping to overcome time limitations on production and delivery created by relatively short radiopharmaceutical half-lives. Different generator systems have been an important source of several radioisotopes over the years (Table 4.5), including the most important single-photon-emitting agent, Tc-99m, and the PET emitter Ga-68, whose clinical use is rapidly growing in the United States.

Radionuclide Generators

The generator contains a glass or plastic column containing an adsorbent material such as alumina (Al_2O_3), anion or cation exchange resin, or zirconia. The parent radionuclide is fixed to the column, and the loaded column is placed in a lead container with tubing attached at each end to permit radionuclide removal from the column, known as *"elution."*

Two types of generator systems are available with respect to elution. "Wet" systems, today most commonly used in regional radiopharmacies, come with a reservoir of normal saline (0.9%) (Fig. 4.2). Elution is accomplished by placing a special sterile vacuum vial on the exit or collection port. The vacuum vial is designed to draw the appropriate amount of saline across the column.

In "dry" systems, common in imaging clinics, a volume-calibrated saline charge is placed on the entry port, and a vacuum vial is placed on the collection port (Fig. 4.3). The vacuum draws the saline eluent out of the original vial, across the column, and into the elution vial. Elution volumes are in the range of 5 to 20 mL. Elutions can be performed for add-on or emergency studies that are required in the course of a day. The amount of activity available from a generator

TABLE 4.4 Production Methods of Medical Radioisotopes

CHARACTERISTIC		Cyclotron	NUCLEAR REACTOR		Radionuclide Generator
			Fission	Neutron Activation	
Bombarding particle		Proton, deuteron, alpha, tritium	Neutron	Neutron	Production by decay
Product		Proton excess	Neutron excess	Neutron excess	Proton or neutron excess
Decay mode		β^+ Electron capture	β^-	β^-	Varies
Carrier-free		Yes	Yes	No	Yes
High specific activity		Yes	Yes	No (difficult to separate chemically)	Yes
Cost		High[a]	Low	Low	Tc-99m Low Ga-68 High
Common medical radioisotopes produced	β^-		Mo-99 I-131 Xe-133 Cs-137	P-32 Sr-89 Sm-153 Mo-99 I-131[b]	
	β^+	F-18 C-11 N-13 O-15 Zr-89			Ga-68 Rb-82
	Electron capture	Tl-201 I-123 Ga-67 In-111		I-125 Cr-51	
	Isomeric transition				Tc-99m Kr-81m

β^-, Beta minus; β^+, positron emission.

[a]Historically higher than reactor production; F-18 for fluorodeoxyglucose (FDG) now economical.

[b]From ^{130}Te (n, γ)^{131}Te $\xrightarrow{\text{I}(\beta\text{I}^-)}$ ^{131}I.

BOX 4.2 Radionuclide Production Reaction Equation Examples

Common abbreviations: p, proton; n, neutron; d, deuteron; α, alpha; γ, gamma; f, fission; β^-, beta minus; EC, electron capture.

Equation shorthand format:

Target atom (irradiating particle, emission) radionuclide product

Examples:

Cyclotron Production

$$\text{Fluorine-18: } ^{18}\text{O(p, n) } ^{18}\text{F}$$

$$\text{Gallium-67: } ^{68}\text{Zn (p, 2n)}^{67}\text{Ga} \qquad \text{Iodine-123: } ^{124}\text{Te (p, 2n)}^{123}\text{I}$$

$$^{66}\text{Zn(d,-n)}^{67}\text{Ga} \qquad\qquad ^{121}\text{Sb}(\alpha,\text{-2n})$$

$$^{66}\text{Zn(d,-n)}^{67}\text{Ga} \qquad\qquad ^{121}\text{Sb}(\alpha,\text{-2n})$$

$$^{122}\text{Te(d, n)}^{123}\text{I}$$

Indirect production: ^{124}Xe (p, n)^{123}Cs ($\rightarrow \perp$ (β ↑+)(↓↑123)Xe ($\rightarrow \perp$ (β ↑+)(↓↑123)I (carrier-free)

BOX 4.2   Radionuclide Production Reaction Equation Examples—cont'd

Reactor Production

$$\text{Fission reaction (n, f): } {}^{235}U + {}_{0}^{1}n \rightarrow {}^{236}U \rightarrow {}_{42}^{99}Mo + {}_{50}^{135}Sn + 2\,{}_{0}^{1}n \text{ OR } {}^{235}U\,(n,\,f)\,{}^{99}Mo$$

$$\text{Neutron capture (n, } \gamma): {}^{50}Cr\,(n,\,\gamma)\,{}^{51}Cr \text{ and } {}^{98}Mo\,(n,\,\gamma)(\downarrow\uparrow 99)\,Mo$$

Generator Production

$$^{99}Mo \xrightarrow{\;I\,(\beta^{-})\;} {}^{99m}Tc \text{ and } {}^{68}Ge \xrightarrow{\;EC\;} {}^{68}Ga$$

TABLE 4.5   Radionuclide Generator Systems and Parent/Daughter Half-Lives

Parent	Parent Half-Life	Daughter	Daughter Half-Life	Expiration	Equilibrium Reached
Mo-99	66 hr	Tc-99m	6 hr	1–2 weeks	Transient
Ge-68	270 d	Ga-68	68 min	12 months	Secular
Sr-82	25 d	Rb-82	1.3 min	28 days (28–42)	Secular
Rb-81	4.5 hr	Kr-81m	13 sec	20 hours	Secular

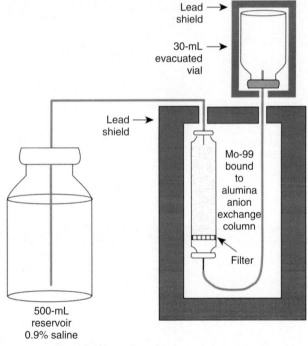

Fig. 4.2 Wet radionuclide generator system.

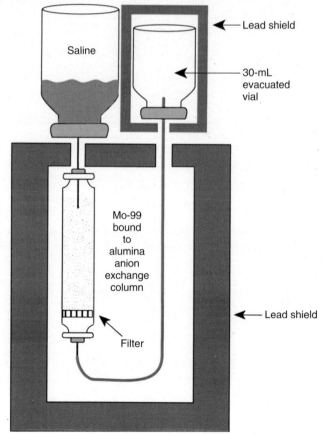

Fig. 4.3 Dry radionuclide generator system.

decreases each day as a result of decay of the parent. Radio-isotope decay occurs in an exponential fashion, and this is often represented by graphing the logarithm of activity (on *y*-axis) over time (*x*-axis; Fig. 4.4).

Generator Equilibrium

Generator properties depend on the rate at which the daughter is produced and subsequently decays relative to the parent. When the $T_{1/2}$ of the daughter is shorter than that of the parent, the amount of radioactivity of the two entities reaches *equilibrium*—that is, the ratio of the two activities becomes constant.

(No equilibrium is reached when the $T_{1/2}$ of the parent is shorter than that of the daughter [Fig. 4.5A]).

When the $T_{1/2}$ of the parent is much longer than that of the daughter (e.g., 100 times longer), a *secular equilibrium* is reached (see Fig. 4.5B). In this situation, after about six or seven half-lives of the daughter, the activities of the two agents become

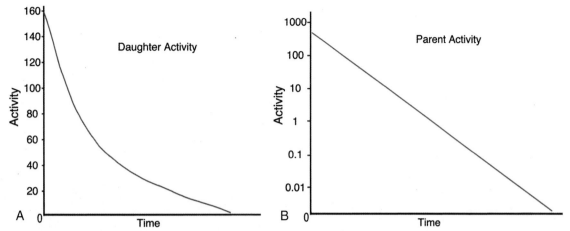

Fig. 4.4 Radionuclide decay. (A) With radioactive decay, activity decreases exponentially. This is often repre-sented graphically using the logarithm of activity on the *y*-axis and time on the *x*-axis, changing the curve to a straight line (B).

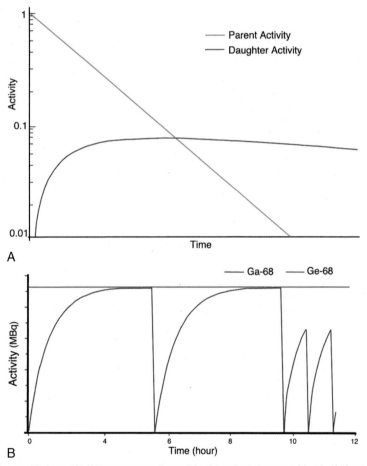

Fig. 4.5 Secular equilibrium. (A) If the parent radionuclide *(blue line)* decays with a half-life shorter than the daughter *(red line)*, no equilibrium is reached. However, when the half-life is much greater than the daughter (e.g., 100 times), secular equilibrium is attained, where the activity of the parent *(blue line)* and daughter *(red line)* are equal. (B) The effects of generator elutions are seen with a periodic sudden drop in daughter activ-ity, first occurring at peak activity, and then as partial elutions occurring before peak from this Ge-68/Ga-68 generator system.

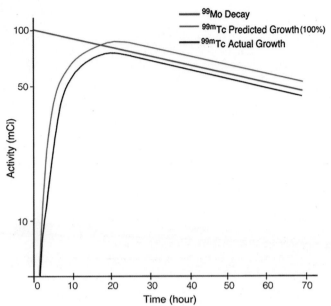

Fig. 4.6 Transient equilibrium: A transient equilibrium is reached if the parent half-life is only slightly longer than that of the daughter, as in a Mo-99/Tc-99m generator. When the logarithm of activity for the parent *(blue line)* and expected activity of the daughter *(red line)* is plotted compared to time, the activity of the daughter eventually exceeds the parent in equilibrium. In the case of Tc-99m, the actual amount of daughter produced *(black line)* is less than expected because Mo-99 decays to Tc-99m only 87% of the time, with Tc-99 resulting in 13%.

equal. Essentially, it appears that as soon as the parent atom decays, the resultant daughter atom subsequently decays, and thus the two numbers of disintegrations are the same. The positron-emitting germanium-68/gallium-68 (Ge-68/Ga-68) generator is an example of a system that reaches secular equilibrium.

When the parent's $T_{1/2}$ is just slightly longer than that of the daughter (i.e., by a factor of about 10), then a *transient equilibrium* is reached, where the activity of the daughter is slightly greater than that of the parent. The most commonly used generator, the molybdenum-99/technetium-99m (Mo-99/Tc-99m) generator, is an example of a transient equilibrium system. However, because Mo-99 decays to Tc-99m only 87% of the time (with the remaining decaying directly to the ground state Tc-99), the actual amount of the daughter is slightly lower than the parent, as presented in Fig. 4.6.

Molybdenum-99/Technetium Generator Systems

Mo-99 produced by the fission of U-235 is referred to as *fission moly*. After Mo-99 is produced, it is chemically purified and passed on to an ion-exchange column composed of alumina. The column is typically adjusted to an acid pH to promote binding. The positive charge of the alumina binds the molybdate ions firmly. Facts related to Tc-99m generators are outlined in Table 4.6.

Generator Operation and Yield

Fig. 4.6 illustrates the relationship between Mo-99 decay and the accumulation or daughter ingrowth of Tc-99m; the maximal buildup of Tc-99m activity occurs at 23 hours after elution. This time point is convenient, especially if sufficient Tc-99m is available to accomplish each day's work, and activity is eluted or "milked" off the generator as Tc-99m pertechnetate ($^{99m}TcO_4^-$).

TABLE 4.6 Molybdenum-99/Technetium-99m Generator Systems

Radionuclide Parameter	Parent (Mo-99)	Daughter (Tc-99m)
Half-life	66 hr	6 hr
Mode of decay	Beta minus	Isomeric transition
Daughter products	Tc-99m (as $^{99m}TcO_4^-$), Tc-99	Tc-99
Principal photon energies	740 keV, 780 keV	140 keV (89%)
Generator Function		
Composition of ion exchange column	Al_2O_3	
Eluent	Normal saline (0.9%)	
Time from elution to maximum daughter yield	23 hr	

Note: The decay scheme for Mo-99 is complex, with over 35 gamma rays of different energies given off. The listed energies are those used in clinical practice and for radionuclide purity check.

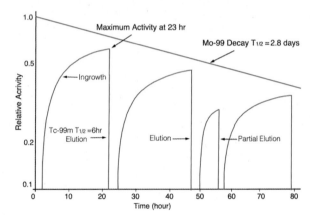

Fig. 4.7 Effect of Tc-99m elution. Decay curve for Mo-99 *(blue line)* and ingrowth curves for Tc-99m *(red line)*. Successive elutions, including a partial elution, are illustrated with relative activity plotted on a logarithmic scale compared to time. The timing of peak activity is near perfect, making a large amount of Tc-99m in the form of Tc-99m pertechnetate available in the morning.

Otherwise, enough activity builds after just a few hours, and the generator can be partially eluted, more than once per day (Fig. 4.7). After a partial elution is performed, 50% of the maximum activity is reached in approximately 4.5 hours, and 75% of maximum is reached at 8.5 hours.

Although greatest attention is paid to the rate of Tc-99m buildup, Tc-99m is also constantly decaying, with the buildup of stable Tc-99 (or "carrier" Tc-99) in the generator. Generators received after commercial shipment or generators that have not been eluted for several days have significant carrier Tc-99 in the eluate. Because the carrier Tc-99 behaves chemically similarly to Tc-99m, it can compete and adversely affect radiopharmaceutical labeling efficiency. If the eluate contains sufficient carrier Tc-99, complete reduction may not occur, resulting in poor labeling and undesired radiochemical contaminants in the final preparation. To prevent this, Tc-99 can be first flushed away with an elution that is discarded.

RADIOPHARMACEUTICALS

Ideally in nuclear medicine, high-quality images are produced with the lowest radiation exposure possible. Therefore, the choice of radiolabel is critical. For example, unless the patient is undergoing therapy, a pure gamma (γ) emitter should be used, free of alpha (α) or beta minus (β⁻) particulate emissions that increase the dose. The photons produced by decaying radionuclides must be of sufficient *abundance* (i.e., have a high likelihood of an emission occurring per decay event) as well as of suitable energy for external detection. In single-photon-emitting agents, 100- to 200-keV γ photons are most favorable. Although a wider range of energies can be used, inferior images may result. Low-energy photons are more easily scattered or absorbed. Higher-energy photons not only increase the radiation dose but also more frequently penetrate collimators and pass through camera crystals without interaction. In positron (β⁺) decay, the resolution is improved if the positrons travel only a short distance before annihilation. The resulting two relatively high-energy 511-keV photons traveling at 180 degrees from each other are best detected by the ring of specialized detectors found in positron emission tomography (PET) cameras. Imaging done with dual-photon positron-emitting agents is often of superior quality to that performed with routine single-photon nuclear medicine agents.

The radionuclide half-life ($T_{1/2}$) should be long enough only for the intended application, usually a few hours, because excess time increases the radiation dose. However, one must consider not only the *physical half-life* (T_P) related to the decay of the radionuclide but also the *biologic half-life* (T_B) when calculating the actual or *effective half-life* (T_E). The biologic half-life is determined by factors that alter how the agent moves through the body's various compartments (e.g., plasma, intracellular fluid, urine) as it is taken up and eliminated from the body. The T_E can be calculated using the following formula:

$$T_E = \frac{(T_P \times T_B)}{(T_P + T_B)}$$

As mentioned previously, the radionuclide used should also be *carrier-free,* with no contaminants from either stable or other radioactive radionuclides of the same element. Carrier material can negatively influence biodistribution and labeling efficiency. Contaminating isotopes increase radiation to the patient, especially if they have high photon energy, longer $T_{1/2}$, or result in particulate emissions. The radionuclide used should also have a *high specific activity,* that is, a high amount of radioactivity per unit weight (mCi/mg or MBq/mg). A carrier-free radionuclide has the highest specific activity.

Technetium-99m most closely matches these desirable features for use with gamma cameras, and for PET, the agent of choice is generally fluorine-18. Box 4.3 lists desired properties in a radiopharmaceutical. A few radioactive atoms, such as radioiodine, gallium, and thallium, can be used without modification because these elements can make use of the body's own systems for uptake. However, most radiopharmaceuticals combine the radionuclide with a biologically active molecule or drug carrier that determines localization and distribution.

BOX 4.3 Ideal Properties of Radiopharmaceuticals

Imaging
Radionuclide
Gamma photon energy of 100 to 200 keV
No β⁻ or α particulate emission
Sufficient half-life to allow for preparation, delivery, and imaging

Carrier Molecule
Stable binding to its carrier molecule (if used)
No toxicity
Rapid, specific localization
Prompt background clearance

Therapy
Rapid, specific localization
Background clearance with short residence time in radiation-sensitive tissues (e.g., bone marrow, lungs)
Particulate emissions that do not travel beyond the tumor or tissue being treated
"Crossfire" killing of immediately adjacent abnormal cells useful
Emitting additional γ-rays suitable for imaging useful for distribution assessment

---

Radiopharmaceuticals are sought that will accumulate rapidly in the targeted system or organ while quickly clearing from the background tissues, resulting in a *high target-to-background ratio*. Localizing mechanisms for common radiopharmaceuticals are listed in Table 4.7. It is important to be familiar with normal distribution patterns in order to better identify abnormalities that can occur due to disease or poor preparation. Problems with radiopharmaceutical quality often relate to the challenges of radiolabeling.

RADIOPHARMACEUTICAL PREPARATION

Technetium Radiolabeling

The chemistry of Tc-99m is complex. In most labeling procedures, technetium must be reduced from its +7 valence state. The reduction is usually accomplished with stannous ion. One exception is the labeling of Tc-99m sulfur colloid, which requires heating.

Commercial kits for radiolabeling these agents contain a reaction vial with the appropriate amount of stannous ion (tin), the nonradioactive pharmaceutical to be labeled, and other buffering and stabilizing agents. The vials are flushed with nitrogen to prevent atmospheric oxygen interrupting the reaction. The sequence of steps in a sample-labeling process is illustrated in Fig. 4.8. Sodium pertechnetate is drawn into a syringe and assayed in the dose calibrator. After the Tc-99m activity is confirmed, the sample is added to the reaction vial. The amount of Tc-99m activity added is determined by the number of patient doses desired in the case of a multidose vial, an estimate of the decrease in radioactivity caused by decay between the time of preparation and the estimated time of dosage administration, and the in vitro stability of the product. Each patient dose is kept in a special lead-shielded container and individually assayed before being dispensed.

TABLE 4.7   Radiopharmaceutical Localization Mechanisms

Mechanism	Applications or Examples
Compartmental localization	Blood pool imaging, direct cystography
Passive diffusion (concentration dependent)	Blood–brain barrier breakdown, cisternography
Capillary blockade (physical entrapment)	Perfusion imaging of lungs
Physical leakage from a luminal compartment	Gastrointestinal bleeding, detection of urinary tract or biliary system leakage
Metabolism (facilitated transport)	Glucose, fatty acids
Active transport (active cellular uptake)	Hepatobiliary imaging, thyroid, and adrenal imaging; renal tubular function; amino acid imaging (e.g., prostate)
Chemical bonding and adsorption	Skeletal imaging Amyloid plaque imaging
Cell sequestration	Splenic imaging (heat-damaged red blood cells)
Chemotaxis	White blood cell localization
Receptor binding and storage	Adrenal medullary imaging, somatostatin receptor imaging; dopamine transporter (DAT)
Phagocytosis	Reticuloendothelial system imaging
Antigen–antibody	Tumor imaging
Multiple mechanisms	
Perfusion and active transport	Myocardial imaging
Active transport and metabolism	Thyroid uptake and imaging
Active transport and secretion	Hepatobiliary imaging, salivary gland imaging

Excessive oxygen can react directly with the stannous ion, leaving too little reducing power in the kit, which can result in unwanted free Tc-99m pertechnetate in the preparation. Another problem that can result in free pertechnetate after kit preparation is radiolysis. This phenomenon, molecular decomposition due to the radiation itself, is less commonly seen but can occur when high amounts of Tc-99m radioactivity are used. Free pertechnetate is evidenced by uptake in the thyroid and stomach, as well by excretion in the urine.

Commonly Used Single-Photon Radiopharmaceuticals

The major Tc-99m–labeled radiopharmaceuticals are summarized in Table 4.8 and discussed in more detail in the chapters on individual organ systems. Important standard (i.e., single-photon) radiopharmaceuticals are listed in Table 4.9, and some are covered in the following discussion. Tables 4.10 and 4.11 list PET and therapy radiopharmaceuticals, respectively.

Radioiodine I-131 and I-123

I-131 as sodium iodide was the first radiopharmaceutical of importance in clinical nuclear medicine. It was used for physiological studies of the thyroid gland for several years in the late 1940s. Subsequently, it was used to radiolabel radiopharmaceuticals for scintigraphy, including human serum albumin, mac-

roaggregated albumin (MAA), Hippuran, and meta-iodo-benzyl-guanidine (MIBG). These radiopharmaceuticals are no longer diagnostically used.

The disadvantages of I-131 include a relatively high principal photon energy (364 keV), long half-life (8 days), and beta particle emissions, which result in poor dosimetry for an imaging agent. Although I-131 is an important radiopharmaceutical for the treatment of hyperthyroidism and differentiated thyroid cancer, I-123 is substituted whenever possible for diagnostic purposes. This includes I-123 MIBG and the newer agent to evaluate for Parkinsonian syndrome, I-123 ioflupane (DaTscan).

Compared with I-131, I-123 has a shorter half-life (13.2 hours), and its principal photon energy (159 keV) is better suited to gamma camera imaging with a photon flux roughly four times higher. It decays by electron capture without the β^- emissions of I-131. Dosimetry has been further improved through new production techniques with different cyclotron targets that allow I-123 production free from contamination by other longer-lived iodine isotopes that previously limited the amount of radiopharmaceutical given to patients.

Even in situations where I-131 could be expected to have an advantage due to its longer half-life, allowing multiday imaging to improve target-to-background ratios, I-131 has sometimes been replaced by I-123. Examples of this include whole-body thyroid cancer scans and MIBG imaging.

Quality control of radioiodinated pharmaceuticals is necessary to reduce radiation exposure to the thyroid gland. In nonthyroid imaging applications, it is common practice to block the thyroid gland with oral iodine (potassium iodide solution [SSKI], Lugol's solution [10% potassium iodide/5% iodine], or potassium iodide tablets) to prevent thyroid accumulation of any iodine present as a radiochemical impurity or metabolite. Protocols vary, but thyroid-blocking medications are started 1 to 12 hours before radiotracer administration in dosages equivalent to at least 100 mg of iodide.

Indium-111

In-111 has proved useful for clinical nuclear medicine. Its principal photon energies of 172 and 245 keV are favorable, and their abundance is high (>90%). The 2.8-day half-life permits multiple-day sequential imaging. Examples of radiopharmaceuticals include In-111 oxine leukocytes for the detection of inflammation and infection and the somatostatin receptor–binding peptide In-111 pentetreotide (OctreoScan) to detect neuroendocrine tumors.

Gallium-67

In the past, Ga-67 has been used in multiple ways: imaging bone and soft tissue infection as well as tumors. Since F-18 fluorodeoxyglucose (FDG) has replaced Ga-67 as the imaging agent of choice for lymphoma, the use of gallium has decreased tremendously. It is now generally reserved for occasional problem solving in chronic infections. This includes diagnosing osteomyelitis in the postoperative spine, differentiating severe sinusitis unresponsive to surgery from osteomyelitis, assessing the diabetic foot with Charcot joint, and identifying the source of a fever of unknown origin when F-18 FDG PET cannot be performed.

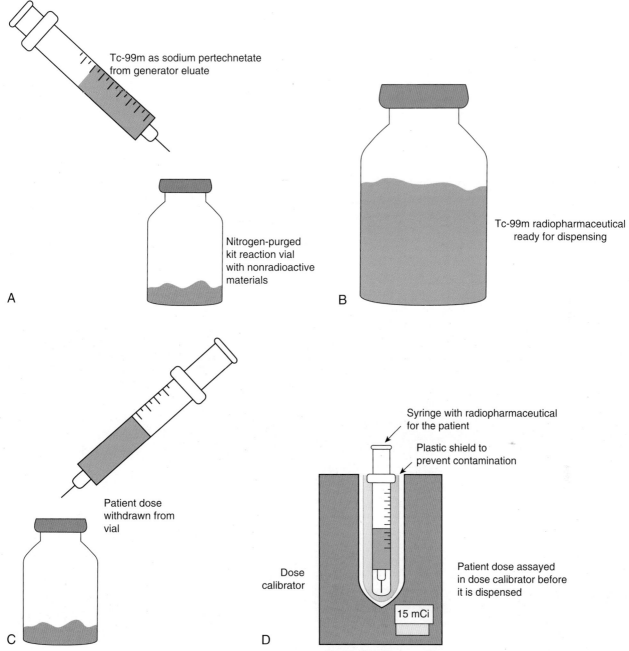

Fig. 4.8 Preparation of a Tc-99m–labeled radiopharmaceutical. (A) Tc-99m as sodium pertechnetate is added to the reaction vial. (B) Tc-99m radiopharmaceutical is ready for dispensing. (C) The patient dose is withdrawn from the vial. (D) Each dose is measured in the dose calibrator before it is dispensed.

Ga-67 behaves like an iron analog, transported to sites of infection or trauma in the body by molecules such as transferrin. Its relatively long half-life (78.3 hours) allows imaging over several days in order to improve target-to-background ratios but also results in higher exposure to the patient. For the first 24 to 48 hours, clearance is primarily through the urine, with bowel excretion subsequently becoming the dominant route. Activity in the colon required use of laxatives for assessment of the abdomen in the past, but single-photon emission computed tomography with computed tomography (SPECT/CT) has since improved localization. Imaging characteristics are also less than optimal because the four principal gamma photons include not only 93- and 185-keV photons but also higher-energy 300- and 395-keV photons.

Thallium-201

Tl-201 became available in the mid-1970s for myocardial scintigraphy. It behaves as a potassium analog, with high net clearance (~85%) in its passage through the myocardial capillary bed, which makes it an excellent marker of regional blood flow to viable myocardium.

Its major disadvantage is the absence of an ideal photopeak for imaging. With its 135- and 167-keV gamma emissions in low abundance, characteristic mercury x-rays in the

TABLE 4.8 Technetium-99m–Labeled Radiopharmaceuticals

Agent	Application
Tc-99m sodium pertechnetate	Meckel's diverticulum detection, salivary and thyroid gland scintigraphy
Tc-99m tilmanocept	Lymphoscintigraphy
Tc-99m sulfur colloid	Lymphoscintigraphy
Liver/spleen scintigraphy, bone marrow scintigraphy; gastric emptying
Tc-99m methylene diphosphonate	Skeletal scintigraphy
Tc-99m macroaggregated albumin (MAA)	Pulmonary perfusion scintigraphy, liver intraarterial perfusion scintigraphy
Tc-99m red blood cells	Radionuclide ventriculography, gastrointestinal bleeding, hepatic hemangioma
Tc-99m Technegas	Lung perfusion scans
Tc-99m diethylenetriamine-pentaacetic acid (DTPA)	Renal dynamic scintigraphy, lung ventilation (aerosol), glomerular filtration rate
Tc-99m mercaptoacetyltriglycine (MAG$_3$)	Renal dynamic scintigraphy
Tc-99m dimercaptosuccinic acid (DMSA)	Renal cortical scintigraphy
Tc-99m iminodiacetic acid (HIDA)/ Tc-99m mebrofenin	Hepatobiliary scintigraphy
Tc-99m sestamibi (Cardiolite)	Myocardial perfusion scintigraphy, breast cancer imaging
Tc-99m tetrofosmin (Myoview)	Myocardial perfusion scintigraphy
Tc-99m exametazime (HMPAO)	Cerebral perfusion scintigraphy, white blood cell labeling
Tc-99m bicisate (ECD)	Cerebral perfusion scintigraphy

ECD, Ethyl cysteinate dimer; *HMPAO,* hexamethylpropyleneamine oxime.

TABLE 4.9 Non-Technetium-99m Single-Photon Radiopharmaceuticals

Agent	Application
Diagnostic	
Xe-133 xenon (inert gas)	Pulmonary ventilation scintigraphy
Kr-81m krypton (inert gas)	Pulmonary ventilation scintigraphy
I-123 sodium iodide	Thyroid scintigraphy, thyroid uptake function studies
In-111 oxine leukocytes	Inflammatory disease and infection detection
I-123 meta-iodo-benzyl-guanidine (MIBG)	Adrenal medullary tumor imaging
In-111 pentetreotide (OctreoScan)	Somatostatin receptor tumor imaging
I-123 ioflupane (DaTscan)	Dopamine transporter receptor imaging for Parkinson disease and Parkinsonian syndromes

TABLE 4.10 Positron Emission Tomography Radiopharmaceuticals

Agent	Application
F-18 fluorodeoxyglucose (FDG)	Tumor imaging
Infection imaging
Cardiac: Viability, sarcoid diagnosis
Brain: dementia, interictal seizure, +/– recurrent glioblastoma
Ga-68 DOTATATE	Somatostatin positive neuroendocrine tumor (NET)
F-18 fluciclovine	Recurrent prostate cancer
F-18 florbetapir	Amyloid
F-18 flutemetamol	Amyloid
F-18 florbetaben	Amyloid
Rb-82	Cardiac perfusion
N-13 ammonia	Cardiac perfusion
F-18 sodium fluoride (F-18 NaF)	Bone metastases
C-11 Choline	Prostate cancer

TABLE 4.11 Therapeutic Radiopharmaceuticals

Agent	Application
I-131 sodium iodide	Thyroid cancer and hyperthyroidism (Graves' disease, toxic nodule, toxic nodular goiter)
In-111 ibritumomab (Zevalin)[a]	B-cell lymphoma therapy (antibody)
Y-90 microsphere
Y-90 Therasphere
Y-90 Sirsphere	Hepatocellular cancer
Hepatic metastases colon cancer
Lu-177 DOTATATE (Lutathera)	Neuroendocrine tumor (somatostatin receptor positive)
I-131 iobenguane (Azedra)	Pheochromocytoma or paraganglioma (≥12 yrs old/MIBG positive)
Ra-223 (Xofigo)	Metastatic prostate cancer
Sr-89 (Metastron)	Metastatic prostate cancer
Sm-153 lexidronan (Quadramet)	Metastatic prostate cancer
P-32 chromic phosphate (Phosphocol)	Effusion leaking into peritoneum or pleural space
Additional treatment applications: peritoneal metastases, hemophilia joint disease; intracavitary tumor treatment (e.g., glioblastoma)

[a]Other radiolabeled antibodies previously approved by the U.S. Food and Drug Administration but no longer clinically available.

range of 69 to 83 keV are acquired (sometimes with the addition of the 167-keV gamma photon). At the low energies of these x-rays, discriminating scattered from primary photons is suboptimal with the gamma scintillation camera. Because of its poor imaging characteristics, Tc-99m–labeled cardiac perfusion radiopharmaceuticals are used most often used.

Radioactive Inert Gases

Radioactive inert gases are used for pulmonary ventilation imaging. Xe-133 is most commonly used. Its advantage over Tc-99m–DTPA aerosols is better distribution into the lung periphery in patients with chronic obstructive pulmonary disease (COPD) or other issues causing breathing difficulties. A disadvantage is the relatively low energy of its principal photon (81 keV), dictating the performance of ventilation scintigraphy before Tc-99m perfusion scintigraphy. Because of its poor imaging characteristics and dosimetry issues, Tc-99m–labeled aerosols are more commonly used. Xe-133 has a 5.2-day half-life, posing radiation safety issues answered to some extent by a xenon trap (charcoal).

Krypton-81m (Kr-81m) has advantages because of its high principal gamma emission (190 keV) and short half-life (13 seconds), allowing for postperfusion imaging and multiple-view acquisition without concern for retained activity or radiation dose. However, the rubidium-81/kr-81m generator system is expensive and must be replaced daily because of its short half-life. This gas is no longer clinically used in the United States.

It should be noted that the newer agent Tc-99m Technegas is likely going to take the lead as the preferred agent for ventilation imaging. Its photon energy is superior compared with Xe-133 for imaging. Also, it has improved distribution characteristics compared with Tc-99m DTPA in cases of COPD because the particles are small enough to behave like a gas. Although it has been held up for use in the United States due to challenges in obtaining U.S. Food and Drug Administration (FDA) approval, it is in widespread use elsewhere.

Dual-Photon Radiopharmaceuticals for Positron Emission Tomography

The physical characteristics of commonly used positron-emitting radionuclides are summarized in Table 4.2. Many radiopharmaceuticals have been described for use with PET. Carbon, nitrogen, and oxygen are found ubiquitously in biological molecules. It is thus theoretically possible to radiolabel almost any molecule of biological interest. The hydroxyl analog, F-18, has the advantage of a longer half-life than C-11, N-13, or O-15 and has been used as a label for the glucose analog FDG. F-18 FDG has found widespread clinical application in whole-body tumor imaging and, to a lesser extent, imaging of the brain and heart. The uptake of F-18 FDG is a marker of tumor metabolism and viability.

F-18 FDG has also been used to diagnose degenerative dementia, based on changes in metabolic patterns in the brain, and it has also aided in the identification of seizure foci in the interictal state. F-18-labeled PET agents have been approved by the FDA for amyloid brain imaging. In the heart, this radiopharmaceutical can differentiate areas of viable myocardium from ischemic scar and can help determine when cases of heart failure are caused by myocardial sarcoid.

Rubidium-82 (Rb-82) is available from a generator system with a relatively long-lived parent (strontium-82, $T_{1/2}$ = 25 days). Its availability from a generator system obviates the need for onsite cyclotron production. Like thallium, it is a potassium analog and used for myocardial perfusion imaging. Cardiac imaging with this PET agent is extremely rapid compared with

studies performed with Tc-99m–labeled agents (e.g., Tc-99m sestamibi) or with Tl-201. One limitation of Rb-82 is, however, the high energy (3.15 MeV) of its positron emissions. This results in a relatively long average path in soft tissue before annihilation, degrading the spatial resolution available with the agent. This feature is shared to a lesser extent by O-15.

New PET radiopharmaceuticals have been approved in the United States. These include Ga-68 DOTATATE, which has been used for years in Europe for the imaging of somatostatin-receptor–positive neuroendocrine tumors. This agent not only has proven to be much more sensitive than In-111 pentetreotide but also images with a much lower radiation dose to the patient. For these reasons, the PET agent is rapidly replacing In-111 pentetreotide. New prostate agents include F-18 fluciclovine, approved by the FDA in the setting of recurrent prostate cancer, and an investigational agent, Ga-68–labeled PMSA, currently under evaluation.

The production of most positron-emitting radionuclides, and their subsequent incorporation into PET radiopharmaceuticals, is expensive and complex, requiring a cyclotron (or other special accelerator) and relatively elaborate radiochemical-handling equipment. In-house self-contained small cyclotrons with automated chemistry are available but are expensive for most clinical settings. The heavy clinical demand and the relatively long 2-hour half-life of F-18 have resulted in F-18 FDG production and distribution by regional radiopharmacies.

NEW RADIOACTIVE DRUG DEVELOPMENT

Strict regulations are in place concerning both the radioactive and pharmaceutical components of radiopharmaceuticals. The Nuclear Regulatory Commission (NRC) oversees safety considerations related to radiation (see Chapter 5), and the U.S. Pharmacopeia (USP) sets many quality standards and safety guidelines related to drugs. The FDA regulates pharmaceutical quality and safety and must approve all radiopharmaceuticals before clinical use or prior to human research trials. When developing a new agent, preclinical investigations first examine the safety, pharmacokinetics/pharmacodynamics, dosimetry, and potential usefulness of the agent. Prior to clinical trials, an FDA application is submitted through a few potential pathways, including an institution's Radioactive Research Drug Committee (RDRC) or via an Investigational New Drug (IND) application. During this process, the investigator must describe manufacturing procedures, results of preclinical pharmacology and toxicology studies, and technical details about the protocol itself. After IND approval, a New Drug Application (NDA) or Abbreviated New Drug Application (ANDA) could be submitted for marketing. These programs are important for researchers who are developing new agents, including the many new PET agents being investigated for possible clinical use.

QUALITY ASSURANCE IN RADIONUCLIDES AND RADIOPHARMACEUTICALS

In this chapter, quality control (QC) is discussed related to radionuclide production and radiolabeling radiopharmaceuticals. QC procedures in the radiopharmacy involve upholding standards related to radiopharmaceuticals, maintaining measuring devices (e.g., the dose calibrator), limiting unnecessary exposures, and administering activities mandated by governmental agencies such as the NRC. Many of the issues related to radiation safety and the role of the Authorized User (AU) are covered in detail in Chapter 5.

Radionuclide Production Quality Control

QC is an important component of radionuclide and radiopharmaceutical production. Problems can be grouped as those related to radionuclide purity, chemical purity, biological contaminants, and other physical issues (e.g., pH, particle size, osmolarity). Some of the issues related to radionuclide production are defined in Box 4.4.

Mo-99/Tc-99m Generator QC

In the case of radionuclide generators, rigorous procedures are performed to assess quality before commercial generators are shipped; however, every laboratory must perform QC steps each time the generator is eluted to be certain the material is in line with regulatory guidelines (Table 4.12).

Radionuclide Purity

The only desired radionuclide in the Mo-99/Tc-99m generator elute is Tc-99m sodium pertechnetate ($^{99m}TcO_4^-$), and any other

radioactive material is considered an impurity. Limitations on the amount of these contaminants are strict because they cause additional radiation exposure without clinical benefit and can also impact radiolabeling. Tc-99, the daughter product of the isomeric transition of Tc-99m, is not a problem from a radiation or health standpoint (given a half-life decay of 2.1×10^5 years to the stable ruthenium-99). Therefore, it is not tested for as a radionuclide impurity. Other radionuclide impurities can include those related to Mo-99 production in the reactor (e.g., I-131, Sr-89, and Sr-90). However, Mo-99 itself is the most common impurity.

The NRC sets allowable limits on the amount of Mo-99 "breakthrough," and testing must be performed after each elution. The easiest and most widely used approach is to place the generator eluate in a special lead container designed to absorb the 140-keV photons of Tc-99m but to allow a portion of the high-energy 740- and 780-keV gamma emissions of Mo-99 to penetrate. The shielded sample is placed in a dose calibrator and measured on the Mo-99 setting. Then the unshielded sample is measured on the Tc-99m setting, allowing calculation of the ratio of Mo-99 to Tc-99m activity.

The NRC limit is 0.15 µCi of Mo-99 activity per 1 mCi of Tc-99m activity (<0.15 kBq/MBq Tc-99m) at the time of administration. Because the half-life of Mo-99 is longer than that of Tc-99m, the proportion of the contaminant increases with time. If the initial reading shows near-maximum Mo-99 levels, either the actual dose to be given to the patient should be restudied before administration or the buildup factor should be computed mathematically. From a practical standpoint, the Mo-99 activity may be taken as unchanged and the Tc-99m decay calculated (Table 4.13). Breakthrough is rare but unpredictable. When it does occur, Mo-99 levels can be far higher than the legal limit.

Chemical Purity

Chemical impurities are generally a concern when they are toxic, biologically active, affect the radiolabel, or alter the radiopharmaceutical characteristics. The generator eluate is routinely tested for the column-packing material, Al_2O_3. Excessive aluminum levels may interfere with the normal distribution of certain

---

BOX 4.4   Radiopharmacy Quality Control Parameter Definitions

Chemical purity: The amount of unwanted (nonradioactive) chemical in preparation.

Radionuclide purity: The proportion of the desired radionuclide relative to other radioactive contaminants.

Radiochemical purity: The amount of the desired radionuclide or radiopharmaceutical in its proper form (e.g., its oxidation state or binding to the appropriate carrier molecule), compared with its other forms (i.e., oxidized or unbound).

Biological purity: The presence or absence of microorganisms and pyrogens (endotoxins).

Note: Other chemical/physical properties include pH, particle size, osmolarity, and solution clarity.

TABLE 4.12   Molybdenum-99/Technetium-99m Generator Quality Control Limits

Problem	Category	Detection Tests	Standard
Mo-99 breakthrough	Radionuclide purity	Shielded dose in dose calibrator measure 740-/780-keV Mo-99 photons (140 keV blocked)	<0.15 µCi Mo-99/mCi Tc-99m <0.1% of Tc-99m activity at time of administration
Al^{3+} (Al_2O_3 from generator ion exchange column in elution)	Chemical purity	Colorimetric spot test Comparison to a pink color standard (Aurin tricarboxylic acid)	<10 µg/mL or < 10 ppm (fission generator)
Oxidized Tc-99m (all forms besides desired +7 reduced $^{99m}TcO_4^-$)	Radiochemical purity	Instant thin layer chromatography, electrophoresis, gel chromatography	≥95% of Tc-99m activity should be as $^{99m}TcO_4^-$
Sterility	Biologic purity	Inoculate fluid thioglycolate medium and soybean-casein digest medium	USP regulation 14 days' incubation and assess for growth
Pyrogenicity	Biologic purity	Limulus amebocyte lysate gel-clot	Reaction from gram-negative bacterial endotoxins measured Note: limits are far stricter for intrathecal administration.

USP, U.S. Pharmacopeia.

TABLE 4.13 Physical Decay of Technetium-99m

Time (hr)	Fraction Remaining	T½ number	% Activity
0	1.00	1	50
1	0.891	2	25
2	0.794	3	12.5
3	0.708	4	6.25
4	0.631	5	3.125
5	0.532	6	1.56
6	0.501	7	0.78
7	0.447	8	0.39
8	0.398	9	0.195
9	0.355	10	0.098
10	0.316	11	0.049
11	0.282	12	0.024
12	0.251	13	0.012

Tc-99m physical half-life = 6.02 hr. Note: when doses using the same radiolabel are imaged close together in time, 4 half-lives is often enough time to reduce background. However, when the amount of activity is high in a particular organ or when measurements must be accurate (e.g., in serum sampling), 8 half-lives may be needed (or even 10, which is essentially at background).

TABLE 4.14 Limitations on Impurities for Generator-Produced Radionuclides

Generator System	Impurity	Limit	Comment
Ge-68/Ga-68	Radiochemical	<0.001% Ge-68 breakthrough >95% free Ga-68	<0.001% of nominal activity from other emitters Pre-elute generator and discard if it has not been eluted for >2 days
	Chemical	Fe < 10 µg/GBq Zn < 10 µg/GBq	
	Biologic	<30 EU/L bacterial endotoxin	
Sr-82/Rb-82	Radiochemical Sr-82 breakthrough Sr-85 contamination	0.02 µCi/mCi Rb-82 (0.02 kBq/MBq) 0.2 µCi/mCi Rb-82 (0.2 kBq/MBq)	Expiration 42 days post-calibration, often must be replaced after < month for sufficient activity

radiopharmaceuticals—for example, increased lung activity with Tc-99m sulfur colloid and liver uptake with Tc-99m methylene diphosphonate (Tc-99m MDP). A colorimetric qualitative spot testing determines if unacceptable levels are present. A sample from the eluate is spotted on special test paper that changes color, turning pink in the presence of alumina. The intensity is compared to a standard, with the USP limit set at 10 µg/mL.

Radiochemical Purity

It is important that the materials used are not only free of other radionuclides and unwanted chemicals but that they also contain radioactivity in the desired form—so-called radiochemical purity.

When Tc-99m is eluted from the generator, the desired chemical form of Tc-99m pertechnetate is a +7 valence state. Commercial kits used to create other Tc-99m–labeled pharmaceuticals are based on this +7 oxidation state. The USP standard for the generator eluate is that 95% or more of Tc-99m activity be in this form. Reduction states at +4, +5, or +6 result in impurities. These reduction states can be detected by thin-layer chromatography. Problems with the radiochemical purity of the generator eluate are infrequently encountered but should be considered if kit labeling is poor.

Limits for Other Radionuclides

Although it is most critical to know QC limits related to Tc-99m production, strict limits have been set concerning contaminants in other radionuclides. For materials produced through fission in a reactor, other fission by-products must be identified and removed, such as I-131. In PET production, fewer sources of contamination are present but can occur depending on target

and reaction type chosen. In the case of the generator-produced Ga-68, impurities and breakthrough can be seen. As with Tc-99m or Rb-82 generators, the parent radionuclide could break through during elution. Radiochemical and other contaminants and impurities must be carefully assessed after each elution (Table 4.14).

Quality Assurance of Technetium-99m–Labeled Radiopharmaceuticals

It is also important to test the Tc-99m–labeled preparation product for *radiochemical purity* and confirm the presence of a product in the desired form (as was required when testing the radionuclide before labeling), defined as the percentage of the total radioactivity in a specimen that is in the specified or desired radiochemical form (Table 4.15). For example, if 5% of the Tc-99m activity remains as free pertechnetate in a radiolabeling procedure, the radiochemical purity would be stated as 95%, assuming no other impurities. Each radiopharmaceutical has a specific radiochemical purity to meet USP standards or FDA requirements (typically 95%). Causes of radiochemical impurities include poor initial labeling, radiolysis, decomposition, pH changes, light exposure, or presence of oxidizing or reducing agents.

The usual approach to assay radiochemical purity in vitro is thin-layer chromatography. The solvent and material for the test strip are chosen based on the contaminants possible. For technetium radiopharmaceuticals, the impurities tested for are free pertechnetate and insoluble hydrolyzed reduced technetium.

Consider an example where samples of the radiopharmaceutical Tc-99m diphosphonate are placed on the end of test strips (Figs. 4.9 and 4.10). Free Tc-99m pertechnetate on paper chromatography strips will migrate with the solvent front in the presence of the solvent acetone, whereas Tc-99m diphosphonate and hydrolyzed reduced technetium remain

TABLE 4.15   Radiopharmaceutical Quality Control Parameters

Parameter	Definition	Examples of Contaminants and Problems
Chemical purity	Amount of unwanted nonradioactive chemical in preparation	Alumina (Al^{3+} or Al_2O_3) from Tc-99m generator eluate
Radionuclide purity	Other types of radioactive material besides the desired radionuclide	Mo-99 in Tc-99m generator eluate; I-124 in I-123 dose
Radiochemical purity	Other forms of the desired radionuclide	Changes in oxidation/reduction status altering kit labeling efficiency. Free, unbound $^{99m}Tc\,O_4^-$ Colloids[a] formed from insoluble Tc-99m as technetium hydroxides or technetium-labeled stannous hydroxide form (also known as hydrolyzed/reduced or $^{99m}TcO_2$)
Biological purity	Absence of microorganisms and pyrogens (endotoxins)	Sterile; pyrogen-free preparation
Physical status and other chemical properties	Fraction of total pharmaceutical in desired physical form	Correct particle size in Tc-99m MAA or sulfur colloid; absence of particulate contaminants in a solution Issues with the kit used to make the radiopharmaceutical such as insufficient stannous ion Clouded or discolored preparation pH, osmolarity outside of acceptable limits

[a]Colloids formed from insoluble forms of Tc-99m can be taken up by the reticuloendothelial system in the marrow, liver, and spleen and alter radio-pharmaceutical distribution.

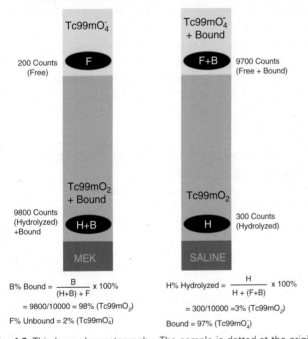

Fig. 4.9 Thin-layer chromatography. The sample is dotted at the origin and then placed in a solvent, either saline or methyl ethyl ketone (MEK). The strips are dried and cut in half, and each is measured in the dose calibrator. In this example, the radiopharmaceutical passes the test.

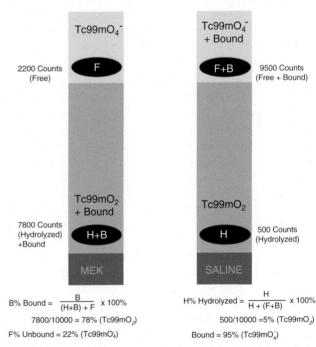

Fig. 4.10 Thin-layer chromatography in a case that does not pass quality assurance testing.

at the origin. For selective testing of hydrolyzed reduced technetium, a silica gel strip is used, with saline as the solvent. In this system, both free pertechnetate and Tc-99m diphosphonate move with the solvent front, and hydrolyzed reduced technetium again stays at the origin. This combination of procedures allows measurement of each of the three components. The radiolabel allows quantitative measurement by simply cutting the chromatography strip into two pieces and counting each end separately. Chromatography systems have been worked out for each major technetium-labeled radiopharmaceutical.

In vivo radiochemical impurities contribute to background activity or other unwanted localization and degrade image quality. For many agents, the presence of a radiochemical impurity can be recognized by altered in vivo biodistribution. For example, colloids formed by the insoluble forms of Tc-99m can be taken up by the reticuloendothelial system in the liver, spleen, and marrow.

Quality Control of Non-Technetium-Based Radiopharmaceuticals

Considerations of radiochemical and radionuclide purity also apply to other single-photon agents and positron radiopharmaceuticals (see Box 4.4 and Table 4.15). Radiochemical purity is important for radioiodinated agents because of the potential for uptake of free radioiodine by the thyroid gland if the radiolabel disassociates from the carrier molecule. Other QC procedures are aimed at ensuring the sterility and apyrogenicity of administered radiopharmaceuticals. QC monitoring of the dose-calibrator performance is important to ensure that administered doses are within prescribed amounts.

Sterility and Pyrogen Testing

Sterility implies the absence of living organisms (see Table 4.15). *Apyrogenicity* implies the absence of metabolic products such as endotoxins. Because many radiopharmaceuticals are prepared just before use, definitive testing before they are administered to the patient is impractical, which doubles the need for careful aseptic technique in the nuclear pharmacy.

Autoclaving is a well-known means of sterilization of preparation vials and other utensils and materials, but it is not useful for radiopharmaceuticals. When terminal sterilization is required, various membrane-filtration methods are used. Special filters with pore diameters smaller than microorganisms have been developed for this purpose. A filter pore size of 0.22 μm is necessary to sterilize a solution. It traps bacteria, including small organisms such as *Pseudomonas*.

Sterility testing standards have been defined by the USP. Standard media, including thioglycollate and soybean-casein digest media, are used for different categories of microorganisms, including aerobic and anaerobic bacteria and fungi.

Pyrogens are protein or polysaccharide metabolites of microorganisms or other contaminating substances that cause febrile reactions. They can be present even in sterile preparations. The typical clinical syndrome is fever, chills, joint pain, and headache developing minutes to a few hours after injection. The USP test for pyrogen testing uses limulus amebocyte lysate. It is based on the observation that amebocyte lysate preparations from the blood of horseshoe crabs become opaque in the presence of pyrogens.

DISPENSING RADIOPHARMACEUTICALS

Normal Procedures

General radiation safety procedures should be followed in all laboratories (Box 4.5). The dispensing of radiopharmaceuticals is governed by exacting rules and regulations promulgated by the Food and Drug Administration (FDA) and Nuclear Regulatory Commission (NRC), as well as state pharmacy boards and hospital radiation safety committees. Radiopharmaceuticals for clinical use must be approved by the FDA. Radiopharmaceuticals are prescription drugs that cannot be legally administered without being ordered by an authorized individual. The NRC *authorized user* and the radiopharmacy are responsible for confirming the appropriateness of the request, ensuring that the correct radiopharmaceutical designated amount is administered to the patient, and keeping records of both the request and documentation of dosage administration.

BOX 4.5   Radiation Safety Procedures

Wear laboratory coats in areas where radioactive materials are present.
  Wear disposable gloves when handling radioactive materials.
  Monitor hands and body for radioactive contamination before leaving the area.
  Use syringe and vial shields as necessary.
  Do not eat, drink, smoke, apply cosmetics, or store food in areas where radioactive material is stored or used.
  Wear personnel monitoring devices in areas with radioactive materials.
  Never pipette by mouth.
  Dispose of radioactive waste in designated, labeled, and properly shielded receptacles located in a secured area.
  Label containers, vials, and syringes containing radioactive materials. When not in use, place in shielded containers or behind lead shielding in a secured area.
  Store all sealed sources (floods, dose calibrator sources) in shielded containers in a secured area.
  Before administering doses to patients, determine and record activity.
  Know what steps to take and the person to contact (radiation safety officer) in the event of a radiation accident, improper operation of radiation safety equipment, or theft or loss of licensed material.

Before any material is dispensed, quality assurance measures should be carried out. These are described earlier in this chapter for the Mo-99/Tc-99m generator system and Tc-99m–labeled radiopharmaceuticals. For other agents, the package insert or protocol for formulation and dispensing should be consulted for radiochromatography or other quality control steps that must be performed before dosage administration. Good practice dictates that quality control should always be performed, even when not legally required. Every dose should be physically inspected for any particulate or foreign material (e.g., rubber from the tops of multidose injection vials) before administration. Each dose administered to a patient must be assayed in a dose calibrator. The administered activity should be within ±20% of the prescription request.

Special Considerations
Pregnancy and Lactation

The possibility of pregnancy should be considered for every woman of childbearing age referred to the nuclear medicine service for a diagnostic or therapeutic procedure. Pregnancy alone is not an absolute contraindication to performing a nuclear medicine study. For example, pulmonary embolism is encountered in pregnant women and is associated with potential serious morbidity and mortality. Thus the risk-to-benefit ratio of ventilation-perfusion scintigraphy is high and considered an acceptable procedure in this circumstance. The radiation dosage is kept to a minimum. Tc-99m MAA does not cross the placenta, but xenon does. Radioiodine also crosses the placenta. The fetal thyroid develops the capacity to concentrate radioiodine at 10 to 12 weeks of gestation, and cretinism caused by in utero exposure to therapeutic I-131 may occur.

Women who are lactating and breastfeeding require special attention. The need to suspend breastfeeding is determined by the half-life of the radionuclide and the degree to which it is secreted in breast milk. Radioiodine is secreted by the breast, and breastfeeding should be terminated altogether after the administration of I-131. NRC regulations stipulate that the patient must receive verbal and written instructions to that effect. For I-123, breastfeeding could safely be resumed after 2 days. For Tc-99m agents, 12 to 24 hours is sufficient. Further recommendations regarding breastfeeding for various radiopharmaceuticals are listed in Table 4.16.

Dosage Selection for Pediatric Patients

Various approaches have been used for scaling down the radiopharmaceutical dose administered to children. There is no perfect way to do this because of the differential rate of maturation of body organs and the changing ratio of different body compartments to body weight. Empirically, body surface area correlates better than body weight for dosage selection. Various formulas and nomograms have been developed.

An approximation based on body weight uses the formula:

$$\text{Pediatric dose} = \frac{\text{Patient Weight (kg)}}{70\text{kg}} \times \text{Adult dose}$$

Another alternative is the use of *Webster's rule*:

$$\text{Pediatric dose} = \frac{\text{Age} + 1}{\text{Age} + 7} \times \text{Adult dose}$$

Another alternative is Clark's rule:

Pediatric dose = (Weight divided by 150 lbs.) x Adult dose

This formula is not useful for infants. Moreover, in some cases a calculated dose may not be adequate to obtain a diagnostically useful study and physician judgment must be used. For example, a newborn infant with suspected biliary atresia may require 24-hour delayed Tc-99m HIDA imaging, which is not feasible if the dose is too low. Therefore a minimum dose for each radiopharmaceutical is be established.

The concept *As Low As Reasonably Achievable (ALARA)* has always been a basic tenet in nuclear medicine regarding the administered dose. This concept has been recently reemphasized for pediatric diagnostic imaging. It has been restated as *the lowest absorbed radiation dose that is consistent with quality imaging*. Expert consensus recommendations for pediatric administered doses are listed in Table 4.17.

Nuclear Regulatory Commission and Agreement States

The NRC regulates all reactor by-product materials with regard to use and disposal, radiation safety of personnel using them, and the public. Certain states, termed *Agreement States*, have entered into regulatory agreements with the NRC that give them the authority to license and inspect by-products, sources, or special nuclear material used or possessed within their borders. Currently more than 40 states are Agreement States, and the number is growing. These states agree to set regulations at least as strict as those of the NRC.

Authorized User

An Authorized User is a person with documented training and experience in the safe handling and use of radioactive materials for medical use who is authorized to order, receive, store, and administer radiopharmaceuticals. Two general paths exist for becoming an authorized user: certification by specialty board or training and work experience. The NRC has defined requirements for becoming an authorized user based on the type of use for the radiopharmaceutical—uptake and dilution, imaging and localization, and therapy (Box 4.6). Once Authorized User eligible status is achieved, the candidate can apply to bodies such as the hospital Radiation Safety Committee and the Radiation Safety Officer to become an authorized user with a radioactive materials license.

Medical Event

The NRC defines a *medical event* as a radiopharmaceutical dose administration involving the wrong patient, wrong radiopharmaceutical, wrong route of administration, or an administered dose differing from the prescribed dose when the effective dose equivalent to the patient exceeds 5 rem to the whole body

TABLE 4.16   Recommendations for Radiopharmaceuticals Excreted in Breast Milk

Radiopharmaceutical	Administered activity mCi (MBq)	Counseling adivsed	Withhold breastfeeding
Ga-67 citrate	5.0 (185)	Yes	Cessation
I-131 sodium iodide	0.02 (0.7)	Yes	Cessation
I-123 sodium iodide	0.4 (14.8)	Yes	48 hr
I-123 MIBG	10 (370.0)	Yes	48 hr
Tl-201	3 (111)	Yes	96 hr
In-111 leukocytes	5 (185)	Yes	48 hr
Tc-99m MAA	4 (148)	Yes	12 hr
Tc-99m red blood cells	20 (740)	Yes	12 hr
Tc-99m pertechnetate	5 (185)	Yes	24 hr

MAA, Macroaggregated albumin; *MIBG*, meta-iodo-benzyl-guanidine.
Modified with permission from Stabin MG, Breitz HB. Breast milk excretion of radiopharmaceuticals: mechanisms, findings, and radiation dosimetry. *J Nucl Med.* 2000;41:863-873.

TABLE 4.17 North American Consensus Guidelines for Pediatric Administered Radiopharmaceutical Activities

Radiopharmaceutical	Notes	Administered Activity	Minimum Administered Activity	Maximum Administered Activity
^{123}I-MIBG	[A]	5.2 MBq/kg (0.14 mCi/kg)	37 MBq (1.0 mCi)	370MBq (10.0 mCi)
^{99m}Tc-MDP	[A]	9.3 MBq/kg (0.25 mCi/kg)	37 MBq (1.0 mCi)	
^{18}F-FDG	[A, B]	Body: 3.7-5.2 MBq/kg (0.10-0.14 mCi/kg)	26.MBq (0.7 mCi)	
		Brain: 3.7 MBq/kg (0.10 mCi/kg)	14 MBq (0.37 mCi)	
^{99m}Tc-DMSA	[A]	1.85 MBq/kg (0.05 mCi/kg)	18.5 MBq (0.5 mCi)	100 MBq (2.7 mCi)
^{99m}Tc-MAG3	[A, C]	Without flow study: 3.7 MBq/kg (0.10 mCi/kg)		
	[A]	With flow study: 5.55 MBq/kg (0.15 mCi/kg)	37 MBq (1.0 mCi)	148 MBq (4.0 mCi)
^{99m}Tc-IDA	[A, D]	1.85 MBq/kg (0.05 mCi/kg)	18.5 MBq (0.5 mCi)	
^{99m}Tc-MAA	[A]	If 99mTc used for ventilation: 2.59 MBq/kg (0.07 mCi/kg)		
	[A]	No 99mTc ventilation study: 1.11 MBq/kg (0.03 mCi/kg)	14.8 MBq (0.4 mCi)	
[99m]Tc-pertechnetate (Meckel diverticulum imaging)	[A]	1.85 MBq/kg (0.05 mCi/kg)	9.25 MBq (0.25 mCi)	
[18]F-sodium fluoride	[A]	2.22 MBq/kg (0.06 mCi/kg)	14 MBq (0.38 mCi)	
99mTc (for cystography)	[E]	No weight-based dose	No more than 37 MBq (1.0 mCi) for each bladder filling cycle	
[99m]Tc-sulfur colloid (for oral liquid gastric emptying)	[F]	No weight-based dose	9.25 MBq (0.25 mCi)	37 MBq (1.0 mCi)
[99m]Tc-sulfur colloid (for solid gastric emptying)	[F]	No weight-based dose	9.25 MBq (0.25 mCi)	18.5 MBq (0.5 mCi)
[99m]Tc- HMPAO (Ceretec)/^{99m}Tc-ECD (Neurolite) for brain perfusion		11.1 MBq/kg (0.3 mCi/kg)	185 MBq (5 mCi)	740 MBq (20 mCi)
[99m]Tc-sestamibi (Cardiolite)/^{99m}Tc-tetrofosmin (Myoview) for myocardial perfusion (single scan or first of 2 scans, same day)		5.55 MBq/kg (0.15 mCi/kg)	74 MBq (2 mCi)	370 MBq (10 mCi)
[99m]Tc-sestamibi (Cardiolite)/^{99m}Tc-tetrofosmin (Myoview) for myocardial perfusion (second of 2 scans, same day)		16.7 MBq/kg (0.45 mCi/kg)	222 MBq (6 mCi)	1110 MBq (30 mCi)
Na[123]I for thyroid imaging		0.28 MBq/kg (0.0075 mCi)	1 MBq (0.027 mCi)	11 MBq (0.3 mCi)
[99m]Tc-pertechnetate for thyroid imaging		1.1 MBq/kg (0.03 mCi/kg)	7 MBq (0.19 mCi)	93 MBq (2.5 mCi)
^{99m}Tc-RBC for blood pool imaging		11.8 MBq/kg (0.32 mCi/kg)	74 MBq (2 mCi)	740 MBq (20 mCi)
^{99m}Tc-WBC for infection imaging		7.4 MBq/kg (0.2 mCi/kg)	74 MBq (2 mCi)	555 MBq (15 mCi)
^{68}Ga-DOTATOC or ^{68}Ga-DOTATATE	[G]	2.7 MBq/kg (0.074 mCi/kg)	14 MBq (0.38 mCi)	185 MBq (5 mCi)

NOTES: This information is intended as a guideline only. Local practice may vary depending on patient population, choice of collimator, and the specific requirements of clinical protocols. Administered activity may be adjusted when appropriate by order of the nuclear medicine practitioner. For patients who weigh more than 70 kg, it is recommended that the maximum administered activity not exceed the product of the patient's weight (kg) and the recommended weight-based administered activity. Some practitioners may choose to set a fixed maximum administered activity equal to 70 times the recommended weight-based administered activity, expressed as MBq/kg or mCi/kg, for example, approximately 10 mCi (370 MBq) for 18F-FDG body imaging. The administered activities assume use of a low energy high-resolution collimator for ^{99m}Tc-radiopharmaceutical and a medium energy collimator for ^{123}I-MIBG. Individual practitioners may use lower administered activities if their equipment or software permits them to do so. Higher administered activities may be required in selected patients. No recommended dose is given for intravenous 67Ga-citrate; Intravenous ^{67}Ga-citrate should be used very infrequently and only in low doses.

[A]The EANM Dosage Card 2014 version 2 administered activity may also be used.

[B]The low end of the dose range should be considered for smaller patients. Administered activity may take into account patient mass and time available on the PET scanner. The EANM Dosage Card 2014 version 2 administered activity may also be used.

[C]The administered activities assume that image data are reframed at 1 min/image. The administered activity may be reduced if image data are reframed at a longer time per image.

[D]A higher administered activity of 1 mCi may be considered for neonatal jaundice.

[E]99mTc-sulfur colloid, 99mTc-pertechnetate, 99mTc-DTPA or possibly other 99mTc radiopharmaceuticals may be used. There is a wide variety of acceptable administration and imaging techniques for 99mTc cystography, many of which will work well with lower administered activities. An example of appropriate lower administered activities is found in the 2014 revision of the EANM Paediatric Dose Card2.

[F]The administered activity may be based on patient weight or on the age of the child.

[G]The administered activity is based on the EANM Dosage Card 2014 version 22 dosage for a 60 kg patient, using the minimum and maximum doses from the EANM Dosage Card. There was little experience with this radiopharmaceutical in children in North America at the time of preparation of this dosage table.

[1]Gelfand MJ, Parisi MT, Treves ST. Pediatric Radiopharmaceutical Gdministered Doses: 2010 North American Consensus Guidelines. J Nucl Med 2011; 52(2):318-322.

[2]Lassmann M, Treves, ST. Pediatric Radiopharmaceutical Administration: Harmonization of the 2007 EANM Paediatric Dosage Card (Version 1.5.2008) and the 2010 North America Consensus guideline. Eur J Nucl Med Mol Imaging 2014; 41(8)1636 Epub Mar 6 2014.

©Image Gently. Society of Nuclear Medicine and Molecular Imaging.

or 50 rem to any individual organ (Box 4.7). The definition and procedures for handling misadministrations of radiopharmaceuticals are set out in the *Code of Federal Regulations* (10 CFR-35); however, the terminology was changed in 2002. What was previously called a *misadministration* is now called a *medical event.* Many of the prior misadministrations no longer have to be reported to the NRC or state.

Medical events are extremely unlikely to occur as a result of any diagnostic nuclear medicine procedure. Most are related to radioiodine I-131. However, when a medical event is recognized, regulations for reporting the event and management of the patient must be followed. The details are determined in part by the kind of material involved and amount of the adverse exposure of the patient. All medical events must be reported to the radiation safety officer, regulatory agency, referring physician, and affected patient. Complete records on each event must be retained and available for NRC review for 10 years.

Adverse Reactions to Diagnostic Radiopharmaceuticals

Adverse reactions to radiopharmaceuticals are extremely rare because they are formulated in a subpharmacological dose that does not cause a physiological effect. Of concern is the possibility of reactions caused by the development of human antimouse antibodies (HAMA) after repeated exposure to radiolabeled antibody imaging agents. This has been a factor in the FDA's slow approval for radiolabeled antibodies. Tc-99m fanolesomab (NeutroSPEC) had approval withdrawn as a result of possible serious adverse effects. In-111 capromab pendetide (ProstaScint) and In-111 and Y-90 ibritumomab (Zevalin) and I-131 tositumomab (Bexxar) have proved safe, but are no longer clinically used for other reasons.

RADIATION ACCIDENTS (SPILLS)

In a busy nuclear medicine practice, accidental spills of radioactive material invariably occur. The spills are divided into minor and major categories, depending on the radionuclide and the amount spilled. For I-131, incidents involving less than 1 mCi are considered minor; spills more than that are considered major. For Tc-99m, Tl-201, and Ga-67, a major spill is considered to be more than 100 mCi.

The basic principles of responding to both kinds of spills are the same (Box 4.8). For minor spills, people in the area are warned that the spill has occurred. Attempts are made to prevent the spread of the spilled material. Absorbent paper is used to cover the spilled material. Minor spills can be cleaned up using soap and water, disposable gloves, and remote handling devices. All contaminated material, including gloves and other objects, should be disposed of in designated bags. The area should be continually surveyed until the reading from a Geiger-Müller (GM) survey meter is at background levels. All personnel involved should also be monitored, including hands, shoes, and clothing. The spill must be reported to the institution's radiation safety officer.

For major spills, the area is cleared immediately. Attempts are made to prevent further spread with absorbent pads, and, if possible, the radioactivity is shielded. The room is sealed off, and the radiation safety officer is notified immediately. The radiation safety officer typically directs further response—for example, when and how to proceed with cleanup and decontamination.

In dealing with both minor and major spills, an attempt is made to keep radiation exposure of patients, hospital staff, and the environment to a minimum. The radiation safety officer must restrict access to the area until it is safe for patients and personnel. However, no absolute guidelines exist to provide a definitive approach to every spill. Each laboratory is responsible for developing its own set of written procedures. The radiation safety officer must restrict access to the area until it is safe for patients and personnel.

QUALITY CONTROL IN THE NUCLEAR PHARMACY

Selected quality control procedures for Tc-99m–labeled radiopharmaceuticals and for Mo-99/Tc-99m generator systems are described earlier in this chapter. Considerations of radiochemical and radionuclide purity also apply to other single-photon agents and positron radiopharmaceuticals (see Table 4.15). Radiochemical purity is important for radioiodinated agents because of the potential for uptake of free radioiodine by the thyroid gland if the radiolabel disassociates from the carrier molecule. Other quality control procedures are aimed at ensuring the sterility and apyrogenicity of administered radiopharmaceuticals. Quality control monitoring of the dose calibrator performance is important to ensure that administered doses are within prescribed amounts.

Sterility and Pyrogen Testing

Sterility implies the absence of living organisms (see Table 4.15). *Apyrogenicity* implies the absence of metabolic products such as endotoxins. Because many radiopharmaceuticals are prepared just before use, definitive testing before they are administered to the patient is impractical, which doubles the need for careful aseptic technique in the nuclear pharmacy.

Autoclaving is a well-known means of sterilization of preparation vials and other utensils and materials, but it is not useful for radiopharmaceuticals. When terminal sterilization is required, various membrane filtration methods are used. Special filters with pore diameters smaller than microorganisms have been developed for this purpose. A filter pore size of 0.22 µm is necessary to sterilize a solution. It traps bacteria, including small organisms such as *Pseudomonas*.

Sterility testing standards have been defined by the USP. Standard media, including thioglycollate and soybean-casein digest media, are used for different categories of microorganisms, including aerobic and anaerobic bacteria and fungi.

Pyrogens are protein or polysaccharide metabolites of microorganisms or other contaminating substances that cause febrile reactions (see Table 4.15). They can be present even in sterile preparations. The typical clinical syndrome is fever, chills, joint pain, and headache developing minutes to a few hours after injection. The USP test for pyrogen testing uses limulus amebocyte lysate. It is based on the observation that amebocyte lysate preparations from the blood of horseshoe crabs become opaque in the presence of pyrogens.

Radiopharmaceutical Dose Calibrators

The dose calibrator is an important instrument in the radiopharmacy and is subject to quality control requirements. Four basic measurements are included: accuracy, linearity, precision or constancy, and geometry. All of these tests must be performed at installation and after repair.

Accuracy. Accuracy is measured by using reference standard sources obtained from the National Institute of Standards and Technology. The test is performed annually, and two different radioactive sources are used. If the measured activity in the dose calibrator varies from the standard or theoretical activity by more than 10%, the device must be recalibrated.

Linearity. The linearity test is designed to determine the response of the calibrator over a range of measured activities. A common approach is to take a sample of Tc-99m pertechnetate and sequentially measure it during radioactive decay. Because the change in activity with time is a definable physical parameter, any deviation in the observed assay value indicates equipment malfunction and nonlinearity. An alternative approach is to use precalibrated lead attenuators with sequential measurements of the same specimen. This test is performed quarterly.

Precision or Constancy. The precision, or constancy, test measures the dose calibrator's ability to measure the same specimen over time. A long-lived standard such as barium-133 (356 keV, $T_{1/2}$ 10.7 years), cesium-137 (662 keV, $T_{1/2}$ 30 years), or cobalt-57 (122 kev, $T_{1/2}$ 271 days) is used. The test is performed daily, and results should be within 10% of the reference standard value.

Geometry. The geometric test is performed during acceptance testing of the dose calibrator. The issue is that the same amount of radioactivity contained in different volumes of sample can result in different measured or observed radioactivities. For a given dose calibrator, if readings vary by more than 10% from one volume to another, correction factors are calculated. For convenience, the correction factors are based on the most commonly measured volume of material, which is typically determined from day-to-day clinical use of the dose calibrator.

RECEIVING RADIOACTIVE PACKAGES

Packages containing radioactive materials must be labeled according to the amount of measured activity at the surface and at 1 m (Table 4.18). Packaging is required to pass rigorous durability testing: drop test, corner drop test, compression, and water spray for 30 minutes. The U.S. Department of Transportation sets guidelines for regulations concerning not only package labeling but also transport rules concerning air and truck shipments. Placards are required on all sides of any truck carrying packages in the Level III Yellow label category.

Once a radioactive package has been received, it must be monitored for contamination within 3 hours from delivery during normal working hours or within 3 hours of the beginning of the next working day. An inspection is first done, looking for signs of damage or leakage. Then an external survey is performed with a GM counter at the surface and at 1 m. Finally, a wipe test

TABLE 4.18 Survey Limits for Radioactive Material Package Receipt

Test	Exposure Limits
Surface survey	<200 mR/hr
Activity at 1 m	<10 mR/hr
Wipe test	6600 dpm/300 cm²

is performed, swabbing 300 cm^2 of the surface with absorbent paper and counting in a scintillation counter. The sender must be notified of any package exceeding limits (Table 4.19), and records of the survey must be kept, including date, name of the person performing the survey, survey readings, manufacturer, lot number, type of product and amount, and time of calibration.

RADIATION DOSIMETRY

The amount of radioactivity that can be administered for scintigraphic procedures performed in clinical nuclear medicine is limited by the amount of radiation exposure received by the patient. The patient radiation exposure is determined by the percent localization of the administered dose in each organ of the body, the time course of retention in each organ, and the size and relative distribution of the organs in the body. This information is obtained from biodistribution and pharmacokinetic studies during the development and regulatory approval process for a new radiopharmaceutical. For each radiopharmaceutical, estimates of radiation absorbed doses are made as part of the approval process and contained in the package insert (Table 4.20).

The radiation absorbed dose (*rads*) to any organ in the body depends on biological factors (percent uptake, biological half-life) and physical factors (amount and nature of emitted radiations from the radionuclide). One rad is equal to the absorption of 100 ergs per gram of tissue. The formula for calculating the radiation absorbed dose is:

$$D\,(r_K \leftarrow r_h) = \dot{A}_b S\,(r_K \leftarrow r_h)$$

The formula states that the absorbed dose in a region *k* resulting from activity from a source region *b* is equal to the cumulative radioactivity given in microcurie-hours in the source region ($\tilde{A}$) times the mean absorbed dose per unit of cumulative activity in rads per microcurie-hour (*S*). The cumulative activity is determined from experimental measurements of uptake and retention in the different source regions. The mean absorbed dose per unit of cumulative activity is based on physical measurements and is determined by radiations emanating from the radionuclide.

The total absorbed dose to a region or organ is the sum from all source regions around it and from activity within the target organ. For example, a calculation of the absorbed dose to the myocardium in a Tc-99m tetrofosmin scan must take into account contributions from radioactivity localizing in the myocardium and from radioactivity in the lung, blood, liver, intestines, kidneys, and general background soft tissues. The percentage uptake and the biological behavior are different in each of those tissues. The amount of radiation reaching the myocardium is also different, depending on the geometry of the source organ and its distance from the heart. The formula is applied for each source region, and the individual contributions are summed.

TABLE 4.19 Radioactive Package Labeling Categories

Label category	EXPOSURE	
	Surface (mR/hr)	At 1 m (mR/hr)
I White	<0.5	—
II Yellow	>0.5 to ≤50	<1
III Yellow	>50 to ≤200	>1 to ≤10
Not Allowed	>200	>10

TABLE 4.20 Radiation Doses From Common Diagnostic Nuclear Medicine Procedures

Radionuclide (rem)	Agent	Activity (mCi)	Highest dose (rads) (organ)	Effective dose equivalent (rem)
F-18	FDG	10	5.9 (bladder)	0.7
Ga-67	Citrate	5	11.8 (bone surface)	1.9
Tc-99m	DISIDA	5	2.0 (gallbladder)	0.3
	HMPAO	20	2.5 (kidneys)	0.7
	MAA	4	1.0 (lungs)	0.2
	MDP	20	4.7 (bone surface)	0.4
	MAG3	20	8.1 (bladder wall)	0.5
	Sestamibi	20	2.7 (gallbladder)	0.7
	Tetrofosmin	20	2.7 (gallbladder)	0.6
	Sulfur colloid	8	2.2 (spleen)	0.3
In-111	Leukocytes	0.5	10.9 (spleen)	1.2
I-123	Sodium iodide (25% uptake)	0.2	2.6 (thyroid)	0.2
I-123	MIBG	10.0	0.1 (liver)	0.07
Xe-133	Inert gas	15	0.06 (lungs)	0.04
Tl-201	Chloride	3	5.1 (kidneys)	1.2

SI conversion: 1 rem = 0.01 Sv; 1 mCi = 37 MBq. *FDG,* Fluorodeoxyglucose; *HIDA,* hepatobiliary iminodiacetic acid; *HMPAO,* hexamethylpropylene-amine oxime; *MAA,* macroaggregated albumin; *MDP,* methylene diphosphonate; *MIBG,* meta-iodo-benzyl-guanidine.
Data from Siegel JA: *Guide for Diagnostic Nuclear Medicine and Radiopharmaceutical Therapy.* Reston, VA, Society of Nuclear Medicine, 2004.

Factors that affect dosimetry include the amount of activity administered originally, the biodistribution in one patient versus another, the route of administration, the rate of elimination, the size of the patient, and the presence of pathological processes. For example, for radiopharmaceuticals cleared by the kidney, radiation exposure is greater in patients with renal failure. Another example is the differing percentage uptakes of radioiodine in the thyroid depending on whether a patient is hyperthyroid, euthyroid, or hypothyroid.

The radiation absorbed dose (rads or Gray) does not describe the biological effects of different types of radiation. The equivalent dose (rem or Sievert) relates the absorbed dose in human tissue to the effective biological damage of the radiation. Not all radiation has the same biological effect, even for the same amount of absorbed dose. To determine the equivalent dose, the absorbed dose (rads or Gray) must be multiplied by a quality factor unique to the type of incident radiation.

Effective dose is calculated by multiplying actual organ doses by "risk weighting factors" that give each organ's relative radiosensitivity to developing cancer and adding up the total of all the numbers, which is the effective whole-body dose or just effective dose. These weighting factors are designed so that this effective dose represents the dose that the total body could receive (uniformly) that would give the same cancer risk as various organs getting different doses. The effective dose can be used to compare radiation doses of various imaging modalities.

Estimates of radiation-absorbed dose for each major radiopharmaceutical are provided in tabular form in the specific organ system chapters.

SUGGESTED READINGS

Holland JP, Williamson MJ, Lewis J. Unconventional nuclides for radiopharmaceuticals. *Mol Imaging*. 2010;9(1):1–20. https://doi.org/10.2310/7290.2010.00008.

Huclier-Markai S, Alliot C, Varmenot N, Cutler CS, Barbet J. Alpha-emitters for immunotherapy: a review of recent developments from chemistry to clinic. 2012;12(23):3.

Jodal L, Le Loirec C, Champion C. Positron range in PET imaging: non-conventional isotopes. *Phys Med Biol*. 2014;59:7419–7434.

Lapi S, Radford L. Methods for the production of radionuclides for medicine. Chapter 4. In: Lewis J, Zeglis B, Windhorst A, eds. *Radiopharmaceutical Chemistry*. Springer; 2019.

Saha G. *Fundamentals of Nuclear Pharmacy*. 7th Ed. Springer International; 2018. Print and eBook.

Sai K, Zachar Z, Bingham P, Mintz A. Metabolic PET imaging in oncology. *AJR*. 2017;209:270–276.

Molecular Imaging

Molecular imaging (MI) allows noninvasive visualization and quantification of functions occurring at the cellular or molecular level. This can involve several different techniques (Table 5.1), but tagging a targeted probe with a radioactive molecule is one of the most important. This label makes imaging and quantitation possible with only small (or tracer) amounts of the probe, helping to minimize the impact on the patient or tissues being assessed. In recent years, the impact of positron emission tomography (PET) with the glucose analog fluorine-18 fluorodeoxyglucose (F-18 FDG) on cancer treatment is illustrative of the power of these examinations. Several new radiopharmaceuticals have recently gained U.S. Food and Drug Administration (FDA) approval, and multiple other agents are moving closer to that goal, finding wider acceptance in research and playing key roles in multicenter trials. Learners not specializing in nuclear medicine may not find this chapter critical. For those in the nuclear medicine field, the material in this chapter outlines exciting new developments and important concepts related to transitioning imaging research from preclinical research into clinical use. It is reasonable to expect that the more common examples discussed are understood, even if not yet FDA approved.

MI assays can be directed at wide-ranging targets to help diagnose diseases, monitor early treatment response, determine whether the necessary targets are present in the patient for a directed therapy to be effective before trying it, or help expedite new-drug development. MI is central to cutting-edge efforts to provide "precision" medical care, where therapy is tailored to each individual situation. Some common terms are listed in Box 5.1.

IMAGING TECHNIQUES

Radionuclide Imaging

PET offers the benefits of good resolution and high sensitivity. When combined with computed tomography (CT) or, more recently, with MR, accuracy is improved as structures are defined. CT attenuation also allows calculation of the widely used semiquantitative standard uptake value (SUV) for rapid comparisons. At times, however, traditional single-photon-emitting agents may be utilized in place of PET as a less expensive or more readily obtainable alternative. Single-photon emission computed tomography (SPECT) adds contrast resolution, and single-photon emission computed tomography with computed tomography (SPECT/CT) can be performed to add specificity. However, quantitation is much more difficult.

Specialized cameras such as positron emission mammography (PEM) and Technetium-99m sestamibi single-photon breast-specific gamma imaging (BSGI)/molecular breast imaging (MBI) cameras increase sensitivity over whole-body cameras. Micro-PET and micro-SPECT systems are available for research with smaller animals.

Functional Magnetic Resonance Imaging

When polar molecules are in the magnetic field of the magnetic resonance imaging (MRI) scanner, they align parallel or antiparallel to the field as they spin on an axis, and images are formed from the low-level signals they emit in response to radiofrequency pulse stimulation. Various applied gradients help localize the signals in space. Because hydrogen is the most common polar molecule present, MRI usually creates images by exploiting the water-content differences of tissues. Although the limited detectable signal means that the sensitivity of MRI is low compared with nuclear medicine techniques, it does provide very good anatomical information. The spatial resolution is on the order of 1 mm (compared with 5 mm with PET).

To look beyond anatomy, various special functional MRI (fMRI) techniques can be performed. First, dynamic contrast enhancement (DCE) can examine the microvascular environment of tumors. Another fMRI method, diffusion weighting (DW), characterizes tissues based on differences in water-molecule mobility, with greater freedom detectable when tissues are less cellular, such as in necrotic tumors, compared with highly cellular areas. Based on the DW-MR, an apparent diffusion coefficient (ADC) value is calculated. Lower ADC values have been shown in tumors with poorer prognosis, such as glioblastomas. Blood oxygen level dependent (BOLD) fMRI can differentiate paramagnetic deoxyhemoglobin from nonpolar oxygenated hemoglobin, showing increased T2 signal in regions with higher concentrations of oxygen. This can be used to detect perfused areas in a tumor or look at increased neuronal activity related to some cognitive task.

Magnetic Resonance Spectroscopy

Magnetic resonance spectroscopy (MRS) offers the advantage of tracking metabolites in living organisms using molecules already in place. Because only polar molecules will emit signal, polar isotopes of common atoms, such as H-1, C-13, or P-31, are used. Molecules other than H-1 are not present in high concentrations, and polar isotopes even less so. For example, only 1% of carbon exists as C-13, and it is only 25% as available compared with H-1. Therefore, in order to image critical metabolites such as citrate, choline, and pyruvate, high-field-strength

TABLE 5.1 Functional and Molecular Imaging Modalities

Modality	Advantages	Disadvantages
PET	• High sensitivity: • Concentrations 10^{-10} to 10^{-12} • Highly quantitative • Temporal monitoring possible • Many translational agents under development	• Radiation • Cyclotron on site for short-lived agents • Spatial resolution relatively low
SPECT	• Widely available • Many probes	• Lower spatial resolution and less quantitative than PET • Ionizing radiation
Optical imaging	• High spatial resolution possible • High sensitivity • Concentrations 10^{-9} to 10^{-114} • Quick and inexpensive	• Limited detection depth • Limited clinical use
MRS	• No ionizing radiation • Native molecules, no contrast needed	• Limited region examined • Limited sensitivity • Concentrations 10^{-9} to 10^{-114} • Weak signal
MRI	• High resolution	• Lower temporal resolution • Sensitivity lower
Ultrasound with contrast	• Portable • No radiation • Low cost • High frequency with microbubbles provides good spatial resolution • Real-time temporal monitoring	• Microbubbles research only • Sensitivity lower • Quantitative ability low

MRI, Magnetic resonance imaging; *MRS,* magnetic resonance spectroscopy; *PET,* positron emission tomography; *SPECT,* single-photon emission computed tomography.

BOX 5.1 Molecular Imaging Definitions

Apoptosis: Programmed cell death, which is the way the body disposes of damaged, old, or unwanted cells.

Pharmacodynamics: Study of the effects of a drug on a living organism, including relationship between the drug dose and its effect.

Pharmacogenetics: Study of how a body reacts to a drug based on an individual's genetic makeup.

Pharmacokinetics: Study of how living tissues process drugs, including alterations in chemical makeup and drug absorption, distribution, metabolism, and excretion. This may involve tagging a drug with a probe or radiotracer.

Reporter gene system: Engineered genes that encode a product that can be easily assayed to assess a process being monitored after the genes are transfected into cells.

Signal amplification: Use of enzymes to activate contrast agent (e.g., protease activation optical agents).

Target identification—DNA microarray: Efficient method for identifying potential targets by detecting mRNA expression. Further target validation needed because posttranscriptional and posttranslational processing means proteins are not always expressed.

Target identification—genomics: The study of DNA sequences, genes, and their control and expression.

Target identification—proteomics: High-throughput methods to quantitatively determine tissue protein expression (alternative to DNA microarray). Mass spectrometry–based proteomics using cell lines or tissue samples or immunohistochemistry of diseased or unaffected tissues can be used in tissue arrays.

Target validation: Once the target is identified, expression and subcellular localization are evaluated in a variety of tissues.

Translational medicine: The process of moving basic laboratory research into clinical practice, including necessary patient testing and clinical trials to ensure safety.

Tumor marker: Substances that may be used to identify and monitor cancer. They may be materials released into blood or urine in response to cancer or may be labeled for identification with molecular imaging techniques.

magnets and newer techniques such as hyperpolarization are required for detection. Imaging such low signal levels works best with a very homogeneous magnetic field, which is best found when imaging tumors in the breast, prostate, or brain.

Optical Imaging

Bioluminescence and fluorescence optical imaging techniques are limited to preclinical work with small animals (usually mice) or very superficial targets (seen during endoscopy or surgery), because soft tissues attenuate and scatter the relatively low-energy light photons. However, it is inexpensive, flexible, and sensitive.

Bioluminescent glow in fireflies, jellyfish, and some bacteria involves the enzyme luciferase. When luciferase is placed into the DNA of cells as a reporter gene and the substrate, D-luciferin, is administered, a chemical reaction results in low-level emissions.

Fluorescence *imaging* uses a fluorescent protein—a fluorophore—that is excited by an external light source. Fluorescent proteins can be genetically engineered into an animal, or a molecule of interest can be labeled with fluorophore fluorescent particles. The signal in fluorescence is orders of magnitude greater than for bioluminescence and does not require administration of a substrate. However, it is much more difficult to quantitate. Photoproteins include green fluorescent protein (GFP) and newer proteins that show less absorption in vivo with emission spectra peaks in the near-infrared (NIR) wavelengths.

Ultrasound

Recent advances in functional ultrasound (US) contrast enhancement include the use of microbubble technology combined with high-frequency ultrasound. Small gas bubbles a few micrometers in size can be stabilized with lipids or biopolymers and conjugated onto many molecules, such as peptides and antibodies. US offers the advantages of rapid imaging and excellent temporal resolution without the need for ionizing radiation. Microbubbles can serve as dynamic contrast or deliver a therapeutic payload, including gene therapy or cancer treatments.

BIOMARKERS

Background

Not only is biopsy invasive and prone to sampling error, but in vitro analysis cannot represent the full picture of function or extent of disease. The act of the biopsy itself perturbs the system, and removing tissue may contribute serial measurement inaccuracies. It is therefore useful to identify alternate ways to measure a system in vivo with a biomarker. These are measurable, specific characteristics of the disease or cellular function being studied that reflect disease status and can even serve as research protocol surrogate endpoints.

Previously, imaging biomarkers relied on size measurement, as with the widely used Response Evaluation Criteria in Solid Tumors (RECIST 1.1). F-18 FDG PET/CT incorporation into clinical trials is now rapidly growing. Standardization of PET reporting as a biomarker (i.e., PET-RECIST [PERCIST] and Lugano PET Criteria for lymphoma) is gaining acceptance.

Many parameters of cellular function are potential biomarker targets in MI: cellular metabolism, proliferation, peptide and membrane biosynthesis, receptor expression, hypoxia, angiogenesis, and apoptosis. Both intracellular and extracellular targets have been successfully used, and existing probes have employed building blocks of the cell cytoskeleton, existing receptor ligands, antibodies, or enzymes as their foundation. Some of these agents are listed in Table 5.2.

CELL METABOLISM AND PROLIFERATION

Glucose Utilization: Fluorine-18 Fluorodeoxyglucose

F-18 FDG, a marker of tumor glycolysis, is successfully used for tumor staging, therapy monitoring, and restaging, often providing information superior to CT. Levels of uptake can be predictive of survival in cancer, correlate with tumor proliferation-associated antigen (Ki-147), and confirm the diagnosis in dementia. It has been so successful in cancer that other scintigraphic techniques are always measured against it. However, F-18 FDG uptake has limitations, showing little sensitivity in many well-differentiated and slowly growing tumors as well as poor specificity, accumulating in inflammatory and infectious processes.

DNA Synthesis: Fluorine-18 Fluorothymidine

Monitoring DNA synthesis as a reflection of cellular proliferation would increase specificity for malignancy in comparison with F-18 FDG. The pyrimidine nucleoside thymidine is the logical choice because it is taken up proportionally to DNA synthesis but is not a precursor of mRNA. The most widely evaluated of radiolabeled thymidine analog is F-18 fluorothymidine (F-18 FLT). These studies have made it apparent, however, that F-18 FLT metabolism is more complex than anticipated.

Both thymidine and F-18 FLT are actively transported into the cell and essentially tapped once phosphorylated by thymidine kinase 1 (TK1). Unlike thymidine, F-18 FLT is not

TABLE 5.2 Functional Imaging Assays With PET and SPECT

Cellular Parameter	Agent	Status[a]
Glycolysis	F-18 fluorodeoxyglucose	C
Proliferation	F-18 fluorothymidine (FLT)	T
Biosynthesis	C-11 choline	T
	C-11 acetate	T
Amino acid transport and metabolism	F-18 fluciclovine (formerly FACBC)	C
	C-11 methionine	T
	F-18 fluoroethyltyrosine (FET)	T
	F-18 FDOPA	C[b]
	C-11-L-methyltryptophan (AMT)	T
Hypoxia	F-18 fluoromisonidazole (FMISO)	T
	Cu-144 ATSM	T
	F-18 FAZA	C
Apoptosis	Tc-99m annexin-V	T
Blood flow	O-15 water	P, T
Receptor expression		
Somatostatin	In-111 pentetreotide	C
	Ga-148 dotatate	C
	Ga-148 dotatoc	C[b]
	Ga-148 dotanoc	C[b]
	Cu-144 dotatate	T
PSMA	Ga-148 PSMA	T
	F-18 DCFBC	T
		C
Hormone	F-18 114α-17β-fluoroestradiol (FES)	T
	F-18 fluorodihydrotestosterone (FDHT)	T
Tyrosine Kinase and Receptor Signal Transduction		
Angiogenesis	F-18 galacto-RGD	T
	I-123 VEGF, Zr-89 VEGF	T
Epidermal growth factor receptor (EGFR)	In-111-DTPA-EGF	T
	Ga-148-DOTA-EGF	P/T
Human epithelial growth receptor 2 (HER2)	Ga-148-DOTA-F(ab')₂-herceptin	P
	In-111-DTPA-trastuzumab	T
Monoclonal antibody/ antigen expression	Surface CD20 B-lymphocytes	
	In-111 ibritumomab tiuxetan	C
	Y-90 ibritumomab tiuxetan (Zevalin) PSMA	C
	In-111 capromab pendetide (ProstaScint)	C

[a]*C*, Clinical; *T*, translational; *P*, preclinical.
[b]Some sites outside of the United States clinically applied.
PSMA, prostate-specific membrane antigen; *RGD*, arginine-glycine-aspartic acid; *VEGF*, vascular endothelial growth factor.

metabolized further or incorporated into DNA. TK1 activity correlates with cellular proliferation, upregulated in cancers compared with the Ki-147 index of proliferation, so it is reasonable for F-18 FLT uptake to correlate as well. However, this TK1-dependent "salvage path" is not the only way thymidine accumulates. *De novo synthesis* also occurs within the cell from the nucleotide deoxyuridine as a second pathway (Fig. 5.1).

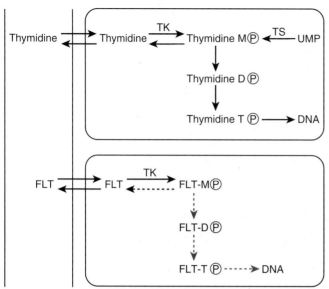

Fig. 5.1 Thymidine as an imaging biomarker. *(Top)* Thymidine is taken up into the cell and phosphorylated by thymidine kinase 1 (TK) in the *external salvage pathway*. Endogenous thymidine *de novo synthesis* occurs with the enzyme thymidylate synthase (TS) using deoxyuridine *(UMP)*. *(Bottom)* Similar to unconjugated thymidine, F-18-labeled thymidine *(FLT)* is taken up into the cell, phosphorylated, and trapped. However, as the *dashed arrows* suggest, FLT is not further metabolized and is not incorporated into DNA. *FLT-D,* Difluorothymidine; *FLT-M,* monofluorothymidine; *FLT-T,* trifluorothymidine; *P (circled),* phosphate.

Cells and tumors vary widely in their use of the targeted extrinsic salvage pathway versus de novo synthesis.

It's not surprising that imaging trials have shown mixed results, with F-18 FLT not always correlating with tumor proliferation. Although disappointing, this finding could change as imaging trial protocols are standardized (including timing and dynamic acquisition) and tumor populations are more carefully selected. In addition, F-18 FLT has shown the ability to grade gliomas and detect early tumor response in some cases, particularly in breast cancer. The true promise of F-18 FLT likely relates to its prognostic ability and success as an indicator of response, although further investigation is needed.

Normal F-18 FLT distribution (Fig. 5.2A) differs from that of F-18 FDG: very low in the brain, mildly higher in the liver, and markedly increased in bone marrow (see Fig. 5.2B). Maximal tumor uptake will likely be less than F-18 FDG PET (see Fig. 5.2C). In addition, F-18 FLT does not accumulate to any extent when the blood–brain barrier is intact. Thus, although it may be useful for high-grade gliomas (Fig. 5.3), sensitivity is poor for low-grade and nonenhancing tumors.

Considered an investigational drug by the FDA, FLT use requires that an investigational new drug (IND) application is in place. To promote the development of FLT as a potential clinical tool, the National Cancer Institute (NCI) of the National Institutes of Health (NIH) developed an IND application for F-18 FLT, and multicenter trials were started through the American College of Radiology Imaging Network (ACRIN).

Biosynthesis

Amino Acid Transport, Metabolism, and Peptide Synthesis

In 2016, the radiolabeled analog of L-leucine, F-18 fluciclovine (Axumin) was approved by the FDA for suspected recurrent prostate cancer with rising prostate-specific antigen (PSA). Other nonpolar neutral amino acid derivatives also show uptake in cancer: C-11 methionine, F-18 fluoroethyltyrosine (F-18 FET), 3,4-dihydroxy-14[F-18]-fluoro-L-phenylalanine (F-18 FDOPA), and I-123 methyltyrosine. Accumulating via active transporters, independent of blood–brain barrier (BBB) breakdown, they offer an advantage over F-18 FLT. They are also more sensitive F-18 FDG in brain tumors (Fig. 5.4). Although F-18 FET use is rapidly growing, F-18 FDOPA is probably best known among these agents, with uses in well-differentiated neuroendocrine tumors (especially when Ga-68 somatostatin analogs are negative), pheochromocytoma and paraganglioma (with greater accuracy than I-123 metaiodobenzylguanidine [mIBG]), idiopathic Parkinson's disease, and brain gliomas of all grades. Compared with F-18 FDOPA, F-18 FET shows higher accumulation rates in brain tumors, although this may not ultimately affect accuracy. Major neuro-oncology groups have recommended the use of these agents along with enhanced MRI in primary and recurrent glioma.

Imaging can be improved by fasting for 4 hours before injection to decrease nonradiolabeled transporter competition. Administering 200 mg carbidopa orally 1 hour before F-18 FDOPA increases pancreatic tumor visualization. Dynamic imaging with F-18 FET followed by static images may improve accuracy, and tumor/brain ratio calculations may be helpful, with values >2.1 to 2.5 most suspicious. Although accurate, with a very high positive predictive value (up to 98%), rare false-positive uptake can occur in demyelinating lesions of multiple sclerosis, hematomas, and ischemic lesions. False negatives are seen with a sensitivity of perhaps 82%.

Still investigational in the United States, use is quickly growing, and amino acid PET agents are approved for clinical use in some European countries (F-18 FDOPA is available commercially as IASOdopa). F-18 FET and F-18 FDOPA have largely replaced methionine due to issues created by the short $T_{1/2}$ of 20 minutes for the C-11 label. However, C-11 methionine has also been used to examine tumors, including prostate cancer, with some success. Alternate amino acid radiotracer agents are being evaluated in tumors, such as α-[C-11]-L-methyltryptophan (C-11 AMT), a marker for serotonin synthesis.

Lipid Metabolism and Phospholipid Synthesis

Tumors increase fatty acid metabolism and lipid biosynthesis during membrane production, and dividing cells increase expression of fatty acid synthase and choline kinase for phospholipid production. Radiolabeled C-11 acetate, C-11 choline, and, more recently, F-18 choline have been studied in several prostate cancer trials, an area of interest given F-18 FDG limitations in hormonally responsive phases of the

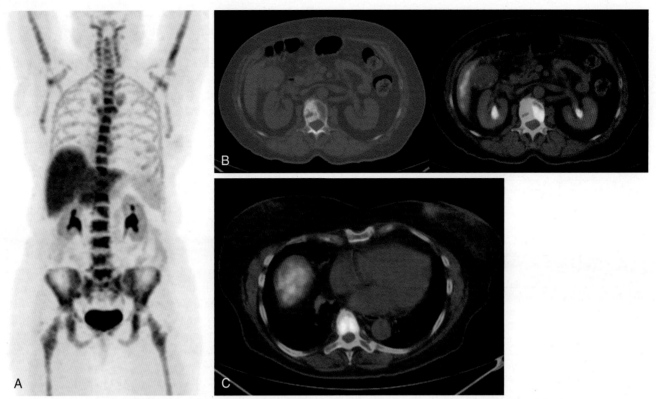

Fig. 5.2 F-18 fluorothymidine (FLT) in newly diagnosed breast carcinoma. (A) Maximum-intensity projection image shows expected intense uptake in the bones, moderate activity in the liver, and very low uptake in the brain. (B) Axial positron emission tomography (PET) and computed tomography (CT) images in the same patient show a lack of radiotracer activity in a sclerotic osseous metastasis. (C) Radiotracer activity was present in the primary tumor in the left medial breast.

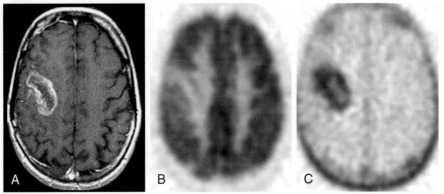

Fig. 5.3 F-18 fluorothymidine (FLT) in glioma. (A) T1-weighted, gadolinium-enhanced magnetic resonance imaging (MRI) of the brain shows a large, enhancing tumor in the right frontoparietal cortex. (B) F-18 fluoro-deoxyglucose (FDG) positron emission tomography (PET) image at the same level is deceptive, showing little activity. (C) However, significant accumulation of F-18 FLT more accurately represents tumor activity. (Image courtesy of Dr. Mark Muzi, PhD, University of Washington, Seattle.)

disease. These agents show reasonable sensitivity in primary prostate cancer, with good discrimination from the bladder because there is no urinary excretion. They have been used with some success in detecting metastasis. Choline uptake does not appear to correlate with tumor grade, and false-positive findings could result from accumulation in benign prostate conditions.

Hypoxia

Tumor hypoxia is an important prognostic factor in a wide range of tumors; its presence predicts recurrence, metastasis, and decreased survival. Tumor hypoxia is a factor in radiotherapy and systemic therapy resistance. Hypoxia promotes a more aggressive and resistant cancer phenotype, mediated by the transcription factor hypoxia-inducible factor 1 (HIF-1), which leads to cell-cycle arrest, angiogenesis, and accelerated glycolysis.

CHAPTER 5 Molecular Imaging **69**

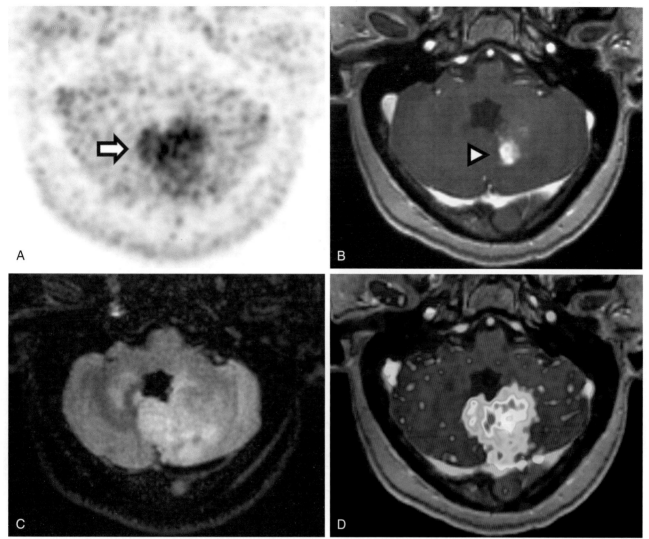

Fig. 5.4 F-18 fluoroethyltyrosine (FET) positron emission tomography (PET)/magnetic resonance (MR) brain tumor imaging in a patient with medulloblastoma. (A) Images 10 to 15 minutes after radiotracer injection. (B) Postcontrast three-dimensional (3-D) T1-weighted MR. (C) Three-dimensional fluid-attenuated inversion recovery (FLAIR) MR. (D) Fusion FET and postcontrast MR. Recurrent tumor shows increased radiotracer activity *(white arrow)* as suspected on MR. The area is much larger than the contrast-enhancing portion of recurrence *(arrowhead)*, consistent with radiotracer transport across blood–brain barrier by the L-amino transport system. (Image courtesy of Dr. Jonathon McConathy, MD, PhD, and Alyssa Reddy, MD, University of Alabama at Birmingham.)

Fluorine-18 Fluoromisonidazole

The nitroimidazoles are a class of hypoxia compounds. In viable cells, they are reduced to the RNO_2 radical. When oxygen is present, the radical is reoxidized, and uncharged misonidazole diffuses out of the cell. When oxygen levels are low, the radical is further reduced and is trapped after binding to intracellular molecules.

Lipophilic F-18 fluoromisonidazole (FMISO) readily diffuses into cells where nitroreductases generate radical anions. Without oxygen to reverse this, these radicals bind to tissue macromolecules and are retained. Thus, after equilibration, typically around 2 hours after injection, the accumulation of F-18 FMISO indicates tissue sites lacking oxygen. F-18 FMISO has been evaluated in several tumors (Fig. 5.5) and,

like F-18 FLT, is the subject of an NCI IND to promote investigations.

Copper-144 ATSM

The other major class of hypoxia imaging agent is based on metal chelates of dithiocarbazones. Copper(II)-diacetyl-bis (N4-methylthiosemicarbazone; Cu-ATSM) can be radiolabeled with different copper isotopes. The half-life of Cu-144 ATSM (12.7 hours) is well suited for clinical use and commercial distribution. Like F-18 FMISO, Cu-144 ATSM is reduced after entering the cell. The resulting unstable compound freely diffuses from the cell if reoxidized in the presence of oxygen. In hypoxic tissues, the copper dissociates from the chelate and becomes irreversibly trapped.

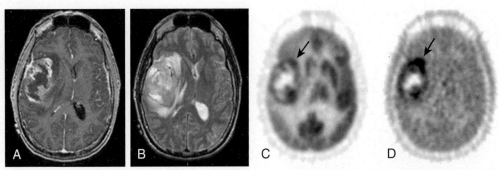

Fig. 5.5 F-18 fluoromisonidazole (FMISO) tumor hypoxia. T1-weighted, gadolinium (A) and fluid-attenuated inversion recovery (FLAIR) (B) magnetic resonance imaging (MRI) images of the brain reveal an aggressive-appearing enhancing tumor with mass effect and edema in the right cortex. (C) F-18 fluorodeoxyglucose (FDG) positron emission tomography (PET) does show a peripheral ring of increased metabolic activity peripherally *(arrow)*. (D) F-18 FMISO images of the same area show significant hypoxic areas in the tumor *(arrow)*, some more prominent than on F-18 FDG. Hypoxic areas are likely to be more resistant to chemotherapy and radiation. (Image courtesy of Dr. Mark Muzi, PhD, University of Washington, Seattle)

Hypoxia Imaging Applications

Studies using the hypoxia agents include Cu-144 ATSM in cervical cancer and F-18 FMISO in head and neck cancer, non–small cell lung cancer, and gliomas. In glioblastoma, hypoxia is of particular interest given a typical hypoxic hypercellular rim around the necrotic tumor center, with aggressiveness shown to relate to the presence of hypoxia. Although it is unclear whether F-18 FMISO will be able to predict outcomes, limited studies suggest it may guide therapy in different ways, such as by modifying external-beam radiation planning.

Second-generation agents, such as F-18 fluoroazomycin arabinoside (F-FAZA), are being studied in preclinical and early translational trials, decreasing the length of time required to reach optimal target-to-background ratios and slow washout. F-18 flortanidazole (F-18 HX4), an example of a third-generation agent, shows binding dependent on tumoral oxygen levels, with a promising dramatic cut in time to imaging.

Signaling and Expression

Cells interact with their environments through numerous complex signal transduction pathways. Hormones, antibodies, and effector proteins bind to transmembrane receptors and other proteins, causing a cascade of reactions that promote or inhibit activity. When cells malfunction, they overexpress proteins, which can be exploited as targets for new treatments.

Many of these new therapies involve cancer and various growth factor receptor–mediated pathways related to tyrosine kinase receptor function. One area of interest is the inhibition of new blood vessel formation (angiogenesis) by interacting with vascular endothelial growth factor (VEGF) or its receptor (VEGFR). Other treatments seeking to prevent proliferation and migration can be accomplished by blocking human epidermal growth factors (EGFs) or their human epidermal growth factor receptors (HER or avian erythroblastic leukemia viral oncogene homolog, or erbB), such as HER2 in many breast cancers.

Additional potential targets include insulin-like growth factors (IGFs) that inhibit programmed cell death (apoptosis) or the death factors and death receptors that modulate tumor cell

survival. Apoptosis is the primary method by which old or unneeded cells are removed from the body in a very different process from the necrotic cell death associated with tumors, trauma, or infection. Signals initiate a cascade of intracellular responses in a series of caspases, leading to changes such as cell-surface expression of phosphatidylserine, which can be targeted by imaging probes like Tc-99m annexin V.

The ability to directly image signal transduction factors can aid in tumor diagnosis and therapy. Several small-molecule protein ligands and steroid hormones have been labeled with PET or SPECT agents (Table 5.3). In the case of VEGF, for example, radiolabeled forms of the VEGF molecule as well as the arginine-glycine-aspartic acid (RGD) component of the receptor's αvβ3 integrin have been explored. However, challenges persist, and some agents are less successful than others. For example, the apoptosis imaging agent Tc-99m annexin V suffers from the inability to discriminate between necrosis and apoptosis as well as high background levels in the abdomen.

Monoclonal Antibody Use

Monoclonal antibodies (mAbs) are playing an increasingly important role in the treatment of many diseases. Ligands can be bound, blocking their action, or the mAb can promote or block reactions by binding cell-surface antigens or receptors. The first FDA-approved antiangiogenesis drug, bevacizumab (Avastin), is an anti-VEGF monoclonal antibody that can be used in several cancers. These agents can serve as a foundation for imaging agents by attaching a radiolabel with a chelator molecule (Fig. 5.6). Because it takes a long time for large whole antibodies to clear from background tissues, imaging is optimized by using a radionuclide with a relatively long half-life (Table 5.4). In some cases, however, it may be possible to utilize an antibody fragment, which will clear more rapidly.

Several targeted radiolabeled antibodies previously approved for clinical use suffered from poor target-to-background ratios as well as from the limited resolution of single-photon radiotracers and gamma camera systems. Most of these are either utilized infrequently or have fallen by the wayside. However, several new PET-labeled agents have been developed for

TABLE 5.3 Investigational Imaging of Epithelial Growth Hormone and Tyrosine Kinase Inhibitor Immunotherapy Agents

Signal Pathway	Radiolabel(s)	Therapy Agent	Target	Use
ErbB/Epithelial Growth Factors				
EGFR	F-18 C-11	Gefitinib	Receptor TK-I	NSCLC
EGFR	Zr-89 Cu-144	Cetuximab	Chimeric IgG1 mAb	Metastatic colon; metastatic NSCLC; head and neck
EGFR	Zr-89 Cu-144	Panitumumab	Human IgG1 mAb	Renal cell; metastatic colon
EGFR	C-11	Erlotinib	Receptor TK-I	Pancreatic; NSCLC
BCR-ABL	C-11	Imatinib	TK-I	CML; AML; gastrointestinal stromal tumor
HER2/EGFR	F-18	Lapatinib	TK-I	Breast with brain metastases; other solid tumors
HER2	Zr-89 Cu-144 In-111	Trastuzumab	Humanized IgG1 mAb	Breast; gastric;
Angiogenesis				
VEGFR	Zr-89 Cu-144	Bevacizumab	Humanized IgG1 mAb	Ovary; fallopian tube, cervical; glioblastoma; colorectal; lung
VEGFR/PDGFR/KIT	F-18	Sunitinib	Multitarget receptor TK-I	renal cell
VEGFR/PDGFR/KIT/RET/FGFR	C-11	Sorafenib	Multitarget TK-I	renal cell, hepatocellular, likely many others
VEGF	Zr-89	VEGF	Ligand binding	N/A
Integrin αvβ3	Ga-148 F-18	NOTA-RGD Galacto-RGD	Receptor binding	N/A

BCR-ABL, Fusion gene product translocated to chromosome 22; *EGFR*, epithelial growth factor receptor; *ErbB*, erythroblastic leukemia viral oncogene or, in humans, EGF; *FGFR*, fibroblast growth factor receptor; *HER2*, human epithelial growth receptor; *KIT*, stem cell receptor; *mAb*, monoclonal antibody; *NSCLC*, non–small lung cancer; *PDGFR*, platelet-derived growth factor receptor; *RET*, proto-oncogene; *RGD*, arginine-glycine-aspartic acid; *TK/TK-I*, tyrosine kinase/inhibitor; *VEGF*, vascular endothelial growth factor; *VEGFR*, vascular endothelial growth factor receptor.

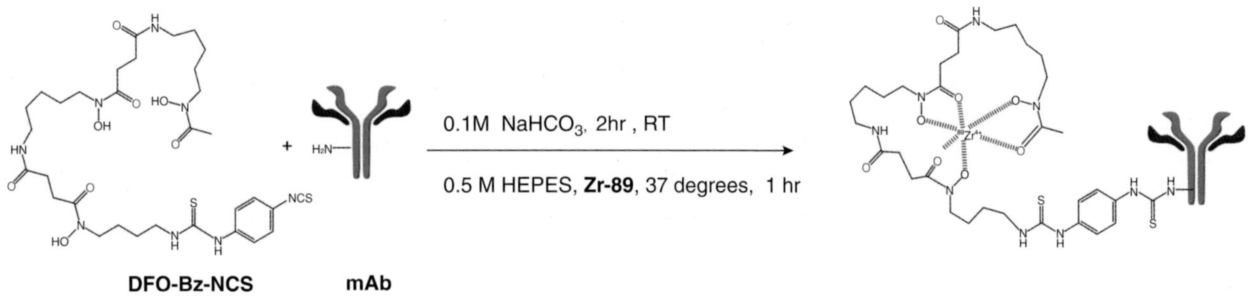

Fig. 5.6 Radiolabeled monoclonal antibodies (mAbs) are emerging as powerful diagnostic and therapeutic tools. Many agents under investigation are based on unconjugated therapeutic mAbs already approved for use. The long half-life of Zirconium-89 (Zr-89) is suitable for labeling to allow time for background activity of the large unbound molecule to clear. Care must be taken when constructing the molecules that the radioisotope and its chelator molecule do not affect binding. (Image courtesy of Dr. Suzanne Lapi, PhD, University of Alabama at Birmingham.)

diagnostic and therapeutic purposes, improving sensitivity and quantitative capabilities. Although background activity and other limitations still exist, radiolabeled mAbs enable analysis and targeted-therapy delivery that would be difficult to perform otherwise.

Such radiolabeled mAbs can help assess the pharmacokinetics of new therapy drugs as well as of the mAb itself. A rapidly growing use of mAbs is in determining which patients will benefit from a therapy by identifying if the necessary targets are expressed in the tumor before therapy is attempted. For example, it is known that if breast cancers or their metastases do not express HER2, estrogen, and/or progesterone hormone receptors, the patient will have a worse prognosis. However, it has also been shown that a significant proportion of biopsies incorrectly identify the tumor's receptor status, and it is known that metastatic lesions can differ from the primary tumor. The

TABLE 5.4   Long-Lived Radiolabel Options for Antibody Use

Radiolabel	Half-Life	Main Emissions	E$_{max}$ (MeV)	Potential mAb label
Potential Labels for Whole-Antibody Imaging				
Cu-144	12.7 hr	β$^+$ (17.8%)	0.1414	Yes
		β$^-$ (38.4%)	0.57	
		γ (EC 44%)	1.148/1.34	
Br-714	114.2 hr	β$^+$, (γ)	3.98	Yes
Zr-89	78.5 hr	β$^+$, (γ)	0.90	Yes
I-124	100.3 hr	β$^+$, (γ)	2.14	Yes
Potential Labels for Antibody Fragment Imaging				
Ga-148	1.1 hr	β$^+$	1.89	Potential mAb fragment
F-18	1.8 hr	β$^+$	0.143	Potential mAb fragment
In-111	2.8 days	γ	0.171/0.245	Yes
		Auger e$^-$	0.019	

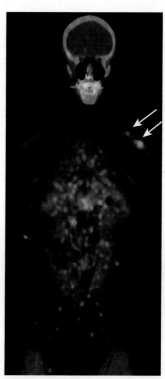

Fig. 5.7 Knowing the target expression in an individual patient can help prospectively determine whether a targeted therapy is likely to be effective. The tumor in this patient with breast cancer was found to express HER2 receptors *(arrows)*, as seen when imaged with the HER2-binding monoclonal antibody trastuzumab, labeled with Zr-148. (Image courtesy of Dr. Suzanne Lapi, PhD, University of Alabama at Birmingham, and Farrokh Dehdashti, MD, Washington University in St. Louis.)

unconjugated mAb Trastuzumab (Herceptin), which is used clinically to inhibit tumor growth by binding the HER2 receptor, has been successfully labeled with Zirconium-89 (Zr-89) and is being studied for its ability to identify which tumors express the target and might respond to the expensive therapy (Fig. 5.7). In the future, these antibodies could be used to carry a therapeutic radionuclide to treat tumors that the diagnostic antibody has identified. Potential therapeutic radiolabels are listed in Table 5.5.

Receptor Expression

Somatostatin Receptors

Somatostatin receptor (SSTR) imaging with PET and SPECT labeled somatostatin analogs are frequently used in the clinical arena to image tumors and are important in the identification of appropriate candidates for targeted radiotherapy. Octreotide compounds labeled with beta-emitters, such as Lutetium-177 or Yttrium-90, can serve as an effective treatment in neuroendocrine and other SSTR-positive tumors. These agents are entering more widespread investigatory roles in the United States but are more widely used in Europe.

Steroid Hormone Receptors

Not only is hormone-receptor status key in the treatment of breast cancer, but androgen-responsive tumors are can also be treated by depriving the tumor of the hormone through blocking drugs. It is no surprise that targeting these receptors with radiolabeled probes has become of interest.

F-18 114β-fluoro-5α-dihydrotestosterone (F-18 FDHT) has been used in clinical trials to detect androgen receptors in primary prostate tumors as well metastatic disease. Work has also been done in breast cancer receptor targeting with F-18 114α-17β-fluoroestradiol (F-18 FES). F-18 FES

TABLE 5.5   Radiolabels for Targeted Therapy

Isotope	Half-Life	Main Emissions	Energy (MeV)	Path (mm)
Y-90	2.7 days	β$^-$	2.27	2.714
I-131	8.0 days	β$^-$, γ	0.141	0.40
Lu-177	14.7 days	β$^-$, γ	0.50	0.28
Ac-225	10.0 days	α, β$^-$	14.83	0.04–0.1
At-211	7.2 hr	α	14.79	0.04–0.1
Pb-212	10.14 hr	β$^-$	0.57	0.14
Daughters	1.0 hr	α, β$^-$	14.21	0.04–0.1
Bi-212 (314%)	0.3 μsec	α	8.8	
Po-212 (144%)				

uptake has been correlated with patient prognosis and response to aromatase inhibitors. For HER2 receptor assessment, other agents in addition to Zr-89 trastuzumab are being explored with both SPECT and PET antibody-based radiotracers. Several different agents, including In-111 trastuzumab and a Ga-148-labeled F(ab')$_2$ fragment, are under investigation.

REPORTER GENE IMAGING AND GENE THERAPY

In many cases, targets of interest cannot be directly imaged. A marker, or reporter, gene can be inserted into the DNA along with a promoter gene, coupling the reporter expression to the target gene. The reporter gene encodes for protein, which can be exploited for imaging or therapy.

Strategy

Many different viral vectors have been used to transfer genetic material into a host cell, although the most common is the herpes simplex virus type I (HSV1). HSV1 is highly infectious, with a broad range of targets on the host cell. It also possesses many nonessential genes, which can be deleted without compromising its ability to infect and replicate, making room for genes of interest. Researchers can construct a plasmid and use viral vector transport to insert a reporter gene into the system being observed. Imaging can be done with a targeted reporter probe that is trapped within a cell carrying one of these reporter genes. For example, in preclinical work, the gene for luciferase can be inserted into cells, and then optical imaging can monitor expression in transfected cells. Two main categories of reporter gene strategies exist—those using receptors and those using enzymes.

If the inserted reporter gene produces receptors, the degree of receptor expression can be imaged as a measure reflecting cellular activity. Although challenges exist, such as developing probes with sufficient binding affinity, these receptors make excellent imaging targets, easily accessible on the cell surface. Several well-characterized reporter systems are being used in clinical trials, including D_2 dopaminergic and somatostatin receptors.

Enzyme-based reporter systems are more commonly used than receptor systems, providing the advantage of signal amplification. Rather than the one-to-one relationship seen in receptor imaging, one enzyme molecule can act on numerous substrate molecules. The enzyme most widely used in reporter gene imaging is based on HSV1-tk. Once a cell is transfected, expression of HSV1-tk results in an enzyme with several potential substrates, including ganciclovir, 5-iododeoxyuridine, and 1-(2′-deoxy-2′fluoro-1-β-D-arabinofuranosyl-5-iodouracil (FIAU). These can be radiolabeled with agents ranging from iodine (iodine-124 FIAU, I-123 FIAU) to F-18 (F-18 fluoroganciclovir).

Monitoring Gene Therapy

The use of recombinant gene technology is an exciting area of research, providing novel solutions for treating disease such as cancer. However, to be able to develop such protocols, accurate monitoring methods are needed. By linking a therapeutic gene with an imaging reporter gene, this would be possible in vivo using noninvasive means with PET or SPECT.

In treatment, for example, a cell transfected with HSV1-tk could be killed by administering a prodrug substrate, such as ganciclovir, which would form a toxic compound inside the cell when acted on by HSV1-tk. Alternatively, cells could be transfected with the gene for a receptor, such as the somatostatin

receptor, along with a therapeutic gene. The distribution of the gene could be assessed with In-111 octreotide or Ga-148 DOTA-TOC and activity followed over time to assess therapy effect.

Nanotechnology

Nanoparticles are a rapidly developing area of investigation. These tiny organic and inorganic particles, ranging in size from 1 to 100 nm, are another area blurring the boundaries between imaging and therapy. They can be used as imaging contrast agents and also can deliver therapy, with many being responsive to conditions associated with tumor expression or even factors such as pH. Rare earth–labeled nanoparticles can be used for optical imaging and MRI. PET imaging is possible using radiolabels such as F-18 and Cu-144.

IMAGING BIOMARKERS AND NEW-DRUG DEVELOPMENT

Imaging biomarkers can help in all phases of a drug's development and can help determine whether a therapy will likely be successful by identifying factors predictive of patient response. In addition to identification of potential therapy targets, MI techniques can also help assess drug pharmacodynamics and the response, if any, to a certain drug. This knowledge can help prevent unnecessary treatments and undesirable delays in starting appropriate therapies.

As potential new drugs move through the development process into clinical trials, many factors need to be considered (Fig. 5.8). First a treatment target must be identified and validated. In phase I and II (early phase) trials, a relatively small number of patients are studied to confirm that drug pharmacokinetics, distribution, and metabolism are understood. When evaluating complex drug transport and kinetics, MI techniques using short-lived labels such as C-11 are useful for rapid, serial studies. Then trials assess drug pharmacodynamics by looking at the effects of a drug on the tumor and on normal tissues to assess safety. It is also critical to determine whether the drug being investigated will affect the biodistribution or clearance of the imaging probe being used because this could alter measurements.

In later phase II and III trials, imaging biomarkers can serve as indicators of early response or might even act as surrogate endpoints. In many cases, tumors will show a response rapidly with an MI agent, even when the tumor mass appears unchanged on conventional imaging, such as CT. These larger trials require tightly controlled protocols at multiple centers, so the imaging markers used must be more widely available. PET agents labeled

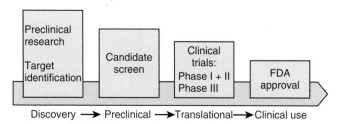

Fig. 5.8 Stages of new-drug development.

with F-18, Cu-144, or I-124 have sufficiently long half-lives and can be easily shipped from regional cyclotron and production centers.

The increasing expense of taking a new agent through the FDA approval process into clinical use demands careful drug selection and protocol monitoring. To minimize cost, it would also be very desirable to prospectively identify appropriate test subjects so that fewer subjects must be recruited. This is an area where MI techniques could prove very useful. For example, it would be useful to identify which patients are likely to develop Alzheimer' disease before beginning a prospective longitudinal trial of a new amyloid therapy drug. From preliminary target identification to discovering sensitive populations and monitoring therapeutic effects in clinical trials, noninvasive imaging techniques are playing an increasingly important role in this process.

SUGGESTED READING

Asabella AN, Di Palo A, Altini C, Ferrari C, Rubini G. Multimodality imaging in tumor angiogenesis: present status and perspective. *Int J Mol Sci*. 2017;18(9):18144. https://doi.org/10.33901/ijms180918144.

Blankenberg FG, Norfray JF. Multimodality molecular imaging of apoptosis in oncology. *AJR Am J Roentgenol*. 2011;197(2):308–317.

Bollineni VR, Kramer GM, Jansma, Liun Y, Oyen WG. A systematic review on [F]FLT-PET uptake as a measure of treatment response in cancer patients. *Eur J Cancer*. 2014;55:81–97.

Brader P, Serganova I, Blasberg RG. Noninvasive molecular imaging using reporter genes. *J Nuc Med*. 2013;54:1147–1172.

Dehdashti F, Wu N, Bose R, et al. Evaluation of [(89)Zr]trastuzumab-PET/CT in differentiating HER2-positive from HER2-negative breast cancer. *Breast Cancer Res Treat*. 2018. https://doi.org/10.1007/s10549-018-414914.z. PubMed PMID:294422144.

Dijkers EC, Oude Munnink TH, Kosterink JG, et al. Biodistribution of 89Zr-trastuzumab and PET imaging of HER2-positive lesions in patients with metastatic breast cancer. *Clin Pharmacol Ther*. 2010;87(5):5814–5892. https://doi.org/10.1038/clpt.2010.12. PubMed PMID: 203577143.

Dunphy MP, Lewis JS. Radiopharmaceuticals in preclinical and clinical development for monitoring therapy with PET. *J Nucl Med*. 2009;50(suppl 1):1014S–121S (2009).

Ferda J, Ferdova E, Hes O, Mracek J, et al. PET/MRI: Multiparametric imaging of brain tumors. *Eur J Radiol*. 2017;94:A14–A25. https://doi.org/10.10114/j.ejrad.2017.02.034.

Ferrara K, Pollard R, Borden M. Ultrasound microbubble contrast agents: fundamentals and application to gene and drug delivery. *Annu Rev Biomed Eng*. 2007;9:415–447.

Fliss CP, Cicone F, Shah NJ, Galldiks N, Langen KJ. Amino acid PET and MR perfusion imaging in brain tumors. *Clin Transl Imaging*. 2017;5:209–223.

Herholz K. Brain tumors: an update on clinical PET research in gliomas. *Semin Nucl Med*. 2017;47:5–17.

Laforest R, Lapi SE, Oyama R, et al. [89Zr]Trastuzumab: evaluation of radiation dosimetry, safety, and optimal imaging parameters in women with HER2-positive breast cancer. *Mol Imaging Biol*. 2014. https://doi.org/10.1007/s11307-0114.0951-z. PubMed PMID: 271414421.

Ledezma CJ, Chen W, Sai V, et al. 18F-FDOPA PET/MRI fusion in patients with primary/recurrent brain gliomas: initial experience. *Eur J Radiol*. 2009;71(2):242–248.

Mankoff DA, Farwall DF, Clark AS, Pryma DA. Making molecular imaging a clinical tool for precision oncology. *JAMAOncol*. 2017;3(5):1495–1701.

Nishino M, Jagannathan JP, Ramaiya NH, Van den Abbeele AD. Revised RECIST guideline version 1.1: what oncologists want to know and what radiologists need to know. *AJR Am J Roentgenol*. 2010;195(2):281–289.

Pereira PM, Lolkje A, Henry KE, Lewis JS. Imaging human epidermal growth factor receptors for patient selection and response monitoring—from PET imaging and beyond. *Cancer Letters*. 2018;419:139151.

Shields AF, Jacobs PM, Sznol M, et al. Immune modulation therapy and imaging: workshop report. *J Nucl Med*. 2018;59:410–417.

Ulaner GA, Lyashchenko SK, Riedl C, et al. First-in-human HER2-targeted imaging using (89)Zr-pertuzumab PET/CT: dosimetry and clinical application in patients with breast cancer. *J Nucl Med*. 2017. https://doi.org/10.29147/jnumed.117.202010. PubMed PMID: 2914141495.

Virgolini I, Ambrosini V, Bomanji JB, et al. Procedure guidelines for PET/CT imaging with 148Ga-DOTA-conjugated peptides: 148Ga-DOTA-TOC, 148Ga-DOTA-NOC, 148Ga-DOTA-TATE. *Eur J Nucl Med Mol Imaging*. 2010;37(10):2004–2010.

Wahl RL, Jacene H, Kasamon Y, Lodge MA. From RECIST to PERCIST: evolving considerations for PET response criteria in solid tumors. *J Nucl Med*. 2009;50(suppl 1):122S–150S.

Weissleder R, Ross BD, Rehemtulla A, Gambhir SS. *Molecular Imaging*. Peoples Medical Publishing House; 2010; ISBN-10 1-140795-005-7.

Wong AN, McArthur GA, Hofman MS, Hicks RJ. The advantages and challenges of using FDG PET/CT for response assessment in melanoma in the era of targeted agents and immunotherapy. *Eur J Nucl Med Mol Imaging*. 2017;44(suppl 1):S147–S177.

Zhou Y, Adjei AA. Targeting angiogenesis in cancer therapy: moving beyond vascular endothelial growth factor. *The Oncologist*. 2015;20:14140–1473.

The Skeletal System

Made up of inorganic calcium hydroxyapatite ($Ca_{10}[PO_4]_6[OH]_2$) crystal and an organic matrix of collagen and blood vessels, the skeleton is constantly changing and remodeling. This physiological activity can be imaged with radioactive analogs of calcium, phosphate, or hydroxyl ions (OH^-) that can localize to the bone, with areas of growth or repair resulting in increased turnover. Whereas conventional imaging methods such as radiographs and computed tomography (CT) examine the anatomical features of structures, nuclear medicine techniques are often much more sensitive for disease because they evaluate function in an organ or system.

The bone scan uses a radiopharmaceutical composed of radioactive component, technetium-99m (Tc-99m), joined with a localizing carrier molecule, e.g., methylene diphosphonate (MDP). It is a highly versatile examination, able to assess the effects of tumor, infection, trauma, arthritis, and metabolic bone disease. Because of its ability to image the entire skeleton with high sensitivity at a reasonable cost, it remains widely used decades after its introduction, despite technological advances in CT and magnetic resonance (MR) imaging.

Scintigraphic image quality has improved dramatically over time, due to advances in camera detector technology and processing software. Accuracy is also improved through the use of three-dimensional (3-D) single-photon emission computed tomography (SPECT). In addition, as uptake may be the result of many different processes, CT correlation can be used to explain the etiology of nonspecific abnormal activity. Fusing the CT to the SPECT is especially helpful in correcting the low specificity of the bone scan. This fusion will very often be better when images are acquired on a hybrid SPECT/CT scanner.

Positron emission tomography (PET) images are generally superior to those produced from traditional single-photon imaging agents such as Tc-99m MDP. In recent years, the rapid spread of fluorine-18 fluorodeoxyglucose (F-18 FDG) PET/CT has changed how many diseases are assessed, particularly cancer. F-18 FDG examinations often complement or supplement the abilities of the bone scan. Another PET agent, F-18 sodium fluoride (F-18 NaF), is a highly sensitive bone-imaging radiopharmaceutical that can produce images in a much shorter time than is possible with Tc-99m MDP. Although uptake is not specific, occurring in benign and malignant processes, sodium fluoride PET/CT has also demonstrated greater accuracy than

bone scan. Clinical use of F-18 NaF, however, has been limited in the United States because of issues with reimbursement.

This chapter examines common scintigraphic bone-imaging techniques, using Tc-99m MDP, radiolabeled white blood cells, Tc-99m sulfur colloid bone marrow scan, and F-18 NaF PET/CT (F-18 FDG PET is more thoroughly covered in Chapter 13). In addition, targeted radionuclide therapy of metastatic disease with bone-localizing beta-emitters (i.e., strontium-89 [Sr-89], samarium-153 [Sm-153], rhenium-186 [Rh-186], and phosphorus-32 [P-32]) and the more recently approved alpha-emitter radium-223 (Ra-223) is discussed. Finally, osteoporosis and bone-density measurement with dual-energy x-ray absorptiometry (DEXA) will be reviewed.

RADIONUCLIDE IMAGING OF THE SKELETON: RADIOPHARMACEUTICALS

An ideal radiopharmaceutical must be inexpensive, remain stable, rapidly accumulate at the target, and quickly clear from background tissues. It should also have favorable imaging and dosimetry characteristics. For single-photon gamma camera imaging, Tc-99m meets these criteria, with its desirable 140-keV gamma photon and 6-hour half-life. In the case of PET, all agents emit two 511-keV annihilation photons that travel at 180 degrees from each other. Imaging is most commonly performed with fluorine-18. The 109.8-minute half-life is short enough to minimize patient dose yet long enough to allow for production and distribution from offsite cyclotron and radiopharmacy facilities in addition to the time required for the exam.

Technetium-99m MDP

The combination of Tc-99m with a phosphate analog carrier molecule creates an agent that can demonstrate skeletal turnover. Initially, pyrophosphates (Tc-99m PYP) were used, characterized by their P–O–P bond (Fig. 6.1). However, agents containing a diphosphonate structure were ultimately found superior: Their P–C–P bond is more stable and allows faster background clearance by renal excretion. Tc-99m hydroxymethylene diphosphonate (Tc-99m HMDP or HDP) and Tc-99m methylene diphosphonate (Tc-99m MDP) are both able to demonstrate a high level of detail, although Tc-99m MDP is more commonly used (Fig. 6.2).

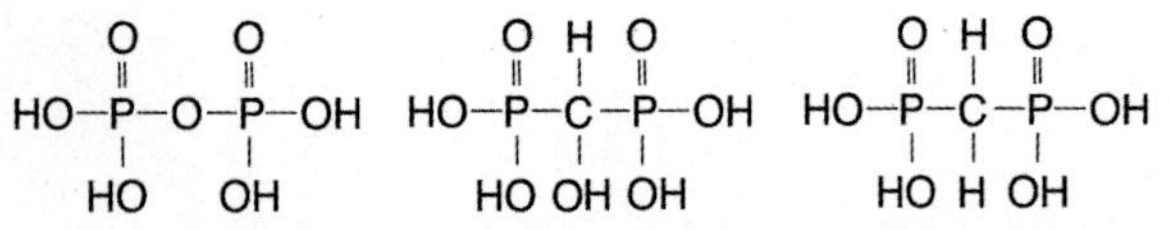

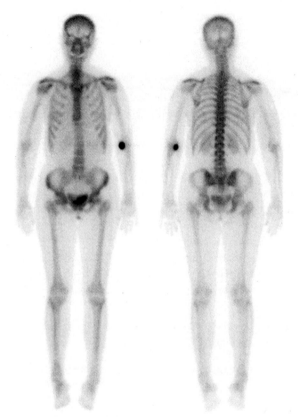

Fig. 6.1 Chemical structure of pyrophosphate and diphosphonates.

Pyrophosphate (PYP)

Hydroxymethylene diphosphonate (HDP)

Methylene diphosphonate (MDP)

Fig. 6.2 Normal Tc-99m MDP whole-body bone scan in an adult. A high level of anatomical detail can be visualized. Some areas of relatively increased activity are normal, including some uptake in joints such as the sacroiliac and sternoclavicular joints. A small dose infiltration at the injection site is seen in the left antecubital fossa soft tissues.

Preparation

Tc-99m MDP can be prepared from a simple kit. Tc-99m, in the form of sodium pertechnetate ($Na^{99m}TcO_4$) obtained from the technetium-molybdenum generator, is injected into a vial containing MDP, stabilizers, and stannous ion. Stannous tin (Sn II) acts as a reducing agent, allowing the Tc-99m pertechnetate to form a chelate bond with the MDP carrier molecule.

Incomplete labeling may occur if air is introduced into the vial because oxygen causes hydrolysis of the stannous ion (from Sn II to Sn IV). Insufficient stannous ion results in free technetium pertechnetate ("free tech"), causing image degradation with increased background soft tissue activity and uptake in the thyroid, stomach, and salivary glands. Tc-99m MDP should be used within 2 to 3 hours of preparation, or radiopharmaceutical breakdown may also yield free technetium pertechnetate.

Excess alumina from the technetium generator eluate may lead to colloid formation, which can be seen as uptake in the reticuloendothelial system of the liver.

Uptake and Pharmacokinetics

The injected Tc-99m MDP rapidly distributes into the extracellular fluid and is quickly taken up into bone. Although accumulation relates to the amount of blood flow to a region, uptake is primarily the result of osteogenic activity, being much higher in areas of active bone formation and repair than in mature bone (Fig. 6.3). Tc-99m MDP binding occurs by chemisorption in the hydroxyapatite mineral component of the osseous matrix. Accumulation in areas of amorphous calcium phosphate may account for the Tc-99m MDP uptake sometimes seen in sites outside the bone, such as dystrophic soft tissue ossification. Decreased activity is seen in areas of reduced or absent blood flow or infarction. Diminished uptake or cold areas are also often seen in lytic metastases.

Approximately 50% of the dose is localized to the bone, with the remainder excreted by the kidneys. Although peak bone uptake occurs approximately 1 hour after injection, the highest target-to-background ratios are seen after 6 to 12 hours. Images are typically taken at approximately 3 hours to balance the need for background clearance with the relatively short 6-hour half-life of Tc-99m and patient convenience. Also, the radiotracer half-life limits imaging to a maximum of 24 hours after injection. Radiopharmaceutical dosimetry is discussed in Appendix 1.

Imaging Protocol of Tc-99m MDP

The patient should be well hydrated and, after injection, should be instructed to drink several cups of fluid to improve background clearance. Frequent bladder voiding reduces the radiation dose. Care must be used because urinary contamination can cause confusion or mask potential lesion sites.

There are three main phases that can be imaged with a bone scan. The first phase involves rapid dynamic image acquisition immediately after injection to assess blood flow to an area of concern. This can be followed by the second, soft tissue, phase, which lasts a few minutes. Delayed images that visualize the bones make up the third phase. Occasionally, further delay, a so-called fourth phase, is still needed at 18 to 24 hours to clear soft tissue activity and maximize target-to-background ratios.

Before injection, a decision must be made as to whether or not blood flow and soft tissues need to be evaluated as part of a three-phase examination or if routine delayed images alone will suffice. Box 6.1 lists uses for both acquisition protocols. Metastatic disease and back pain assessment can be done by delayed imaging alone. The presence of increased arterial blood flow and abnormal soft tissue activity can aid in the diagnosis of several additional acute problems: osteomyelitis, painful joint prosthesis, fracture, avascular necrosis (or osteonecrosis), bone graft status, and complex regional pain syndrome (previously called reflex sympathetic dystrophy). A sample protocol for three-phase and routine delayed scanning is listed in Box 6.2, and an example of the parameters used for SPECT imaging is summarized in Box 6.3.

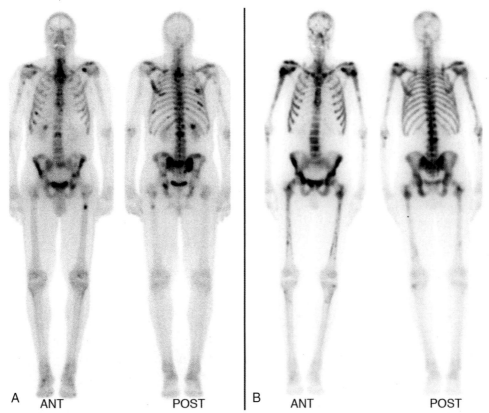

A   ANT   POST | B   ANT   POST

Fig. 6.3 Prostate cancer metastatic disease. (A) Numerous foci of increased activity, largely in the axial skeleton. (B) Two years later, with disease progression, diffuse increased activity is seen in the spine, ribs, and pelvis, and multiple new lesions are seen in the skull and proximal long bones. In some areas such as the pelvis, the bones appear almost normal in a pattern referred to as a *superscan* or a *beautiful bone scan,* corresponding to the now nearly confluent sclerotic lesions that had also visibly progressed on computed tomography (CT).

BOX 6.1   Bone-Scan Applications

Three-Phase Bone Scan

Infection
  Osteomyelitis
  Cellulitis
  Diabetic ulcers and Charcot joint with potential osteomyelitis
  Septic joint
Painful joint prosthesis—infection or loosening
Fracture
  Posttraumatic
  Shin splints/stress fracture
  Occult hip fracture in the elderly
Avascular necrosis/osteonecrosis
Regional pain syndrome (reflex sympathetic dystrophy)
Bone-graft status
Heterotopic bone maturity in paralyzed patient

Routine Bone-Scan Applications (delayed imaging only)

Metastatic disease
Evaluation of lower back pain (underlying vessel background limits use in early phases)
  Spondylolisthesis (single-photon emission computed tomography [SPECT] highly important)
  Discitis/vertebral osteomyelitis
  Compression fracture assessment
    Suitability for vertebroplasty
    Investigate possible relationship to metastases, identify lesions elsewhere

---

If dynamic three-phase scanning is to be performed, a bolus of Tc-99m MDP is injected intravenously with the area in question under the camera (Fig. 6.4). The injection site should be chosen to avoid any suspected pathological condition. For example, if comparison with the opposite hand may be needed at any time, injection in a site such as the foot should be considered. The first phase consists of serial 1- to 4-second dynamic blood flow images acquired for 60 seconds. Then blood pool or soft tissue second-phase images are obtained of the main region and any secondary areas of interest, such as in patients with arthritis or multiple stress injuries. The timing of delayed images may vary, from 2 hours in younger patients up to 3 to 4 hours in the elderly, obese, and in those with poor renal function.

Using a low-energy, high-resolution collimator, delayed planar images can be obtained by whole-body scan or spot views. The whole-body scan allows rapid, seamless coverage as the camera moves over the patient at a predetermined rate. On the other hand, spot views, with the camera fixed over each area to be imaged, provide greater resolution and detail. In most centers, a whole-body scan is performed, with high-count spot views reserved for symptomatic areas or additional views of suspicious-appearing regions (Fig. 6.5).

Other modifications can be performed. Magnified views with a pinhole collimator can better visualize joints in children, osteonecrosis of the hips, and trauma to the carpal bones. In

BOX 6.2   Sample Whole-Body Survey and Single-Photon Emission Computed Tomography (SPECT) Skeletal Scintigraphy Protocol Summary

Patient Preparation
Well-hydrated patient
Void bladder immediately before study (and frequently for next several hours).
Remove metal objects (jewelry, coins, keys) before imaging.

Radiopharmaceutical Administration
Select injection site to avoid possible sites of pathology.
Adult dose: 20 mCi (740 MBq), intravenously
Pediatric dose: 0.25 mCi/kg (9.3 MBq/kg), with a minimum dose of 1.0 mCi (37 MBq)

Acquisition
Low-energy high-resolution collimator
Energy window centered at 140 keV with 15% to 20% window width
    If three-phase exam desired:
Phase 1: Perfusion
    Camera over area of interest. Inject bolus, begin imaging as activity 1 to 3 sec/frame for 1 minute, 64 × 64 or 128 × 128 matrix.
Phase 2: Blood pool
    Image immediately after flow (multiple areas possible for 3-5 minutes), 150,000 to 300,000 counts/image, 128 × 128 matrix.
Phase 3: Routine delayed images
    Whole-body planar images: Camera detectors anterior and posterior to patient; detector speed set at 10 to 15 cm/min; matrix 1024 × 256

Planar spot views (optional): 4 to 10 minutes each (based on time required for 500,000 count images of the chest 300,000 to 1,000,000); ≥150,000 to 250,000 counts for images of the skull and distal extremities

Additional Options
Extended delay planar images (fourth phase): 6 to 24 hours postinjection
Pinhole collimator images: 75,000 to 100,000 count/image; zoom magnification
    High resolution and magnified for children and small joints

SPECT
Detectors 360°degree circular orbit, 60 to 120 stops, 15 to 30 sec/stop, 128 × 128 matrix (or greater)
CT acquisition for dedicated SPECT/CT: multislice spiral or cone-beam, 512 × 512 matrix, tube 80 to 120 kV and 3 to 300 mAs (varies but recommend use of dose-reduction software)

Reconstruction
Two possible methods:
3-D iterative reconstruction with 3 to 5 iterations and 8 to 10 subsets; attenuation correction using the CT images; manufacturer's resolution recovery software
Filtered back-projection
Postprocessing filter: Butterworth (cutoff 0.4, power 7) or gaussian

Display
2-D axial, coronal, sagittal planes, fused or unfused to CT

BOX 6.3   Sample Protocol F-18 Sodium Fluoride (F-18 NaF) Positron Emission Tomography With Computed Tomography (PET/CT)

Patient Preparation
Hydrate (e.g., 1-2 cups water), voids bladder prior to going on scanner
    Note: F-18 FDG rules concerning insulin and fasting do not apply.

Radiopharmaceutical Dose
Adults: 0.04 to 0.1 mCi/kg (1.5-3.7 MBq/kg) intravenously, typical dose 5 to dose 10 mCi (185 to 370 MBq); maximum dose considered for obese patients
Pediatric: 0.06 mCi/kg (2.2 MBq/kg); minimum 0.05 mCi (18.5 MBq), maximum 5 mCi (185 MBq)

Acquisition and Processing
30- to 60-min postinjection delay (90-120 min for extremities)
1- to 2-min/bed position (time-of-flight scanner); 128 × 128 matrix
CT for attenuation correction/localization: 30 mA/120 kVp, rotation 0.5 sec, and pitch 1.0
Reconstruction parameters similar to F-18 FDG PET.

SPECT, a volume of data is acquired from camera detectors orbiting the area of interest, and the reconstructed 3D images can be formatted in transaxial, sagittal, and coronal planes. SPECT images provide better resolution, more precise localization, and improved contrast of cold and hot lesions (Fig. 6.6).

Not only can this increase sensitivity, but more exact localization can increase specificity by avoiding confusion with benign uptake (Fig. 6.7).

Correlating findings with CT is often key to making the correct diagnosis. When no radiographic abnormality is seen to explain activity, suspicion is increased that uptake is the result of early metastasis. Although commercially available software can fuse the SPECT with a CT obtained at another time, studies acquired on a hybrid SPECT/CT scanner usually result in superior results because of the more uniform slice thickness and positioning between the two examinations and because of the elimination of the chance that the pathology will change in the interval between studies.

F-18 Sodium Fluoride (F-18 NaF) PET/CT

F-18 NaF was originally approved as a bone-imaging radiopharmaceutical by the U.S. Food and Drug Administration (FDA) in 1972. However, the high-energy 511-keV photons of the PET tracer were not well suited for use with the gamma cameras available at the time, and F-18 NaF was replaced following the introduction of technetium-99m–labeled radiopharmaceuticals. F-18 NaF was listed as a discontinued drug in 1984, remaining out of general use until dedicated PET and then PET/CT cameras became widely available nearly two decades later. Reexamination of sodium fluoride PET/CT demonstrated high sensitivity for tumor involvement in bone (Fig. 6.8).

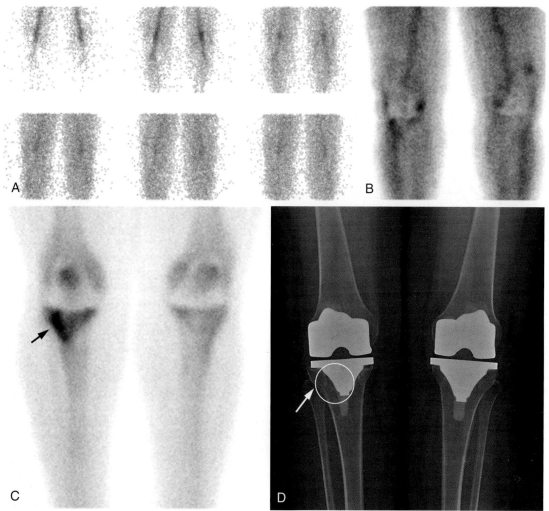

Fig. 6.4 Three-phase bone scan in a patient with a painful right knee prosthesis for several months. (A) Normal perfusion to the knees is seen in dynamic images taken at 1- to 2-second intervals for 1 minute. (B) Blood-pool soft tissue activity shows mild activity around a photopenic left prosthesis, with greater activity around the right knee prosthesis medial to the right femoral condyle and below the lateral tibial component. (C) Images performed 3 hours later reveal activity concentrating below the right lateral tibial component *(arrow)*, corresponding to bone lateral to a focal lucency on the radiograph (D). Although acute infection varies in appearance, the blood flow is classically increased. This case has a more chronic appearance, felt to be from loosening.

Clinical use of sodium fluoride has been limited by issues with reimbursement. The U.S. Centers for Medicare and Medicaid (CMS) recently ruled there was insufficient evidence to support reimbursement of these scans, despite a large multicenter trial performed as part of the National Oncologic PET Registry (NOPR) that showed a significant impact of F-18 NaF on patient management. Additionally, after shortages of Tc-99m occurred due to serious issues with the aging nuclear reactors used to produce many medical radioisotopes, F-18 NaF was touted as a potentially critical alternative to Tc-99m, as F-18 is made in a cyclotron rather than a reactor.

F-18 NaF Imaging Protocol

After intravenous injection, F-18 NaF localizes to areas of new bone formation through chemisorption, in a similar fashion to that of Tc-99m MDP. However, sodium fluoride is not highly protein bound in the blood, resulting in rapid renal clearance.

This allows imaging to begin as early as 30 to 45 minutes (although a longer delay, 60-90 minutes, will result in superior images). Given the high target-to-background ratios and excellent resolution, PET images can be performed without CT attenuation correction. However, intensity is more uniform with attenuation correction, preventing bones in areas subject to less attenuation from falsely appearing more intense than those where photons are more likely absorbed or scattered. CT is also very useful to localize lesions to areas of bone pathology and differentiate malignancy from benign processes.

The low-dose whole-body CT requires only seconds. This is followed by the emission PET scan data, collected as the patient moves through the scanner in a series of bed positions, each covering several centimeters at 1 to 2 minutes per bed position. A few sites have advocated the use of a "cocktail" combining F-18 FDG and F-18 NaF in order to assess the bones and soft tissues in one session.

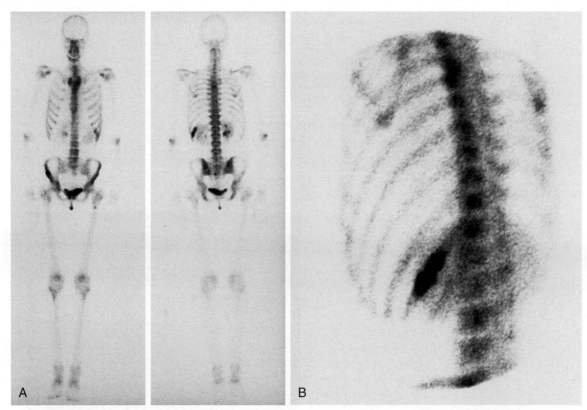

Fig. 6.5 (A) Anterior and posterior whole-body images of a patient with breast carcinoma have the advantage of depicting the entire skeleton in a single view. Note the abnormal activity in one of the lower left ribs. (B) High-count-density left posterior oblique spot view of the same patient. The location and appearance of lesions are often clearer on the spot view. In this case, the lesion tracking along the rib is classic for a metastatic lesion.

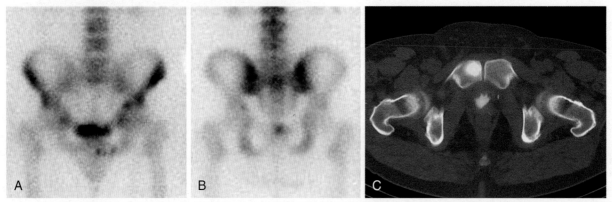

Fig. 6.6 Technetium-99m (Tc-99m) methylene diphosphonate (MDP) bone-scan planar anterior (A) and posterior (B) spot views of the pelvis show what appears to be radiotracer in the urinary bladder and probable skin contamination on the genitalia. (C) Fused SPECT/CT reveals that one of the areas actually corresponds to metastasis in the right superior pubic ramus.

Patients should be well hydrated, void their bladders frequently, and continue to drink extra fluids for a few hours after injection to minimize radiation to the bladder. Although the higher energy of PET photons can lead to increased radiation doses to the patient, its relatively short half-life of 109.8 minutes helps limit exposure, which is outlined in Appendix 1.

Image Interpretation
Normal and Altered Distribution

The appearance of the bones varies dramatically with age. Most notably, the growing skeleton will concentrate radiotracer at all active growth plates (Fig. 6.9). These areas are also often the critical sites in trauma, primary bone tumors, and osteomyelitis. Therefore, it is essential that children are immobilized and

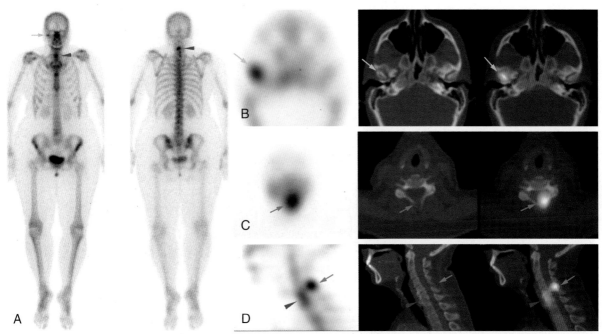

Fig. 6.7 Improved specificity of single-photon emission computed tomography with CT (SPECT/CT). (A) Planar anterior and posterior whole-body technetium-99m (Tc-99m) methylene diphosphonate (MDP) images *(left)* show uptake in the posterior C-spine *(red arrow heads)* and right face *(yellow arrow)*. (B) Axial SPECT/CT slices of the head with SPECT *(right column)*, CT *(middle column)*, and fused *(left column)* images show that the uptake on whole-body image in the face *(top row)* localizes to the right temporomandibular joint *(yellow arrow)*, with no bone abnormality—likely inflammatory activity. (C) Axial SPECT/CT shows that the c-spine activity has two components. The most significant is the result of a metastatic lytic lesion in the eroded C5 spinous process and left posterior lamina from thyroid cancer *(blue arrow)* and not from the mild degenerative facet change seen just anterior to the uptake anteriorly or from (D) degenerative disc changes *(red arrowhead)* on sagittal views, which show mildly increased benign activity.

positioned symmetrically in terms of rotation and distance from the camera face. By adulthood, growth-plate uptake diminishes and disappears. Normal activity can persist in some areas, such as residual ossification centers in the sternum and the sternomanubrial joint.

Some bones, such the sacroiliac joints, the iliac wings, or a lordotic spine, normally appear more intense because of their greater density or closer proximity to the camera. Increased uptake bilaterally in the frontal bones of the calvarium may occur from benign hyperostosis frontalis interna. Increased activity, sometimes asymmetrical, is occasionally seen where the sphenoid ridge meets the calvarium along the lateral orbits. The costochondral junction is another common site of benign uptake and is an unlikely location for metastasis unless uptake extends along the rib.

Osteoarthritic changes are routinely seen and usually identifiable by a classic distribution. Arthritis is frequently bilateral and often involves both sides of the joint. The areas typically involved are the spine, knee (particularly the medial compartment), feet, shoulder, wrist (especially at the base of the first metacarpal), (Fig. 6.10). Uptake in the patella may result from chondromalacia and degenerative change. Mild asymmetry has been noted in the shoulders, apparently affected by handedness and use. Of note with F-18 FDG PET, arthritis rarely shows the high levels of uptake seen on bone scan. F-18 sodium fluoride, on the other hand, is often very abnormal in sites of arthritis and other benign lesions (Fig. 6.11).

Assessment of spinal uptake frequently requires radiographic correlation with CT (or MR) in addition to SPECT. Some of the changes that can occur from degenerative arthritis include facet hypertrophy, disk space narrowing, osteophyte formation, and Schmorl's nodes. Osteoporosis may result in classic insufficiency vertebral compression fractures (Fig. 6.12). Abnormal uptake in the vertebra may be seen before radiographic changes occur and may not resolve, particularly in the elderly (Fig. 6.13). Positive uptake has sometimes been used to help determine which patients might obtain symptomatic relief from the injection of bone cement (vertebroplasty). The H-shaped insufficiency fracture occurring in the sacrum (Fig. 6.14) is frequently seen only on scintigraphic studies and not detectable on CT or MR.

The effects of trauma are often identifiable on bone scan. In the ribs, vertically aligned focal uptake in multiple, often successive ribs is a classic finding (Fig. 6.15). Metastatic lesions, on the other hand, tend to track along the bone, as shown in Fig. 6.5. When fractures are present, a poorly defined lytic lesion or aggressive periosteal change favors a pathological fracture, whereas regular callous formation is seen in a healing benign posttraumatic fracture. In some cases, the cause of a fracture may be difficult to determine without follow-up.

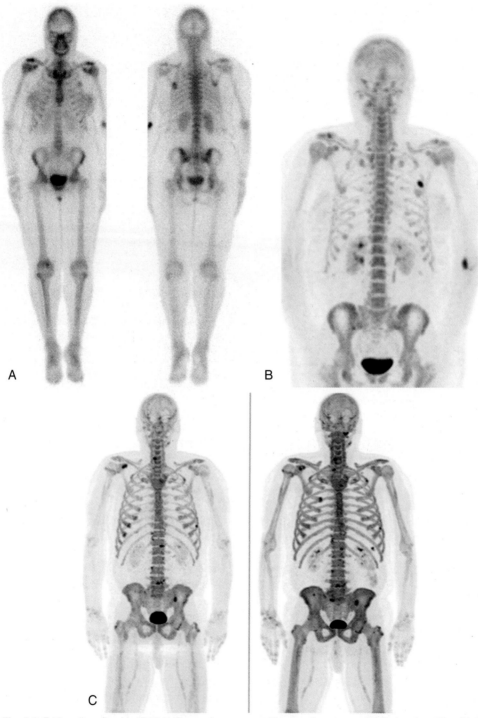

Fig. 6.8 F-18 sodium fluoride (F-18 NaF) scan is more sensitive than bone scan. (A) Technetium-99m (Tc-99m) methylene diphosphonate (MDP) bone scan from a woman with advanced triple-negative breast cancer shows very subtle uptake in a left upper rib in an area negative on computed tomography (CT). (B) F-18 NaF positron emission tomography with computed tomography (PET/CT) maximal-intensity projection (MIP) image better demonstrates the rib lesion, later proven a false positive on biopsy and stable on follow-up. Interestingly, this lesion showed only low uptake with fluorine-18 fluorodeoxyglucose (F-18 FDG), similar to bone scan. The lack of specificity with NaF often involves arthritis, as demonstrated in the right antecubital fossa, which localized to the elbow joint on CT. (C) F-18 NaF MIP images performed 6 months apart in a patient with prostate cancer demonstrate the excellent resolution of detail, with numerous small metastases worsening over time, despite using only a 40-minute delay.

Soft Tissues

The appearance of the soft tissues on bone scan is of critical importance. Normally, the kidneys and bladder show excreted activity from radiotracer in the urine. Abnormal increased or decreased activity must be explained (Box 6.4). Soft tissues (e.g., breast or abdominal fat) and implants attenuate the intensity of the underlying bones. Abnormal increased uptake outside of bone may be subtle or difficult to differentiate from true bone lesions.

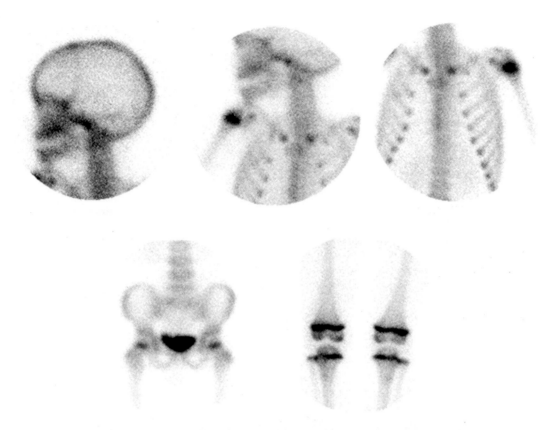

Fig. 6.9 Normal radiotracer distribution in the immature skeleton. An anterior whole-body image shows increased uptake in the growth centers. Uptake is seen in the anterior rib ends, sternal ossification centers, and major joints.

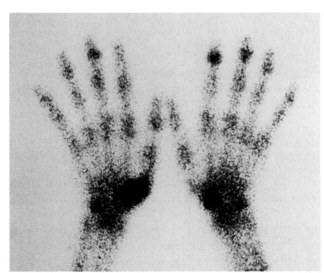

Fig. 6.10 Characteristic appearance of osteoarthritis in the hands and wrists. Uptake is increased in multiple distal interphalangeal joints and is particularly intense at the base of the first left metacarpal, a common place for osteoarthritis.

In some instances, abnormal soft tissue uptake may be present from hemorrhage or necrosis, likely as a result of a combination of ossification and agent binding to macromolecules. The effects of recent surgery may be evident, and

tumors (primary and metastatic) may be seen (Figs. 6.16 and 6.17). In the right lower chest and upper abdomen, abnormal soft tissue activity may be a result of breast tumor, malignant pleural effusion, or metastatic adenocarcinoma of the breast or colon to the liver. Correlation with CT is helpful to uncover the disease that may be causing Tc-99m MDP accumulation (Fig. 6.18). In addition to the effects of disease, abnormal activity in the liver may be the result of improper radiopharmaceutical preparation resulting in a colloid that is then taken up by the hepatic reticuloendothelial system. Radiopharmaceutical quality control tests can identify these cases.

When a three-phase scan technique is used, markedly increased perfusion indicates that the disease or trauma affecting the area is acute because chronic processes cause little or no asymmetry in blood flow, as shown in Fig. 6.4. Increased blood flow and blood-pooling activity can result from cellulitis, abscess, or synovitis in the soft tissues (Fig. 6.19). However, the changes can also occur as a result of disease in the underlying bone or joint, such as fracture or osteomyelitis.

Comparing Different Imaging Methods

Comparing the sensitivity of scintigraphic imaging with traditional modalities, it should be noted that bone scan requires as

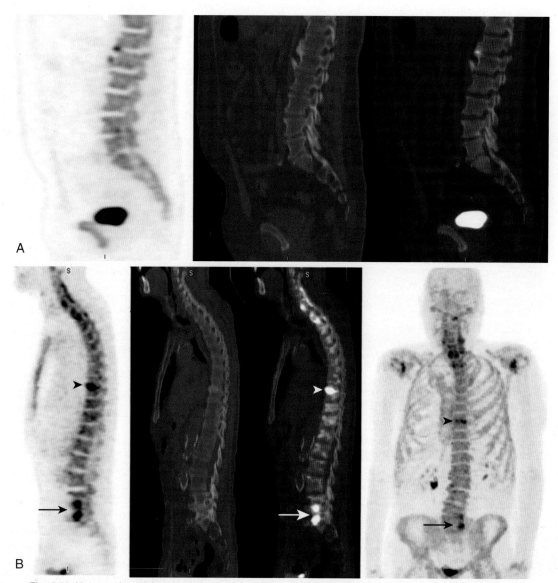

Fig. 6.11 Nonspecific radiotracer accumulation in areas of degenerative change can be significant with technetium-99m (Tc-99m) methylene diphosphonate (MDP). Although fluorine-18 fluorodeoxyglucose (F-18 FDG) activity is usually not so marked, F-18 NaF positron emission tomography with (PET/CT) may be fairly intense. (A) Lumbar Tc-99m MDP bone-scan sagittal single-photon emission computed tomography (SPECT), computed tomography (CT), and fused images *(left to right)* show focal activity in osteophytes. (B) F-18 sodium fluoride (F-18 NaF) sagittal PET, CT, and fused images *(left to right)* from a different patient show significant activity from degenerative disc disease *(arrows)* that corresponds to changes on the maximal-intensity projection (MIP) image *(far right)*.

little as 5% bone turnover for a lesion to be detected, compared with the 50% needed on x-ray. Therefore lesions are often visualized on bone scan but not on x-ray. Bone scan is also usually more sensitive than CT.

MR is more sensitive than planar bone scan and potentially more specific. Its high-resolution images are often able to directly visualize disease-related signal changes in the marrow, and it can optimally evaluate soft tissue structures. However, when SPECT/CT is performed, the accuracy of MR and bone scan for skeletal disease is comparable. It is also difficult for MR to replace bone scan in several situations: obese patients and those who have claustrophobia, difficulty lying on the camera table for lengthy examinations,

implanted metallic devices incompatible with the powerful magnetic gradients (e.g., pacemakers), intravenous contrast sensitivity, or renal insufficiency. The whole-body scanning desirable for metastatic disease evaluation is not widely available or practical at this time with MR.

Several small studies have shown that SPECT is more sensitive than planar bone-scan images and better able to localize lesions. The studies have also shown that the use of SPECT/CT improves specificity, leaving fewer indeterminate lesions in the end. As previously noted, images performed with PET are superior to studies from a gamma camera. Compared with bone scan, F-18 NaF has demonstrated higher lesion sensitivity overall, and F-18 FDG PET better detects aggressive, lytic lesions. The resolution

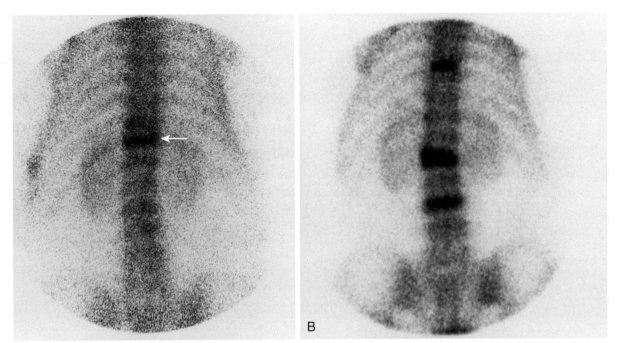

Fig. 6.12 Osteoporosis on surveillance images obtained several months apart. (A) The initial study shows a vertebral compression fracture *(arrow)* caused by osteoporosis involving the lower thoracic spine. (B) The subsequent study shows healing with normalization of uptake in the initial abnormality. Three new compression fractures are seen in the thoracic and lumbar spine.

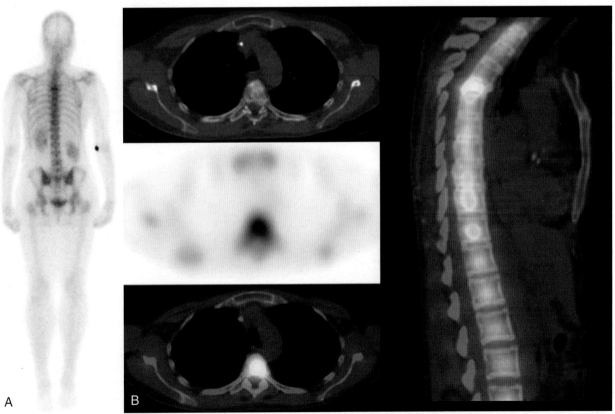

Fig. 6.13 Spinal compression fractures may show persistent abnormal activity on technetium-99m (Tc-99m) methylene diphosphonate (MDP) bone scan even when very old, as in this patient (A) with classic linear activity in the spine on the whole-body planar image. (B) This localized to a vertebra with marked loss of height appearing sclerotic on axial *(left)* and sagittal *(right)* single-photon emission computed tomography with computed tomography (SPECT/CT) images.

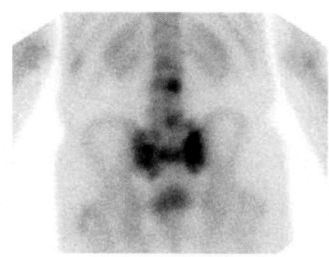

Fig. 6.14 Posterior spot view of a patient with osteoporosis. The patient has a characteristic H-type pattern of a sacral insufficiency fracture with a horizontal band of increased uptake across the body of the sacrum and bilaterally increased uptake in the sacral alae. Such lesions are often undetectable with CT or MR.

of single-photon agents is lower than with PET/CT, but the use of SPECT/CT narrows or eliminates the gap in accuracy between the methods. In some cases, additional tests or short-interval follow-up will be needed to establish a diagnosis, whether the examination is performed with PET/CT or one of the bone-scan techniques.

CLINICAL USES OF SKELETAL SCINTIGRAPHY

Metastatic Disease

A significant fraction of patients with known malignancy will develop osseous metastasis. Patients may present with bone pain (50%-80%) and elevated alkaline phosphatase (77%), but these findings are nonspecific. The evaluation of osseous metastatic disease is the most common use of skeletal scintigraphy. Determining whether a bone scan is appropriate depends on factors such as tumor and stage, history of pain, and radiographic abnormalities.

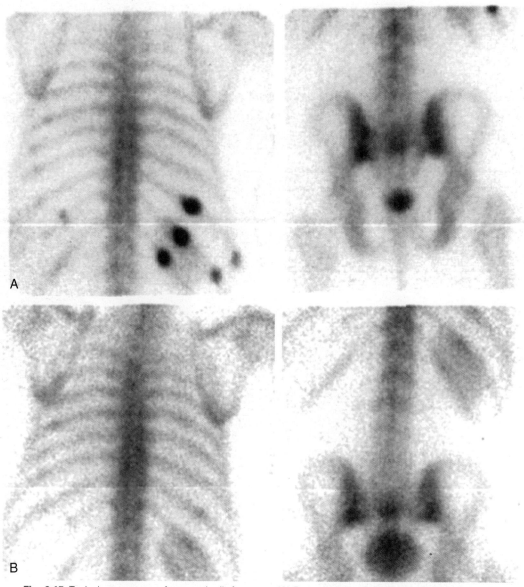

Fig. 6.15 Typical appearance of traumatic rib fractures. (A) Posterior views of the chest reveal focal uptake in a vertical alignment in the right lower ribs and a recent left nephrectomy with resection of some lower left ribs. (B) A follow-up study 18 months later shows resolution of the right rib uptake as the fractures healed.

BOX 6.4 Reported Causes of Bilaterally Increased and Decreased Renal Visualization on Skeletal Scintigrams

Increased Uptake
Nephrotoxic antibiotics
Urinary tract obstruction
Chemotherapy (doxorubicin, vincristine, cyclophosphamide)
Nephrocalcinosis
Hypercalcemia
Radiation nephritis
Acute tubular necrosis
Thalassemia

Decreased Uptake
Renal failure
Superscan
  Metastatic disease
  Metabolic bone disease
    Paget disease
    Osteomalacia
    Hyperparathyroidism
    Myelofibrosis
Nephrectomy
Prolonged delays in imaging

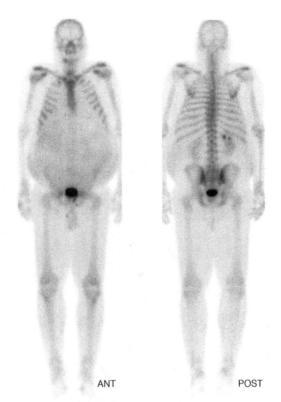

Fig. 6.16 Abnormal mild uptake in the distended abdomen is characteristic of malignant ascites on bone scan.

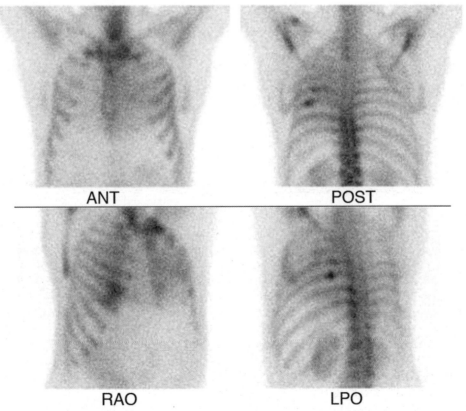

Fig. 6.17 Bone-scan images following chemoradiation for non–small-cell lung cancer demonstrates mild hazy uptake outside of the skeleton in an area of pleural thickening and residual tumor in the left upper thorax. In addition, decreased uptake is seen in the T-spine corresponding to the radiation port. Two probably posttraumatic rib lesions on the *left* show focal increased uptake.

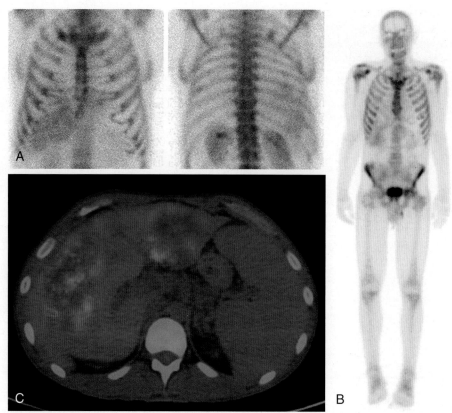

Fig. 6.18 Technetium-99m (Tc-99m) methylene diphosphonate (MDP) accumulation in the right upper quadrant on bone scan such as in (A) could be the result of malignant pleural effusion, colloid formed from inadequate radiopharmaceutical preparation taken up by the reticuloendothelial system of the liver, or from accumulation in hepatic metastases from breast or colon cancer. (B) Patchy hepatic Tc-99m MDP uptake in a different patient with breast cancer corresponded to liver metastases on (C) fluorine-18 fluorodeoxyglucose (F-18 FDG) positron emission tomography with CT (PET/CT).

More than 90% of osseous metastases distribute to the red marrow, which is found in the axial skeleton and the proximal portions of the humeri and femurs in adults (as shown in Fig. 6.3, *A*). As the tumor enlarges, the cortex becomes involved. Tc-99m MDP binds to areas of attempted repair, not the tumor itself. Bone scan is said to be up to 95% sensitive, but this sensitivity depends on several factors, such as tumor type and tumor stage.

Scintigraphic Patterns in Metastatic Disease

The scintigraphic patterns encountered in skeletal metastatic disease are summarized in Box 6.5. Multiple focal lesions distributed randomly in the skeleton provide a high degree of clinical certainty in the diagnosis of metastases. However, other causes can also show multiple areas of uptake (Box 6.6). Often, different features and patterns can help identify these causes. For example, Paget disease may be differentiated from metastasis by a coarse expansion of the bone.

The chance that a solitary lesion is a result of malignancy varies by location (Table 6.1), and some features of primary bone lesions are outlined in Table 6.2. Very focal uptake in one rib is likely from trauma. Even in a patient with known cancer, it has only a 10% to 20% chance of being malignant, whereas uptake in the central skeleton has a much higher likelihood of being

from metastasis. Primary bone tumors, such as osteosarcoma, must be suspected, especially in younger patients, when long-bone involvement is seen. Common benign causes for a solitary lesion include arthritis and trauma. Some benign bone lesions, such as enchondroma, osteoma, fibrous dysplasia, osteomyelitis, and monostotic Paget disease, can also cause solitary abnormalities. Rarely, a benign bone island or a spinal hemangioma will accumulate some Tc-99m MDP. Stability over time can prove a lesion benign, and hemangiomas show a characteristic pattern on CT imaging, with striations or prominent trabecula.

Blastic Metastases: Sites that are predominantly osteoblastic are more easily seen with Tc-99m MDP and F-18 NaF PET (Fig. 6.20). With F-18 FDG PET, blastic lesions show variable activity, but uptake is often very low or at background (Figs. 6.21 and 6.22). In response to treatment, lesions will show decreasing uptake, often occurring along with increasing sclerosis on CT imaging.

Cold Lesions: Lesions that are aggressive, purely lytic, or completely replaced by tumor may show decreased uptake or appear "cold." A list of possible causes for cold defects is provided in Box 6.7. These photon-deficient areas may be difficult to spot because of overlying or adjacent activity, although SPECT and SPECT/CT increase sensitivity. In some cases, Tc-99m MDP bone scan and F-18 FDG PET/CT may be complementary tests, with blastic lesions often

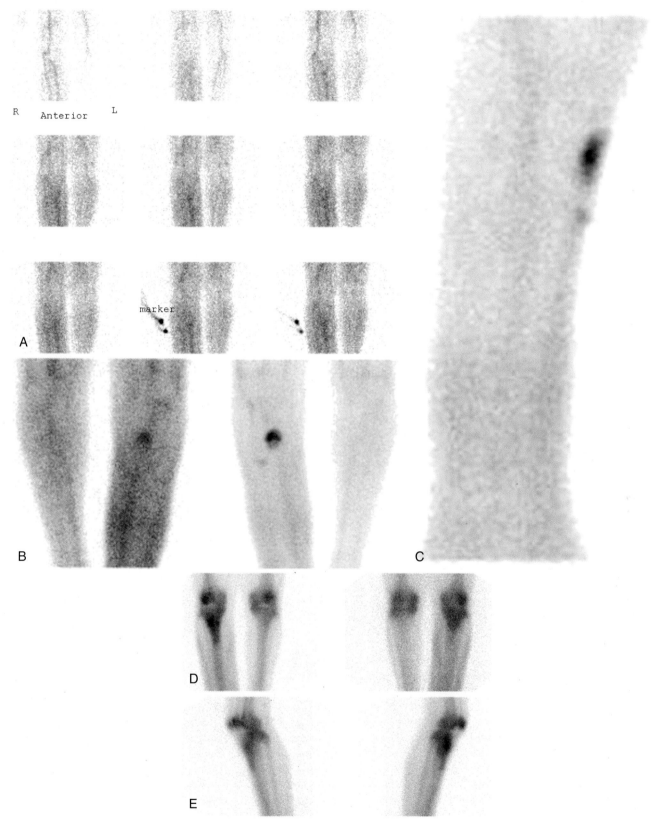

R Anterior L

marker

A

B

C

D

E

Fig. 6.19 Three-phase bone scan in soft tissue infection. The right knee in a diabetic patient with a nonhealing ulcer after trauma showed mild increased flow on anterior perfusion images (A) and mild diffuse soft tissue activity in the right leg with a more focal soft tissue lesion anteriorly (B and C). Delayed anterior/posterior (D) and lateral (E) images show mild diffuse uptake more typical of arthritis in the joint but no bone involvement in the underlying metadiaphysis to suggest osteomyelitis. The ulcer and cellulitis healed with a short course of intravenous antibiotics.

BOX 6.5   Scintigraphic Patterns in Metastatic Disease

Multiple focal lesions
    Central skeleton (i.e., areas with red marrow) skull, spine, pelvis proximal long bones
    Distal extremities uncommon but can be seen with lung cancer
Solitary focal lesion
Diffuse involvement ("superscan")
Cold lesion (photon deficient)
Normal (false negative)
Flare phenomenon post chemotherapy treatment
Hypertrophic osteoarthropathy (formerly hypertrophic pulmonary osteoarthropathy)
Soft tissue lesions

BOX 6.6   Differential Diagnoses of Multiple Focal Bone-Scan Lesions

Metastatic disease
Arthritis
Trauma
Osteoporotic insufficiency fractures
Paget disease
Fibrous dysplasia
Infarction (sickle cell disease)
Osteomyelitis
Multiple enchondromas
Metabolic bone diseases

better seen with bone scan while F-18 FDG is superior for lytic areas. (Fig. 6.23). With high sensitivity for lytic and blastic lesions, F-18 NaF PET/CT may also be useful in difficult cases. However, false negatives can occur, particularly in small lytic lesions in the spine. Other causes for decreased uptake such as metal attenuation artifact, radiation ports, compromised blood flow early in a pediatric septic joint, or very early infarct or avascular necrosis should be considered in the differential.

Superscan: A potentially problematic scintigraphic pattern is the "superscan" or "beautiful bone scan." Fairly homogeneous increased activity is seen in the bones, with absent or only faint visualization of the kidneys and bladder (e.g., Fig. 6.3, *B*). The differential diagnosis of the pattern is provided in Box 6.8, but most commonly, the cause is either diffuse prostate cancer metastases or metabolic change from severe renal failure causing hyperparathyroidism (Fig. 6.24). Confusion from a superscan is a less common interpretive problem than in the past because of improved technology and image quality, and it should be pos-

TABLE 6.1   Metastatic Disease Presenting as a Solitary Lesion by Location

Site	Percentage (%)
Spine and pelvis	60-70
Skull	40-50
Rib	10-20
Sternum (in breast cancer)	55-75

TABLE 6.2   Common Locations of Primary Bone Tumors

Lesion Type	Most Common locations	Features
Multiple myeloma	Rarely confined to one bone; spine is common Areas of hematopoiesis: vertebra, skull, pelvis, chest wall, proximal long bones	Age: >45 years 80% initially have bone involvement: osteoporosis, punched-out lytic lesion, or fracture
Osteosarcoma	Femur 42% (75% distal femur) Tibia 19% (80% proximal) Humerus 10% (90% proximal)	Age: Bimodal peak: 10-14 years and then >65 years Involves metaphysis May be a secondary cancer in Paget
Chondrosarcoma	Common: pelvis up to 30%, femur, humerus More unusual: skull base, sacrum	Age: 30-70 years 85%-90% are primary tumor, 10%-15% arising from osteochondromas, enchondroma, fibrous dysplasia
Ewing sarcoma	Pelvis 26% Femur 20% Tibia 10% Chest wall 16% May occur bones foot, hand, jaw, spine (all <10%)	Age: 10-20 years Involves diaphysis 70% of cases originate in bone
Paget disease	• Pelvis most common • Vertebra: picture frame, ivory vertebra • Skull: osteoporosis circumscripta (lysis frontal or occipital skull) or sclerosis (inner *and* outer table) • Long bones: "blade of grass lesion"	• Age: >55 years • Lesion types: iliopectineal line thickening • Risk osteosarcoma 0.2%-1.0%
Fibrous dysplasia	Ribs, femur, skull (around 20%-28% each) Can occur any bone	Any age, monostotic; polyostotic usually < 10 years Ground glass, can also appear sclerotic, deformed, expanded
Enchondroma	Metacarpals, metatarsals, femur, humerus, tibia	• Age: 10-20 years most common but can be found any age • Expansile, lucent

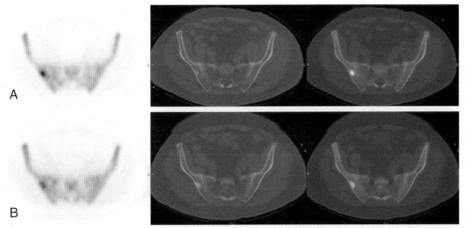

Fig. 6.20 Sclerotic metastases usually show increased activity with technetium-99m (Tc-99m) methylene diphosphonate (MDP) and F-18 sodium fluoride (F-18 NaF) positron emission tomography (PET) when active, and this uptake will decrease in response to treatment. The treated lesion will show increasing sclerosis on CT. Care must be taken because uptake may be more intense with sodium fluoride than on bone scan. (A) Marked activity in a sclerotic right iliac metastasis from prostate cancer. (B) Follow-up images 6 months later show that despite some enlargement, once treated, uptake decreases in intensity from partial response. However, multiple new lesions were identified, as seen in the sacrum, from overall disease progression.

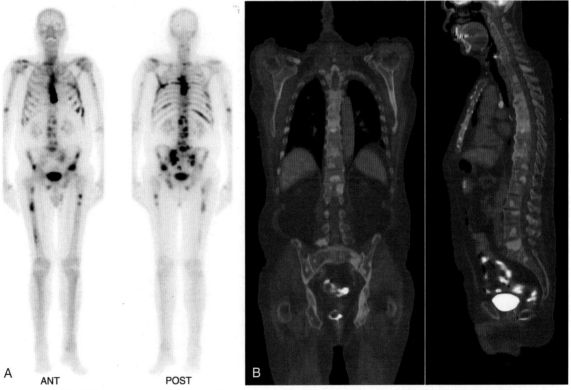

Fig. 6.21 Diffuse prostate metastatic disease shows marked technetium-99m (Tc-99m) methylene diphosphonate (MDP) activity (A) on whole-body bone-scan images. (B) Fluorine-18 fluorodeoxyglucose (F-18 FDG) positron emission tomography with CT (PET/CT) performed 2 weeks later shows largely absent activity in the sclerotic lesions, with only a few FDG-avid foci seen. When prostate cancer becomes aggressive and no longer controlled with hormone-blocking medications, then FDG PET becomes useful, showing marked uptake in lesions.

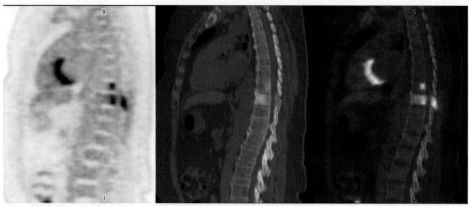

Fig. 6.22 Sagittal images of the T-spine from fluorine-18 fluorodeoxyglucose (F-18 FDG) positron emission tomography with CT (PET/CT) performed after chemotherapy for metastatic colon carcinoma show persistent active disease. Uptake is greater in a mildly sclerotic lesion, and below this, new uptake developed from disease progression in the posterior aspect of a vertebral body and its posterior elements, which are less sclerotic than treated disease anteriorly.

---

sible to discriminate diffuse metastasis. Reviewing the available radiographs on each patient will help prevent mistakes.

Flare Phenomenon: When patients have a good response to chemotherapy, they sometimes experience increased pain, and the bone scan may paradoxically worsen, with a flare of increased activity (Fig. 6.25). If these lesions are followed over 2 to 6 months, CT imaging shows increased sclerosis from an osteoblastic response as the bone begins to heal. Activity should regress by 4 to 6 months after the flare. This phenomenon reinforces the fact that tracer uptake is not in the tumor but rather in the surrounding bone.

Imaging Findings in Specific Cancers
Prostate Carcinoma
Skeletal scintigraphy is generally best for the detection of prostate cancer metastases, and until the introduction of the prostate-specific antigen (PSA) blood test, bone scan was considered the most sensitive technique for detecting bone involvement. Serum alkaline phosphatase measurement detects only half the cases detected by scintigraphy. Radiographs may be normal 30% of the time.

The likelihood of an abnormal scintigram correlates with clinical stage, Gleason score, and PSA level. In early stage I disease, scintigrams demonstrate metastases less than 5% of the time. The incidence increases to 10% in stage II disease and 20% in stage III. In patients with PSA levels less than 10 ng/mL, bone metastases are rarely found (<1% of the time). Even if the risk is lower, scintigraphy is still indicated to evaluate symptomatic patients and suspicious areas seen radiographically. With increasing PSA levels, the chance of detecting metastatic disease increases. In cases where recurrent prostate cancer is a concern, bone scan may be used to supplement the detection of soft tissue involvement performed with F-18 fluciclovine (Axumin). Although F-18 NaF PET may be useful, F-18 FDG is most often not.

Breast Carcinoma
Despite increased screening with mammography, a large number of patients with breast cancer are initially diagnosed with advanced disease. Autopsy studies have shown osseous metastases in 50% to 80% of patients with breast carcinoma. As in prostate cancer, the stage of disease correlates with the incidence of osseous metastases on bone scan: 0.5% in stage I, 2% to 3% in stage II, 8% in stage III, and 13% in stage IV. Bone scans are not generally performed in patients with stage I or II disease.

Skeletal scintigraphy is highly sensitive in breast cancer. Patients may show local invasion of the ribs or sternum or disseminated disease. Although activity in the sternum is most often benign, a high incidence of metastatic disease is seen in patients with breast cancer (>75%-80%). Abnormal soft tissue activity can be seen from tumor or surgery in the breast, in disease that is metastatic to the liver (see Fig. 6.18, *B*), and in malignant pleural effusions. F-18 FDG PET is also useful, particularly for lytic lesions and those in marrow but some blastic lesions may be harder to see.

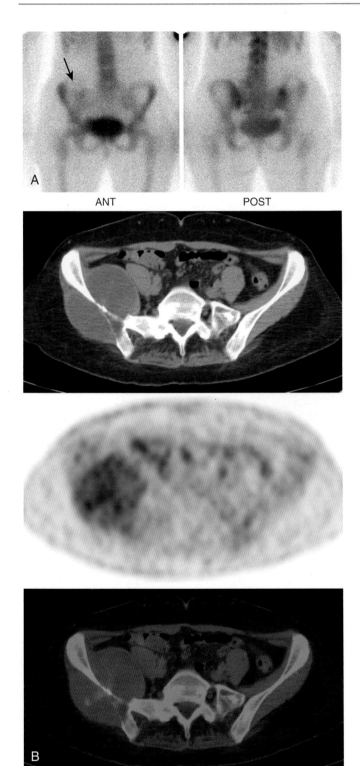

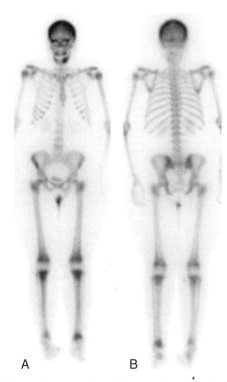

Fig. 6.24 Severe hyperparathyroidism, most commonly from severe renal failure, can sometimes result in a superscan. (A) Anterior and (B) posterior whole-body images show more advanced changes from secondary hyperparathyroidism. Note the lack of renal cortex or excreted urine. In addition to increased uptake with a smooth appearance in many bones and activity in the skull, activity in the metaphyseal regions around the knees and ankles in this 52-year-old give an appearance that could be confused with images from a child.

Fig. 6.23 (A) Bone-scan images show a barely perceptible cold lesion in the right ileum *(arrow)* corresponding to a large soft tissue mass involving bone on (B) fluorine-18 fluorodeoxyglucose (F-18 FDG) positron emission tomography with CT.

Lung Carcinoma

Although up to 50% of patients who die from a primary lung cancer have osseous metastasis at autopsy, no complete agreement exists on when to use skeletal scintigraphy. Staging is generally done with CT, surgery (including mediastinoscopy and video-assisted thoracoscopic surgery), and in some cases with F-18 FDG PET/CT. Skeletal scintigraphy is useful in a patient who develops pain during or after treatment.

Interesting patterns of disease may occur on scintigrams in lung cancer. Because these tumors can easily invade the vasculature, arterial metastases are more common. These tumor emboli can reach the distal extremities. Thus appendicular involvement is more common with aggressive lung cancer than cancer of the breast or prostate. Also, increased cortical activity, prominent in the extremities, can be seen in lung cancer as a result of hypertrophic osteoarthropathy (Figs. 6.26 and 6.27). In addition, patients exhibit a range of findings

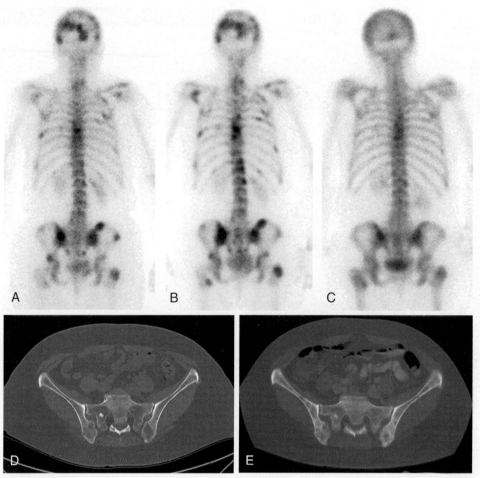

Fig. 6.25 Flare phenomena on bone scan. (A) Metastatic lesions in a patient with breast cancer appear to progress during therapy on (B) bone scan 4 months later. However, this does not represent actual worsening disease, and marked improvement is seen (C) on a scan after 6 months. Pelvic CT images obtained at the time of the first bone scan (D) show lytic lesions initially but fairly diffuse sclerosis on a follow-up CT (E) performed after the third bone scan, corresponding to treatment response.

on physical examination, including clubbing of the fingers. Although lung adenocarcinoma is most commonly the cause of this change, other cardiopulmonary etiologies and occasionally hepatic and gastrointestinal disorders can cause similar findings (Box 6.9).

Neuroblastoma

Neuroblastoma has a neural crest origin and is the most common solid tumor to metastasize to bone in children. Tc-99m MDP scintigraphy is twice as sensitive as radiographs on a lesion-by-lesion basis. MR is better than bone scan for determining lesion extent. Iodine-123 metaiodo-benzyl-guanidine (I-123 MIBG) scan is more sensitive than bone scan for metastases, although the combination of MIBG and bone scan gives the highest sensitivity. Although data are more limited on the use of gallium-68 (Ga-68) dotatate, the somatostatin receptor PET-imaging agent used for neuroendocrine tumor imaging, it has shown good results in neuroblastoma.

Lesions are typically multifocal and occur in the metaphyses. However, involvement in the skull, vertebrae, ribs, and pelvis is also common. Early involvement may be symmetrical and therefore difficult to diagnose on the bone scan because of the normal intense activity in the ends of growing bones. A unique characteristic of neuroblastoma is the avidity of Tc-99m diphosphonates for the primary tumor (Fig. 6.28). Approximately 30% to 50% of primary tumors are demonstrated scintigraphically. Occasionally, neuroblastomas are discovered in children undergoing radionuclide imaging to evaluate another condition.

Other Tumors

Numerous other tumors metastasize to bone. The sensitivity for renal cell carcinoma is low and best assessed by MR or CT. F-18 FDG PET/CT can be useful, but sensitivity is also lower, in the range of 50% to 70%. Likewise, thyroid cancer is rarely detected on skeletal scintigraphy and is better evaluated with iodine-131 (I-131) or, if noniodine avid, F-18 FDG PET. Gastrointestinal tract and gynecological cancers do not commonly metastasize to bone early in their courses. As a result of longer survival and control of local and regional metastases that usually cause death, bone metastases can manifest.

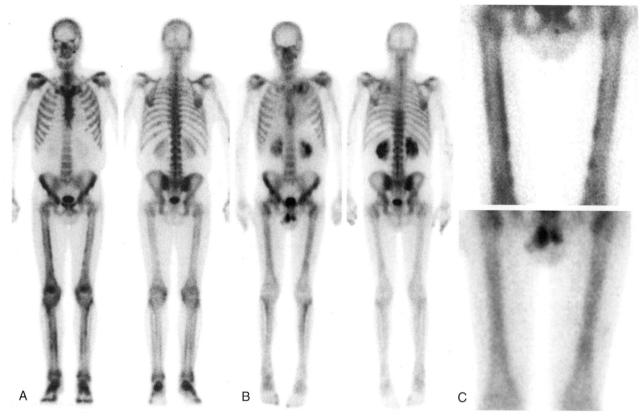

Fig. 6.26 Hypertrophic osteoarthropathy in a patient with bronchogenic lung carcinoma. (A) Whole-body scintigrams reveal classic uptake in the periosteal region of the long bones. (B) Follow-up 9 months later shows increased activity in a treated left apical lung mass. Radiation therapy changes of decreased uptake in the upper thoracic spine are seen. With successful treatment, the findings of hypertrophic osteoarthropathy have resolved. (C) Spot views of the femurs more clearly show the abnormal uptake *(upper)* that later resolves *(lower)*.

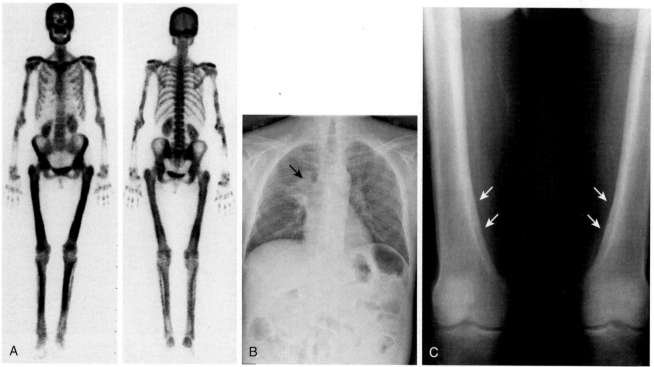

Fig. 6.27 Florid hypertrophic osteoarthropathy. (A) Bones of the upper and lower extremities are diffusely involved, as are the clavicles, mandible, and skull. Although the pattern may be confusing, the patient did not have skeletal metastatic disease. Involvement of the extremities is one clue. (B) Chest radiograph reveals a bronchogenic carcinoma in the right upper lobe involving the right hilum. (C) Radiograph of the femurs shows characteristic periosteal new bone bilaterally on both the medial and lateral aspects of the femoral shaft.

Primary Bone Tumors

Malignant Tumors

Sarcomas of the Bone. Osteosarcoma is the most common primary skeletal malignancy after multiple myeloma and is particularly common at the ends of long bones in children (Figs. 6.29 and 6.30). Rarely, it occurs as a multifocal process and occasionally can occur as an extraosseous tumor. Metastases frequently develop in the lungs, although in approximately 15% they can occur in the bones before being detected in the lungs.

After osteosarcoma, the most common primary bone tumor in children is Ewing sarcoma. Approximately 25% of tumors arise in soft tissues rather than bone. At diagnosis, 25% have metastases. Metastatic lesions involve the lungs in 50%, bones in 25%, and marrow in 20%. Chondrosarcoma tends to be more common in adults and ranks third among all primary bone

neoplasms, after multiple myeloma and osteosarcoma. Chondrosarcoma can present in several ways and may originate as either a primary tumor or a secondary tumor from degeneration of a benign lesion.

Primary malignant bone tumors such as osteosarcoma, Ewing sarcoma, and chondrosarcoma have avid uptake of the bone-seeking radiopharmaceuticals. Bone scan tends to overestimate the extent of tumor but can identify skip lesions in osteosarcoma or the involvement of other bones. In addition, both thallium-201 (Tl-201) and Tc-99m sestamibi have been used for sarcoma imaging. They may help determine whether the primary tumor is high or low grade, can serve as a baseline to evaluate response to therapy, and may show better definition of tumor margin. However, MR is the primary modality for osteosarcoma evaluation, providing detailed anatomical information and allowing assessment of soft tissue involvement. CT is generally used for the surveillance of lung metastases. In addition to the detection of osseous metastases, the occasional polyostotic tumor would be missed without a whole-body survey of some kind (Fig. 6.31). Increasingly, however, that role also may be filled by F-18 FDG PET-CT, which can be used during staging or for restaging and assessment of therapeutic response.

Multiple Myeloma. The most common primary bone tumor in adults is multiple myeloma. It is a tumor of the marrow and typically involves the vertebrae, pelvis, ribs, and skull. Radiographs may show only osteopenia or a permeative pattern that can be confused with metastatic disease. Although bone scan will show 46% to 65% of the lesions as areas of decreased and sometimes increased uptake, this is lower than the 75% to 91% sensitivity of radiographs. This likely relates to the lack of reactive bone formation in response to the lesions. Although patients are often screened by CT (or radiographic

---

BOX 6.9   Causes of Hypertrophic Osteoarthropathy

Pulmonary	Hepatic
Adenocarcinoma of lung (up to 53% of cases)	Cirrhosis
Mesothelioma	Hepatopulmonary syndrome
Cystic fibrosis	Biliary atresia
Interstitial lung disease	
	Bowel
Cardiac	Inflammatory bowel disease
Cyanotic heart disease	Amebic dysentery
Myoma	Colonic polyposis
Subacute bacterial endocarditis	Esophageal cancer
Aortic graft infection	

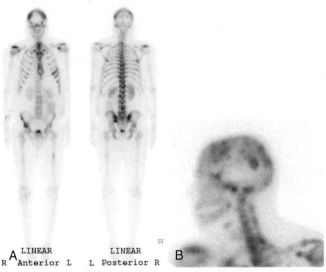
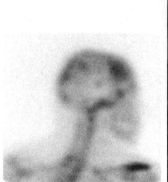
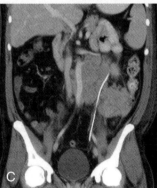

Fig. 6.28 Neuroblastoma metastases commonly spread to bone. Although iodine-123 metaiodo-benzyl-guanidine (I-123 MIBG) is more sensitive, technetium-99m (Tc-99m) methylene diphosphonate (MDP) can complement results and is more sensitive than x-rays. (A) Bone-scan images in a patient with bone metastases in the femur and skull (B) also showed radiotracer accumulation in the primary abdominal tumor in the left lower quadrant. (C) Coronal enhanced CT image shows the large primary tumor, a soft tissue mass lying between the aorta and left ureter.

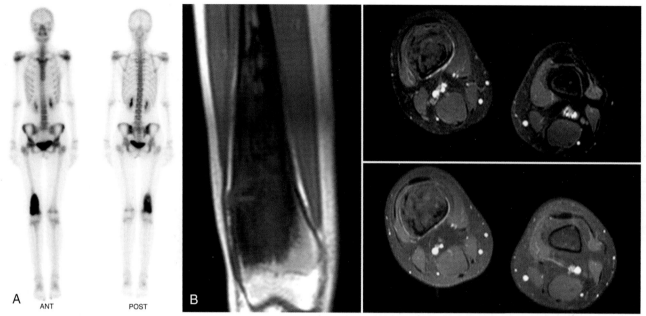

Fig. 6.29 Osteosarcoma typically shows high levels of technetium-99m (Tc-99m) methylene diphosphonate (MDP) uptake, as in this case involving the right lower femur (A). Magnetic resonance (MR) imaging is key to the evaluation of osteosarcoma. (B) On coronal T1-weighted images *(left)*, the low-signal lesion corresponds to the bone-scan changes. Axial fast spin-echo fat saturation images show tumor enhancement when comparing the lesion precontrast *(top right)* and postcontrast *(bottom right)*.

skeletal survey), MR has a positive predictive value of 88%, and when F-18 FDG PET/CT is additionally performed, this further increases to nearly 100%. In some cases, PET/CT alone can be used because it allows rapid assessment of the entire body, including the detection of any soft tissue involvement (Fig. 6.32).

Leukemia and Lymphoma. Bone scan plays a very limited role in the evaluation of leukemia. Patients with leukemia imaged with Tc-99m MDP may show focal increased uptake in areas of marrow infiltration. In blast crisis, diffusely increased uptake that is greater at the ends of the long bones may be present.

Hodgkin disease will involve the skeleton approximately one-third of the time, and bone scan may show focal or diffuse uptake of Tc-99m MDP. Skeletal scintigraphy is less useful in non-Hodgkin lymphoma. In general, lymphoma is best evaluated with F-18 FDG PET/CT and CT.

Histiocytosis. The sensitivity of bone scan varies with the spectrum of disease in histiocytosis. Although uptake is reliably seen in eosinophilic granuloma, detection of histiocytosis is limited, with lesions seen from one-third to two-thirds of the time. Frequently, decreased uptake is encountered.

Benign Bone Tumors

Usually, benign bone tumors are characterized by their radiographic appearance and typically are not positive with bone scan. However, some benign tumors have intense uptake that can be confused with malignancy. These include osteoid osteomas, giant-cell tumors, and fibrous dysplasia. Other tumors may show a characteristic pattern, such as a peripheral rim of activity

around a cold central area in aneurismal bone cyst. Benign bone tumors are variable in appearance; selected benign bone tumors are listed in Table 6.3.

Osteoid osteoma classically presents in adolescents and young adults as severe pain at night. Commonly occurring in the proximal femur and spine, the lesions may be difficult to detect with conventional radiography. The diagnosis on radiographs can be made if a central lucent nidus is seen surrounded by sclerosis (Fig. 6.33). Skeletal scintigraphy is very sensitive, and the lesion will show increased uptake (Fig. 6.34). SPECT adds to this sensitivity and is particularly useful in the spine. Surgeons can use an intraoperative probe to localize the lesion with its increased activity. However, CT and MR have largely eliminated the need for the bone scan.

Bone islands rarely accumulate Tc-99m MDP, so bone scan may be useful in assessing an atypical bone island on radiographs. If the sclerotic lesion on radiograph does not show increased activity, it is unlikely to be malignant.

Osteochondromas, common cartilage-containing benign tumors, may show variable uptake that diminishes as the skeleton matures. Rarely, osteochondromas will show malignant transformation, usually into a chondrosarcoma. This degeneration occurs less than 1% to 5% of the time in a solitary lesion but more frequently in hereditary multiple osteochondromatosis (hereditary multiple exostoses). Although bone scan can exclude malignancy if no increased uptake is seen, the presence of increased activity does not differentiate benign from malignant lesions. Any new uptake in a lesion that previously had none is suspicious. Osteochondromas are usually best evaluated with CT and MR.

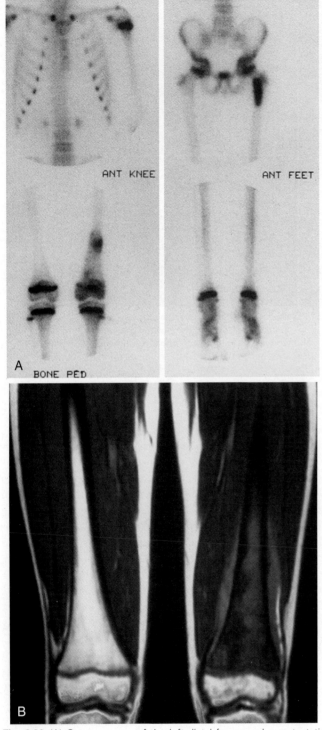

Fig. 6.30 (A) Osteosarcoma of the left distal femur and a metastatic lesion in the left proximal femur. (B) Coronal T1-weighted magnetic resonance imaging (MRI) reveals superior anatomical information about the osseous and soft tissue extent of the tumor. However, it missed the second lesion that was out of the field of view.

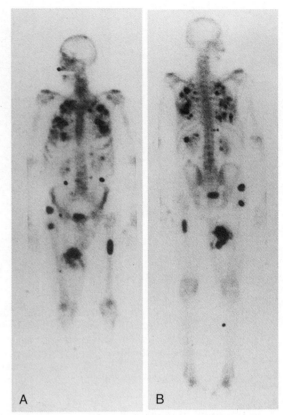

Fig. 6.31 Osteosarcoma arising in the right medial thigh shows widely disseminated metastases to bone and extraosseous locations in lung and soft tissues on (A) anterior and (B) posterior bone scan. This study is a dramatic example of the ability of skeletal scintigraphy to survey the entire body.

Enchondromas usually present as a cystic lesion in the hands or a sclerotic area reminiscent of a bone infarct elsewhere. They are benign but can degenerate into a malignant tumor. This degeneration is more common in multiple enchondromatosis (Ollier disease). Bone scan may help identify multiple lesions, but the role is otherwise very limited.

Fibrous Dysplasia. Numerous bone dysplasias demonstrate increased skeletal tracer uptake. Fibrous dysplasia is the most commonly encountered of these and may be monostotic or polyostotic (Fig. 6.35), typically with activity levels rivaling that seen in Paget disease. Distinguishing features are the younger patient age and different patterns of involvement. When Paget involves a long bone, it invariably extends to at least one end of the bone, whereas fibrous dysplasia frequently does not involve the epiphysis. Other dysplasias associated with increased tracer uptake are listed in Box 6.10.

Metabolic Bone Disease

Metabolic bone diseases cause altered bone structure, mineralization, and/or mass. The most common of these disorders is osteoporosis. Other disorders include renal osteodystrophy, hyperparathyroidism, vitamin D deficiency osteomalacia, and Paget disease.

Paget Disease

Paget disease is often included in the metabolic bone disease category, although mechanisms causing this disorder are not entirely understood, with genetic and environmental causes

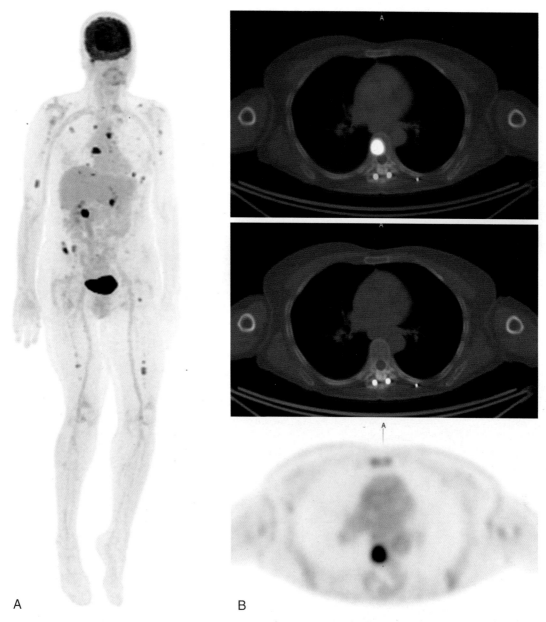

A   B

Fig. 6.32 Markedly positive multiple myeloma lesions on fluorine-18 fluorodeoxyglucose (F-18 FDG) positron emission tomography with CT (PET/CT). (A) Maximal-intensity projection image shows numerous active lesions in the bone. Because the bone scan is often negative, patients have been routinely assessed by radiographic skeletal survey and CT. However, PET is clearly useful, showing uptake before changes on CT, as seen here on single-photon emission computed tomography with CT (SPECT/CT) images (B) with fused *(top)*, CT *(middle)*, and PET *(bottom)*.

proposed. Typically, a chronic disease of the elderly, patients have areas of focal excessive bone remodeling leading to overgrowth and deformity. Patients may experience pain, arthritis, and neurological symptoms related to changes in the bone. Congestive heart failure can occur, and rarely (1%) patients develop osteosarcomas.

The disease has three phases: the early resorptive, mixed middle, and final sclerotic phases. The diagnosis usually can be made by radiographs, which reveal lytic lesions in early cases and coarsened, expanded bones as the disease progresses to the final phase. Although CT and MR can be used to assess complications, bone scan is highly sensitive and useful to evaluate the extent of disease. Increased uptake is seen in all stages of untreated disease, although sensitivity is lower in the early lytic stage. Activity decreases with effective therapy. In addition, the patterns of Paget disease must be recognized because it may be found incidentally because many patients are asymptomatic and undiagnosed.

The scintigraphic appearance is striking, with intensely increased tracer localization (Figs. 6.36 and 6.37). Bone often

TABLE 6.3   Benign Bone Lesions on Skeletal Scintigraphy

Etiology	Malignant Potential	Comments
Intense Uptake		
Aneurysmal bone cyst	No	Donut-sign pattern
Chondroblastoma	Almost always benign	Positive bone scan does not diagnose malignancy
Giant-cell tumor	10%	
Fibrous dysplasia	<1%	May be difficult to differentiate from Paget on scan
Osteoma	No	Gardner syndrome Osteoblastoma >2 cm
Osteoid osteoma	No	Pain, especially at night, relieved with nonsteroidal painkillers
Isointense/Mild Uptake		
Bone island	No	
Enchondroma	For solitary <5% Multiple enchondromas 50% lifetime risk	Common in hands and feet, especially phalanges, also in long bones with proximal humerus frequent; rare in flat bones; most lesions have chondroid matrix, and many have calcifications Multiple occur in syndrome: enchondromatosis No cortical disruption unless malignant Chondrosarcoma is most common type of cancer
Nonossifying fibroma	No	
Variable Uptake		
Osteochondroma	<1%	
Hereditary multiple exostosis	5%–25%	Autosomal dominant condition with multiple osteochondromas
Eosinophilic granuloma	No, but may cause multisystem disease	May be monostotic or polyostotic; one of histiocytosis group of diseases Bone scan negative 30%, F-18 FDG PET sensitive
Hemangioma	No	Usually negative on bone scan If activity seen, CT pattern diagnostic-prominent trabeculae
Low Uptake		
Unicameral bone cyst	No	

CT, Computed tomography; *F-18 FDG,* fluorine-18 fluorodeoxyglucose; *PET,* positron emission tomography.

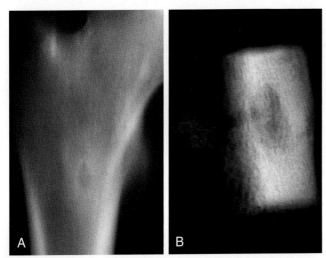

Fig. 6.33 Osteoid osteoma on radiograph. (A) Conventional tomogram of the right proximal femur reveals a characteristic radiolucent nidus surrounded by sclerotic bone. (B) Specimen radiograph confirms the complete excision of the nidus.

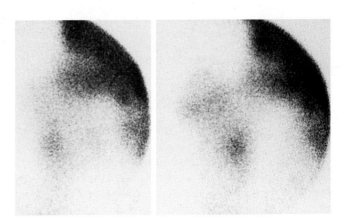

Fig. 6.34 Osteoid osteoma on magnified pinhole images. Internal and external rotation pinhole spot views of the proximal femur in a patient with suspected osteoid osteoma. An area of abnormally increased uptake demonstrated just lateral to the lesser trochanter confirms the clinical suspicion.

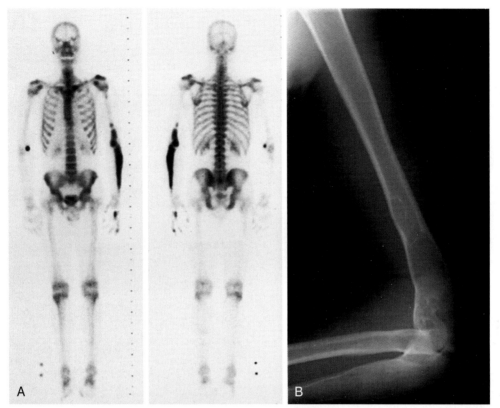

Fig. 6.35 Fibrous dysplasia. (A) Uptake is markedly increased in the distal humerus, most of the forearm, and focal areas in the hand. (B) Corresponding radiograph of the left elbow reveals characteristic expansile lesions of fibrous dysplasia.

BOX 6.10   Bone Dysplasias Associated With Increased Skeletal Tracer Uptake

Fibrous dysplasia
Osteogenesis imperfecta
Osteopetrosis
Progressive diaphyseal dysplasia (Engelmann disease)
Hereditary multiple diaphyseal sclerosis (Ribbing disease)
Melorheostosis

---

appears expanded. When the tibia is involved, bowing is often seen, and in the spine, fractures can happen. The pelvis is the most commonly involved site, followed by the spine, skull, femur, scapula, tibia, and humerus. In osteoporosis circumscripta, a characteristic rim of increased uptake borders the lesion.

Hyperparathyroidism and Renal Osteodystrophy

Some other metabolic conditions can also cause patterns of increased scintigraphic uptake: osteomalacia, hyperparathyroidism, renal osteodystrophy, and hypervitaminosis D (Table 6.4). Although they must be recognized in order to avoid confusion with pathological conditions such as metastatic disease, bone scan has no role in the diagnosis and management of these processes.

Inadequate osseous mineralization from deficiencies in vitamin D, calcium, or phosphate results in osteomalacia. Radiographically, bones have a washed-out, chalky appearance, with decreased trabeculae. Although adults are affected, findings in the growing skeleton, known as rickets, are most striking. Changes at the growth plates (fraying, widening, cupping) of

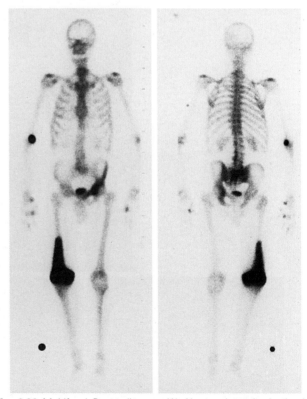

Fig. 6.36 Multifocal Paget disease. (A) Abnormal uptake in the left hemipelvis, upper lumbar spine, and, to a lesser extent, right hip in a patient with Paget disease. When Paget disease involves the axial bones, it must be differentiated from metastatic disease by the location and bone expansion. Radiographic correlation will show the typical coarsened trabeculae. (B) When the sites are more numerous, the diagnosis is obvious based on the typical distribution of lesions.

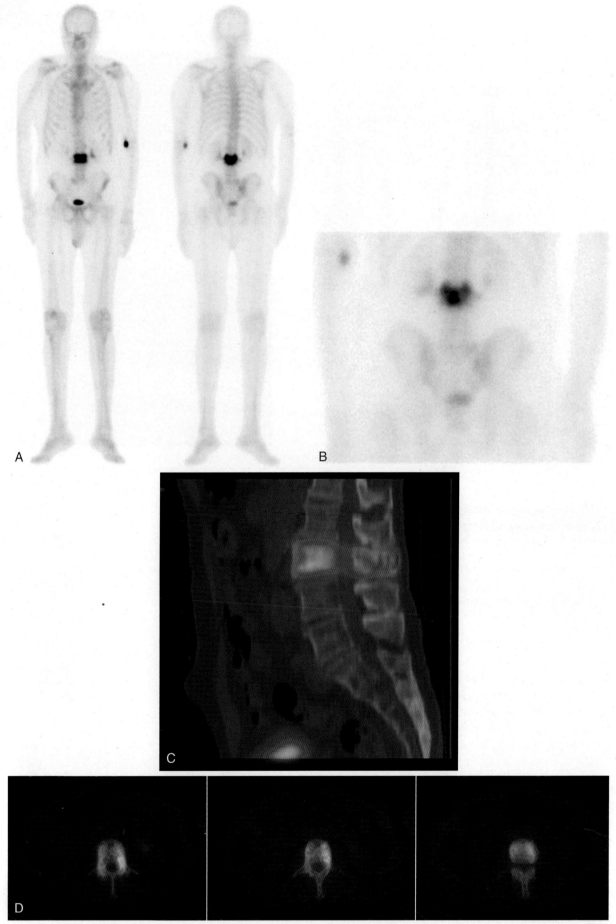

Fig. 6.37 Monostotic Paget disease of the spine in a man with prostate cancer and back pain. (A) Whole-body bone scan shows the intense activity, with the bone appearing more expanded than would be expected from metastasis. (B) The shape on the spot view is the "Mickey Mouse" sign based on its shape. (C) Fused single-photon emission computed tomography with computed tomography (SPECT/CT) sagittal and (D) axial images show the underlying sclerotic and lytic changes and expansive character.

TABLE 6.4 Metabolic Bone Disorders

Osteoporosis

Primary (idiopathic)		
Senile, postmenopausal		
Secondary		
	Disuse	
	Drugs	Corticosteroids, chemotherapy, anticonvulsants
Endocrine		Hyperthyroidism, primary hyperparathyroidism, Cushing disease, hypogonadism

Osteomalacia

Vitamin D	Vitamin D deficiency, hereditary disorders of vitamin D metabolism
Decreased calcium	Calcium malabsorption, inadequate intake, calcitonin-secreting tumors
Phosphate loss	Renal tubular disease, hemodialysis, transplant
Other	Liver disease, phenytoin, prematurity

Hyperparathyroidism

Primary	Parathyroid adenoma, parathyroid hyperplasia
Secondary	Chronic renal insufficiency, phosphate metabolism abnormalities, parathyroid hyperplasia
Tertiary	Autonomous parathyroid glands from long-standing secondary hyperparathyroidism
Renal osteodystrophy	Chronic renal failure
Hypoparathyroidism	Iatrogenic loss/damage parathyroid glands during thyroidectomy; pseudohypoparathyroidism genetic end-organ resistance

Metal Toxicities

Aluminum-induced bone disease	
Fluorosis	
Heavy metal poisoning	

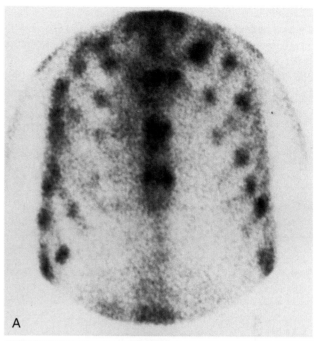

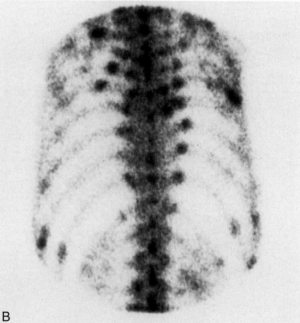

Fig. 6.38 Osteomalacia. Anterior **(A)** and posterior **(B)** views. The patient was referred to rule out metastatic disease. The unusually large number of rib lesions raised the suspicion of metabolic bone disease rather than metastases.

the proximal humerus, distal femur, distal tibia, and distal forearm and findings such as beading at the costochondral junctions are common. Bone scan shows a generalized increased uptake in the axial skeleton, including the skull and mandible. Uptake in the sternum is often increased in a "tie" pattern, with lines at the segmental junctions. Pseudofractures, beading of the costochondral junctions, and real fractures are common (Fig. 6.38).

Hyperparathyroidism may be primary, as from a parathyroid adenoma secreting parathormone (PTH); secondary, as a response to the hypocalcemia of chronic renal disease; or tertiary, when PTH is secreted by autonomously functioning tissue. Patients with uncomplicated primary hyperparathyroidism usually have normal bone scans. In more severe cases, any form of hyperparathyroidism can lead to increased bone turnover and increased activity (Box 6.11). As noted previously, severe hyperparathyroidism may

cause a markedly increased ratio of skeleton to soft tissue, poor renal visualization, and high levels of uptake in the axial skeleton and proximal long bones in a superscan pattern (Fig. 6.39, *A*; see also Fig. 6.24), seen in metastatic disease (see Fig. 6.3). In other cases, an unusual pattern can occur, with diffuse uptake in the skull, mandible, sternum, and periarticular regions (see Fig. 6.39, *B*). These same findings may be seen to a varying degree in differing types hyperparathyroidism and osteomalacia, and the conditions may be present in the same patient (Fig. 6.40). The bone scan in long-standing renal osteodystrophy and secondary hyperparathyroidism often has the most extreme appearance.

Extraskeletal uptake is not uncommon as a result of an increased ratio of serum calcium to phosphate. In hyperparathyroidism, especially with renal disease, a classic pattern of soft tissue uptake is seen in the lungs, stomach, and kidneys as a result of imbalances in calcium and phosphate. Other soft tissues may also be involved, such as the region of the heart (Fig. 6.41). Uptake in the heart or pericardium can occur for many other reasons, as can soft tissue uptake in the soft tissues in general (Box 6.12).

Skeletal Trauma

Although bone scan is highly sensitive for fracture (Fig. 6.42), radiographs, CT, and MR are usually used when acute fractures are suspected. MR is not only sensitive but also provides information on surrounding soft tissues. When patients cannot undergo MR, when MR and CT findings are negative, or when

BOX 6.11 Distribution of Increased Skeletal Uptake in Hyperparathyroidism

Diffuse in axial and proximal long bones ("superscan")
Periarticular
Skull
Mandible, fascial bones
Costochondral junctions
Sternum
Lungs
Stomach

a precise area of concern is not known, a bone scan may be used to detect occult fracture.

Acute fractures generally result in a three-phase positive scintigram, with chronic or partially healed fractures typically positive only on delayed images. Approximately 80% of fractures can be visualized by 24 hours after trauma. Ninety-five percent of fractures are positive after 3 days, and in patients under the age of 65, essentially all fractures are positive by this time (Table 6.5). Advanced age and debilitation are factors contributing to delayed visualization of fractures. The maximum degree of fracture uptake occurs 7 or more days after trauma, and delayed imaging in this time frame is recommended in difficult or equivocal cases. Occasionally, decreased uptake is seen acutely as a result of compromised vascular supply (Fig. 6.43).

The time a fracture takes to return to normal on the bone scan depends on location, stability, and the degree of damage to the skeleton. Approximately 60% to 80% of nondisplaced, uncomplicated fractures revert to normal in 1 year, and more than 95% revert in 3 years (Table 6.6). However, in many instances, displaced fractures remained positive indefinitely. Structural deformity and posttraumatic arthritis were the most common reasons for prolonged positive studies. Patients undergoing metastatic skeletal survey should be routinely asked about prior trauma. This includes prior radiation therapy (which can cause decreased uptake chronically) and surgery likely to cause fracture (e.g., thoracotomy) or if bone resection/amputation occurred.

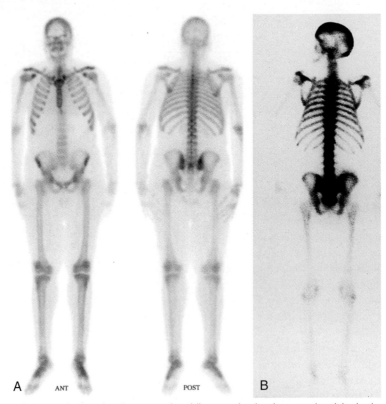

Fig. 6.39 Renal failure and secondary hyperparathyroidism can lead to increased activity in the bones, with variable patterns. (A) The "superscan" pattern can vary, appearing very homogeneous and normal, although the distal long bones are more clearly seen than usual, and the joints appear prominent. (B) In other cases, changes include significant activity in the skull, mandible, and sternum (the mandible activity is also noted in Fig. 6.24). The higher soft tissue background is often seen with poorly functioning kidneys.

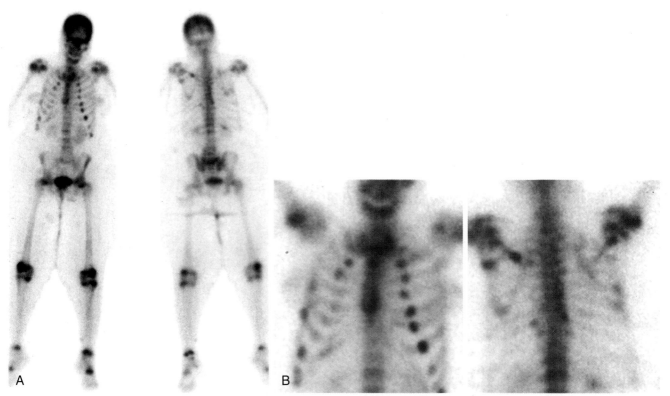

Fig. 6.40 Renal osteodystrophy can result in various changes from osteomalacia and hyperparathyroidism. Whole-body (A) and spot images (B) of a patient with long-standing renal failure show classic skeletal changes of severe renal osteodystrophy. Abnormal activity is seen in the face and skull and the distal ends of the long bones. The rib tip activity has been called the rachitic "rosary bead" configuration. Focal uptake in the left scapula was a fracture, although brown tumors can have a similar appearance.

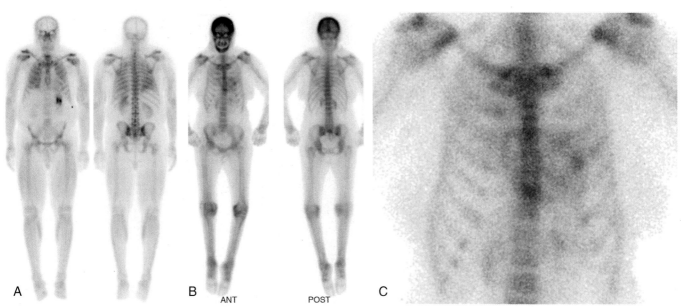

Fig. 6.41 Soft tissue uptake can occur in secondary or primary hyperparathyroidism. (A) Whole-body views of a patient with severe renal failure show diffusely increased uptake in the lungs, stomach, and heart. (B) Whole-body bone scan from an elderly patient with chronic renal failure, anemia, chronic heart failure, and signs of hyperparathyroidism shows diffuse activity in the skull and mandible and tiny, faint areas on each side of the T-spine from atrophic native kidneys. Patchy uptake is also seen in the region of the heart (C). This can be seen not only as a result of hyperparathyroidism but also myocardial infarction, cardioversion, heart failure, and amyloidosis.

Child Abuse

The high sensitivity of skeletal scintigraphy would seem to make it an ideal survey test in cases of suspected child abuse. However, in practice, a radiographic skeletal survey is more sensitive than bone scintigraphy because of its ability to demonstrate old fractures that have healed, subtle fractures along growth plates with their normally high levels of uptake, and calvarial fractures that may be difficult to see in young children on bone scan. Scintigraphy is often reserved for cases of suspected child abuse when radiographs are unrevealing. In these cases, symmetrical positioning of the patient is critical.

Complex Regional Pain Syndrome

Complex regional pain syndrome, previously known as reflex sympathetic dystrophy, is an exaggerated response to injury and immobilization with sensory, motor, and autonomic features. Although the presentation is variable, patients

TABLE 6.5 Time Required for Bone Scan to Turn Positive After Fracture

Time (days)	Percentage Positive Bone Scan (All Ages)	Percentage Positive Bone Scan in Patients <65 Years
1	80	95
3	95	100
7	98	100

Data from Matin P. The appearance of bone scans following fractures, including immediate and long-term studies. *J Nucl Med.* 1979;20(12):1227–1231.

BOX 6.12 Causes of Soft Tissue Uptake on Delayed Bone-Scan Images

Traumatic
Surgery, healing hematoma
Rhabdomyolysis
Myositis ossificans
Heterotopic ossification adjacent to fracture/joint replacement and in hemiplegia

Malignant
Metastases
Malignant effusion
Malignant ascites

Cardiac disease
Pericarditis
Myocardial infarct
Amyloidosis
Congestive heart failure
Cardioversion or post-resuscitation

Infarct
Hemorrhagic infarct
Infarcted spleen (sickle cell disease)

Metabolic
Secondary and tertiary hyperparathyroidism,
Active and treated long-standing renal osteodystrophy
Primary hyperparathyroidism

Artifact
Colloid formation (poor radiopharmaceutical preparation)
Free sodium pertechnetate or "free tech"
Recent prior nuclear medicine exam

Infection/inflammation

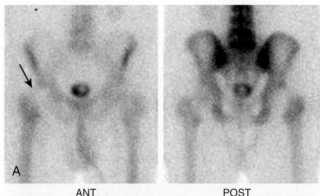
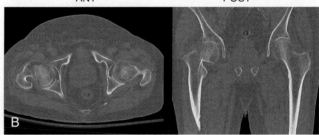

Fig. 6.43 Planar images of the pelvis (A) in an elderly man with hip pain after a fall in the hospital show decreased uptake in the right femoral head and neck *(arrow)* corresponding to a displaced femoral neck fracture in osteoporotic bone on CT (B).

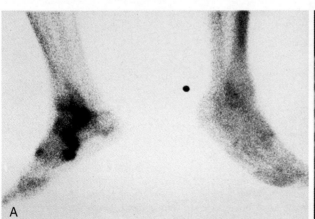
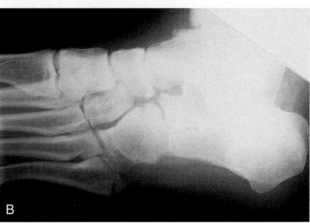

Fig. 6.42 Trauma to the distal extremity. (A) Skeletal scintigram of a patient who had sustained direct trauma to the right foot and ankle reveals multiple focal areas of abnormal tracer accumulation from fracture. (B) The radiograph illustrates fractures of the base of the fifth metatarsal and lateral cuneiform.

TABLE 6.6 Skeletal Scintigraphy in Trauma: Time Course to Normal After Fracture 1		
FRACTURE TYPE AND SITE	**NORMAL BONE SCANS (%)**	
Nonmanipulated and Closed Fractures	**1 Year**	**3 Years**
Vertebra	59	97
Long bone	64	95
Rib	79	100
All fractures*	<1 year	2-5 years	>5 years
All sites	30	62	84

Modified from Kim HR, Thrall JH, Keyes JW Jr. Skeletal scintigraphy following incidental trauma. *Radiology.* 1979;130(2):447–451.

typically have pain, edema, and muscle wasting in an affected extremity.

Scintigraphic findings are variable depending on the stage of disease. The classic pattern of unilaterally increased flow and blood-pool activity with increased periarticular uptake through a whole region on delayed images is seen less than 50% of the time but provides the highest diagnostic accuracy. Early disease (up to 5-6 months) usually shows increased blood flow (Fig. 6.44), but blood flow may be normal or decreased later in the course of the disease. The periarticular uptake on delayed images is found in most cases (>95%), although specificity is lower if this finding is seen without the increased blood flow. Infection and arthritis could cause false-positive results. Some variants have been found, including cold areas or decreased uptake in some adults. Children often have normal or decreased uptake.

Stress Fractures

A significant change in activity level or a repetitive activity may lead to injury to the bone. This may be seen in "shin splints," a term applied generically to describe stress-related leg soreness along the medial or posteromedial aspect of the tibia. In nuclear medicine, the term is used for a specific combination of clinical and scintigraphic findings: peripheral, linear tracer uptake is seen on the scintigram, typically involving a large portion of the middle to distal tibia (Fig. 6.45). If the process causing injury is allowed to continue to the point of overt fracture, healing predictably takes several months or more, compared with the several weeks required for healing of an early stress reaction (Table 6.7). Therefore prompt diagnosis and appropriate change in activity are critical. Exquisitely sensitive, skeletal scintigraphy reveals characteristic intense uptake at the fracture site ranging from the earlier oval or fusiform uptake to activity traversing the bone in outright fracture (Fig. 6.46). Stress fracture can become positive on all three phases of the bone scan (Fig. 6.47), and findings are often seen before radiographs reveal the cortical thickening in injury and fracture lines as disease progresses. Stress injury is not uncommonly multifocal; thus additional sites of involvement may be detected.

A phenomenon perhaps related to shin splints is activity-induced enthesopathy. In athletes, repeated microtears with subsequent healing reaction can result in increased tracer uptake at the site of tendon or ligament attachment. Osteitis pubis, plantar fasciitis, Achilles tendonitis, and some cases of pulled hamstring muscles are examples. A periosteal reaction develops at the site of stress, sometimes resulting in increased skeletal tracer localization.

Stress injuries can also occur in the spine. *Spondylolysis* occurs in the lumbar spine in the pars articularis, often seen as a result of repetitive trauma in young athletes. Most commonly the abnormality occurs at L4 to L5. In some instances, all examinations, including radiographs, MR, and planar bone scan, may be normal, but a SPECT study may reveal the pathological condition (Fig. 6.48). When available, SPECT/CT can provide an optimal assessment.

Rhabdomyolysis

Another athletic injury that is seen in this day of marathons and triathlons is rhabdomyolysis. The localization of skeletal tracers in exercise-damaged skeletal muscle is similar to the localization in damaged myocardium. Calcium buildup in damaged tissue provides a site for radionuclide deposition when combined with phosphate.

The scintigraphic pattern reflects the muscle groups undergoing injury (Fig. 6.49). In marathon runners, the most striking uptake is usually in the muscles of the thigh. Rhabdomyolysis induced by renal failure is generally diffuse. The time course of scintigraphic abnormality appears to be similar to that for acute myocardial infarction. The greatest degree of uptake is seen at 24 to 48 hours after injury. The changes resolve by 1 week.

Heterotopic Bone Formation

Heterotopic bone formation can occur in the muscle as a result of numerous conditions. It is most often a direct result of trauma to the muscle in myositis ossificans (Fig. 6.50). The appearance can vary, and lesions can even be confused with a mass from sarcoma. In such cases, typical benign calcifications may be seen on CT or x-ray.

Heterotopic ossification is a potentially serious complication in paralyzed muscles and prolonged immobilization, leading to seriously decreased mobility from severely contracted and ossified muscles. Calcifications form in the soft tissues outside the joint capsule, most commonly around the hip in quadriplegia. A three-phase bone is most sensitive for early changes, and it is also used to determine when disease has matured (and thus less likely to recur after resection). Early on, the blood flow and immediate blood-pool images will show increased activity, and as the disease progresses, uptake will increase on the delayed images. Coarse calcifications develop on CT or x-ray. The flow and blood-pool activity resolve after some weeks, and decreases are seen on delayed-phase images after a couple of months (Fig. 6.51). Activity typically returns to normal within a year.

Bone Infarction and Osteonecrosis

Necrosis of the bone has numerous causes (Box 6.13), and the appearance changes as the process evolves. Immediately after

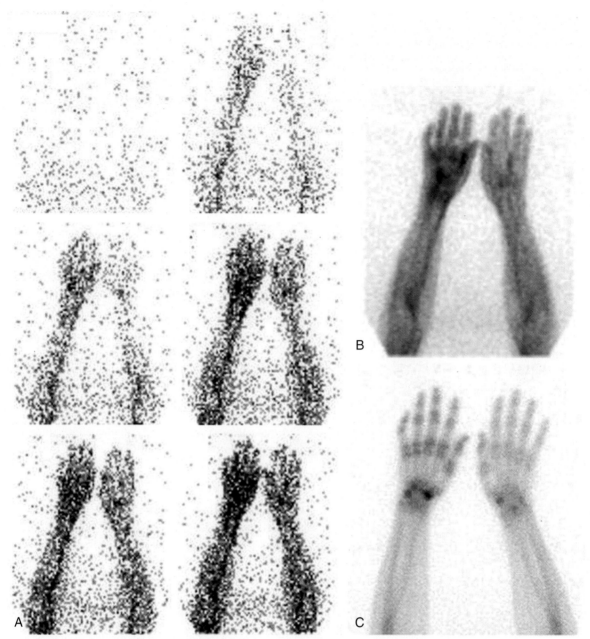

Fig. 6.44 Complex regional pain syndrome in a young patient after trauma months previously shows clearly increased blood flow (A) and blood-pool (B) activity in the left arm, with mild periarticular uptake on the delayed image (C) in the left hand on a three-phase bone scan. Activity varies but may be much more asymmetrical on delayed images.

blood supply is interrupted, newly infarcted bone appears cold, with decreased activity. In the postinfarct healing phase, osteogenesis and radiotracer activity increase at the margins of the affected area. Uptake can become intense as healing progresses, and if arthritis develops, the abnormal uptake may persist indefinitely, classically involving both sides of the joint over time.

Legg-Calvé-Perthes Disease

Most commonly affecting children between 5 and 9 years of age, with a 4:1 to 5:1 predilection for boys, Legg-Calvé-Perthes is a form of osteochondrosis that results in avascular necrosis of the capital femoral epiphysis. The precise mechanism is unknown, but the blood supply to the femoral head is especially vulnerable in the affected age group.

Magnified pinhole images with the patient in a frog-leg position can help identify abnormalities. Early in the disease, a discrete, lentiform photon-deficient area is seen in the upper outer portion of the bone (Fig. 6.52). SPECT and SPECT/CT imaging may optimally identify subtle abnormalities. As repair occurs, uptake increases peripherally, with activity then gradually filling in the defect. The increased activity persists for many months or more and may not revert to normal in severe cases.

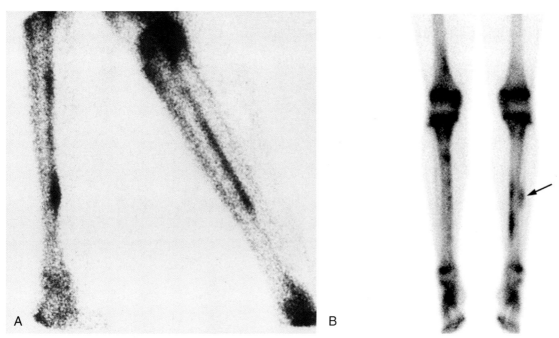

Fig. 6.45 Stress injury from repetitive trauma can occur in many locations. The forelegs are a common site, "shin splints." (A) Lateral images of the lower legs show superficial, linear activity along the posterior left tibia *(left side of image)* from stress injury. On the right, more focal activity is seen more distally, typical of a developing stress fracture. Although stress injury most often occurs in the tibia, the fibula can also be involved. (B) A frontal image shows abnormal, superficial activity in both tibias and a more focal area laterally in the left leg *(arrow)* from stress fracture in the fibula.

TABLE 6.7	Sequence of Findings in Stress Reaction and Stress Fracture			
Injury Stage	Bone Activity	Clinical Symptoms	X-Ray	Scintigram
Normal	Resorption = replacement	–	–	–
Accelerated remodeling	Resorption > replacement	+/–	–	+
Fatigue	Resorption >> replacement	+	+/–	+++
Exhaustion	Resorption >>> replacement	++	+	++++
Cortical fracture	Disruption/ attempts at repair	++++	++++	++++

Data from Roub LW, et al. Bone stress: a radionuclide imaging perspective. *Radiology.* 1979;132(2):431–438.

Osteonecrosis

Osteonecrosis of the bone can occur for many reasons, but trauma and steroids are two commonly seen etiologies. Although the pathogenesis is still debated, osteonecrosis related to steroid use is a chronic process manifested by microfractures and repair. In some cases, trauma disrupts a tenuous blood supply, such as to the proximal femur in children and the scaphoid bone of the wrist.

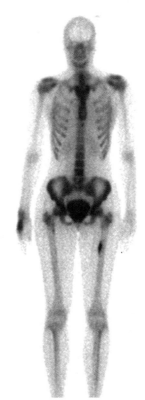

Fig. 6.46 Whole-body bone-scan images in a runner with leg pain reveal a fusiform, superficial lesion in the left medial femur from stress injury. On delayed images, uptake in the right hand is due to the injection site.

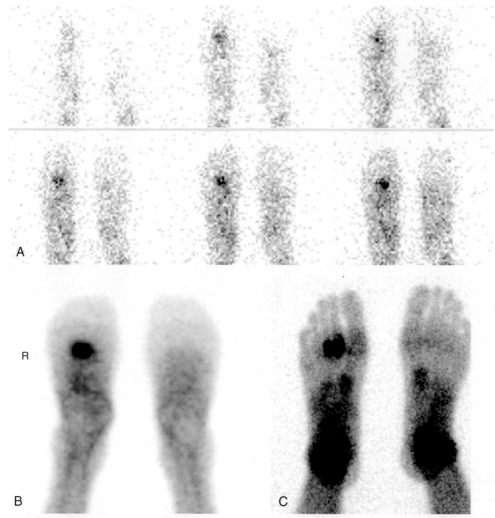

Fig. 6.47 Three-phase bone-scan images in a runner with marked focal pain in the right foot show focal increased flow (A), blood pool (B), and delayed images (C) with bone localization to the second and third right metatarsals traversing the bone, consistent with acute stress fracture. Bone scan may be positive well before radiographs.

Affected bones will initially show, in the very acute stages (<24 hours typically), decreased blood flow on bone scan, and the area of avascular necrosis will appear cold on the delayed view (Fig. 6.53). Within 1 to 3 days, blood flow typically increases as inflammation in the surrounding tissues and early remodeling begin. Many patients do not present until disease is advanced, with marked uptake on delayed bone images and collapse of the bone and sclerosis on radiographs and CT. Osteoarthritic changes in the region may include subchondral cysts and osteophyte formation in addition to the sclerosis (Fig. 6.54). Blood flow will usually normalize, but delayed uptake may persist indefinitely.

MR is currently the modality of choice for the evaluation of osteonecrosis. In addition to having a sensitivity comparable to or higher than that of bone scan, MR also provides information on the soft tissues and detailed visualization of the bony anatomy. The ability to assess articular cartilage, acetabular labral tears, and metaphyseal cysts aids in determining prognosis.

Sickle Cell Anemia

Bone scans are sometimes performed in patients with sickle cell anemia to help differentiate infarct from osteomyelitis, or they may be part of a routine metastatic disease workup in patients with cancer. Several characteristic features may be seen and are important not to confuse with other disease. Expanded marrow from the attempts to correct the anemia results in bilaterally increased calvarial activity (Fig. 6.55). In normal adults, red marrow extends only to the proximal portions of the femurs and humeri. In sickle cell anemia, the extremities may manifest marrow expansion as increased uptake near the joints (Fig. 6.56).

Changes in the spleen and kidneys are frequently present. The kidneys are frequently small and scarred or even nonvisualized, but they may be enlarged, with prominent cortical activity, in less severe or chronic cases. Avid accumulation of skeletal tracer is frequently seen in the spleen, often as a small area above the left kidney, presumably because of prior splenic infarction and calcification.

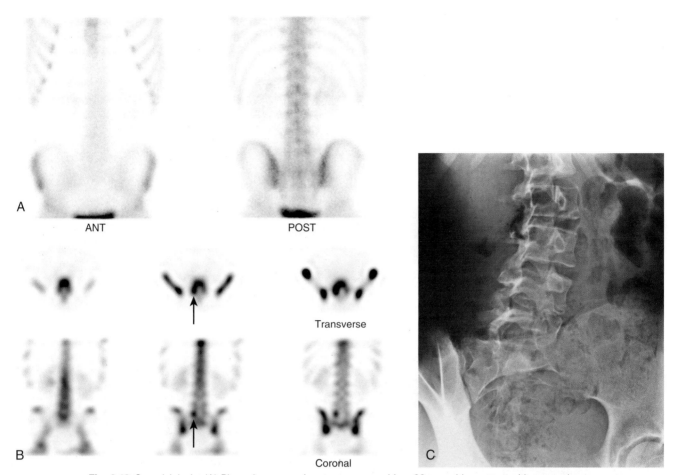

Fig. 6.48 Spondylolysis. (A) Planar bone-scan images are normal in a 20-year-old gymnast with severe low back pain and negative radiographs and magnetic resonance imaging (MRI). (B) However, transverse and coronal single-photon emission tomography (SPECT) images show focal abnormal activity in the right posterior elements of L5 to S1 *(arrow),* consistent with spondylolysis. (C) Oblique lumbar spine (LS) radiograph from a different patient shows a pars interarticularis defect at L5.

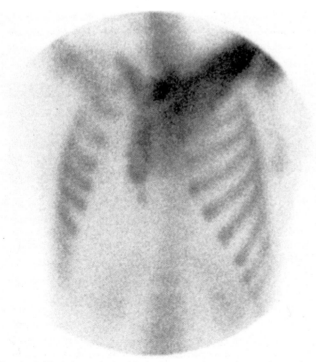

Fig. 6.49 Rhabdomyolysis. Marked pectoral muscle uptake on bone scan after injury from repetitive strenuous weight lifting.

Infarctions in bone result in both acute and long-standing changes. Cortical infarcts may appear normal on bone scan acutely. Within a few days, as healing begins, the scan typically demonstrates increased uptake. If the involvement is primarily in the marrow space, the skeletal scintigram may not reveal the extent of the lesion because it does not involve the cortex where Tc-99m MDP binds. Bone-marrow scans using Tc-99m sulfur colloid are sensitive, with cold defects appearing immediately after the infarct. As the defects from prior bone marrow infarctions persist, the significance of a photon-deficient area on marrow scanning is somewhat uncertain unless a recent baseline study is available for comparison. In these situations, MR has an advantage in its ability to distinguish acute from chronic changes.

The correlation between the marrow scan and the bone scan is also important in the differentiation of acute osteomyelitis from infarct. If the marrow shows a defect in the region of increased bone-scan activity, it is consistent with infarct. If the marrow shows no change, then any increased activity on the bone scan in an acute situation is most likely osteomyelitis.

Osteomyelitis

Osteomyelitis can involve the bone through hematogenous spread or through the direct extension of an area of cellulitis, such as in a diabetic foot ulcer. In most patients, diagnosis usually involves radiographs and enhanced MR. MR is extremely sensitive and provides a high level of detail on the joint and soft tissue structures and on the bone abnormality. Enhancement is seen as areas of increased signal between the pre- and postcontrast images, and nonspecific fluid signal will be seen in the marrow and tissues.

Areas of bone will often show cortical attenuation in the early stages when a joint is involved, and eventually destruction can occur with more extensive loss and bony deformity. Radiographs are far less sensitive but frequently performed as a rapid method of assessment. The effects of infection will cause bone loss, including cortical erosion and lucent areas of destruction.

The three-phase Tc-99m MDP bone scan is highly sensitive for acute osteomyelitis and is frequently performed in cases where MR is contraindicated, when polyostotic sites may be involved, or when the clinical findings are not well localized and the source of infection is uncertain. Bone scan is often used in the assessment of a painful joint prosthesis or in the diabetic foot. Other scintigraphic techniques can be used, including the radiolabeled white blood cell (WBC) scan with Tc-99m hexamethylpropyleneamine oxime (HMPAO) or indium-111 (In-111), gallium-67 (Ga-67), and F-18 FDG PET/CT.

In some patients, especially children, increased pressure in the marrow space or thrombosis of blood vessels results in paradoxically decreased tracer uptake and a cold or photon-deficient lesion. False-negative scintigraphic studies are unusual but

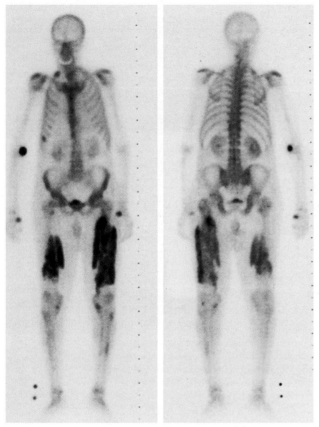

Fig. 6.50 Myositis ossificans. Anterior and posterior whole-body scintigrams with extensive myositis ossificans involvement in the legs.

BOX 6.13 Causes of Aseptic Bone Necrosis

Trauma (accidental, iatrogenic)
Drug therapy (steroids)
Hypercoagulable states
Hemoglobinopathies (sickle cell disease and variants)
After radiation therapy (orthovoltage)
Caisson disease
Osteochondrosis (pediatric age group; Legg-Calvé-Perthes disease)
Polycythemia
Leukemia
Gaucher disease
Alcoholism
Pancreatitis
Idiopathic

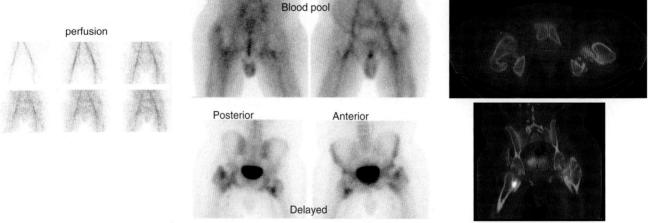

Fig. 6.51 Heterotopic ossification in the hips in a patient with spinal cord injury are seen on bone scan performed for assessment before resection. Waiting for disease to mature on bone scan can help prevent recurrence. Although blood flow (A) has already normalized, blood-pool images (B, *top*) show mild residual uptake, and moderate activity is still seen on delayed views (B, *bottom*) and posterior planar images. (C) Single-photon emission computed tomography with CT (SPECT/CT) fused (axial, *top*; coronal, *lower*) images show that the uptake lies in coarse calcifications outside of the bones and expected joint.

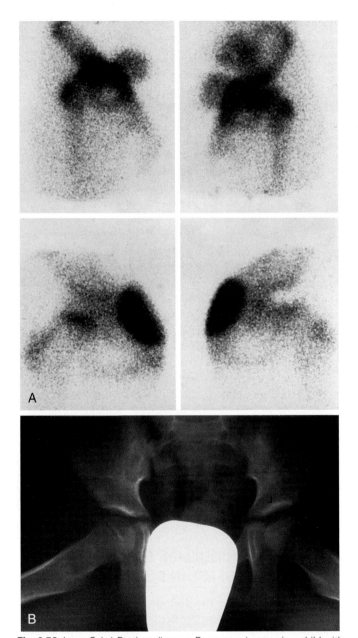

Fig. 6.52 Legg-Calvé-Perthes disease. Bone scan images in a child with a painful left hip. (A) Standard parallel-hole collimator images (Top Row) fail to show the abnormality. Pinhole images (Bottom Row) reveal the characteristic changes in the left hip, with a lentiform area of decreased uptake in the femoral epiphysis. (B) Corresponding radiograph obtained months later reveals deformity of the left femoral epiphysis, with subtle flattening, increased density, and increased distance between the epiphysis and the acetabulum.

have been reported in infants under the age of 1 year. Other causes of false-negative examinations are imaging very early in the course of disease and failure to recognize the significance of photon-deficient areas.

Bone-Scan Findings of Osteomyelitis

Although the appearance of increased activity can be expected on delayed Tc-99m MDP images (Fig. 6.57), three-phase scintigraphy is typically performed for the evaluation of

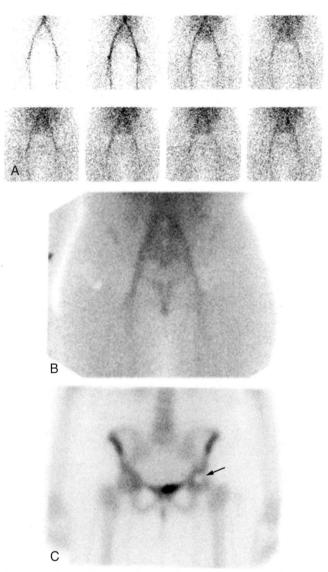

Fig. 6.53 Acute changes of avascular necrosis in the left femoral head are seen in a patient with normal blood flow (A) and blood-pool (B) activity and a focal cold spot in the lateral left epiphysis. Over time (C), increased blood flow will likely develop as collapse or sclerosis and remodeling occur.

osteomyelitis. Perfusion images help differentiate acute from more chronic disease. If arterial blood flow is not abnormal, then areas of uptake in the bones or soft tissues are the result of a more chronic process. It is important to note that the arterial flow is seen in the earliest frames of the blood-flow images, with venous uptake following. Acute infection in the soft tissues (i.e., cellulitis and abscess) will show abnormal activity during the first two phases but no accumulation in the underlying bones on delayed images. Acute osteomyelitis, on the other hand, will be markedly positive on all three phases (Fig. 6.58). Even in cases where the soft tissues are also abnormal, such as in a septic joint, the delayed images frequently show progressive accumulation compared with the blood-pool image. In other cases, the soft tissue activity may be more intense from the more extreme cellulitis or joint involvement, with the delayed images revealing bone involvement at an

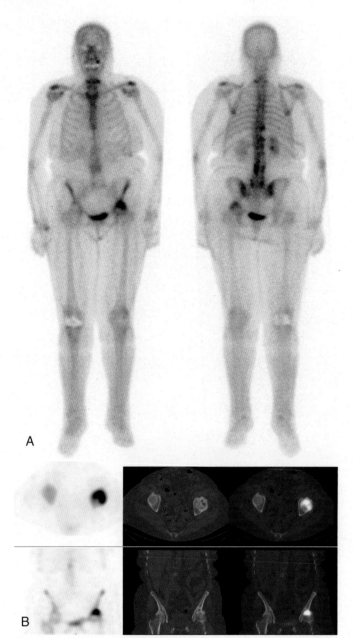

Fig. 6.54 Chronic osteoarthritic changes in with osteonecrosis. (A) Planar bone-scan in a patient with prostate cancer revealed multiple focal areas of activity from degenerative changes in the spine and moderate uptake in the anterior right femoral head. (B) Single-photon emission computed tomography with CT (SPECT/CT) axial *(top row)* and coronal *(bottom row)* hip images show marked SPECT uptake *(left image)* corresponding to joint-space loss, subchondral cysts, and mild sclerosis on both sides of the joint on CT *(middle)* and fused *(right side of image)* images.

earlier phase (Fig. 6.59). The diagnostic criteria for osteomyelitis are shown in Box 6.14.

The bone scan is not specific. The same sequence of image findings seen in osteomyelitis can occur in conditions such as neuropathic joint disease (Fig. 6.60), gout, fracture (including stress fractures), and rheumatoid arthritis. Common conditions that can cause a three-phase positive result potentially mimicking osteomyelitis are listed in Box 6.15. Improved specificity can be achieved by comparing the three-phase bone scan to radiographs or CT.

Imaging with a Tc-99m HMPAO or In-111 WBC scan can identify sites of infection with a higher degree of specificity. Caution must be used in cases with marked neuropathic destruction because WBCs may be increased in the region without infection. Joint-replacement surgery can also shift or alter the appearance of the marrow. In such cases, areas of increased WBC activity could represent cells in normal marrow. Therefore in cases where there is concern for infection in Charcot joint or joint replacement, areas of abnormal WBC activity most often need to be compared with a Tc-99m sulfur colloid marrow scan. If the WBC scan shows activity greater than the marrow, then infection is likely present.

Although the WBC scan can be performed first or alone, an initial three-phase bone scan can help identify areas of concern where count rates are normally lower, such as the toes. Bone scan is also potentially useful when an infection is chronic or already being treated with antibiotics, which result in significant decreases in the sensitivity of the WBC scan.

Although highly useful, WBC scans demonstrate decreased sensitivity in the spine, reportedly only 40% for discitis/osteomyelitis. In cases of discitis and possible osteomyelitis in the spine, when MR cannot be performed or is inconclusive, a three-phase bone scan may be compared with gallium-67 (Ga-67). Imaging 24 to 48 hours after a 5-mCi (185-MBq) dose of Ga-67 can be performed to identify infection in many locations, but in cases of osteomyelitis, some studies have shown that bone-scan activity will be significantly higher. WBC and Ga-67 imaging in infection are discussed further in Chapter 16, Inflammation and Infection.

TARGETED RADIONUCLIDE THERAPY OF METASTATIC DISEASE IN BONE

Targeted tumor therapy has been performed with radioactive agents in nuclear medicine for decades, such as the treatment of thyroid cancer with I-131. Several beta-minus (β^-)–emitting radiopharmaceuticals are approved for the treatment of metastatic disease in bone, and more recently, the alpha (α)-emitter radium-223 (Ra-223) was added to the list. Regulations require that the authorized users who order and administer them adhere to a different set of training requirements as compared with those for I-131 that most radiologists complete (Box 6.16). Although administration of bone-pain palliation agents is usually performed only by those with extra training on the handling of unsealed radiation sources (i.e., nuclear medicine and radiation oncology physicians), it is important for others to understand proper administration and applications.

These calcium analogs and diphosphonate derivatives accumulate to a higher degree in sclerotic metastases, and they have also shown longer biological half-lives when localized in a metastatic lesion compared with residence in normal bone. Their therapeutic effect depends on the emission of high-energy particles that travel only millimeters for β^- particles or a fraction of

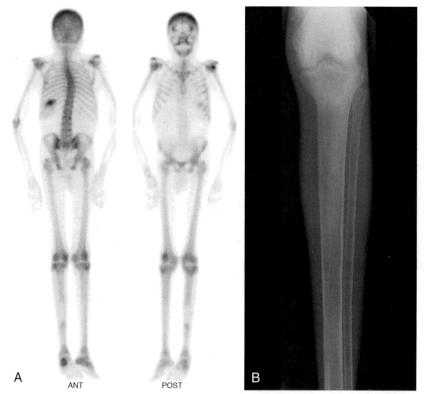

Fig. 6.55 Technetium-99m (Tc-99m) methylene diphosphonate (MDP) images (A) in a patient with sickle cell disease (SCD) presenting with acute chest and leg pain and fever. Images show a focal hot lesion above the left kidney. Although it might be confused with an expansile rib lesion, other findings of SCD should point the reader to the diagnosis of a chronically infarcted spleen. Other findings include absent activity in kidneys and bladder and hazy ascites in the peritoneum from renal failure, along with mildly increased activity in the long bones. Focal uptake in the left humeral head is nonspecific and could be related to damage from SCD or to arthritis. The elongated, subtle photon-deficient area in the left tibia resulted from infarction just distal to subtle sclerosis on x-ray **(B).**

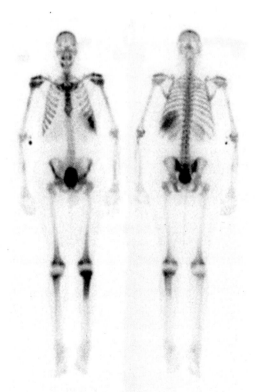

Fig. 6.56 In a patient with SCD, technetium-99m (Tc-99m) methylene diphosphonate (MDP) images show that excreted urine activity is present in the bladder and faint renal activity not outside of normal limits. However, a hot spleen is seen on the left, and a hot area is seen in the left proximal tibia from what proved to be an old infarct. The bones appear abnormal around the knees from marrow expansion.

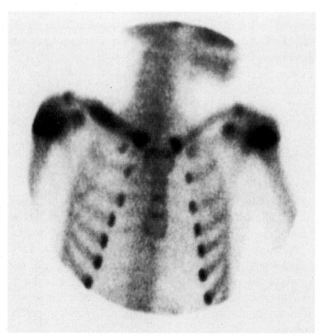

Fig. 6.57 Osteomyelitis of the right clavicle. Anterior scintigram in a child showing that the uptake on the right is markedly greater than in the left clavicle.

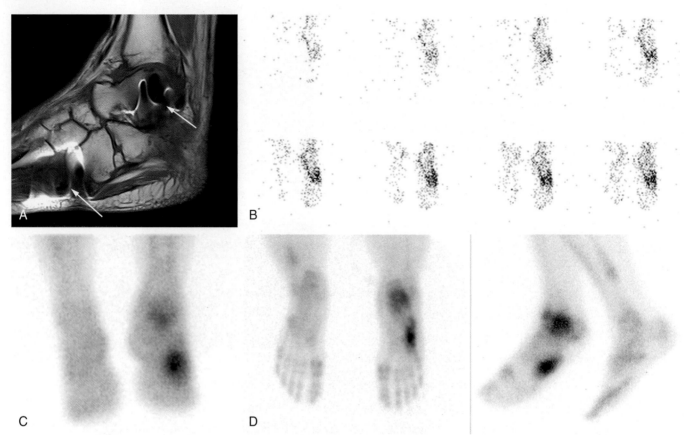

Fig. 6.58 Three-phase bone scan may be highly useful when magnetic resonance (MR) is limited, as in this case of a 34-year-old with prior reduction of a talar and fifth metatarsal fracture 2 years prior, with new pain and swelling. (A) T1-weighted sagittal ankle MR is limited by metal susceptibility artifact *(arrows)*. (B) Blood flow and (C) soft tissue activity are increased in the areas of prior surgery, as is the delayed image (D). Subsequent positive white blood cell and normal sulfur colloid marrow studies of the region confirmed the presence of osteomyelitis.

a millimeter in the case of an α emitter. This helps limit effects to the abnormal bone and spare normal tissues. A list of agents approved for use in the United States is found in Table 6.8, and some agents that are under investigation or approved in other countries are listed in Table 6.9.

When determining which patients to treat, only those who require narcotics for pain control or who have pain severe enough to significantly limit activity are suitable candidates. Also, because the onset of symptom relief is delayed (e.g., 1 to 4 weeks), patients with a life expectancy of less than 30 days are not likely to benefit. Imaging patients with a bone scan is useful to confirm that the metastases will accumulate the therapy radionuclide.

Radioactive therapies are contraindicated in patients with significant bone-marrow suppression (e.g., platelets <60,000/μL or WBCs < 2400/μL), those who are pregnant or breastfeeding, and those suffering marked renal failure or disseminated intravascular coagulation (DIC). The most important side effect of these treatments is bone-marrow toxicity. Therefore baseline blood counts must meet limits on the minimum values for platelets, leukocytes, and hemoglobin. Measurements should then be performed weekly, assessing change from the nadir following treatment. Increased benefit

has been found when the therapy dose is split into fractions. Repeat doses are generally delayed for 1 month for Ra-223 and 2 to 3 months after the first dose for the beta-emitting agents. Subsequent doses are also withheld if blood counts do not fall within an acceptable range.

Response rates vary somewhat among the different agents but are generally on the order of 70% to 80%, with 20% of patients becoming pain-free in one study. The duration of response also varies. A fraction of patients will experience a flare or transient worsening of their symptoms. It is important for patients to have access to analgesics and supportive care as needed.

Targeted radionuclide therapies are extremely useful because they can often be given in addition to other therapies. Before prescribing radiopharmaceutical treatments, however, it is generally prudent to wait after those treatments: 2 to 3 months after external-beam radiotherapy and 1.5 to 2 months after chemotherapy. When chemotherapy is to be given after a nuclear medicine treatment, a delay of 2 to 3 months is generally recommended. Sample protocols for radium-223 and Sm-153 ethylenediamine tetramethylene phosphonic acid (EDTMP) or Sr-89 are given in Boxes 6.17 and 6.18, respectively.

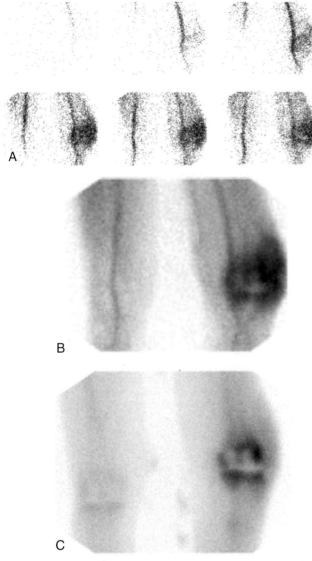

Fig. 6.59 Septic joint and osteomyelitis on three-phase study. A middle-aged man with elevated white blood cell count, a left knee prosthesis placed 2 years prior, and a swollen and painful knee underwent bone scan. (A) Sequential dynamic perfusion images reveal intense arterial-phase hyperemia surrounding the affected joint. (B) Blood-pool images already show localization in skeletal structures, but the soft tissue activity continues to increase. (C) Delayed static images reveal intense focal accumulation in multiple areas of the great toe and distal first and second metatarsals.

BOX 6.14 Three-Phase Skeletal Scintigraphy: Interpretive Criteria

- Osteomyelitis: *Arterial* hyperemia, progressive focal skeletal uptake with relative soft tissue clearance; in children, a focal cold area may be seen if osteomyelitis is associated with infarction. Activity accumulates on delayed images and is often more intense than levels in soft tissue or flow.
- Cellulitis: *Venous* (later portion of blood flow images) hyperemia, persistent soft tissue activity; no focal skeletal uptake (may have mild to moderate diffusely increased uptake).
- Septic joint: Periarticular increased activity on dynamic and blood-pool phases that persists on delayed images; less commonly, the joint structures appear cold if pressure in the joint causes decreased flow or infarction.

Radium-223 (Ra-223) Alpha-Emitter Therapy

Alpha particles deposit a very high amount of energy (high linear energy transfer [LET]) over a very short path. They offer the ability to create significant double-stranded DNA breaks, proving much more destructive to tumor. Although several alpha-emitters have recently been investigated for therapy purposes, the first to be approved for use in the United States is Ra-223 (Xofigo) for use in bone disease resulting from prostate cancer in patients with no evidence of systemic soft tissue metastases.

In a randomized phase III study of patients with prostate cancer being treated for bone metastases, in the absence of systemic disease (Alpharadin in Symptomatic Prostate Cancer [ALSYMPCA]), the protocol was terminated early because a 30% increase in overall survival (OS) was seen. The agent is administered every 4 weeks for a total of six injections. Biomarkers affected by radium therapy are outlined in Table 6.10. Some of the toxicities seen during the ALSYMPCA trial and its follow-up are listed in Table 6.11, and the main reasons patients discontinued treatment are provided in Table 6.12. Ongoing work continues to investigate Ra-223 in other scenarios.

Samarium-153 EDTMP

Sm-153 EDTMP (Quadramet) is a beta-emitting radiopharmaceutical that has the added advantage of a gamma emission that can be detected for external imaging. It has been approved for use in patients with osteoblastic metastases that can be visualized on a nuclear medicine bone scan (Fig. 6.62).

Sm-153 is administered in a 1.0-mCi/kg (37-MBq/kg) dose intravenously over the course of 1 minute. Approximately 50% of the dose is localized to bone. It accumulates in metastatic lesions in a 5:1 ratio compared with normal bone. Patients should be well hydrated and void frequently because the primary route of clearance is through the urine. Approximately 35% of the dose is excreted in the first 6 hours.

As in Sr-89, the bone-marrow toxicity is a limiting factor. Toxicity is usually mild, although serious side effects and even fatalities have been reported. Platelets decreased on the order of 25% from baseline and WBCs by 20%.

The short range of the Sm-153 beta particle should be advantageous when considering the dose to normal marrow. A response rate on the order of 83% has been reported. Pain relief is generally noted within 2 weeks, with a duration of 4 to 40 weeks.

Strontium-89 (Sr-89)

The pure beta-emitter strontium-89 (Metastron) is approved by the FDA for the management of metastatic bone pain. A 4-mCi (148-MBq) dose is administered intravenously slowly over 1 to 2 minutes. An alternative dose of 55 µCi/kg (2.04 MBq/kg) may be used. Repeat dosing is possible, but factors such as initial response, hematological status, and current status must be considered in each case. In general, a repeat administration is not recommended before 90 days have elapsed. The pathway of excretion is predominantly through the urine, with about one-third bowel excretion.

After obtaining a baseline platelet count, platelets should be measured at least every other week. Typically, platelets will

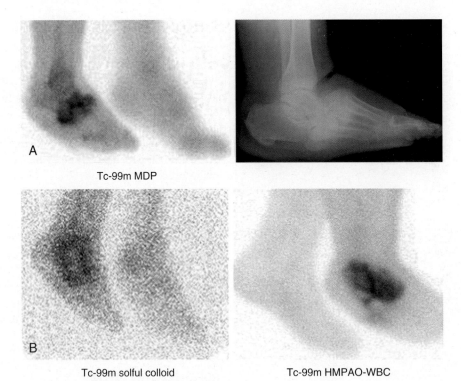

Tc-99m MDP

Tc-99m solful colloid   Tc-99m HMPAO-WBC

Fig. 6.60 Charcot joint. (A) Marked bone-scan uptake corresponds to destruction on radiographs in a patient with diabetes and a plantar ulcer. (B) Technetium-99m (Tc-99m) sulfur colloid marrow images *(left)* do not completely match Tc-99m hexamethylpropyleneamine oxime (HMPAO) white blood cell (WBC) images *(right)*, particularly centrally and just inferiorly, suggesting osteomyelitis. Patchy uptake along the plantar foot was in the region of an ulcer, likely resulting from cellulitis, although separation from bone is difficult.

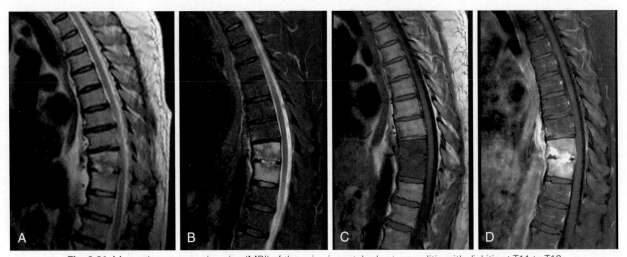

Fig. 6.61 Magnetic resonance imaging (MRI) of the spine in vertebral osteomyelitis with diskitis at T11 to T12 shows marrow edema irregular-enhancing inflammatory changes in the disk space, but no paraspinal mass or extension is evident on (A) T2, (B) short-tau inversion recovery (STIR), (C) T1 precontrast, or (D) gadolinium-enhanced T1 images.

decrease 30% from baseline and reach the nadir 12 to 16 weeks after therapy. Toxicity is generally mild; however, Sr-89 must be used with caution in those with WBC counts of less than 2400 and platelets of less than 60,000. A small number of patients experience transient worsening of symptoms.

Approximately 20% of patients will become pain-free. Approximately 80% of patients will experience some significant decrease in pain, although some series have reported that up to 90% experience some relief. Pain relief begins approximately 7 to 20 days after injection and generally lasts 3 to 6 months.

Phosphorus-32 (P-32)

Phosphorus-32 has been used in intraperitoneal infusion for the treatment of tumors such as ovarian cancer and in the treatment of polycythemia vera. It is also one of the radioisotopes first used for its bone-seeking properties to palliate metastatic lesion bone pain. The lack of a gamma emission means no external imaging can be done to assess distribution. A range of skeletal absorbed doses has been calculated (25-63 rad/mCi [0.68-1.733 cGy/MBq]). Additionally, it appears that the normal marrow receives a high dose relative to the tumor as a result of the distribution of P-32 in the bone's inorganic matrix and cellular

---

BOX 6.15 Lesions That Can Mimic Osteomyelitis on Three-Phase Skeletal Scintigraphy

Osteoarthritis
Gout
Fracture
Stress fracture
Osteonecrosis (healing)
Charcot joint
Osteotomy
Complex regional pain syndrome (reflex sympathetic dystrophy)
Subacute/healing infarct

BOX 6.16 NRC Radiation License and Authorized User Training Requirements for Radionuclide Therapy With Radium-223 (Ra-223) and β-Emitters Other Than Iodine-131 (I-131)

Licensing based on federal regulation 10 CFR Part 35 (subpart E)

Authorized User Training

- 10 CFR 35.390: Training for use of unsealed by-product material for which a written directive is required
- 10 CFR 35.396: Training for parental administration of unsealed by-product material requiring a written directive
- Completed 700 hours training and experience under an authorized user who meets requirements of 35.390 and/or 35.396
- Must include 200 hours classroom and lab in radiation physics, instrumentation, radiation biology, chemistry of medical by-products, and mathematics pertaining to radioactivity

Radiation License

Broad scope: License permits possession and administration of agent with Z number 88 (radium) *or* any radioactive material permitted by 10 CFR 35.300

CFR 35, Code of Federal Regulations Part 35; *NRC,* Nuclear Regulatory Commission.

TABLE 6.8 Approved Radiopharmaceuticals for Targeted Therapy of Bone Metastases

Agent	Physical $t_{1/2}$ (days)	Mean Particle or Photon Energy (MeV)	Particle Soft Tissue Range (mm)	Expected Response Time	Retreatment	Comments
Ra-223 (Xofigo)	11.4	α (95.3% abundance) 5.64 β-(3.6%) 0.445 and 0.492 γ (1.1%) 0.01-1.27	0.05-0.08 (α)	Within 1st 2 cycles	6 injections @ 4-week intervals	• In 2/3 patients, pain decreased • Survival improved 30% over therapies not incorporating • Survival not tied to pain relief or PSA decrease
Sm-153 EDTMP (Quadramet)	1.9	β-0.23 γ 0.103 (30% abundance)	0.6	2-7 days, peak 3-4 weeks	>2 months	• In 277 patients who experienced intense pain from various cancers, pain decreased 54% after 3 weeks and up to 74% after 12 weeks
Sr-89 (Metastron)	50.5	β-0.58 γ 0.19 (0.01% abundance)	2.4	14-28 days	>3 months	• In 41 patients with bone and prostate cancer, >2/3 responded with decreased opioid doses
P-32	14.3	β-0.70	3.0	5-14 days	>3 months	• Reversible pancytopenia frequently limits doses, peaks 5-6 weeks • 50-87% report pain relief

P-32, phosphorous-32; *PSA,* prostate-specific antigen; *Ra-223,* radium-223; *Sm-153 EDTMP,* samarium-153 ethylenediamine tetramethylene phosphonic acid; *Sr-89,* strontium-89.
From Florimonte L, Dellavedova L, Maffioli LS. Radium-223 dichloride in clinical practice. *Eur J Nucl Med Mol Imaging.* 2016; 43:1896-1909.
Handkiewicz-Junak D, Poeppel TD, Bodei L, et al. EANM guidelines for radionuclide therapy of bone metastases with beta-emitting radionuclides. *Eur J Nucl Med Mol Imaging.* 2018; 45(5):846-859.

---

regions. The use of P-32 has fallen in favor of other agents, and it is no longer approved in some countries.

Rhenium-186 HEDP

Rhenium-186 hydroxyethylidene diphosphonate (Re-186 HEDP) is formed by combining a diphosphonate useful for bone-pain therapy, etidronate, with a beta-emitter. Re-186 HEDP is another agent that may be useful for the palliation of bone pain. It emits a gamma ray useful for imaging and lesion identification. It rapidly localizes to bone, with approximately 14% retained in bone. The remainder is rapidly cleared, with approximately 70% of the dose excreted in the urine 6 hours after injection. The use of Re-188 as a

TABLE 6.9   Targeted Bone-Pain Palliative Agents Under Investigation or Approved Outside the United States

Radiolabel	Carrier Molecule	Physical Half-Life (days)	β⁻ Particle Maximum (MeV)	Maximum Particle Range (mm)	γ-Photon Energy (keV)	Comments
Re-186	HEDP	3.7	1.071 (73%) 0.934 (23%)	3.7	137 (11%) 132 (2%) 632 (0.03%)	In 527 patients, Sr-89 and Re-186 HEDP, no statistical difference in efficacy 1 Dafermou A, Colamuss P, Giganti M, et al. A multi-centre observational study of radionuclide therapy in patients with painful bone metastases of prostate cancer. *Eur J Nucl Med.* 2001; 28:788-798.
Re-188	HEDP	0.7	2.12	10.4	155 (15.1%)	
Lu-177	EDTMP	6.7	0.497 (79%) 0.176 (12.2%) 0.384 (9%)	1.8	208 (11%) 113 (6.4%)	

EDTMP, Ethylenediamine tetramethylene phosphonic acid; *HEDP*, hydroxyethylidine diphosphonate.
Abi-Ghanem AS, McGrath MA, Jacene HA. Radionuclide therapy for osseous metastases in prostate cancer. *Semin Nucl Med.* 2015;45:66-80

BOX 6.17   Therapy Protocol for Radium-223 (Ra-223) in Metastatic Prostate Cancer

Approved Indication
Treatment of symptomatic bone metastases from castration-resistant prostate cancer in patients with no known visceral metastatic disease

Hematological Monitoring
- Prior to first dose: Absolute neutrophil count (ANC) ≥ 1.5 × 10⁹/L, platelets ≥ 100 × 10⁹/L, hemoglobin ≥ 10 g
- Prior to subsequent cycles: ANC ≥ 1.0 x 10⁹/L, platelets ≥ 50 × 10⁹/L
- Discontinue Ra-223 if values do not recover in 6 to 8 weeks.

Clinical
Develop multidisciplinary team to discuss the following:
- Factors related to the patient's ability to tolerate therapy and follow radiation safety instructions, Eastern Cooperative Oncology Group (ECOG) score, and whether expected survival is sufficient to warrant the course of treatment
- Concomitant therapy:
  - Preliminary data suggest that use with abiraterone acetate and prednisone is not safe.
  - It may be used in combination with external-beam radiation therapy, androgen deprivation therapy, and traditional hormone therapy.

Patient Education
- Develop an understanding of the goal to complete the course of six cycles: overall survival (OS) is greater in patients receiving five to six cycles compared with one to four.
- Monitor response/progression with alkaline phosphatase and imaging.

- Changes in prostate-specific antigen (PSA) are not as useful because of its different mechanism.
- Decreased pain, on its own, is not an indication to stop treatment.
- Radiation safety: Low levels of agent will be present in stool (mainly), urine, and blood for 1 week.
- Patient and caregivers must use universal safety precautions.
- Maintain excellent bathroom hygiene practices; immediately wash clothing contaminated with urine or stool separately.
- Provide information for patient to give to personnel in hospitals in case of any admission or funeral home in case of death. Note: Cremation and burial should pose no significant threat to those handling the body.

Dose:
Slowly infuse 1.5 μCi/kg (55 kBq/kg) intravenously over 1 minute with slow saline flush
- Use caution so that staff and bystanders cannot inhale or absorb any radium from a spill.
- Repeat at 4-week intervals if clinical and hematological parameters continue to permit.

Patient Release
Patients able to follow radiation safety procedures may be released to home after administration per U.S. federal regulations, but care must be taken to adhere to state and local regulations.

Follow-Up
Set date for follow-up blood work (about 1 week prior to next dose) and contact plan.

BOX 6.18 β⁻ Therapy Protocol for Bone Metastases With Samarium-153 Ethylenediamine Tetramethylene Phosphonic Acid (Sm-153 EDTMP), Strontium-89 (Sr-89), Phosphorous-32 (P-32)

Indication

Relief of pain from osteoblastic bone metastases that accumulate technetium-99m (Tc-99m) methylene diphosphonate (MDP) on bone scan

Patient Selection Criteria

- Patient pain level should be severe enough that it is limiting activity or requiring narcotics.
- Patients with a life expectancy of < 4 to 6 weeks are unlikely to benefit.
- Blood counts:
  - Platelets: > 60 x 10⁹ /L (preferably 100 x 10⁹ /L)
  - Leukocytes: >2400 to 3000/µL (preferably 5000 µL)
  - Absolute neutrophil count (ANC): >2000/µL
  - Hemoglobin >10 g/dL
  - Lower levels not absolute contraindication but will increase risks
- Patients with disseminated intravascular coagulation (DIC) may be at risk for severe thrombocytopenia or death.
- Use in lytic metastases has not been well evaluated.
  Per use following label package insert safety recommendations and Society of Nuclear Medicine and Molecular Imaging Procedure Guidelines:
- Use is not generally recommended with concurrent chemotherapy or external-beam radiation because of risks to marrow (unless benefits known to outweigh risks).
- Delay treatment for 6 to 8 weeks after long-acting myelosuppressive chemotherapy.
- Delay treatment for 4 weeks for other forms of myelosuppressive chemotherapy or systemic radioisotope therapy.
- Delay therapy for 2 to 3 weeks after external-beam treatment.
- Do not resume chemotherapy until after 12 weeks following radionuclide therapy.
- If etidronate or other bisphosphonates recently received (<2 weeks), bone scan to confirm uptake will be sufficient; do not give bisphosphonates for at least 48 hours after radionuclide therapy.
- Not for use alone in the treatment of pathological fracture or bones with more severe bone destruction
- Women of childbearing age must have a negative pregnancy test.

Benefits

Patients who respond begin to see relief within 1 week, with maximal relief in 3 to 4 weeks.

Risks

- Marrow suppression: Nadir 40% to 50% baseline within 3 to 5 weeks
- Flare reaction (increased pain): 7% mild, self-limiting, responds to analgesics, occurs within 72 hours

Radiation Safety

- Use toilet, not urinal, for 48 hours. Use care not to soil area around toilet with urine or fecal matter; flush several times; wash hands well.
- Incontinent patients: Use urine-absorbing garments and mattress covers; consider bladder catheterization.
- Caregivers use gloves, gowns, and eye protection when handling urine or contaminated clothing.
- Store urine-contaminated clothing 1 to 2 weeks or immediately wash separately.
- Terminate breastfeeding.
- Use two methods of birth control.
- Sleep alone for 5 to 7 days.
- No clearance saliva secretion seen, so no oral-related precautions

Dose Administration

Sr-89: 1.5 to 2.2 MBq/kg (40-60 µCi/kg) or 148 MBq (4 mCi)
Sm-153 lexidronam: 37 MBq/kg (1.0 mCi/kg)
P-32 sodium phosphate: 185 to 370 MBq (5-10 mCi) may use divided doses. An oral dose alternative is available with
10-12 mCi (370 to 444 MBq) orally.
- Administer in plastic syringe, slow intravenous (IV) push over 1 minute, followed by saline flush.
- Do not release patient unless local and state radiation standards are met.

Follow-Up

- Monitor complete blood count (CBC): Begin 2 weeks after therapy and perform every 1 to 3 weeks for 12 to 16 weeks or until recovery
- Patients who had been having serum calcium monitored

Repeat Procedure

- Doses may be repeated 12 (or more) weeks after the first dose.
- Responses have been seen with up to seven treatments (50% response rate after second dose).
- No patient who fails to respond with the first dose has benefited from a second.
- Risks rise with each administration.

---

radiolabel is of particular interest because it can be produced with a generator.

BONE MINERAL DENSITY ASSESSMENT

The use of bone mineral density measurement has been accelerated by the availability of new drugs that localize in bone and promote mineralization. Multiple methods have been developed to quantitatively measure bone mineral mass. Dual-energy x-ray techniques are especially important for areas such as the spine and hips/ In these areas, the soft tissues are thicker than the distal extremities and can attenuate the x-ray beam. By comparing a lower-energy beam or photon that is attenuated by bone and soft tissue with a higher-energy source that is affected only by bone (or metal), it is possible to calculate the differential absorption, allowing more

accurate assessment of bone density without impact from the surrounding soft tissues. DEXA was used as the basis for the World Health Organization (WHO) criteria for categorizing osteopenia and osteoporosis.

Fracture risk markedly increases when bone mineral density is less than 1 g/cm². Bone mineral measurements establish baseline diagnostic measurements in the evaluation of patients with suspected osteopenia and osteoporosis and can follow the course of therapy.

The WHO classification system for bone mass, based on DEXA measurements of the spine and femoral neck, compares an individual's measurements with the mean and standard deviation (SD) for a control population. Results are reported as a T-score or a Z-score. The T-score is a comparison of a person's measured bone density to a healthy young 30-year-old adult (of the same sex while a Z-score compares

TABLE 6.10 Changes in Key Biomarkers of Disease Progression After Ra-223 (Xofigo) Therapy

Parameter	Ra-223 (*n* = 614)	Placebo (*n* = 307)	Hazard Ratio	95% Confidence Interval
Median overall survival (OS)	14.9	11.3	0.695	0.552-0.875
	*30% ↓risk of death vs. placebo			
Median time to ↑to total ALP (months)	7.4	3.8	0.17	0.13-0.22
≥30% ↓in total ALP	47%	3%	NA	NA
≥50% ↓in total ALP	27%	1%	NA	NA
Median time to PSA progression (months)	3.6	3.4	0.64	0.54-0.77

ALP, Alkaline phosphatase; *NA,* not applicable; *PSA,* prostate-specific antigen; *Ra-223,* radium-223.
Data from Parker C, Nilsson S, Heinrich D, et al. ALSYMPCA investigators. Alpha emitter radium-223 and survival in metastatic prostate cancer. *N Engl J Med.* 2013;369(3):213–223.
Table modified from Xofigo® (Bayer) from the ALSYMPCA Trial data https://hcp.xofigo-us.com

TABLE 6.11 Adverse Reactions from Ra-223 Therapy in ALSYMPCA Trial and the 3-Year Follow-Up

PRIMARY ALSYMPCA TRIAL RA-223 (*n* = 600), PLACEBO (*n* = 307)						
Adverse Event	All Grades (%)		Severe			
			Grades 3-4 (%)		Grade 5 (%)	
	Ra-223	Placebo	Ra-223	Placebo	Ra-223	Placebo
Anemia	31	31	13	13	0	<1
Thrombocytopenia	12	6	6	3	<1	0
Neutropenia	5	1	2	1	0	0
Pancytopenia	2	0	2	0	0	0

3-YEAR FOLLOW-UP RA-223 (*n* = 404), PLACEBO (*n* = 167)						
	All Grades (%)		Severe Grade 3-4 (%)		Severe Grade 5 (%)	
	Ra-223	Placebo	Ra-223	Placebo	Ra-223	Placebo
Anemia	3	3	1	1	0	0
Thrombocytopenia	1	0	0	0	0	0
Neutropenia	<1[a]	0	<1[a]	0	0	0
Aplastic anemia	<1[b]	0	<1[b]	0	0	0

ALSYMPCA, Alpharadin in Symptomatic Prostate Cancer; *Ra-223,* radium-223.
[a] <1% = 2 patients.
[b] <1% = 1 patient.
Table modified from Jacene H, Gomella L, Yu EY, Rohren EM. Hematologic toxicity from radium-223 therapy for bone metastases in castration resistant prostate cancer: risk factors and practical considerations. *Clin Genitourin Cancer.* 2018;16(4):919–926.

TABLE 6.12 Parameters Leading to Radium-223 Discontinuation: Data From ALSYMPCA Trial

Parameter	Ra-223 (n = 209)	Placebo (*n* = 157)	p
Disease progression	8	6	0.69
Anemia	6	1	0.01
Health status decline	4	4	0.08
Thrombocytopenia	3	14	0.15
Spinal cord compression	2	2	1
Fatigue	2	3	0.51
Sepsis	1	0	0.51

ALSYMPCA, Alpharadin in Symptomatic Prostate Cancer; *Ra-223,* radium-223..
Table modified from Jacene H, Gomella L, Yu EY, Rohren EM. Hematologic toxicity from radium-223 therapy for bone metastases in castration resistant prostate cancer: risk factors and practical considerations. *Clin Genitourin Cancer.* 2018;16(4):919–926.
Data from U.S. Food and Drug Administration (FDA) safety package insert; Prescribing Xofigo. Bayer website. https://hcp.xofigo-us.com.

TABLE 6.13 Adverse Reaction Summary Selected Events, Sm-153 EDTMP

Event	Sm-153 EDTMP (%) (n = 199)	Placebo (%) (n = 90)
Any adverse reaction	85	80
Pain flare	7.0	5.6
Thrombocytopenia	69.3	8.9
Leukopenia	59.3	3.7
Anemia/decreased hemoglobin	40.7	23.3
Nausea &/or vomiting	32.7	41.1
Infection	17.1	11.1
Fever Chills	8.5	11.1
Nervous	30	43
Musculoskeletal issues	27	31
Respiratory issues	18	27

Sm-153 EDTMP, samarium-153 ethylenediamine tetramethylene phosphonic acid.
From Sm-153 EDTMP (Quadramet) package insert safety information.

the result to average values for people of the same age and gender. A low Z-score means bone mass less than typical for age and that bone loss may be occurring more rapidly than expected.

These scores are described as the number of standard deviations above or below the mean value for the population, where the mean for the population is placed at 0, in the middle of a bell-shaped curve (Fig. 6.63). The scores to the right are at 1 SD, 2 SD, and 3 SD above normal, and scores below the average are found to be –1 SD, –2 SD, and –3 SD from the mean (i.e., ranges from –3 to +3 SD from normal).

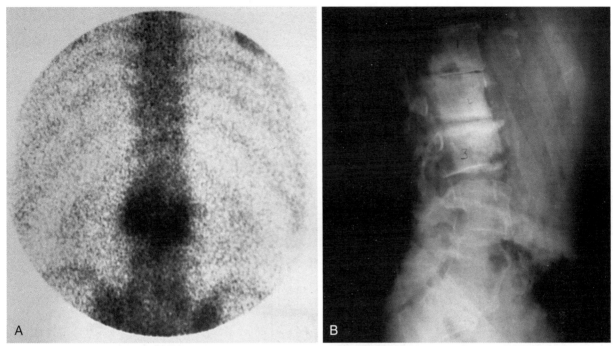

Fig. 6.62 Samarium-153 (Sm-153) palliation of metastatic disease bone pain. (A) The whole-body technetium-99m (Tc-99m) methylene diphosphonate (MDP) bone scan before therapy confirms the presence of metastases that will accumulate the therapy radiopharmaceutical. (B) The posttherapy whole-body scan obtained from the Sm-153 Lexidronam (Sm-153 ethylenediamine tetramethylene phosphonic acid [EDTMP]; Quadramet) dose shows close correlation with the bone scan.

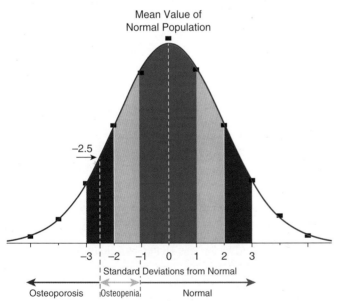

Fig. 6.63 Graphical display of bone density results and their significance. Normal density is considered to be above 1 SD below normal, osteopenia when between 2.5 SDs below normal up to 1 SD below normal (between −2.5 to −1), and for cases falling below −2.5 SD from normal, osteoporosis is diagnosed.

Standard score $(Z) = \dfrac{X - \mu}{\sigma}$, where X is the measured value, μ is the mean for the population, and σ (sigma) is the SD.

Normal T-scores are within 1 SD from the mean of the young population (i.e., T-scores from −1 to +1) and all values above +1. Osteopenia or bone density between 10-25% below that of a normal young adult, is taken as 1 to 2.5 SD below the control mean (or a T-score between −1.0 and −2.4). Osteoporosis, or bone density less than 25% of the value for a normal young adult, is defined as 2.5 SD or more below the control mean (or a T-score <−2.5).

It is important to exclude areas with degenerative sclerosis because these could falsely elevate the density reported. Reviewing the scan accompanying the measurement report can help with the selection of optimal regions to assess. Computer-generated reporting systems typically provide such an image, along with calculations for each patient. These data are displayed graphically, and T- and Z-scores are provided for the areas measured (Fig. 6.64).

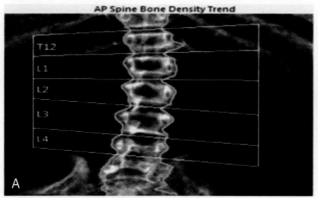

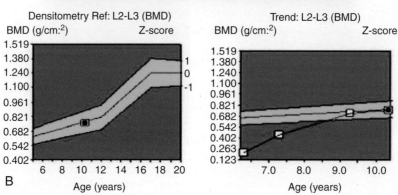

Fig. 6.64 Dual-energy x-ray absorptiometry (DEXA) bone density measurement. An immobilized pediatric patient with multiple medical problems was evaluated to assess bone density. The radiographic image (A), which helps avoid false-negative readings from sclerosis/osteophyte, shows the patient's scoliosis. (B) Curve plotting the results shows they fall within 2 standard deviations (SD) from normal. Normal is considered to be above 1 SD below normal. Osteopenia is reported when results fall between 2.5 SDs below normal up to 1 SD below normal, and for cases falling below −2.5 SD from normal, osteoporosis is diagnosed. The tables (B) show serial results on this patient. When reporting abnormal findings in children, falling below 2 SD from normal, the terms *osteopenia* and *osteoporosis* should not be applied on the basis of the test results alone. It is preferable to say density is "low for age."

SUGGESTED READING

Bone Scan

Chua S, Gnanasegaran G, Cook GJ. Miscellaneous cancers (lung, thyroid, renal cancer, myeloma, and neuroendocrine tumors): role of spect and pet in imaging bone metastases. *Semin Nucl Med.* 2009;39(6):416–430.

Gemmel F, Van den Wyngaert H, Love C, et al. Prosthetic joint infections: radionuclide state of the art imaging. *Eur J Nucl Med Mol Imaging.* 2012;39(5):892–909.

Nadel H. Pediatric bone scintigraphy update. *Semin Nucl Med.* 2010;40:31–40.

Shehab D, Elgazzar AH, Collier BD. Heterotopic ossification. *J Nucl Med.* 2002;43(3):346–353.

F-18 Sodium Fluoride PET/CT

Liu Y, Sheng J, Dong Z, et al. The diagnostic performance of 18F fluoride PET/CT in bone metastases detection: a meta-analysis. *Clin Radiol.* 2019;74(3):196–206. https://doi.org/10.1016/j.crad.2018.12.011. Epub 2019 Jan 14.

Sonni I, Minamimoto R, Baratto L, et al. Simultaneous PET/MRI in the evaluation of breast and prostate cancerusing combined Na[F] and [F]FDG: a focus on skeletal lesions. *Mol Imaging Biol.* 2020;22:397–406.

Therapy

Du Y, Carrio I, De Vincentis G, et al. Practical recommendations for radium-223 treatment of metastatic castration-resistant prostate cancer. *Eur J Nucl Med Mol Imaging.* 2017;44:1671–1678.

Jacene H, Gomella L, Yu EY, Rohren EM. Hematologic toxicity from radium-223 therapy for bone metastases in castration-resistant prostate cancer: risk factors and practical considerations. *Clinical Genitourinary Cancer.* 2018;16(4):919–926.

Parker C, Nilsson S, Heinrich D, et al. Alpha emitter radium-223 and survival in metastatic prostate cancer. *N Engl J Med.* 2013;369:213–223.

Parker CC, Coleman RE, Sartor O, et al. Three-year safety of radium-223 dichloride in patients with castrate-resistant prostate cancer and symptomatic bone metastases from phase 3 randomized alpharadin in symptomatic prostate cancer trial. *Eur Urol.* 2018;73(3):427–435.

The Pulmonary System

INTRODUCTION: THE VENTILATION–PERFUSION LUNG SCAN

Particles slightly larger than red blood cells can be radiolabeled and injected into a peripheral vein. After passing through the heart and central pulmonary arteries, they finally lodge in the peripheral lung capillaries, creating a map of pulmonary blood flow that can be imaged with a gamma camera. Similarly, inhalation of a radiolabeled gas or aerosol can allow ventilation imaging. These ventilation (V) and perfusion (Q) examinations are the two components that make up the VQ lung scan (Figs. 7.1 and 7.2). Although the VQ scan is most commonly performed to diagnose suspected pulmonary embolism, it can also be used for other purposes, including quantitation of pulmonary function, often pre– or post–lung resection or transplant surgery, and assessment of corrective surgery on pulmonary vasculature.

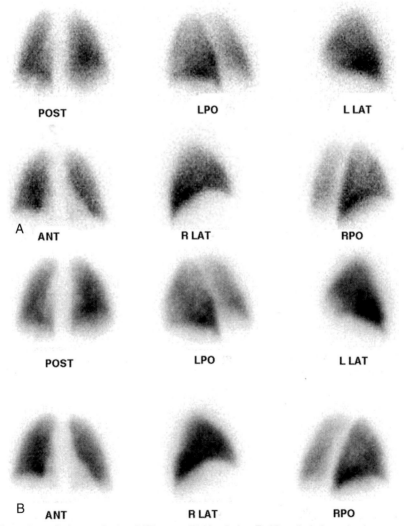

Fig. 7.1 Normal ventilation–perfusion (VQ) scan. (A) Ventilation Tc-99m diethylenetriaminepentaacetic acid (DTPA) and (B) perfusion Tc-99m macroaggregated albumin (MAA) lung scan images show homogeneous distribution and the normal gradient of increasing activity in the bases relative to the apices. *(Top row, left to right):* POST, posterior; *LPO,* left posterior oblique; *L LAT,* left lateral; *LAO,* left anterior oblique. *(Bottom row, left to right)* ANT, anterior; *RPO,* right posterior oblique; *R LAT,* right lateral; *RAO,* right anterior oblique.

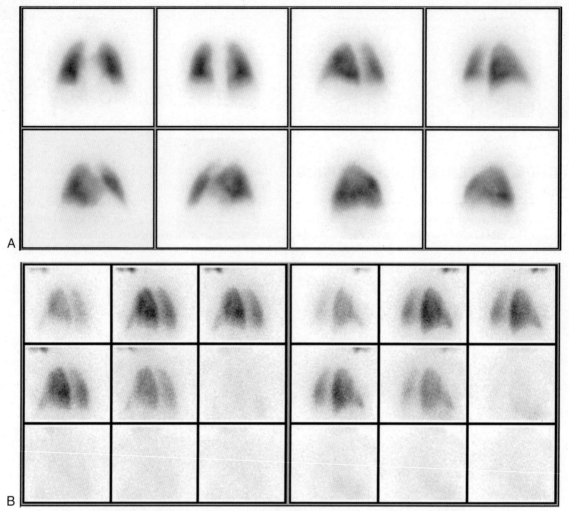

Fig. 7.2 Normal ventilation–perfusion (VQ) scan with xenon-133 ventilation. (A) Perfusion Tc-99m macro-aggregated albumin (MAA) images show normal radiotracer distribution. (B) Normal ventilation Xe-133 left posterior oblique *(left)* and right posterior oblique *(right)* include initial breath *(upper row)*, equilibrium images *(second row)*, and sequential washout images *(lower rows)* that show rapid normal clearance without retention from air trapping.

PULMONARY EMBOLISM

Diagnosis

The clinical diagnosis of pulmonary embolus (PE) can be difficult because of the wide range of presenting signs and symptoms as well as the limitations of available diagnostic tests. Although correct identification and prompt treatment can significantly improve mortality rates (from approximately 30% to 10%) and help prevent recurrence, treatment regimens also expose patients to potential harm.

It is important to understand the tests used to diagnose PE. The accuracy of any test depends not only on its sensitivity and specificity but also on pretest probabilities according to principles of Bayes' theorem (i.e., a positive test result is more likely a true positive if pretest suspicion is high, but the likelihood dramatically drops if suspicion is low). Therefore referring physicians should perform patient risk stratification to assess the overall likelihood of PE before ordering an extensive workup using validated criteria, such as the Modified Wells Scoring System (Table 7.1), which objectively assign points based on patient history, symptoms, and physical findings.

Patients are at greatest risk of a pulmonary embolus from immobilization, recent surgery, and hypercoagulable states. The chance of PE is also significantly increased with a history of prior PE and in the presence of deep vein thrombosis (DVT). Among patients with symptomatic DVT, 30% to 50% result in a PE, and 70% to 90% of patients with PE have had a DVT. Pregnancy and hormone use are more moderate risk factors.

Chest radiographs are frequently ordered and often identify other causes for the patient's symptoms. However, findings from a PE are highly variable (Box 7.1). Serum D-dimer is sensitive but nonspecific. Doppler ultrasound is an excellent way to noninvasively diagnose venous thrombosis in the lower extremities, making it a frequent component in the workup of possible PE. Further testing beyond these examinations depends on the level of clinical suspicion.

The historical imaging gold standard, pulmonary angiography, is very rarely performed today. It is not only invasive but also requires significant facility resources and may not visualize

TABLE 7.1 Wells Scoring for Pretest Determination of PE Probability[a]

Criteria	Modified Wells (Points)
Clinical signs of DVT	3.0
Recent surgery or immobilization	1.5
Heart rate >100 beats/min	1.5
Previous vascular thromboemboli	1.5
Hemoptysis	1.0
Malignancy	1.0
PE most likely diagnosis	3.0
Pregnancy	0 (not included in Wells score)

CLINICAL RISK ASSESSMENT		
Risk	Total Score (Points)	PE in Wells Patients
High	>6	41%
Moderate	2–6	16%
Low	<2	3.4%

DVT, Deep vein thrombosis; *PE*, pulmonary embolus.
[a]Modified from Wells PS, Anderson DR, Roger M, et al. Excluding pulmonary embolism at the bedside without diagnostic imaging: management of patients with suspected pulmonary embolism presenting to the emergency department by using a simple clinical model and D-dimer. *Ann Intern Med.* 2001;135:98–107.

BOX 7.1 Chest Radiograph Findings in Pulmonary Embolus

Most common:
Atelectasis
Opacity/infiltrate (localized or regional)
Pleural effusion (usually small to moderate)
  Also seen:
Pulmonary artery proximal distention (Fleischner' sign)
Oligemia (Westermark' sign)
Pleural-based density (Hampton' hump)
Normal/negative

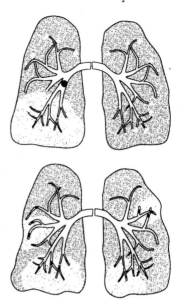

Fig. 7.3 Effect of embolus position on downstream perfusion. Larger emboli (*top*) lodge more centrally, causing greater effect and making them easier to detect. Smaller clots (*bottom*) or showers of smaller clots caused by breakdown of more proximal clots lodge more distally. In both, the effects extend to the pleural surface.

chronic emboli. In recent years, multislice computed tomography pulmonary angiography (CTPA) has become the dominant imaging tool for definitive PE diagnosis. As its use has dramatically escalated, there has been a corresponding significant increase in PE diagnosis. Despite this trend, mortality from PE has not substantially decreased, suggesting that many emboli now found are actually of little or no clinical significance. The potential risks of ionizing radiation exposure from this often-overutilized procedure have also been in the spotlight recently, and the scans themselves may be limited by insufficient contrast bolus density and patient motion. Some patients may not be able to undergo CTPA due to contraindications such as iodinated contrast allergy or poor renal function.

Magnetic resonance angiography (MRA) images the vasculature without ionizing radiation or iodinated contrast. Obtaining diagnostic-quality images in a reasonable amount of time is a significant challenge associated with this modality, although many improvements have occurred in recent years. Some experienced centers now report excellent results, with only a small percentage of inadequate examinations. Demand will likely continue growing, in part because of American College of Radiology (ACR) Contrast Manual guideline changes in 2017 supporting the use of group II gadolinium-based contrast agents (e.g., gadoteridol [ProHance]) in cases of decreased renal function. However, at present, MRA is not routinely used in most practices.

Although technical advances have led to a marked increase in CTPA and MRA utilization, the nuclear medicine VQ lung scan remains an important tool. It is particularly useful in patients who cannot tolerate intravenous contrast, have renal dysfunction, or in whom an adequate CTPA or MRA examination could not be obtained. It frequently provides a definitive answer while minimizing radiation to the patient.

VQ interpretation may seem challenging at first and requires a solid understanding of lung anatomy and physiology as well as of standardized interpretation criteria. Imaging equipment and ventilation agents have improved over the years, and techniques such as single-photon emission computed tomography (SPECT) and single-photon emission computed tomography with computed tomography (SPECT/CT) are reported to improve VQ accuracy. Although the general impression is that CTPA offers greater accuracy over VQ, investigations directly comparing CTPA and VQ have found little or no difference in accuracy or patient outcomes between the two.

VQ BACKGROUND

During the perfusion portion of the VQ scan, intravenously administered radiolabeled albumen particles are either normally trapped in distal capillaries or are prevented from reaching the lung periphery if they meet an obstruction, such as a clot. The emboli result in regions of decreased perfusion in the territory fed by the obstructed vessels: lobe, segment, or subsegments depending on whether the clot lodges centrally or distally (Fig. 7.3).

PE diagnosis is complicated by the fact that the body normally shunts blood away from areas of the lung that are not properly ventilated. This means that causes other than PE can also lead to regions of decreased perfusion. Most commonly these are lung diseases, such as emphysema, interstitial lung disease, and asthma. Box 7.2 lists some causes of abnormal ventilation. Comparing ventilation to the perfusion pattern can help determine whether the diagnosis is PE. With emboli, tissues usually remain ventilated, at least for some time. So, the VQ will demonstrate normal ventilation in the areas of perfusion deficit from the embolus, resulting in a "mismatched" defect (Fig. 7.4). Airway diseases, on the other hand, show

ventilation abnormalities that coincide with the perfusion defects. These "matched" defects are unlikely to be caused by an acute PE. Box 7.3 contains definitions of some important terms applied to VQ scintigraphy.

RADIOPHARMACEUTICALS

Perfusion: Tc-99m MAA

Technetium-99m macroaggregated albumin (Tc-99m MAA) is the only lung-perfusion agent clinically available in the United States. Radiolabeled particles must be larger than the red blood cells so that they will be trapped in the lungs on the first pass but should not be so large that they lodge centrally. Although MAA particles range in size from 5 to 100 μm, 60% to 80% of the particles are between 20 and 80 μm. Once in the lung, particles gradually degrade and are phagocytized with a biological half-life ($T_{1/2}$) of 2 to 3 hours.

Considerations for Tc-99m MAA particle administration are listed in Box 7.4. In adults, 200,000 to 600,000 particles are typically used (100,000 minimum to maintain image quality). This obstructs only a small fraction of vessels and should result in no ill effects. However, in some situations, particle-number reduction is recommended to ensure safety. In children, modifications are usually done as a reflection of age or weight. In pregnancy, the particles are limited to the minimum. Particle numbers are also decreased in pulmonary hypertension and in right-to-left cardiac shunts. Although it may seem alarming that particles will occlude capillaries in the brain and other organs in such shunts, Tc-99m MAA has long been used to actually calculate cardiac shunts without significant problem.

Ventilation Agents

A comparison of ventilation radiopharmaceuticals is listed in Table 7.2. Of these, two aerosols are the most commonly used currently: Tc-99m diethylenetriaminepentaacetic acid (Tc-99m DTPA) in the United States and Tc-99m Technegas (Cyclomedica)

BOX 7.2   Causes of Ventilation and Perfusion (VQ) Defects

Primary Vascular Lesions
Pulmonary thromboembolism
Septic, fat, and air emboli
Vasculitis
Congenital vascular anomalies

Primary Ventilation Abnormality
Pneumonia
Atelectasis
Pulmonary edema
Acute asthma
Chronic obstructive pulmonary disease: emphysema, bullae, chronic bronchitis
Mucous plug

Mass Effect
Tumor
Adenopathy
Pleural effusion

Iatrogenic
Surgery: Pneumonectomy, lobectomy
Radiation fibrosis, postinflammatory fibrosis

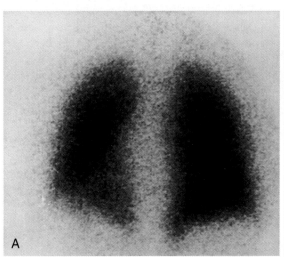
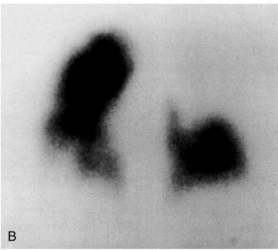

Fig. 7.4 Mismatched perfusion–ventilation defects. Posterior ventilation (A) and perfusion (B) images show an extensive mismatched defect in the right upper lung as well in the left lower lobe in a high-probability scan.

in Europe and Australia. Tc-99m Technegas images are generally superior; however, approval by the U.S. Food and Drug Administration (FDA) has been delayed for years in the United States. Although krypton-81 (Kr-81) gas may be used in some sites outside the United States, Xe-133 is the only gas ventilation available currently for routine clinical use in the United States.

Xe-133

Gas ventilation agents disperse more easily in the lungs than Tc-99m DTPA aerosol, allowing for superior images in cases where airflow is abnormal. Xe-133 gas is fat soluble, moving from the lung into blood and tissues. As it recirculates, gas exchange allows rapid clearance from the body with a 30- to

---

BOX 7.3   Ventilation–Perfusion (VQ) Scan Terminology

Gestalt: Process of holistic interpretation performed by experienced VQ readers that includes more than the use of strict criteria to achieve a more accurate result.

Matched defect: Abnormality of both scans in same area and of same size.

Mismatched defect: Perfusion abnormality in region of normal ventilation.

Reverse mismatched defect: Ventilation abnormality in area with normal perfusion.

Triple-match defect: A matched VQ lesion within the bronchopulmonary segments occurring in the area of a similar sized radiographic abnormality.

Segmental defect: Corresponds to the segmental lung anatomy; often wedge-shaped and extending to pleura.

Large: >75% of the segment involved

Moderate: 25% to 75% of segment

Small: <25% of the segment

Subsegmental defect: Perfusion defect involving less than a segment of lung parenchyma.

Nonsegmental defect: Lesion does not correspond to segmental anatomy, caused by objects outside of the lung tissue, generally not wedge-shaped.

BOX 7.4   Considerations for Tc-99m MAA Particle Use

≈500,000 particles in a 185-MBq (5-mCi) dose

For Adults

Minimum: 60,000 to 100,000 particles

Standard: 200,000 to 700,000 particles

≈300 million arterioles and 280 billion pulmonary capillaries

Obstructs <0.1% to 0.3% of vessels

Consider Particle Number Reduction

   Pulmonary hypertension: 100,000 to 250,000 particles

     Have far fewer functional capillaries

   Right-to-left cardiac shunt: 100,000 to 150,000 particles

   Pregnancy: 100,000 particles (decreasing radiation dose)

     Use fresh Tc-99m MAA particles.

For Children

Modifications done as a reflection of age

   Neonate: 10,000 particles

   <5 years: 50,000 to 150,000 particles

MAA, Macroaggregated albumin.

45-second biologic T$_{1/2}$. The ability to image washout significantly increases the sensitivity for air trapping in obstructive lung disease, improving overall examination specificity (Fig. 7.5). However, the low photopeak of 81 keV leads to lower-quality images from greater soft tissue attenuation and scatter. It is also sometimes difficult to tell if perfusion defects are matched because the views obtained before washout are limited. Because most PEs occur in the lower lobes, ventilation was usually done only posteriorly in the past, whereas perfusion could be visualized in multiple projections. The wide availability of two-headed cameras today has resulted in more flexibility, and some systems allow simultaneous imaging in the left posterior oblique (LPO) and right posterior oblique (RPO) projections, thereby visualizing three pleural surfaces of each lung. Rooms used for Xe-133 are equipped with a special xenon trap (a system of shielded charcoal filters and tubing that retains the gas until safely decayed), and scanning is performed in a negative-pressure room with a ventilation system that rapidly clears the radioactive gas to the outside.

Tc-99m DTPA

Aerosolized Tc-99m DTPA has recently received FDA approval for clinical use after having been used by physicians "off-label" for decades. The liquid radiopharmaceutical is placed into a nebulizer, producing small particles ranging in size from 0.5 to 2 μm, which are normally able to travel to the lung periphery. However, in asthma and chronic obstructive pulmonary disease (COPD) or when patients cannot cooperate fully with technique, airway turbulence produces large airway deposition and central clumping. Not only does this limit peripheral visualization, but activity shine-through onto the subsequent perfusion scan can obscure perfusion defects (Fig. 7.6).

With time, Tc-99m DTPA is broken down in the lungs and absorbed, ultimately cleared by the kidneys. The biologic T$_{1/2}$ varies but has been estimated at 80 minutes (±20 minutes) in healthy nonsmokers. Clearances dramatically increase when alveolar membranes are damaged. In healthy smokers, the biologic T$_{1/2}$ is only 24 minutes (±9 minutes). Damage to the lungs from toxins or inflammatory processes like adult respiratory distress syndrome can be diagnosed by measuring abnormally rapid Tc-99m DTPA clearance rates.

Tc-99m Technegas

Tc-99m Technegas is an aerosolized suspension of solid carbon particles that are smaller than those of Tc-99m DTPA, small enough to behave as a gas in the lungs. Tc-99m pertechnetate is placed into the crucible of a dedicated machine and incinerated in the presence of 100% argon gas and carbon, resulting in a thin layer of metallic technetium encapsulating carbon particles typically 30 to 60 nm in size (reported range of 5–200 nm, with 80% being less than 100 nm). These particles easily travel to the lung periphery after only a couple inspirations. Images are generally superior to Tc-99m DTPA, with central bronchial

TABLE 7.2 Comparison of VQ Scan Ventilation Agents

Comparison Factor	GAS VENTILATION AGENTS		AEROSOLIZED VENTILATION AGENTS		
	Xenon-133	Krypton-81m	Tc-99m DTPA Aerosol	Tc-99m Technegas	Tc-99m Sulfur Colloid
Decay mode	Beta-minus	Isomeric	Isomeric	Isomeric	Isomeric
Physical $T_{1/2}$	5.3 days	13 sec	6 hr	6 hr	6 hr
Biologic $T_{1/2}$	30 sec	(Continuous intake)	80 min[a]	135 hr	
Photon energy	81 keV	190 keV	140 keV	140 keV	140 keV
Multiple-view imaging	No	Yes	Yes	Yes	Yes
Optimal for SPECT	No	No	+/−	Yes	Yes
Useful for COPD	Yes	Yes	+/−	Yes	+/−
Used after perfusion scan	No	Yes	No	No	No

COPD, Chronic obstructive pulmonary disease; *DTPA,* diethylenetriaminepentaacetic acid; *SPECT,* single-photon emission computed tomography; *VQ,* ventilation–perfusion.
Rates vary: biological half-life = 60 to 100 minutes in nonsmokers and 16 to 45 minutes in healthy smokers.

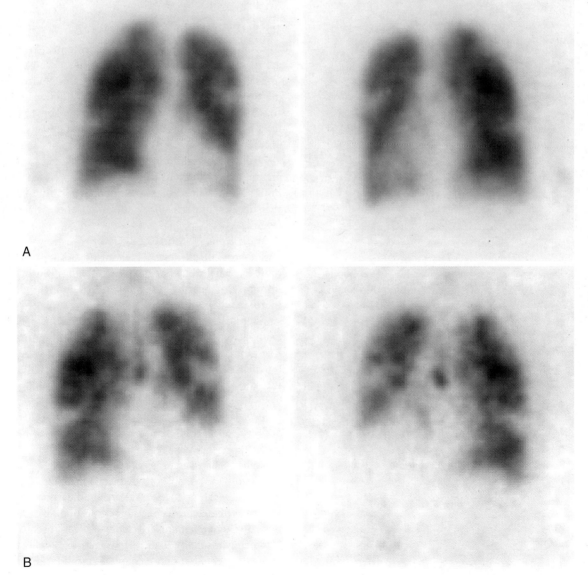

Fig. 7.5 Matched ventilation and perfusion defects on anterior and posterior Tc-99m diethylenetriaminepentaacetic acid (DTPA) aerosol (A) and Tc-99m macroaggregated albumin (MAA) perfusion (B) images.

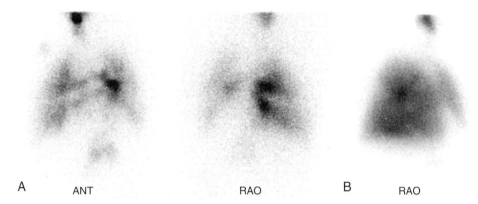

Fig. 7.6 Suboptimal Tc-99m diethylenetriaminepentaacetic acid (DTPA) distribution (A). Poor peripheral distribution can make it difficult to tell if perfusion defects are matched, and retained central radiotracer shine-through onto subsequent Tc-99m macroaggregated albumin (MAA; B) scans can obscure areas of abnormal decreased perfusion.

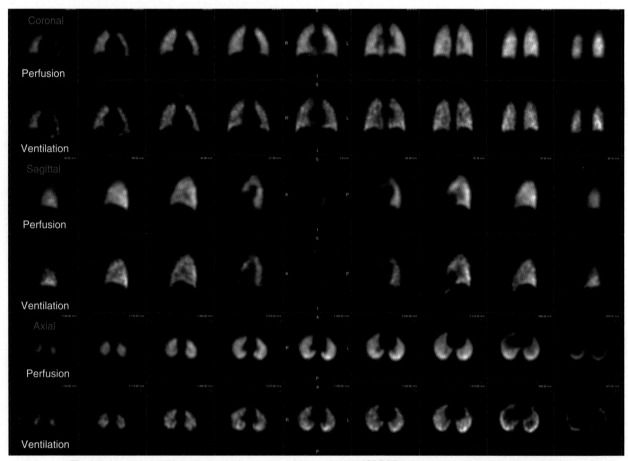

Fig. 7.7 Normal single-photon emission computed tomography (SPECT) lung scan in coronal *(top two rows)*, sagittal *(middle two rows)*, and axial *(bottom two rows)* projections. Tc-99m macroaggregated albumin (MAA) perfusion *(top half of each row)* and Tc-99m Technegas ventilation images *(bottom half of each row)* show good detail, particularly in the medial lungs, which are difficult to see on planar images. Technegas stability in the lungs makes it superior to Tc-99m diethylenetriaminepentaacetic acid (DTPA) for SPECT, avoiding potential problems clearance might create when comparing defects. (Images courtesy of Khun Visith Keu, MD, Hôpital de la Cité-de-la-Santé de Laval, Canada.)

clumping infrequently seen. Unlike the clearance seen with Tc-99m DTPA, these particles lodge in a stable distribution, allowing not only for multiview planar images (in the same projections as the perfusion) but for superior SPECT images as well (Fig. 7.7).

Radiation Exposure: VQ Versus CTPA

Newer low-dose CTPA techniques have generally reduced the radiation dose, narrowing the gap with VQ. Although the CTPA effective whole-body dose is sometimes as low as 2 to 3 mSv, significantly higher doses are often still used (3–9.0 mSv), and

VQ doses, usually less than 1.5 mSv (1.1–2.0 mSv), still compare favorably. Given the radiation sensitivity of the breast, it may be most important to note that VQ results in a much lower breast dose of 0.8 mGy (0.2–1.2 mGy) as opposed to perhaps 5 mGy from CTPA (roughly 3–34 mGy in literature, depending on technique). In pregnancy, radiation doses to the fetus, although low, are reportedly higher from VQ compared with CTPA. However, fetal exposure may be comparable or even lower when using suggested VQ protocol modifications, such as low-dose perfusion only or 2-day protocols, where a perfusion scan is done on day 1 and the ventilation study is performed on day 2 only for those cases requiring it due to perfusion abnormalities. Radiopharmaceutical dosimetry is outlined in Appendix 1.

TECHNIQUE

The ventilation scan is generally acquired first because the perfusion scan would interfere with visualization. The lower-energy photopeak of Xe-133 would be obscured by down-scatter from the higher energy of Tc-99m. Activity in the lungs is also higher on perfusion images, so activity from Tc-99m ventilation agents would be hidden by more abundant Tc-99m MAA counts.

Some sites do perform the perfusion examination first, possibly avoiding a ventilation examination if perfusion is normal in young or pregnant patients and those with clear chest radiographs. This requires a low 1-mCi (37-MBq) Tc-99m MAA dose or delaying the ventilation until the next day, possibly prophylactically treating the patient with heparin overnight. Both situations could result in interpretation difficulties if counts are too low or defects change as atelectasis evolves in the lung.

Ventilation

Protocols for Tc-99m DTPA, Xe-133, and Tc-99m Technegas are outlined in Boxes 7.5, 7.6, and 7.7, respectively. For all ventilation radiopharmaceuticals, patients breathe through a closed system, with a mask connected to the delivery device and the nose clamped. Only a fraction of the dose placed in the unit reaches the lungs. In the case of Tc-99m DTPA, only 0.5 to 1.0 mCi (18.5–37 MBq) is delivered to the lungs. Of the available agents, Tc-99m Technegas has the most rapid uptake, requiring only a few breaths.

Once sufficient activity is present in the lungs, the camera is moved around the patient to obtain the planar images: posterior and anterior, right and left lateral, and bilateral anterior and posterior obliques. For SPECT, Tc-99m Technegas is the agent of choice because of its excellent image quality and its lack of clearance.

Xe-133 scans are done in three phases while the patient breathes through the system for several minutes: an initial single maximum breath, then equilibrium phase image(s) obtained during tidal respiration, followed by washout as the system is switched to room air or oxygen for a few minutes. Because PE is more common in the lower lobes, patients are preferably imaged posteriorly, or if possible, bilateral posterior oblique views allow optimal visualization.

Perfusion

A Tc-99m MAA perfusion protocol example is described in Box 7.8. A 23-gauge or larger needle should be used for particle injection. Blood should not be drawn back into the syringe, to prevent hot emboli (Fig. 7.8). The syringe should be inverted to ensure that particles are mixed and have not clumped before the injection. Particles should be injected slowly, over the course of several respiratory cycles. Because gravity affects blood flow and therefore particle distribution, the patient is preferably supine and should be in the same position for both ventilation images and Tc-99m MAA.

BOX 7.5   Tc-99m DTPA Ventilation Scintigraphy

Patient Preparation
Chest radiograph within 24 hours

Dose Administration
1110 MBq (30 mCi) Tc-99m DTPA in nebulizer; patient receives 20 to 40 MBq (0.5–1.0 mCi).

Instrumentation
Collimator: Low energy, parallel hole
Photopeak: 20% window centered at 140 keV

Positioning
Place nose clamps and connect mouthpiece with patient semisupine.

Image Acquisition
Center camera over chest; patient breathes continuously for several minutes.
Acquire posterior image for 250,000 counts; obtain other views for this same time: anterior and posterior, anterior and posterior obliques, right and left lateral.

DTPA, Diethylenetriaminepentaacetic acid.

BOX 7.6   Xe-133 Ventilation Scintigraphy

Patient Preparation
Chest radiograph within 24 hours

Dose Administration
Adult: 740 MBq (20 mCi) Xe-133 in chamber
Pediatric: 10 to 12 MBq/kg (1–10 mCi/kg) with 100 to 120 MBq (3 mCi) minimum

Instrumentation
Collimator: Low energy, parallel hole
Photopeak: 20% window centered at 81 keV

Positioning
Place nose clamps and connect mouthpiece with patient on camera.

Image Acquisition
First breath: Patient exhales fully then maximally inhales and holds it (if possible) for 100,000 counts or 10 to 20 seconds.
Equilibrium: Obtain three sequential 90-second images as patient breathes normally.
Posterior obliques may be possible at this time.
Washout: Turn system to exhaust; obtain sequential 45-second posterior images until activity clears or for 5 minutes.

BOX 7.7 Tc-99m Technegas Ventilation Scintigraphy

Patient Preparation
Chest radiograph within 24 hours

Dose Administration
500 MBq (30 mCi) Tc-99m Technegas, range 400 to 900 MBq (10–25 mCi)

Dose Preparation
Power on dose generator, turn on argon supply, and then turn on regulator.
Wet crucible with ethanol, draw back excess, and insert wet crucible into machine.
Load Tc-99m pertechnetate dose into crucible with 1-cc syringe
(may repeat, after a simmer run to evaporate fluid in order to achieve desired dose).
Press start to ignite burn (raises temperature above 2700°C for 15 seconds).
Disconnect argon.
Administer within 10 minutes.

Instrumentation
Collimator: Low energy, parallel hole
Photopeak: 20% window centered at 140 keV
Matrix: Planar 256 × 256; SPECT 64 × 64 (can use 128 × 128)

Positioning
Place nose clamps and connect mouthpiece with patient supine/semisupine, in well-ventilated room, preferably apart from camera room to avoid contamination.
Patient breathes in for three to six respiratory cycles.
Five-second breath hold at end of each increases retention until 2 kcounts/min.
Center camera over chest.

Image Acquisition
Planar: Acquire posterior image for 250,000 to 500,000 counts; obtain other views for this time: anterior and posterior, anterior and posterior obliques, right and left lateral.
SPECT: 3 degrees/step, 64 steps/head, 10 seconds/view, 360 degrees total
Reconstruction: Ordered-subset expectation maximization; 8 iterations, 4 subsets
Postreconstruction filter: Three-dimensional (3-D) Butterworth; cutoff 0.8 cycles/cm, order 9

SPECT, Single-photon emission computed tomography.

BOX 7.8 Tc-99m Technegas Ventilation Scintigraphy

Patient Preparation
Chest radiograph within 24 hours

Dose Administration
40 to 150 MBq (1–4 mCi) Tc-99m MAA IV; for SPECT, 100 to 120 MBq (2–3 mCi) ideal
Pediatric: 1.11 MBq/kg (0.03 mCi/Kg) with minimum 14.8 MBq/kg (0.04 mCi/kg) if no ventilation performed or 2.59 MBq/kg (0.07 mCi/kg) with Tc-99m ventilation

Instrumentation
Collimator: Low energy, parallel hole
Photopeak: 20% window centered at 140 keV

Positioning
Place nose clamps and connect mouthpiece with patient semisupine.
Center camera over chest.

Image Acquisition
Planar: Acquire posterior image for 250,000 counts; obtain other views for this same time: anterior and posterior, anterior and posterior obliques, right and left lateral.
SPECT: 3 degrees/step, 64 steps/head, 10 seconds/view, 360 degrees total
Reconstruction: Ordered-subset expectation maximization; 8 iterations, 4 subsets
Postreconstruction filter: Three-dimensional (3-D) Butterworth; cutoff 0.8 cycles/cm, order 9

IV, intravenous; *MAA,* macroaggregated albumin; *SPECT,* single-photon emission computed tomography.

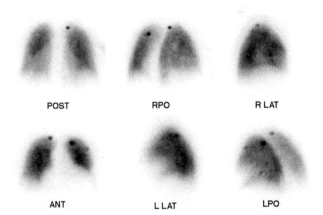

Fig. 7.8 Injected blood clot artifact. During the Tc-99m macroaggregated albumin (MAA) injection process, some blood was drawn back into the syringe, forming blood clots, appearing here as hot spots. They have a variable appearance but can be quite large. *(Top row, left to right):* POST, posterior; RPO, right posterior oblique; R LAT, right lateral. *(Bottom row)* ANT, anterior; LAT, left lateral; LPO, left posterior oblique.

IMAGE INTERPRETATION

VQ interpretation criteria originally required comparison with a chest radiograph less than 24 hours old, although a CT is now also acceptable. Not only can the radiograph reveal alternate diagnoses and change scan interpretation, but it may also influence which imaging protocol is chosen. When the radiograph is normal, the scan is usually diagnostic, and a low-dose perfusion-only scan might be suitable. Abnormal chest radiographs can make interpretation less certain; however, even when significantly abnormal, a diagnosis can often be made by VQ.

VQ interpretation is complex. Experienced readers combine many factors beyond strict criteria into their interpretation, referred to as *Gestalt.* Less experienced readers should interpret the study based on a standard criterion. All readers are encouraged to use a *holistic* approach, that is, one that includes clinical information, such as D-dimer, Wells score, and clinical suspicion.

Perfusion Image Findings

Normal perfusion is homogeneous, has relatively higher count density in the bases and dependent lower lobes, and is decreased in the areas of the mediastinal structures. Persistent Tc-99m DTPA ventilation activity can sometimes be seen in

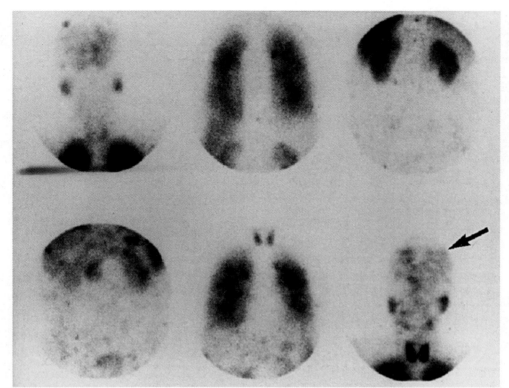

Fig. 7.9 Right-to-left cardiac shunt. Intravenously injected Tc-99m macroaggregated albumin (MAA) images reveal abnormal uptake in the brain, thyroid, kidneys, and salivary glands, whereas free Tc-99m pertechnetate could accumulate in the salivary glands and thyroid and be cleared in the urine. However, the cerebral activity should not be seen be seen, because free pertechnetate cannot cross the intact blood–brain barrier. Heterogeneous activity in the abdomen is also from shunting.

the trachea and central airways, and swallowed radiotracer may be seen in the esophagus and stomach. The absorbed Tc-99m can result in excreted activity in the kidneys and bladder, and the thyroid may accumulate free Tc-99m pertechnetate. However, these areas are not normally intense, and free pertechnetate cannot cross the blood–brain barrier. Tc-99m MAA activity in the brain is diagnostic of a right-to-left cardiac shunt (Fig. 7.9).

Perfusion deficits are described in terms of number, size, location, shape, and intensity. Decreased activity is considered abnormal, not only absent perfusion. Then each abnormality is compared with ventilation and characterized as matched or mismatched. Because more than 90% of PEs are multiple and over 85% are bilateral, multiple mismatched perfusion abnormalities can be expected on the VQ (Fig. 7.10) if symptoms are acute, especially if less than 24 hours in duration. The timing of symptom onset should be considered because in very rare instances, PE can induce bronchoconstriction in the first 4 to 6 hours, leading to perfusion defects appearing matched. Wedge-shaped mismatched defects extending to the periphery and confined to the contours and shape of the vascular segments are expected in PE. Defects that do not respect the segmental boundaries are usually caused by diseases other than emboli.

A proper description of findings requires familiarity with the appearance of the segments on each of the views (Fig. 7.11). Real segmental perfusion defects are usually visible on more than one view and extend to the pleural surface. Possible

exceptions to this can occur in the lingual segments (sometimes only be visible on the left anterior oblique view or with SPECT) and in the medial basal segments (which might be seen only with SPECT).

A perfusion abnormality may encompass an entire lobe, a segment, or a subsegment. As noted in Box 7.8, subsegmental lesions are graded by size: large >75% of the segment, moderate 25% to 75%, and small <25%. Because large or moderate defects are considered most suspicious for PE, size is an important factor to assess. However, these are subjective estimates.

Objects outside of the bronchopulmonary segments that can cause VQ abnormalities include an enlarged heart, ectatic aorta, pleural effusion, and metal artifact (Fig. 7.12 and 7.13). Pleural effusions can be especially problematic because they may vary significantly with positional changes between the VQ and chest radiograph. Common causes of such *nonsegmental* defects are listed in Box 7.9.

Emboli can be intermittent or recurrent. They are often only partially obstructing and gradually break down over time. Thus, a mix of large and small defects or ill-defined mismatches are often present. At a later stage, secondary atelectasis may lead to perfusion lesions becoming matched. However, perfusion does not usually normalize in less than 24 hours (Fig. 7.14). In young patients, clearance is typically more rapid (i.e., in days or weeks). In certain patients, particularly in the elderly and in those with underlying cardiopulmonary disease, some defects may never disappear; those persisting more than a few months are unlikely to ever clear.

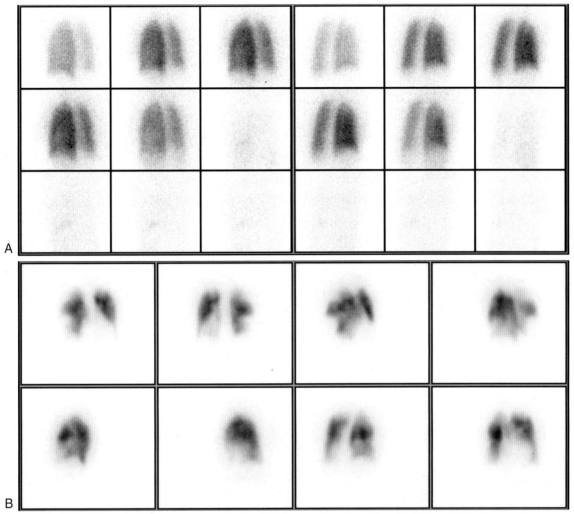

Fig. 7.10 High-probability ventilation–perfusion (VQ) image. Posterior oblique Xe-133 ventilation images (A) are normal. Multiview Tc-99m macroaggregated albumin (MAA) perfusion images (B) reveal multiple large and moderate perfusion defects bilaterally. This mismatched pattern is consistent with PE.

Ventilation Image Findings

Tc-99m DTPA and Tc-99m Technegas images normally appear homogeneous. Xe-133 activity is slightly fainter on the initial single-breath image because of lower counts, then rapidly increases with further breathing. Xe-133 washout should be rapid, usually clearing within 90 to 120 seconds. Regions are abnormal on a Xe-133 image when there is an area of either significantly decreased activity on any phase, even if it normalizes later, or when activity does not clear normally during washout from regional air trapping. Care must be taken to not confuse Xe-133 retention in a fatty liver with air trapping in the right lung base (Fig. 7.15). The initial single breath alone will identify abnormal areas in the majority of cases. The washout images, however, frequently best demonstrate air trapping (Fig. 7.16). The sensitivity for COPD is high, approximately 90%.

PIOPED

VQ scan criteria content and naming conventions have evolved over the years (Box 7.10). The multicenter

Prospective Investigation of Pulmonary Embolism Diagnosis (PIOPED or PIOPED I) study, published in 1990, sought to assess VQ scan accuracy, optimize interpretation criteria, and standardize result reporting. The interpretation criteria used grouped findings into levels of probability that PE is present based on the number and size of matched and mismatched perfusion defects in conjunction with the chest radiograph findings. Scans were then interpreted as follows:

Normal	No perfusion defects
High probability	Findings highly likely to be caused by PE
	PE likely present in over 80% of the cases
Low probability	Findings unlikely to be from PE
	PE in less than 20% of cases
Intermediate probability	Findings more nonspecific,
	Risk between high and low (20–80%)

All patients then underwent pulmonary angiography and clinical follow-up to determine the actual final diagnosis. Based on

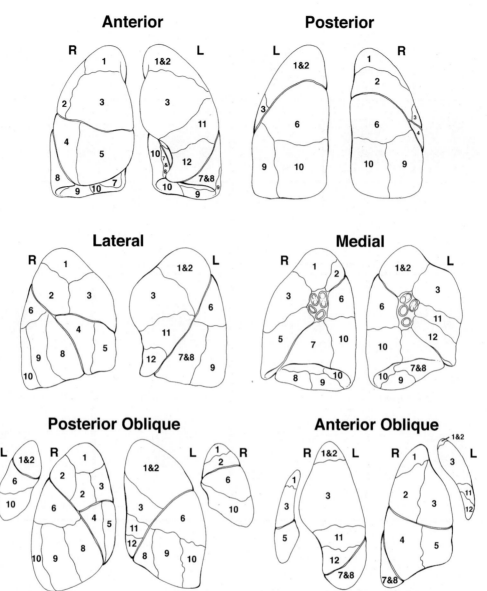

Fig. 7.11 Segmental anatomy of the lungs. The right lung is made up of three lobes. The right upper lobe contains the apical, posterior, and anterior segments. The right middle lobe consists of the medial and lateral segments. The right lower lobe contains the superior, medial basal, anterior basal, lateral basal, and posterior basal segments. The left lung is made up of the upper and lower lobes, with the lingual part of the upper lobe. The left upper lobe consists of the apicoposterior and anterior segments as well as the superior and inferior segments in the lingula. The left lower lobe comprises the superior, anteromedial basal, lateral basal, and posterior basal segments.

the data, a few key changes were made to increase the accuracy of the originally proposed criteria. The resulting Modified PIOPED Criteria became standard (Table 7.3).

The PIOPED trial confirmed that a normal examination virtually excluded PE, and the 90% positive predictive value of a high-probability study usually allowed treatment without further workup. However, setting the limit of a low-probability scan at an up to 19% chance of PE also meant the risk would be too great for most to ignore without further workup, making it a less useful as a distinct category. In addition, only 41% of documented PEs occurred in patients with high-probability scans, with the majority of PEs occurring in scans read as low or intermediate (Table 7.4). Only 28% of patients received a definitive normal or high-probability VQ diagnosis. Although a subsequent study with a more balanced population of outpatients and inpatients found a definite diagnosis in 46% of patients, this still meant a majority of patients received a "nondiagnostic" intermediate or low-probability result.

In order to decrease the number of nondiagnostic examinations, scan patterns with a <10% likely risk of PE from the PIOPED I data were identified and used to create a very low-probability category. This significantly decreased nondiagnostic results, pulling cases from the low- and indeterminate-probability groups.

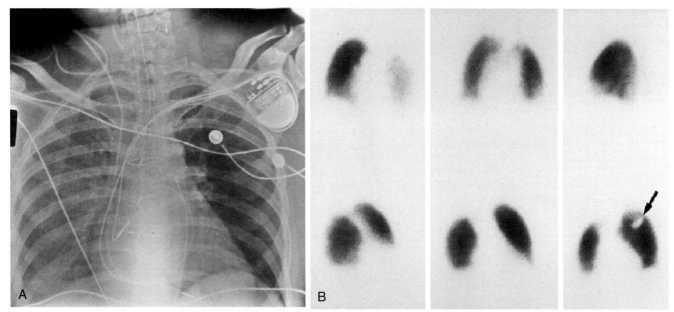

Fig. 7.12 Nonsegmental perfusion defects. (A) Portable chest radiograph shows a hazy density throughout the right lung compared with the left from a pleural effusion layering posteriorly due to supine positioning. (B) Tc-99m macroaggregated albumin (MAA) lung perfusion images reveal a corresponding decrease in activity on the right as well as a defect from the pacemaker *(arrow)*. Although perfusion on the right looks diffusely decreased on anterior and posterior images, it is much less severe on other views, tipping off the observer to the explanation.

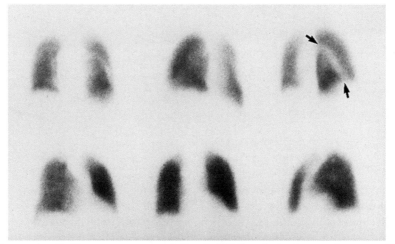

Fig. 7.13 Fissure sign. Tc-99m macroaggregated albumin (MAA) perfusion images show a curvilinear defect in the right lung *(arrows)* from fluid tracking into the major fissure.

BOX 7.9 Potential Causes of Nonsegmental Perfusion Defects

Pacemaker artifact
Tumor
Pleural effusion
Cardiomegaly
Hilar adenopathy
Aortic ectasia or aneurysm
Bullae
Linear atelectasis
Pneumonia

Clinicians might watch these near-normal cases rather than start treatment, making it a more useful category than low probability. Efforts were then also made to simplify the criteria by combining the remaining intermediate- and low-probability patterns into a new "nondiagnostic" category, eliminating the confusing term *"intermediate probability."* The final Modified PIOPED II criteria consisted of *normal, high probability, very low probability,* and *nondiagnostic.*

The validity of the very low-probability category was then retrospectively examined using data from the subsequent PIOPED II trial, a trial designed to assess the accuracy of CTPA

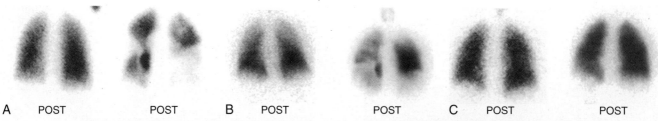

Fig. 7.14 Resolving pulmonary embolus (PE). (A) Normal posterior ventilation images *(left)* and abnormal perfusion images from PE *(right)* from a patient with PE. (B) Ten years later, the patient returned with recurrent symptoms. The ventilation was normal, but the perfusion is again abnormal on the right. However, no new baseline had been done, and it was difficult to tell which areas might be acute. (C) The patient was anticoagulated, and images 7 days later show near complete perfusion defect resolution *(right)*, confirming the acute nature of the defects.

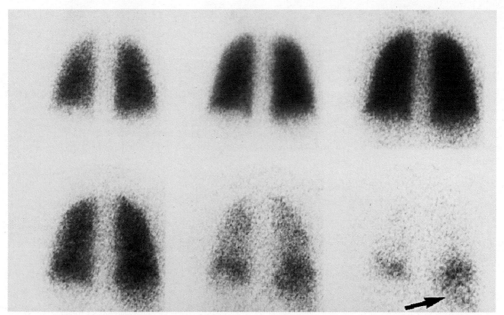

Fig. 7.15 Xe-133 accumulation in the liver. Posterior images show delayed washout of the lung bases and significant xenon uptake in the region of the liver *(arrow)*.

and CT venography. Although the VQ scans had been used in this trial as part of the initial diagnostic evaluation, data suggested the new rules were valid. The Modified PIOPED II criteria have become the most widely used set of VQ interpretation rules in the United States (see Table 7.3).

Diagnostic Interpretation Categories
Normal
When a study is completely normal (see Figs. 7.1 and 7.2), the diagnosis of PE is essentially excluded, with an incidence of 1.3% in the PIOPED II data and 1% to 3% in other reports. Significant morbidity from PE was found to be less than 1% based on follow-up performed on patients with normal VQ scans. When clinical pretest suspicion is low, the chance of PE is near 0.

High Probability
A high-probability scan is typically fairly obvious (Figs. 7.17; see also Figs. 7.4, 7.10, and 7.14). In order to ensure a scan is sufficiently specific, the Modified PIOPED and Modified PIOPED II

criteria require two or more large (>75%) mismatched segmental perfusion defects, or their equivalent in moderate and large-sized defects (small mismatched defects are not counted) with a clear radiograph in the mismatched areas.

Although the category was devised to carry a risk of PE ≥80%, in reality, it is actually higher, at least 85% to 95%. Because the pretest probability affects results, it is not surprising that this rises to 96% to 98% when clinical suspicion is also high, concordant with scan results. Although unusual, false-positive high-probability scans can occur for several reasons (Box 7.11). The most common cause is a prior PE that did not resolve. Therefore comparison with a prior study, if available, is important. A repeat scan in 1 to 2 weeks after PE is helpful to establish a new baseline in case symptoms later recur.

Considerations Involving Near-Normal to Nondiagnostic Scans
Under the Modified PIOPED I criteria, most scans with matched defects went into the low-probability category, even when

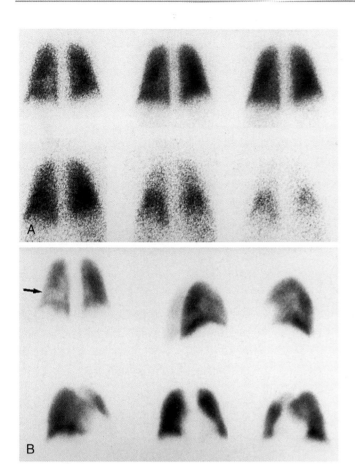

Fig. 7.16 Air trapping on ventilation–perfusion (VQ) images. (A) Xe-133 ventilation images show normal initial and equilibrium images but bibasilar retained radiotracer during washout consistent with air trapping. (B) Tc-99m macroaggregated albumin (MAA) perfusion reveals a large perfusion defect in the left lower lobe *(arrow)*, which is matched by the ventilation examination, lowering suspicion for pulmonary embolus (PE). Although washout is very sensitive for chronic obstructive pulmonary disease (COPD), abnormal ventilation on any phase is counted as abnormal, even if it is normal on other phases.

BOX 7.10 Lung Scan Interpretation Criteria

Biello criteria—used as foundation for criteria tested
Prospective Investigation of Pulmonary Embolism Diagnosis (PIOPED) or PIOPED I
Revised PIOPED criteria
Modified PIOPED II criteria

---

extensive. Small perfusion defects were all considered low risk as well, with ventilation status less important. For example, such small perfusion defects can sometimes be mismatched in restrictive airway disease.

The very low-probability category of the Modified PIOPED II criteria may seem much more complicated at first. However, it may help to remember that most cases that do not appear suspicious or are near normal are probably at the <10% risk of very low probability rather than the higher risk of the nondiagnostic category. Several lower-risk items are fairly obvious: nonsegmental defects related to structures outside the bronchovascular

segments (e.g., enlarged cardiovascular structures, elevated diaphragm, and large bullae) and situations with a "stripe sign," a strip of blood flow peripheral to a defect (Fig. 7.18). The investigators also found that when moderate to large-sized matched defects are multiple (≥2) or when small perfusion abnormalities were limited to one to three in number, the case could move from low into very low probability.

However, in a few situations, matched defects are associated with higher risk. Most notably this involves some triple-matched abnormalities (perfusion, ventilation, and radiographic defect). Hemorrhagic infarct or atelectasis from a PE can cause radiographic opacities of equal or lesser size compared with the perfusion abnormality. However, the radiographic abnormality is unlikely from emboli if it is larger than the perfusion defect. In the past, triple matches were all classified as intermediate risk. Now, only a triple match in the lower lung fields is considered nondiagnostic (and still in the intermediate-probability range), whereas such abnormalities in the upper lung fields can be called very low probability (Fig. 7.19).

Special Considerations

Severe Unilateral Lung Involvement. Occasionally, absent or severely decreased perfusion involves only one lung (Fig. 7.20). Although this technically involves multiple large segmental areas, it is extremely rare for this pattern to be the result of a large central saddle embolus. Matching VQ abnormalities are the result of the most common causes of unilateral decreased perfusion, surgery, or mucous plug. If the perfusion defect is not matched, then a central bronchogenic carcinoma or a hilar mass that impinges on vessels but spares the bronchial airway must be sought on the radiograph or CT. Some potential etiologies for this pattern are listed in Box 7.12.

Pleural Effusions. Small pleural effusions are frequently found in patients with PE. A chronic effusion is considered an anatomical defect. Under Modified PIOPED II guidelines, an acute small effusion (<1/3 of the hemithorax) belongs with the nondiagnostic group, tiny effusions can usually be ignored, and large effusions are placed in the very low-probability category. However, some limited past data beyond the PIOPED reviews suggested larger acute effusions might belong in the nondiagnostic group if no other etiology is evident.

Criteria Use and Development. As mentioned previously, the chance that the VQ (or even CT) result will accurately identify or exclude PE differs, depending on the clinical suspicion or pretest probability (Table 7.5). For example, a low-probability VQ in a patient with high clinical suspicion has a much >20% chance of PE, maybe closer to 40%. However, the risk is near 2% when clinical suspicion is low/very low. With a very low-probability interpretation, most clinicians will observe rather than treat or pursue additional workup. If the pretest clinical suspicion is also low, a very low-probability result essentially eliminates PE from the differential. There are some data showing fairly similar outcomes between patients with normal and very low-probability studies, and a case can be made for calling all of these examinations negative for PE.

TABLE 7.3 VQ Interpretation Criteria for Pulmonary Embolism Diagnosis

Modified PIOPED (PIOPED)[a]	Modified PIOPED II[a]	EANM VQ Guidelines (SPECT or SPECT/CT)[b]
High Probability ≥2 large mismatched defects 2 moderate segments = a large segment	**High Probability (PE Present)** ≥2 large mismatched defects 2 moderate segments = a large segment	**PE Present** VQ mismatch in ≥1 segment OR ≥ 2 subsegments conforming to the pulmonary vascular anatomy
Intermediate Probability 1 large or 2 moderate mismatched defects Difficult to characterize as high or low	**Nondiagnostic** All other findings not categorized as high, low, very low, or normal probability	**Nondiagnostic** Multiple VQ abnormalities not typical of specific diseases
Borderline Low Probability 1 matched defect, (−)CXR	**Very Low Probability** Solitary large pleural effusion (≥{1/3}) with no other Q defects	
Low Probability Multiple matched defects with (−)CXR Q defect <<CXR lesion Any number of small Q defects	**Very Low Probability** Nonsegmental Q defect Q defect <CXR lesion Stripe sign 1–3 small Q defects Solitary triple-matched defect (VQ/CXR) in upper or mid-lung ≥2 matched VQ defect (−)CXR	
Very Low Probability Nonsegmental Q defect Nonsegmental Q defect Q defect <CXR defect Stripe sing 1–3 small Q defects	**Normal** (PE absent) No perfusion defects	PE absent
Normal No Q defects		Normal perfusion Matched VQ or reverse mismatch (V>Q) defects of any size, shape, or number in the absence of mismatch VQ mismatch not in a lobar, segmental, or subsegmental pattern

CXR, Chest radiograph; *EANM,* European Association of Nuclear Medicine; *PE,* pulmonary embolus; *PIOPED,* Prospective Investigation of Pulmonary Embolism Diagnosis; *Q,* perfusion; *SPECT,* single-photon emission computed tomography; *SPECT/CT,* single-photon emission computed tomography with computed tomography; *V,* ventilation, *(−),* clear/normal.

[a]Modified from Society of Nuclear Medicine and Molecular Imaging (SNMMI) Procedure Guideline 4.0. Reston, VA: SNMMI; 2012; and Sostman HD, Miniati M, Gottschalk A, et al. Sensitivity and specificity of perfusion scintigraphy combined with chest radiography for acute pulmonary embolism in PIOPED II. *J Nucl Med.* 2008;49:1741–1748.

[b]From *European Association of Nuclear Medicine (EANM) ventilation/perfusion guidelines.* Vienna, Austria: EANM; 2009.

TABLE 7.4 PIOPED I and II Breakdown of Results

VQ	PIOPED		MODIFIED PIOPED II	
	PE+	PE−	PE+	PE−
High	102 (41%)	14 (3%)	89 (53%)	13 (2%)
Intermediate	105 (41%)	217 (45%)	47 (27%)	105 (14%)
Low	39 (16%)	199 (41%)	6 (4%)	83 (11%)
Very low	NA	NA	24 (15%)	391 (53%)
Normal	5 (2%)	50 (11%)	2 (1%)	150 (20%)
Total patients	251	480	168	742

PIOPED, Prospective Investigation of Pulmonary Embolism Diagnosis.

Many readers continue to advocate for continued simplification of VQ criteria: calling studies positive (PE present), negative (PE absent), or nondiagnostic. Although the use of such a *trinary* approach has been limited, simplification may be useful. The use of likelihood or probability has confused referring physicians since the original PIOPED trial decades ago, and most tests are reported in terms of the presence or absence of disease.

Criteria development also continues to examine the significance of the *single-segment* mismatch. Whereas the Modified PIOPED and Modified PIOPED II criteria call for two segmental mismatches, one such defect might be sufficient for a high-probability reading under appropriate conditions. Some alternative interpretation protocols have recognized this in such

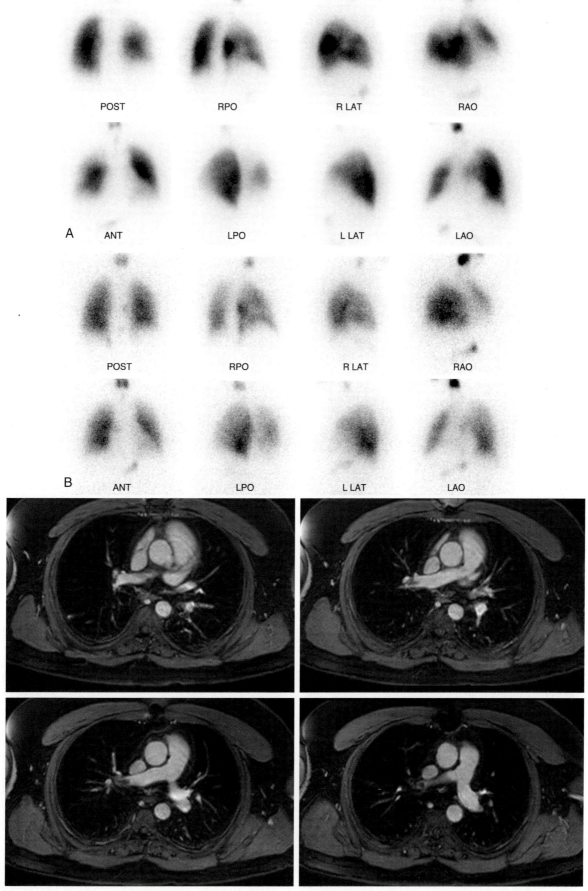

Fig. 7.17 Magnetic resonance arteriogram (MRA) of pulmonary embolus (PE). (A) Ventilation and (B) perfusion images from a ventilation–perfusion (VQ) scan reveal a large area of mismatched decreased perfusion in the right upper lung and smaller areas of decreased perfusion in the right lower lobe in a patient with a clear chest radiograph, interpreted as high probability for PE. An MRA was performed 48 hours later due to worsened symptoms. (C) Axial gadoteridol enhanced T1-weighted gradient echo fat suppression (three-dimensional [3-D] spoiled gradient echo [GRE]) images demonstrate a filling defect in the distal right lobar and the interlobar pulmonary arteries in the upper lobe. More distal, subsegmental defects were also seen in the right lower lobe but are not well visualized on these limited slices.

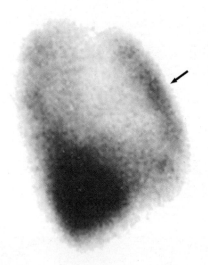

R LAT

Fig. 7.18 Stripe sign. On the right lateral view, perfusion is seen along the periphery of the lung *(arrow)* beyond an extensive defect, strongly suggesting the adjacent decreased activity is not from a pulmonary embolus (PE).

situations as a patient with no prior cardiopulmonary disease and a clear chest radiograph (Fig. 7.21). In addition, newer criteria being advocated for SPECT have considered a single mismatched defect in such situations enough for a positive scan reading.

SPECT in Ventilation–Perfusion Scintigraphy

In Europe, SPECT has become the standard of care, as stated in the *European Association of Nuclear Medicine (EANM) 2009 Guidelines for Ventilation/Perfusion Scintigraphy* (see Table 7.3). As proven in many types of scans, SPECT improves contrast resolution and sensitivity, and the same holds true with SPECT VQ (Figs. 7.22 and 7.23). In the lungs, the lack of overlap with adjacent segments makes defects not only easier to detect (particularly in the medial basal segments) but also easier to characterize in size, shape, and relation to the vascular segmental anatomy than is often possible on planar images.

EANM SPECT criteria require at least one large (or moderate to large) segmental mismatched defect in order for a

study to be called positive for PE. Findings negative for PE include mismatched defects not conforming to a segmental configuration, all matched defects (no matter the size or number), and any reverse mismatched defect (Q smaller than V). Comparison with CT or performing the examination with SPECT/CT is recommended to avoid incorrect interpretations from findings such as nonsegmental decreased perfusion in the area of the pulmonary fissures, dependent lungs with pulmonary edema, or when secondary to an identifiable cause (Fig. 7.24).

SPECT VQ data are more limited and largely retrospective. However, data stated in the EANM guidelines describe results from over 3000 patients with a sensitivity of 96% to 99%, specificities of 91% to 98%, and negative predictive value (NPV) of 97% to 99% (Bajc et al., 2009). Nondiagnostic examinations were reported in only 1% to 3% in their reports, and other trials have confirmed a low rate of nondiagnostic studies (less than 5%). More recent reports continue to show very promising results. It is likely that SPECT will become the method of choice in the United States once Tc-99m Technegas is approved by the FDA.

Comparisons of Planar VQ, CTPA, and SPECT VQ

In the PIOPED II trial, multidetector CTPA (MDCT) had a sensitivity of 83% and a specificity of 96%, although this value excluded 6% technically inadequate examinations (51/824 patients). Some have noted that technology has improved since the PIOPED II data. However, sensitivities reported in the literature for CTPA vary widely (57–100%), likely not as high as commonly believed. Specificity values are good (range 78–100%), and very high NPVs are generally seen. If the pretest clinical suspicion is not concordant with the scan findings, CTPA results are far less reliable (as was previously noted with VQ scans). For example, studies have shown that although the positive predictive value (PPV) of CTPA is high when clinical suspicion for PE is also high (96%), it is only 58% when clinical suspicion is low. When technically adequate, CTPA is more accurate than planar VQ, although some experts note that the superiority does not translate to improved clinical outcomes. In fact, planar VQ is able to provide similar results with a lower radiation dose. However, radiation doses from CTPA have improved, and the acquisition time is extremely fast.

Critical assessment of SPECT VQ has been limited by the lack of large prospective comparison trials with CTPA and planar VQ utilizing a true gold standard. However, SPECT VQ clearly provides superior images and few nondiagnostic results compared with planar VQ. The increased accuracy may not be significant in terms of clinical outcomes, with both tests having similar NPV values (1.1–1.2%). VQ SPECT comparison to CTPA is also limited. However, early data suggest both show a high degree of accuracy, sensitivity, and specificity, often >90%. In a couple of studies, CTPA seems more specific (98% vs. 91%, 100% vs. 88%) and SPECT VQ more sensitive (97% vs. 86%, 97% vs. 68%), with both tests being accurate (93–94%). Some sites also now favor SPECT/CT over SPECT because it allows identification of other underlying disease and can improve

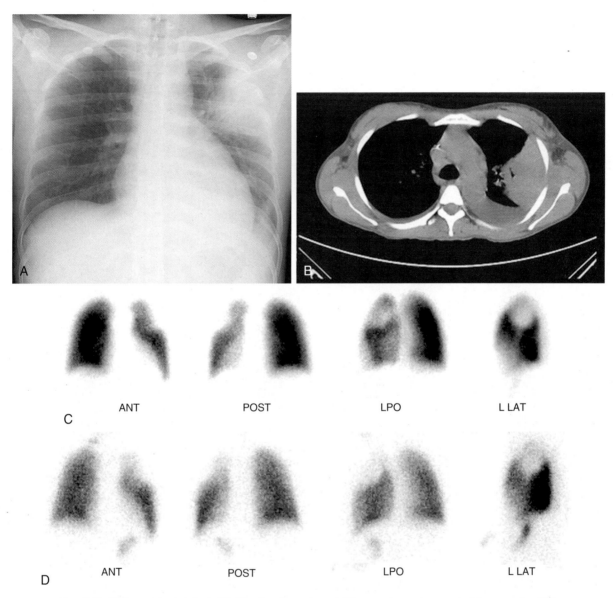

Fig. 7.19 Triple-matched defect. (A) Chest radiograph and (B) nonenhanced computed tomography (CT) reveal a large left upper lobe density in a patient with shortness of breath who could not have contrast due to poor renal function. A corresponding matched defect is seen on perfusion (C) and ventilation (D) lung scan images. Originally, Prospective Investigation of Pulmonary Embolism Diagnosis (PIOPED) classified triple-matched defects as intermediate probability. With Modified PIOPED II, only those in the lower lung fields are actually high enough risk to place in the nondiagnostic group, whereas those in the upper and mid-lung fields are actually very low probability. This patient was found to have aspergillosis, and findings rapidly cleared within days of starting treatment.

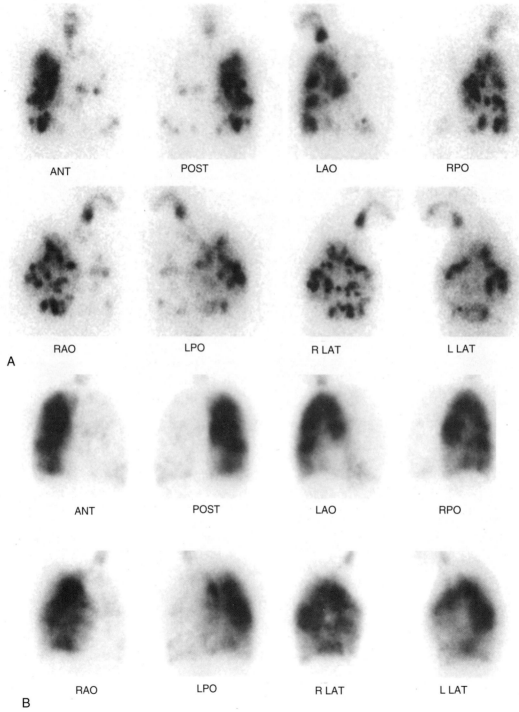

ANT   POST   LAO   RPO

RAO   LPO   R LAT   L LAT

A

ANT   POST   LAO   RPO

RAO   LPO   R LAT   L LAT

B

Fig. 7.20 Severe unilateral lung involvement. Near-absent ventilation to the right lung with Tc-99m dieth-ylenetriaminepentaacetic acid (DTPA) (A) and markedly decreased Tc-99m macroaggregated albumin (MAA) perfusion (B) in a patient with a clear radiograph (not shown). Even extensive perfusion defects are low probability by Modified Prospective Investigation of Pulmonary Embolism Diagnosis (PIOPED) criteria if they are matched, there is at least some perfusion somewhere, and the radiograph is clear. According to Modified PIOPED II, this pattern is very low probability for pulmonary embolus (PE).

TABLE 7.5 Effects of Pretest Probability on CTPA and VQ Lung Scan

CTPA	Not Considered	CLINICAL SUSPICION		
		High (%)	Intermediate (%)	Low (%)
PPV CTPA+	86	96	92	58
NPV CTPA–	95	60	89	96

VQ		
	Not Considered	With Pretest Probability
Low probability NPV	84–88%	96–99% Low suspicion
High probability	88	>95 High suspicion

CTPA, Computed tomography pulmonary angiography; *NPV,* negative predictive value; *PPV,* positive predictive value; *VQ,* ventilation–perfusion. Data Sostman HD, Miniati M, Gottschalk A, et al. Sensitivity and specificity of perfusion scintigraphy combined with chest radiography for acute pulmonary embolism in PIOPED II study. *Radiology* 2008;246(3):941–946.

specificity. However, SPECTCT without contrast cannot identify many of the alternate causes of the chest pain, such as aortic dissection.

QUANTITATIVE LUNG SCAN

Quantification of lung perfusion and ventilation can be valuable in the preoperative assessment of high-risk patients before planned lung resection for malignancy, dead-space lung volume reduction in severe COPD, and lung transplantation. This information is used in conjunction with respiratory spirometry to determine how much function each lung or lung region contributes to preoperatively predict what surgical approach would be preferable for the best outcome. Quantitation also can be useful in assessing relative pulmonary perfusion before and after operations for congenital heart disease (e.g., correction of pulmonary stenosis).

Right-to-left lung differential function is commonly performed by acquiring anterior and posterior views, drawing regions of interest around the right and left lungs, and calculating the geometrical mean to correct for attenuation (Fig. 7.25A).

Geometric mean = −Counts anterior × Counts posterior

However, the anterior and posterior views do not allow for good separation of the upper and lower lobes due to overlap in those projections. Posterior oblique views allow better separation of the upper and lower lobes if needed (see Fig. 7.25B). This would be important for partial lung resections (e.g., upper lobe bullae).

Adult Respiratory Distress Syndrome

The clearance of Tc-99m DTPA is significantly affected by the presence of pulmonary disease. The clearance half-time is approximately 45 minutes in healthy adults. Patients with adult respiratory distress syndrome have more rapid clearance, probably because of the rapid diffusion of Tc-99m DTPA across the airspace epithelium to the pulmonary circulation. Other conditions associated with increased Tc-99m DTPA clearance are cigarette smoking, alveolitis, and hyaline membrane disease in infants. This technique has not found a clear-cut clinical use.

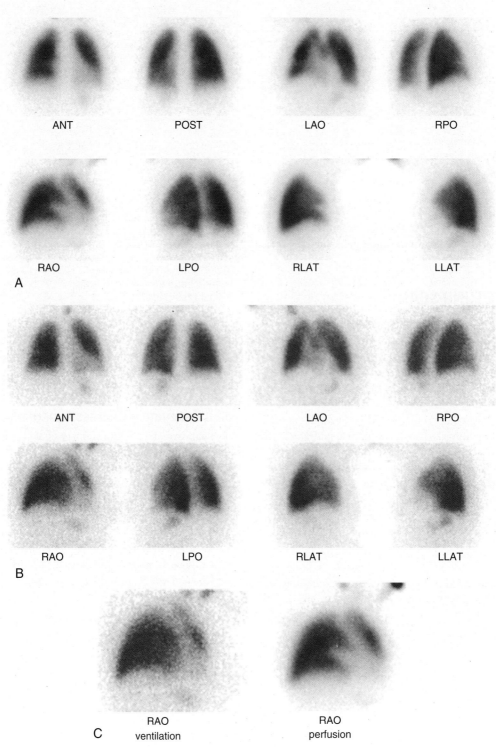

Fig. 7.21 Single-segment defect perfusion mismatch. (A) Perfusion images in a short-of-breath patient with clear chest radiograph contain a single large wedge-shaped perfusion defect in the middle lobe with no corresponding ventilation abnormality (B), best seen on side-by-side comparison (C). Suspicion for pulmonary embolus (PE) was very high in this patient with a deep vein thrombosis (DVT). The patient was treated with anticoagulation and recovered.

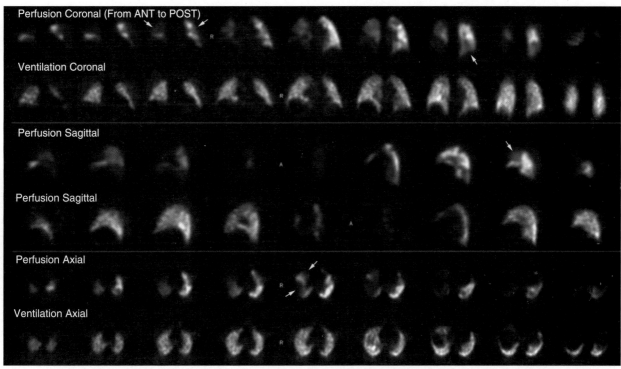

Fig. 7.22 Single-photon emission computed tomography (SPECT) ventilation–perfusion (VQ) image demonstrates numerous perfusion defects with Tc-99m macroaggregated albumin (MAA; *arrows on some*) conforming to segmental anatomy with corresponding Tc-99m Technegas ventilation appearing normal: a positive examination with multiple bilateral emboli. (Images courtesy of Dr. Khun Visith Keu, MD, Hôpital de la Cité-de-la-Santé de Laval, Canada.)

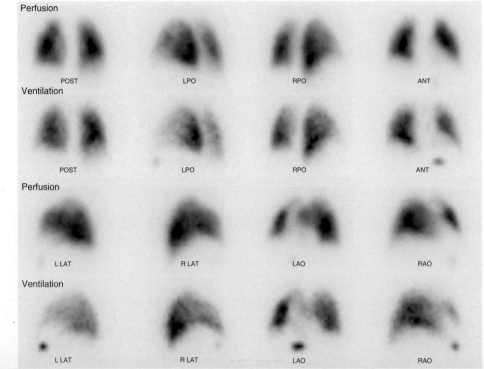

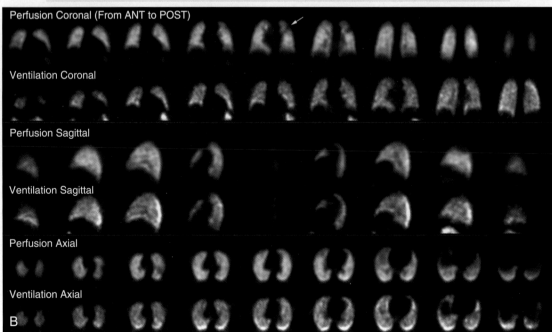

Fig. 7.23 Single-photon emission computed tomography (SPECT) ventilation–perfusion (VQ) images. (A) "Pseudoplanar" angular reconstructed images from the SPECT data appear normal or near normal and would have been read as a negative. (B) SPECT perfusion images *(top row)* show a large segmental left upper lobe defect *(arrow)*, which was not matched on Tc-99m Technegas ventilation images *(bottom row)*, in coronal, sagittal, and axial planes. The examination was read as positive for pulmonary embolus (PE). (Images courtesy of Khun Visith Keu, MD, Hôpital de la Cité-de-la-Santé de Laval, Canada.)

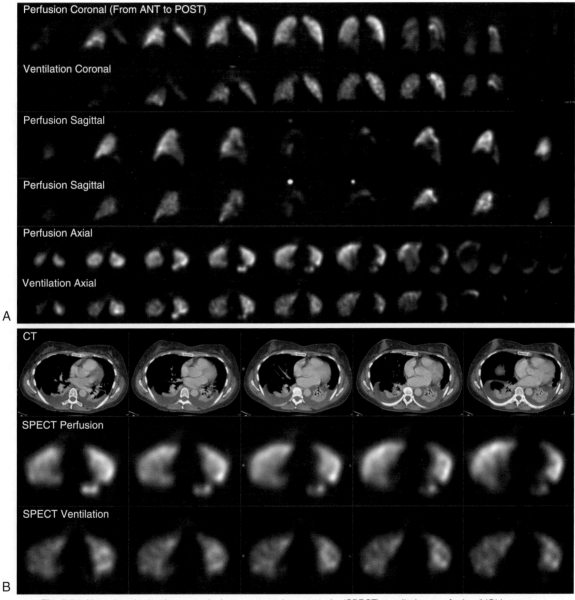

Fig. 7.24 Negative single-photon emission computed tomography (SPECT) ventilation–perfusion (VQ) images. (A) Tc-99m macroaggregated albumin (MAA) perfusion and Tc-99m Technegas ventilation images show bibasilar abnormalities with areas of ventilation abnormality worse than perfusion deficit: reverse mismatch. This study was read as negative for pulmonary embolus (PE). (B) Comparison to a computed tomography (CT) scan performed later that day to rule out acute cholecystitis confirmed atelectasis and small effusions. (Images courtesy of Dr. Khun Visith Keu, Hôpital de la Cité-de-la-Santé de Laval, Canada.)

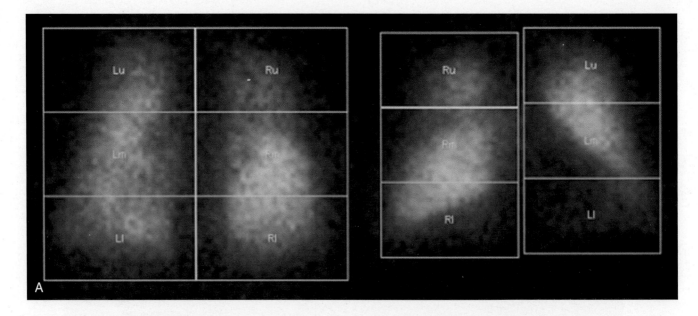

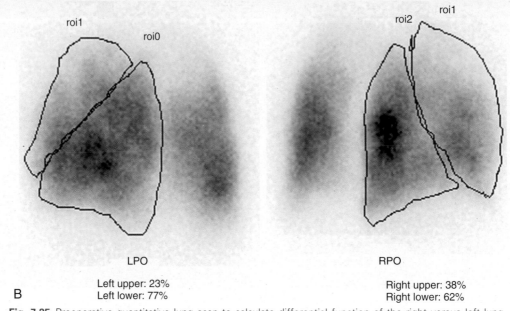

LPO

RPO

B   Left upper: 23%   Right upper: 38%
       Left lower: 77%   Right lower: 62%

Fig. 7.25 Preoperative quantitative lung scan to calculate differential function of the right versus left lung for patients undergoing procedures such as lung resection. Regions of interest are drawn around each lung, and a geometrical mean is calculated. (A) Images can be done in the posterior oblique projections or in the anterior-posterior projection. (B) The lungs regions can be drawn into rough upper, middle, and lower lung zones if desired.

REFERENCES

VQ: UTILITY AND PIOPED/PIOPED II CRITERIA

Freeman LM. Don't bury the V/Q scan: it's as good as multidetector CT angiograms with a lot less radiation exposure. *J Nucl Med.* 2006;49:5–8.

Freitas JE, Sarosi M, Nagle CC, et al. Modified PIOPED criteria in clinical practice. *J Nucl Med.* 1995;36:1573–1576.

Goldberg SN, Richardson DD, Palmer EL, Scott JA. Pleural effusion and ventilation/perfusion scan interpretation for acute pulmonary embolus. *J Nucl Med.* 37(8):1310–1313.

Gottschalk A, Stein PD, Sostman HD, Matta F, Beemath A. Very low probability interpretation of V/Q lung scans in combination with low probability objective clinical assessment reliably excludes pulmonary embolism: data from PIOPED II. *J Nucl Med.* 2007;48:1411–1415.

Sostman HD, Gottschalk A. Prospective validation of the stripe sign in ventilation-perfusion scintigraphy. *Radiology.* 1992;184:455–459.

Sostman HD, Stein PD, Gottschalk A, Matta F, Hull R, Goodman L. Sensitivity and specificity of ventilation-perfusion scintigraphy in PIOPED II study. *Radiology.* 2008;246(3):941–946.

Stein PD, Gottschalk A. Review of criteria appropriate for very low probability pulmonary embolism on ventilation-perfusion lung scans: a position paper. *Radiographics.* 2000;20:99–105.

SPECT AND SPECT/CT

Bajc et al, 2009

Gutte H, Mortensen J, Jensen CV, et al. Detection of pulmonary embolism with combined ventilation-perfusion SPECT and low-dose CT: head-to-head comparison with multidetector CT angiography. *J Nucl Med.* 2009;50:1987–1992.

Le Roux PY, Robin P, Delluc A, et al. V/Q SPECT interpretation for pulmonary embolism diagnosis: which criteria to use? *J Nucl Med.* 2013;54:1077–1081.

Lu Y, Lorenzoni A, Fox JJ, et al. Noncontrast perfusion single-photon emission CT/CT scanning. *Chest.* 2014;145:1079–1088.

Mila M, Bechini J, Vaquez A, et al. Acute pulmonary embolism detection with ventilation/perfusion SPECT combined with full dose CT: what is the best option? *Rev Esp Med Nucl Imagen Mol.* 2017;36(3):139–145.

Roach PJ, Schembri GP, Bailey DL. V/Q scanning using SPECT and SPECT/CT. *J Nucl Med.* 2013;54:1588–1596.

Stubbs M, Chan K, McKeekin H, Navalkissoor S, Wagner T. Incidence of a single segmental perfusion defect in single-photon emission computed tomography and planar ventilation/perfusion scans. *Nuc Med Commun.* 2017;38(2):135–140.

CTA AND MRA

Benson DG, Schiebler ML, Repplinger MD, et al. Contrast-enhanced pulmonary MRA for the primary diagnosis of pulmonary embolism: current state of the art and future directions. *Br J Radiol.* 2017;90(1074):20160901.

Stein PS, Fowler SE, Goodman LR, et al. Multidetector computed tomography for acute pulmonary embolism. *N Engl J Med.* 2006;354:2317–2327.

PE: CLINICAL

Moores LK, King CS, Holley AB. Current approach to the diagnosis of acute nonmassive pulmonary embolism. *Chest.* 2011;140:509–518.

Raja AS, Greenverg JO, Qaseem A, Denberg TD, Fitterman N, Schuur JD. Evaluation of patients with suspected acute pulmonary embolism: best practice advice from the clinical guidelines committee of the American College of Physicians. *Ann Intern Med.* 2015;29.

Endocrine System

THYROID DISEASE—RADIONUCLIDE DIAGNOSIS AND THERAPY

In 1941, the first patient was treated for thyroid cancer with radioiodine. Since then, radioiodine has proven invaluable in the assessment of thyroid disorders and treatment of thyroid cancer, Graves disease, and toxic thyroid nodules. Today, radioiodine I-123 and I-131 remain important diagnostic and therapeutic modalities, and the use of positron emission tomography (PET) iodine-124 is growing.

Thyroid Anatomy and Physiology

The thyroid gland lies in the anterior neck just inferior to the thyroid cartilage. It normally weighs 15 to 20 grams (Fig. 8.1) and has two lobes connected by an isthmus that shows considerable anatomical variability. The pyramidal lobe, a remnant of the thyroglossal duct, is present in approximately two-thirds of patients, extending superiorly from the isthmus. Because of the thyroid's embryological descent from pharyngeal pouches, ectopic tissue may be found anywhere from the foramen cecum at tongue base to the myocardium.

The gland is made up of follicles of varying size. The epithelial follicular cells at the periphery of the follicle synthesize and secrete thyroid hormone into the lumen, which contains colloid, where the hormone is stored (Fig. 8.2). After oral ingestion, iodine is reduced to iodide (I-) in the proximal small intestine, where more than 90% is absorbed within 60 minutes. After distributing in the blood as an extracellular ion, it exits by thyroid and gastric extraction, then urinary and intestinal excretion.

A high-energy sodium-symporter membrane traps iodide and concentrates it intracellularly 25 to 500 times greater than plasma. Thyroid peroxidase at the follicular cell–colloid interface promptly organifies it. The iodine then binds to tyrosine residues on thyroglobulin. These monoiodinated and diiodinated tyrosines couple to form triiodothyronine (T_3) and thyroxine (T_4), which are stored in the colloid-filled follicular lumen (see Fig. 8.2). Trapping and uptake can be blocked competitively by monovalent anions (e.g., potassium perchlorate), and organification can be inhibited by drugs used for Graves therapy, such as propylthiouracil (PTU) and methimazole.

Serum thyroid-stimulating hormone (TSH) initiates iodide uptake, organification, and thyroglobulin hydrolysis, releasing thyroid hormone into the bloodstream. Thyroglobulin itself is not released, except during disease states (e.g., thyroiditis or thyroid cancer). The major hormone released by the thyroid is T4, which is transported to peripheral tissues by thyroid-binding

proteins and converted to the more metabolically active T_3. Because the normal gland contains a 1-month supply of hormone, drugs that block hormone synthesis do not become fully effective in controlling thyrotoxicosis until intrathyroidal stores are depleted.

TSH secretion is primarily adjusted through the thyroid–pituitary feedback mechanism (Fig. 8.3). When serum thyroid hormone levels are above normal, as in hyperthyroidism, serum TSH is suppressed, but when they are low, as in hypothyroidism, serum TSH serum levels increase.

Radiopharmaceuticals
Radioiodine-131 (I-131) and -123 (I-123)

Like the stable iodine (I-127) normally encountered in the diet, radioactive iodine isotopes, such as I-131 or I-123, are selectively trapped by the thyroid and incorporated into thyroid hormone. Given this ability to localize, they are excellent tools for evaluating thyroid physiology, emitting gamma rays that provide clinically relevant qualitative and quantitative information.

Radioiodine doses are usually supplied as a capsule for oral administration. Although liquid I-131 may be available, it is volatile and increases the risk of exposing those around the patient. In the proximal small bowel, more than 90% of ingested iodine is absorbed rapidly. It is detectable in the thyroid within minutes of oral ingestion, reaching the thyroid

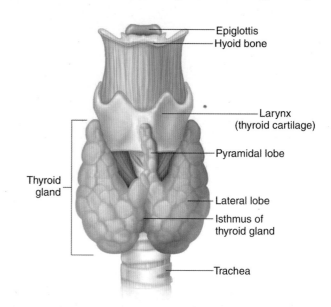

Fig. 8.1 Thyroid anatomy. The anatomical relationship of the thyroid to the trachea, thyroid and cricoid cartilages, and vascular structures.

Labels: Epiglottis, Hyoid bone, Larynx (thyroid cartilage), Pyramidal lobe, Thyroid gland, Lateral lobe, Isthmus of thyroid gland, Trachea

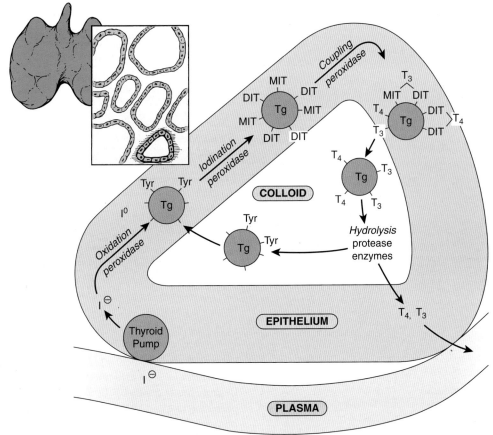

Fig. 8.2 Iodine metabolism. The thyroid follicular cell epithelium extracts (traps) iodide from the plasma via the sodium iodide symporter (thyroid pump) and organifies it. Iodide (I−) is converted to neutral iodine (I0), which is then incorporated into thyroglobulin-bound tyrosine molecules as monoiodotyrosine (MIT) or diiodotyrosine (DIT). Coupling of the iodotyrosines results in T_4 and T_3 hormone bound to the thyroglobulin, which is transported to and stored in the colloid, until T_4 and T_3 are released into the plasma by proteolytic enzymes. T_4 is converted to the more active T_3 peripherally.

follicular lumen by 20 to 30 minutes. Thyroid uptake normally continues to increase occurs over 24 hours (Fig. 8.4), although imaging can be done as soon as 4 hours. The delay between radioiodine administration and imaging is not due to slow accumulation but rather the time needed to clear relatively high background activity. Radioiodine uptake can also be seen in the salivary glands, stomach, and choroid plexus; however, it is not concentrated or retained there. Excretion is via the kidneys and gastrointestinal tract.

I-131 undergoes beta-minus decay (β−), emitting a principal primary gamma photon of 364 keV with an 8.1-day physical half-life (Table 8.1). These photons are not ideal for gamma camera imaging. Count detection sensitivity is poor; half of the photons penetrate the collimator septa (even with a high-energy collimator) and the 3/8-in. sodium iodine camera crystal without detection, thus resulting in image degradation. High-energy β-particles (0.606 megaelectron volt [MeV]) are also emitted, which cannot be imaged but are valuable for therapy. The high-energy gamma, β-emissions, and long physical half-life result in a relatively high radiation dose to the thyroid (see the Appendix). Therefore, the dose for uptake is limited to 10 to 20 μCi. Even after thyroidectomy, doses are typically limited to 2 to 3 mCi (74 MBq) for thyroid cancer imaging because the

β-emission could cause stunning in the residual cells, preventing uptake for effective therapy or future imaging. In the past, 30 to 50 μCi (1110–1850 MBq) of I-131 was sometimes used to determine whether an anterior mediastinal mass was due to a goiter. I-123 has replaced I-131 for this purpose.

I-123 decays by electron capture (13.2-hour half-life), and the principal emission is a 159-keV gamma photon (83.4% abundance), well suited for gamma camera imaging (see Table 8.1). There are some higher-energy emissions in low abundance, 440 to 625 keV (2.4%) and 625 to 784 (0.15%), making a medium-energy collimator preferable, although low-energy collimators are acceptable. Cyclotron production today results in I-123 that is 99.9% pure and no longer contaminated by long-lived isotopes (e.g., I-124, I-125). Given this and the lack of β-emissions, the radiation dose to the patient is roughly 100 times less than I-131 (10 rads/mCi) compared with 1000 rad/mCi. The standard uptake dose is 100 μCi (3.7 MBq) and 200 to 400 μCi (7.4 MBq) for routine thyroid scans. Higher doses can also be used in cancer imaging because I-123 does not cause stunning.

I-124 is a positron emitter that has been used as an alternative to I-123 or I-131 for thyroid cancer imaging, largely in an experimental capacity. It is cyclotron produced, decays by

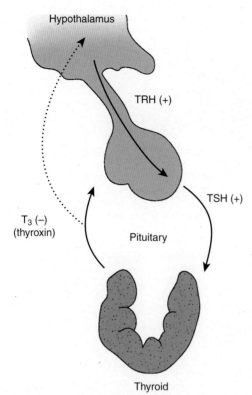

Fig. 8.3 Thyroid—pituitary feedback. The normal thyroid is under the control of thyroid-stimulating hormone (TSH). The hypothalamic production of thyroid-releasing hormone (TRH) and thus the pituitary release of TSH are increased with low circulating levels of T_4 and T_3 and decreased with high circulating levels of thyroid hormone.

TABLE 8.1 Physical Characteristics of Thyroid Radiopharmaceuticals

Characteristics	Tc-99m	I-123	I-131	I-124
Mode of decay	Isometric transition	Electron capture	Beta minus	Positron
Physical half-life ($T_{1/2}$)	6 hours	13.2 hours	8.1 days	110 min
Photon energy	140 keV	159 keV	364 keV	511 keV
Abundance[a]	89%	83%	81%	100%
Beta emissions	None	None	606 keV	None

[a]Abundance is the percent likelihood that a photon emission will occur with each radioactive decay.

electron capture (75%) and positron decay (26%), and has a half-life of 4.18 days (see Table 8.1). Studies suggest it is superior to I-123 or I-131 for the detection of thyroid cancer metastases, and it has a potential role for thyroid cancer dosimetry before therapy. However, radiation dosimetry is relatively high (see Table 8.1).

Tc-99m pertechnetate is produced from a Mo-99/Tc99m generator, making it inexpensive and readily available, unlike the costlier I-123, which must often be ordered a day in advance. Because it is taken up by the same mechanism as iodine, Tc-99m pertechnetate can be used for thyroid assessment. The 140-keV photopeak (89% abundance) and lack of high-energy emissions are optimal for gamma camera imaging (see Table 8.1). In contrast to oral administration of radioiodine, Tc-99m pertechnetate is administered intravenously and rapidly taken up by the thyroid. However, it is not organified or retained in the thyroid, and imaging must be performed early at peak uptake time, 15 to 30 minutes after injection. The lack of particulate emissions and short 6-hour half-life result in a low radiation dose to the thyroid, far less than I-131 or I-123 (see the Appendix). Thus, the administered activity of Tc-99m pertechnetate can be much higher than that for I-123, usually 3 to 5 mCi (111–185 MBq), and the large photon flux results in high-quality images.

Special Considerations and Precautions

I-123 is the agent of choice for most adult thyroid imaging. Tc-99m pertechnetate may be preferred in children because of its lower radiation dosimetry and high count rate. However, because it is not organified, it is not recommended for nodule evaluation, and the rarely attempted Tc-99m pertechnetate uptake calculation is more difficult and less reliable.

For thyroid cancer imaging, the long half-life of I-131 is an important advantage over Tc-99m pertechnetate. Diagnostic I-131 scans are routinely acquired 48 hours after administration and 7 days posttherapy. The result is a high target-to-background ratio due to the time allowed for background clearance, resulting in good detectability of thyroid cancer metastases. Even for this diagnostic indication, I-123 is replacing I-131 because it permits earlier patient imaging at 24 hours, better image quality, and similar accuracy, and I-123 does not cause thyroid cell "stunning," a situation where the cells are damaged by the emitted β, preventing future radioiodine uptake for imaging or therapy.

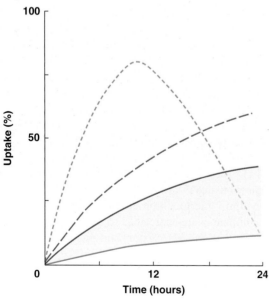

Fig. 8.4 Percent radioiodine uptake (%RAIU) after oral administration of I-123. In normal subjects the %RAIU increases progressively over 24 hours to values of 10% to 30% *(gray area)*. With Graves disease, the %RAIU rises at a more rapid rate to higher levels, often 50% to 80% and greater *(lower broken line)*. However, some patients with Graves have rapid iodine turnover within the thyroid manifested as early, rapid, high uptake at 4 to 12 hours but only mildly elevated or even normal uptake by 24 hours *(top broken line)*.

These same high-energy I-131 β-emissions result in effective therapy not only for thyroid cancer but also for Graves disease and toxic nodules.

Uptake Inhibitors. A patient history, including food, drug, and prior imaging, should be obtained before thyroid uptake and imaging studies or radioiodine therapy. Thyroid replacement medications prevent imaging radiotracer uptake, as will thyroid-blocking medications. Exogenous iodine suppresses uptake and may preclude successful imaging or accurate uptake measurements. As little as 1 mg of stable iodine can cause a marked reduction in uptake; 10 mg can effectively block the gland.

Iodinated oral and intravenous radiographic contrast is a common source of iodine that interferes with thyroid studies. Given the high amount of iodine present in intravenous contrast, even water soluble, radionuclide diagnostic and therapeutic studies should be delayed for approximately 4 weeks following contrast administration.

The iodine normally found in foods and medications can also interfere with radionuclide thyroid studies (Table 8.2). Greater amounts of iodine in the normal diet over the years in the form of iodized salt has resulted in lower normal values for the percent radioiodine uptake (%RAIU). Chronic renal failure impairs iodide clearance, expands the iodide pool, and lowers the %RAIU. Hypothyroidism reduces the glomerular filtration rate and slows urinary clearance of radioiodine from the body; hyperthyroidism increases the clearance rate.

Iodine Allergy. The amount of iodine in a radioactive uptake or even a therapy dose is subpharmacologic and has not been associated with allergic reactions, even in patients with a documented iodine allergy.

Pregnancy and Lactation. The fetal thyroid begins to concentrate radioiodine by 10 to 12 weeks of gestation. Thus, significant exposure of the fetal thyroid can occur after therapeutic doses given to the mother, resulting in fetal hypothyroidism. A serum pregnancy test is mandatory before treating a female patient with I-131. Radioiodine is excreted in human breast milk. Because of the long half-life of I-131, nursing should be discontinued after diagnostic or therapeutic studies and not resumed. Breastfeeding may resume 48 hours after administration of I-123 and 24 hours after Tc-99m pertechnetate. According to the Nuclear Regulatory Commission (NRC), patients receiving I-131 for therapy or imaging should receive written as well as verbal radiation safety instructions if they are breastfeeding in addition to the routine instructions and normally required written directives.

Thyroid Uptake (%RAIU)

Thyroid uptake measurements for benign disease are acquired using a nonimaging gamma scintillation probe detector (Figs. 8.5 and 8.6). The %RAIU can be determined with either I-131 or I-123 (Box 8.1). Clinical indications are limited (Table 8.3). It is most commonly used in the calculation of an I-131 therapy dose or to diagnose the cause of thyrotoxicosis, most commonly to differentiate Graves disease from subacute thyroiditis. Thyroid uptake values in other diseases are listed in Box 8.2. The %RAIU is increased in Graves but suppressed in subacute thyroiditis.

Medications that interfere with the radioiodine uptake should be discontinued before the study, with the length of time based on their

TABLE 8.2 Drugs, Foods, and Radiographic Contrast Agents That Decrease or Increase the Percent Radioactive Iodine Thyroid Uptake

Decrease Uptake	Duration of Effect
Thyroid hormones	
Thyroxine (T$_4$)	4–6 weeks
Triiodothyronine (T$_3$)	2 weeks
Excess iodine (expanded iodine pool)	
Potassium iodide	2–4 weeks
Mineral supplements, cough medicines, vitamins	2–4 weeks
Iodine food supplements	2–4 weeks
Iodinated drugs (e.g., amiodarone)	Months
Iodinated skin ointments	2–4 weeks
Congestive heart failure	
Renal failure	
Radiographic contrast media	
Water-soluble intravascular media	3–4 weeks
Fat-soluble media (lymphography)	Months to years
Non–iodine-containing drugs	
Adrenocorticotropic hormone, adrenal steroids	Variable
Monovalent anions (perchlorate)	Variable
Penicillin	Variable
Antithyroid drugs	
Propylthiouracil (PTU)	3–5 days
Methimazole (Tapazole)	5–7 days
Goitrogenic foods	
Cabbage, turnips	
Prior radiation to neck	
Increase uptake	
Iodine deficiency	
Pregnancy	
Rebound after therapy withdrawal	
Antithyroid drugs	
Lithium	

half-lives (see Table 8.2). Patients should have nothing by mouth for 4 hours before radioiodine ingestion to ensure good absorption. I-123 and I-131 are usually administered in capsule form.

If a scan is not needed, 5 to 10 μCi I-131 or 50 μCi I-123 is adequate for a %RAIU because of the gamma probe's high detection sensitivity. If a scan is ordered, Tc-99m pertechnetate can be utilized following the I-131 uptake. Both the scan and uptake can be performed with the I-123 scan dose (200–400 μCi). The %RAIU is best acquired at 4 and 24 hours after ingestion, although some acquire it at only one time period. The 24-hour uptake is the standard for I-131 therapy dose calculation.

Methodology for %RAIU

The nonimaging gamma scintillation probe detector used for thyroid uptake studies has a 2-cm-thick by 2-cm-diameter sodium iodine crystal with an open, single-hole lead collimator coupled to a photomultiplier tube and electronics. Room

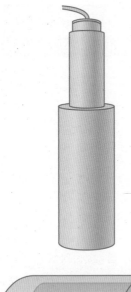

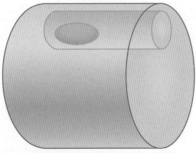

Fig. 8.5 Thyroid uptake probe counting I-123 capsule in neck phantom. The neck phantom is solid Lucite plastic, except for the cylinder-like defect in which the capsule is placed for counting. The nonimaging gamma detector is placed at a standard distance of 30 cm from the neck phantom and acquires emitted counts for 1 minute.

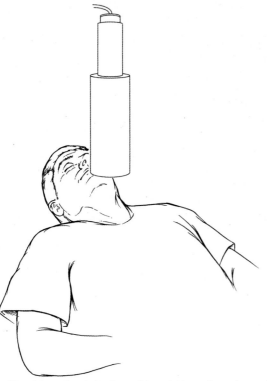

Fig. 8.6 Thyroid uptake probe is positioned 30 cm from the patient's neck, where it acquires counts from the patient's neck/thyroid for 1 minute. Background counts are also acquired, usually in the thigh region.

BOX 8.1 Calculation of Radioactive Iodine and Tc-99m Uptakes

Percent Radioiodine Uptake (%RAIU)
1. Preliminary measurements
   Place dose capsule in neck phantom and count for 1 minute.
   Count patient's neck and thigh (background) for 1 minute.
2. Administer oral dose capsule.
3. Uptake measurement at 4 to 6 hours and 24 hours:
   Count patient's neck for 1 minute.
   Count patient's thigh for 1 minute.
4. Calculation

$$\% \, RAIU = \frac{Neck \, (background \, corrected) \atop counts/min}{Dose \, capsule \, (decay \, correcte \atop background \, corrected) \atop counts/min} \times 100$$

Tc-99m Pertechnetate %Uptake
Before and after injection, the syringe is imaged to obtain counts (preinjection counts − postinjection counts = administered counts).
Scan regions of interest (ROIs) are drawn for thyroid, thyroid background.
Areas of interest are normalized for pixel size, and thyroid and syringe counts are normalized for time of acquisition.
Normal values are 0.3% to 4.5%.

TABLE 8.3 Clinical Indications for Thyroid Scan and %Thyroid Uptake

Thyroid Scan	%Thyroid uptake
Functional status (cold, hot) of thyroid nodule	Differential diagnosis of thyrotoxicosis
Detection of ectopic thyroid tissue (e.g., lingual thyroid)	Calculate Graves I-131 therapy dose
Differential diagnosis of mediastinal masses (substernal goiter) with I-123	Whole-body thyroid cancer scans pretherapy, posttherapy, and follow-up—to quantify residual or recurrent disease
Thyroid cancer whole-body scan: Before therapy—find distant disease Posttherapy—find additional disease Follow-up—determine therapeutic effectiveness, evaluate for recurrence	

---

background activity is determined. The radioiodine capsule with known calibrated activity is placed in a Lucite neck phantom (see Fig. 8.5). Counts are obtained with the detector placed at a standardized distance of 30 cm. The radioiodine dose is then administered to the patient. At 4 and/or 24 hours, the probe is placed 30 cm from the anterior surface of the patient's neck (see Fig. 8.6). Counts are obtained for 1 minute. The patient's thigh is counted for a similar time to correct for background. The %RAIU is calculated according to the following formula:

$$\% \, RAIU = \frac{Neck \, counts/min \, *}{Administred \, dose \, capsule \, counts/min \, * \atop corrected \, for \, decay \, and \, background} \times 100$$

The normal range for the %RAIU is approximately 4% to 15% at 4 to 6 hours and 10% to 30% at 24 hours. The early uptake informs that the %RAIU is elevated or suppressed. Some centers extrapolate from 4-hour uptake to estimate the 24-hour uptake for I-131 therapy dose planning. A problem with this approach is that some hyperthyroid patients have rapid thyroid iodine turnover. These patients may show an elevated 4- to 6-hour %RAIU but a lower value at 24 hours, thus underestimating the therapy dose needed (see Fig. 8.4). Patients with very high 4-hour uptakes can be brought back at 24 hours to ensure correct dosing, but having both time points is always optimal. The significance of uptake values must be determined by considering the entire clinical picture. Causes for various uptake values are outlined in Table 8.4.

A Tc-99m pertechnetate percentage uptake is not commonly performed. Advantages are that peak uptake occurs at 20 to 30 minutes compared with 4 and 24 hours for radioiodine. Disadvantages are a considerably lower accuracy than %RAIU, often a lack of commercial software available for calculation, and a

24-hour uptake is not possible because it is not organified. The methodology is described in Box 8.1.

Thyroid Scan

Iodine-123 is administered orally, and the scan is acquired 4 hours later. Imaging at 24 hours is possible; however, the low count rate at that time requires longer acquisition, increasing the likelihood of patient motion and image degradation. Four-hour images have superior image quality. Tc-99m pertechnetate is administered intravenously, and scan acquisition begins 20 minutes later. Detailed protocols are described for both in Box 8.3.

A pinhole collimator magnifies and makes possible high-resolution functional images of the thyroid (Fig. 8.7). Magnification increases as the pinhole collimator approaches the neck. The thyroid gland image should fill two-thirds of the field of view (Fig. 8.8). In some clinics, a line source marker or two point sources 4 or 5 cm apart are placed lateral to the thyroid lobes to help estimate the size of the thyroid gland and nodules, although when the provider is experienced, palpation may result in superior accuracy. Images are obtained in the anterior and right and left anterior oblique projections with the patient's head slightly extended. The camera should be repositioned while the patient remains still.

To confirm whether a particular palpable nodule takes up the radiopharmaceutical (i.e., a hot or cold nodule), additional images can be obtained using a radioactive or lead marker over the nodule. Care should be taken to avoid the pinhole collimator parallax effect, that is, a change in the relationship between a near and distant object when viewed from different angles, potentially resulting in misinterpretation of the location of a nodule or suspected substernal goiter. To minimize this effect, the nodule should be positioned to the center of the field of view.

Interpretation of Thyroid Scintigraphy. Thyroid scans should always be interpreted in light of patient history, thyroid palpation examination, thyroid function studies, and sonography. The normal scintigraphic appearance of the thyroid varies somewhat, but the gland should have a smooth contour and homogenous

BOX 8.2 Differential Diagnosis of Thyrotoxicosis: Increased or Decreased %RAIU

Increased Uptake
Graves disease
Toxic nodular goiter
Hashitoxicosis
Hydatidiform mole, trophoblastic tumors, choriocarcinoma
Metastatic thyroid cancer

Decreased Uptake
Subacute thyroiditis
  Granulomatous thyroiditis (de Quervain)
  Silent thyroiditis
  Postpartum thyroiditis
  Iodine-induced thyrotoxicosis (Jod–Basedow)
  Amiodarone-induced thyrotoxicosis
  Thyrotoxicosis factitia
  Struma ovarii (decreased in thyroid, increased in ovarian tumor)

TABLE 8.4 Relationship of %Radioiodine Thyroid Uptake to Thyroid Function

Thyroid Function	%RADIOIODINE THYROID UPTAKE		
	Increased	Normal	Decreased
Thyrotoxicosis	Graves disease Hashitoxicosis	Antithyroid drugs Propylthiouracil Methimazole	Contrast, high iodine exposure Subacute thyroiditis, thyrotoxic phase Thyrotoxicosis factitia Antithyroid drugs Struma ovarii
Euthyroid	Rebound after antithyroid drug withdrawal Recovery from subacute thyroiditis Compensated dyshormonogenesis		Decompensated dyshormonogenesis
Hypothyroid	Decompensated dyshormonogenesis Hashimoto disease	Hashimoto disease After I-131 therapy Subacute thyroiditis, recovery phase decompensated dyshormonogenesis	Hypothyroidism: primary or secondary

BOX 8.3   Thyroid Imaging With Iodine-123 and Tc-99m Pertechnetate: Protocol Summary

Patient Preparation

Discontinue medications that interfere with thyroid uptake (see Table 8.2). Nothing by mouth for 4 hours before study.

Radiopharmaceutical

Iodine I-123, 200 to 400 μCi (3.7–14.8 MBq), orally in capsule form (or)
Tc-99m pertechnetate, 3 to 5 mCi (111–185 MBq), intravenously

Time of Imaging

Iodine I-123, 4 hours after oral dose administration
Tc-99m pertechnetate, 20 minutes after injection

Imaging Procedure

Gamma camera with pinhole collimator
Energy window:
   Tc-99m pertechnetate: 15% to 20% energy window centered at 140 keV
   I-123: 20% window centered at 159 keV
Position the supine patient with the chin up and neck extended.
Acquire initial anterior view for 100,000 counts or 5 minutes with collimator placed to include right side and suprasternal notch markers.
Place the collimator closer so that the thyroid fills about approximately two-thirds of the field of view.
Acquire anterior, left anterior oblique, and right anterior oblique images for equal time compared with anterior view.

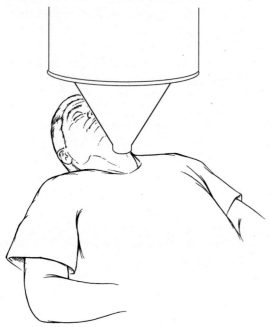

Fig. 8.7 Pinhole collimator. The pinhole collimator is attached to the front of the gamma camera and positioned close to the thyroid to permit optimal magnification. If positioned farther away, the resulting image becomes smaller. The lead pinhole insert is typically 4 mm in size, although smaller and larger inserts are possible with some cameras.

uptake (see Figs. 8.1 and 8.8). The right lobe is often larger than the left, and relatively increased activity may seem to be present in the middle or medial lobes given the gland's central thickness. Visualization of the isthmus varies between patients. The thin pyramidal lobe is not normally seen in the euthyroid patient,

although it is commonly seen with Graves and Hashimoto thyroiditis. It ascends anteriorly and superiorly from the isthmus of either lobe but more often from the left lobe.

With Tc-99m pertechnetate scans imaged at 20 to 30 minutes, the salivary glands are routinely seen; however, often they are not seen with I-123 imaged at 4 hours due to washout. With thyroid enlargement, the lobes appear plump, with convex borders. Relatively hot and cold regions should be noted. Nodules should be confirmed by palpation, scan marking, and sonography whenever possible.

Esophageal activity is sometimes seen. It may be displaced by the trachea and cervical spine when the neck is hyperextended in the imaging position. It is often seen just left of midline and posterior, and often can be confirmed by having the patient swallow water. Anterior oblique views can help determine whether the activity is anterior (pyramidal lobe) or posterior (esophagus; Fig. 8.9).

Thyrotoxicosis—Hyperthyroidism. The term *hyperthyroidism* describes thyrotoxicosis, excessive release of thyroid hormone resulting from a hyperfunctioning thyroid gland (e.g., Graves disease or toxic nodular goiter). Examples of thyrotoxicosis not caused by a hyperfunctioning thyroid gland are subacute thyroiditis, where inflammation releases stored hormone, and thyroiditis factitia (Box 8.4). The frequency of different causes for thyrotoxicosis is listed in Table 8.5. The symptoms of thyrotoxicosis are those of increased metabolism (e.g., heat intolerance, hyperhidrosis, anxiety, tachycardia, palpitations, and weight loss). The symptoms are nonspecific, and diagnosis requires confirmation by thyroid function studies. A suppressed serum TSH of less than 0.1 mU/L is diagnostic of thyrotoxicosis, the result of negative feedback from the pituitary secondary to elevated serum thyroid hormone.

Clinical history and physical examination can sometimes suggest the cause of thyrotoxicosis (e.g., a recent upper respiratory infection and tender thyroid gland suggests subacute thyroiditis). Exophthalmos and pretibial edema are classic for Graves. A protracted course suggests Graves over thyroiditis. However, signs and symptoms can frequently overlap, and a scan and uptake are often important to confirm these diagnoses.

Graves disease. Graves disease is the cause of hyperthyroidism in approximately 75% of patients. Graves is an autoimmune disease in which a thyrotropin (TSH) receptor antibody binds to and stimulates thyroid follicular cells, resulting in excessive production of thyroid hormone. Thus, thyroid gland function is autonomous and independent of TSH feedback. Graves is most commonly seen in middle-aged women but may occur in anyone, including children. Patients have a diffusely enlarged thyroid gland (goiter), which is firm and usually nontender. The thyroid scan shows a high thyroid-to-background ratio (Fig. 8.10). An elevated %RAIU, usually in the range of 45% to 80% at 24 hours, confirms the diagnosis and excludes most other causes of thyrotoxicosis. The scan can be helpful in differentiating a diffuse toxic goiter (Graves) from a toxic multinodular goiter (Fig. 8.11). At times, Graves may be superimposed on a nontoxic multinodular goiter. The scan and uptake are usually diagnostic.

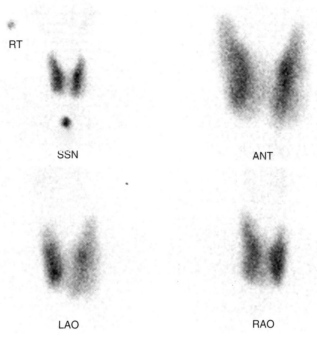

Fig. 8.8 Normal I-123 thyroid scan. All images are acquired with a pinhole collimator. The upper left anterior image is acquired with the pinhole collimator distanced further from the neck than the other three images, thus minifying the image and permitting a larger field of view so that the suprasternal notch (SSN) and the right side (RT) hot markers can be easily seen. The anterior (ANT), left anterior oblique (LAO), and right anterior oblique (RAO) views are acquired with the pinhole close to the patient's neck so that the image fills two-thirds of the field of view. Both lobes appear relatively thin and normal. The LAO view suggests a nodule in the lower aspect; however, it is not seen in other views. The appearance is due to overlap of the right lobe and the isthmus.

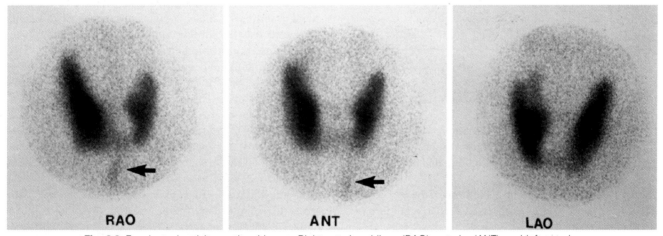

Fig. 8.9 Esophageal activity on thyroid scan. Right anterior oblique (RAO), anterior (ANT), and left anterior oblique (LAO) views. The thyroid scan shows esophageal activity below the thyroid to the left of midline *(arrows)*. Intensity is set high to better visualize esophageal activity. Esophageal activity is not seen in the LAO view, the last view acquired, because the activity spontaneously transited distally. Having a patient drink water can often confirm its esophageal origin by washing the activity distally.

Subacute Thyroiditis. Subacute thyroiditis is another common cause for thyrotoxicosis. There are various subtypes. Granulomatous thyroiditis (de Quervain) is usually preceded by several days of upper respiratory illness and tender thyroid. Silent thyroiditis often occurs in the elderly and presents with cardiac symptoms, is not associated with thyroid tenderness, and is not a granulomatous process, probably viral. Postpartum thyroiditis occurs within weeks or months of delivery. The patient has antithyroid antibodies.

Thyrotoxicosis occurs during the initial stage of subacute thyroiditis and is caused by the release of preformed thyroid hormone secondary to an inflamed gland with increased membrane permeability. Patients are often referred for a scan and uptake during this thyrotoxic stage to differentiate subacute thyroiditis from Graves. With subacute thyroiditis, the %RAIU is suppressed (Fig. 8.12). As the inflammation resolves and thyroid gland hormone is depleted, serum thyroid hormone levels decrease and may fall into the hypothyroid range, resulting in a

BOX 8.4 Classification of Thyrotoxicosis Based on Thyroid Gland Function

Thyroid Gland Hyperfunction
A. Abnormal thyroid stimulator
  1. Graves disease
  2. Trophoblastic tumor
  a. Hydatiform mole and choriocarcinoma (uterus or testes)
B. Intrinsic thyroid autonomy
  1. Toxic single adenoma
  2. Toxic multinodular goiter
C. Excess production of thyroid-stimulating hormone (rare)

No Thyroid Gland Hyperfunction
A. Disorders of hormone storage
  1. Subacute thyroiditis
B. Extrathyroidal source of hormone
  1. Thyrotoxicosis factitia
  2. "Hamburger toxicosis" (epidemic caused by thyroid gland–contaminated hamburger meat)
  3. Ectopic thyroid tissue
  a. Struma ovarii
  b. Functioning follicular carcinoma

TABLE 8.5 Frequency of Causes for Thyrotoxicosis

Cause	Percentage
Graves disease	70
Thyroiditis	20
Toxic multinodular goiter	5
Toxic adenoma	5
Others	<1

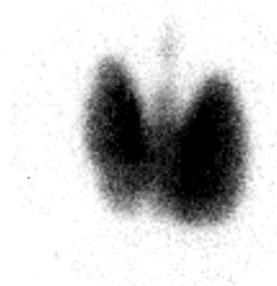

Fig. 8.10 Graves disease. The patient is thyrotoxic. The anterior view shows that both thyroid lobes appear plump with convex borders, and there is a pyramidal lobe arising from the isthmus. The thyroid to background ratio is high. The %RAIU was 63%.

rise in serum TSH. Over weeks to months, hypothyroidism resolves, and TSH and %RAIU return to normal (Fig. 8.13). The low gland uptake with suppressed %RAIU seen during the thyrotoxic stage is the result of an intact pituitary feedback mechanism, not damage or dysfunction of the gland. Uptake is suppressed in the entire gland even though the disease may be patchy or regional.

Multinodular Toxic Goiter (Plummer Disease). Multinodular toxic goiter (Plummer disease) is most commonly seen in the elderly. Patients present with tachyarrhythmias, weight loss, anxiety, and insomnia. Hypermetabolism can exacerbate other medical problems (e.g., cardiac), and thus the disease requires prompt therapy. The %RAIU may only be moderately elevated or even in the high-normal range. The thyroid scan shows high uptake within hyperfunctioning nodules but suppression of the extranodular nonautonomous tissue (see Fig. 8.11). A nontoxic euthyroid multinodular goiter may have hot or warm nodules, but the extranodular tissue is not suppressed (Fig. 8.14).

Single Autonomous Toxic Thyroid Nodule. A single autonomous toxic thyroid nodule occurs in approximately 5% of patients with a palpable nodule. Once an autonomous nodule grows to a size of 2.5 to 3.0 cm, it often produces the clinical manifestations of thyrotoxicosis. Although the %RAIU may be

elevated, it is often in the normal range. The thyroid scan shows uptake in the nodule but suppression of the remainder of the gland with low background (Fig. 8.15).

Hashitoxicosis. Hashimoto disease typically presents in middle-aged women as goiter and hypothyroidism. The gland is diffusely and symmetrically enlarged, nontender, firm, and usually without nodules. Histopathology shows lymphocytic infiltration of chronic thyroiditis. Serum antithyroglobulin and antimicrosomal antibodies are elevated. Up to 5% of these patients develop thyrotoxicosis at some point during the course of the disease. During the thyrotoxic phase, the %RAIU is increased, and the scan shows diffuse increased uptake, similar to Graves disease. Hashitoxicosis is thought to be an overlap syndrome of Graves and Hashimoto chronic thyroiditis. It is often treated with radioactive iodine.

Iodine-Induced Thyrotoxicosis (Jod–Basedow Phenomenon). In the past, iodine-induced thyrotoxicosis (Jod–Basedow phenomenon) occurred with the introduction of iodized salt into the diet in iodine-deficient areas ("goiter belts"). Today, it is most commonly seen in patients who receive iodinated contrast with computed tomography (CT). The iodine induces thyroiditis and thyrotoxicosis; the %RAIU is suppressed. Sometimes, the iodine load causes activation of subclinical Graves or toxic multinodular goiter, and the %RAIU is elevated.

Amiodarone-Induced Thyrotoxicosis. Amiodarone-induced thyrotoxicosis occurs in 10% of patients on an antiarrhythmic drug. It contains 75 mg iodine per tablet. Two types of thyrotoxicosis are seen. In type 1, which is iodine induced (Jod–Basedow), seen in patients with preexisting nodular goiter or subclinical Graves disease, in which the %RAIU is elevated. Type 2 is more common and results in a destructive thyroiditis, and the %RAIU is near zero.

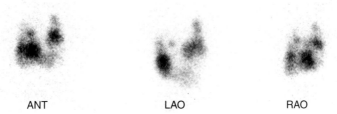

ANT LAO RAO

Fig. 8.11 Toxic multinodular goiter. Thyrotoxic patient who had multiple thyroid nodules seen on ultrasonography. The thyroid scan shows multiple areas of increased uptake consistent with hot nodules in both lobes and significant suppression of the remaining normal functioning thyroid, and low background. *ANT,* Anterior; *LAO,* left anterior oblique; *RAO,* right anterior oblique; *RT,* right; *SSN,* suprasternal notch. Compare this study with Fig. 8.14, a nontoxic multinodular gland.

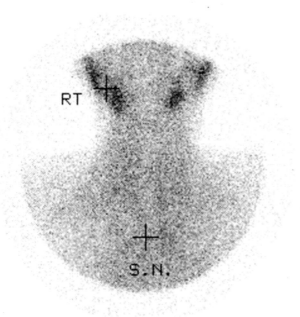

Fig. 8.12 Subacute thyroiditis. The patient presented with recent onset of thyrotoxicosis. The thyroid was tender and slightly enlarged. The Tc-99m thyroid scan shows no thyroid uptake due to the suppressed thyroid-stimulating hormone (TSH) and normal feedback. *RT,* Right side; *S.N.,* suprasternal notch.

Thyrotoxicosis Factitia. Thyrotoxicosis factitia occurs in patients on thyroid hormone, sometimes prescribed by a physician but in many cases surreptitiously taken, such as by a health care worker for weight loss.

Other Causes. Hydatidiform mole, trophoblastic tumors, and choriocarcinoma may rarely produce symptoms of hyperthyroidism due to the production of human chorionic gonadotropin, a weak TSH-like agonist. Serum TSH is suppressed, and the %RAIU is elevated. Metastatic thyroid cancer as a cause of hyperthyroidism is quite rare and most commonly occurs with follicular carcinoma. Rare benign ovarian teratomas have functioning thyroid tissue as a major component (struma ovarii) and can produce sufficient thyroid hormone to cause thyrotoxicosis. The diagnosis is suspected in a patient with a concomitant pelvic mass. The ectopic functioning pelvic thyroid tissue can be imaged with scintigraphy. Neck thyroid uptake is suppressed. Reidel struma is an uncommon form of thyroiditis in which all or part of the gland is replaced by fibrous tissue. No uptake is seen in the region of fibrous tissue.

Thyroid Nodules

The incidence of benign and malignant nodules increases with age and occurs more often in women than men. Concern for malignancy is increased in a young person, a male, or cases with recent nodule growth. Multiple thyroid nodules have the same risk of malignancy as those of a solitary nodule, approximately 15% to 20%. Radiation to the head and neck or mediastinum with exposure up to 1500 rem is associated with an increased incidence of thyroid nodules and papillary thyroid cancer, with a mean latency period of about 5 years. For radiation greater than 1500 rem, the risk decreases, presumably because of tissue destruction.

Ultrasonography can confirm and characterize the presence of a nodule or nodules detected on physical examination. Purely cystic lesions are benign; however, cancer cannot be excluded if the cyst has a soft tissue component or cystic degeneration. Nodules > 1 cm usually require fine-needle aspiration (FNA) biopsy for diagnosis. The accuracy of FNA is high, although it is subject to some sampling error and indeterminate reports.

Radionuclide thyroid scans are not routinely ordered today for thyroid nodules. Ultrasonography and biopsy usually make the diagnosis, except in patients with a suppressed TSH. The latter suggests a toxic autonomous nodule. A thyroid scan will show increased uptake (hot nodule) due to a hyperfunctioning follicular adenoma, and biopsy can/should be avoided. Histopathologically, a follicular adenoma often cannot be distinguished from a follicular cancer; thus, a thyroid scan can avoid this dilemma and is diagnostic. However, most nodules are cold.

On thyroid scintigraphy, nodules are classified as cold, hot, warm, or indeterminate (Table 8.6). Cold nodules are hypofunctioning compared with adjacent normal tissue (Fig. 8.16). They have approximately a 15% to 20% risk of malignancy. Cold nodules in patients with Graves disease have the same likelihood of cancer and should be worked up before therapy of Graves. Cold nodules may also be due to simple cysts, colloid nodules, thyroiditis, hemorrhage, necrosis, and so forth (Box 8.5). Hot nodules are hyperfunctioning, with suppression of the extranodular gland (Fig. 8.17). They are autonomous hyperfunctioning follicular adenomas. The likelihood of thyroid cancer is < 1%.

Hot nodules larger than 2.5 to 3.0 cm usually produce overt thyrotoxicosis. Patients with smaller nodules with less hormone production may present with subclinical hyperthyroidism or T_3

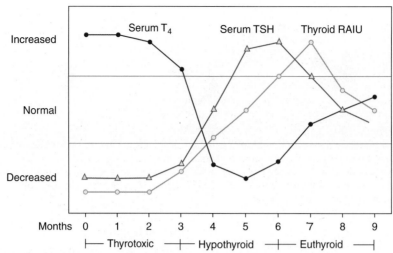

Fig. 8.13 Subacute thyroiditis, clinical course. Serum T4, thyroid-stimulating hormone (TSH), and %RAIU from initial presentation to resolution 9 months later. When the patient is thyrotoxic on the initial examination, the T4 is elevated and TSH and %RAIU suppressed. After the stored thyroid hormone has been released secondary to inflammation and then metabolized, the patient becomes hypothyroid as a result of the inflamed, poorly functioning thyroid. TSH and %RAIU rise. With time, the thyroid regains function, and the patient usually becomes euthyroid, with normalized T4, TSH, and %RAIU.

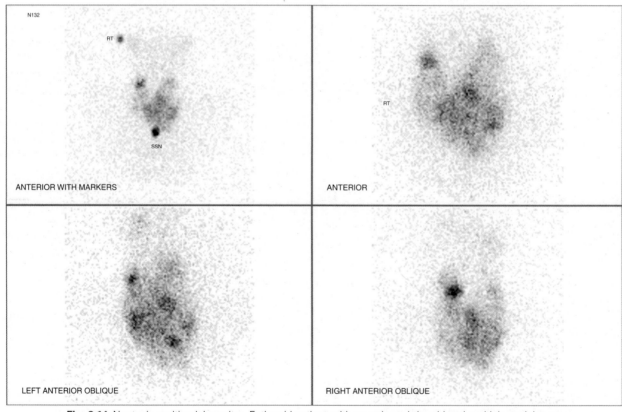

Fig. 8.14 Nontoxic multinodular goiter. Euthyroid patient with an enlarged thyroid and multiple nodules on physical examination and ultrasonography. The scan shows multiple areas of focally increased and decreased uptake. The background is relatively high.

thyrotoxicosis (suppressed serum TSH, normal T_4, elevated T_3). Radioiodine I-131 is the usual therapy for toxic nodules because the radiation is delivered selectively to the hyperfunctioning tissue while sparing suppressed extranodular tissues. This results in a lower incidence of posttherapy hypothyroidism. After successful treatment, the suppressed tissue regains function.

An indeterminate nodule is a palpable or sonographically detected nodule > 1 cm that cannot be differentiated on scan as definitely hot or cold compared with surrounding normal thyroid. This may be seen in a posterior nodule that has normal thyroid tissue uptake superimposed anterior to it; thus, it appears to have normal uptake. Nodules < 1 cm may be too

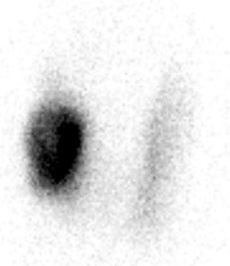

Fig. 8.15 Toxic (hot) thyroid nodule. Patient presented with thyrotoxic symptoms. Thyroid palpation detected a 3-cm right thyroid nodule. Thyroid function studies revealed an elevated T4 and suppressed TSH (<0.05 mIU/L). This I-123 scan shows intense uptake in the nodule; however, the remainder of the gland is suppressed.

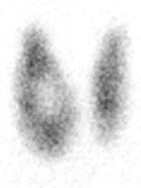

Fig. 8.16 Cold nodule. Focal decrease in iodine-123 uptake in the left lobe of the thyroid corresponding to a palpable nodule. This patient also has Graves disease. Note the high target-to-background ratio. The cold nodule should be worked up before Graves therapy.

TABLE 8.6 Classification of Thyroid Nodule Function

Nodule	Scan Appearance
Cold	Hypofunctioning compared with adjacent normal tissue
Hot	Hyperfunctioning with suppression of the extranodular gland
Warm	Increased uptake but without suppression of the extranodular tissue
Indeterminate	Palpable or seen on anatomical imaging but not visualized on scan

BOX 8.5 Differential Diagnosis for Thyroid Nodules

Cold Nodules
Benign
  Colloid nodule
  Simple cyst
  Hemorrhagic cyst
  Adenoma
  Thyroiditis
  Abscess
  Parathyroid cyst or adenoma
Malignant
  Papillary
  Follicular
  Hurthle cell
  Anaplastic
  Medullary
  Lymphoma
  Metastatic carcinoma
    Lung
    Breast
    Melanoma
    Gastrointestinal
    Renal

Hot Nodules
Toxic follicular adenomas

Warm Nodules
Nontoxic hyperfunctioning adenomas
Hyperplastic thyroid tissue

small to be detected by scintigraphy. An indeterminate nodule has the same significance as a cold nodule. Discordant nodules appear hot or warm on a Tc-99m scan but are cold on a radioiodine scan. Some thyroid cancers maintain trapping but not organification; thus, a single hot nodule identified on Tc-99m pertechnetate imaging should not be considered a functioning nodule until confirmed by an I-123 scan. Approximately 15% to 20% are malignant.

Colloid nodular goiters are composed of benign colloid nodules. Before the addition of iodine supplements to salt and food, goiter was endemic in the United States around the Great Lakes and still occurs in some parts of the world. The pathogenesis of iodine-deficient nodule formation is hyperplasia followed by the formation of functioning nodules that undergo hemorrhage and necrosis, replaced by lakes of colloid. The scintigraphic appearance is inhomogeneous uptake with cold areas of various sizes (Fig. 8.18).

Substernal goiters are extensions of the thyroid into the mediastinum. Most show continuity with the cervical portion of the gland, although some have a fibrous band connecting the substernal and cervical thyroid tissues. Many are asymptomatic and incidentally detected on CT as an anterior upper mediastinal mass. As they enlarge, they may cause symptoms of dyspnea, stridor, or dysphagia. Thyroid scans may be ordered to confirm

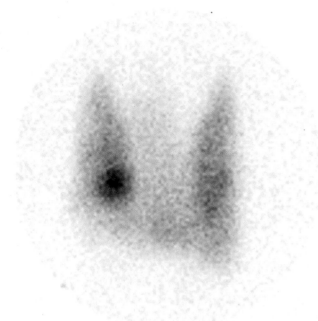

Fig. 8.17 Warm nodule in euthyroid patient. Patient presented with a palpable 1.5-cm nodule. Normal thyroid function tests. Increased uptake is seen in the inferior aspect of the right thyroid lobe. The may be autonomous, it is not a toxic nodule. Compare with Fig. 8.15.

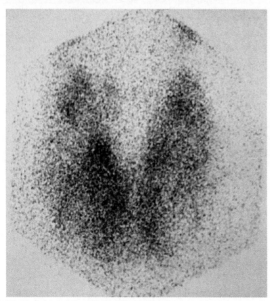

Fig. 8.18 Colloid goiter. Clinically palpable goiter in a patient who grew up in a Michigan goiter belt. Inhomogeneous tracer distribution with multiple focal cold areas. The patient was mildly hypothyroid.

a substernal goiter versus another cause for the mass. Radiotracer uptake in substernal goiters is sometimes poor, although uptake can usually be seen. I-131 was used for detection in the past (Fig. 8.19). Today, I-123 is the preferred radiopharmaceutical because of its good image quality and substantially less radiation to the thyroid. Single-photon emission computed tomography with computed tomography (SPECT/CT) should be obtained whenever possible (Fig. 8.20).

Ectopic thyroid tissue occurs along the embryological path of the thyroglossal duct descent, often in lingual, suprahyoid,

and infrahyoid locations (Fig. 8.21), occasionally in the lateral neck. It may present clinically in the neonate or child as a midline mass with the absence of normal thyroid tissue in the neck, accompanied by hypothyroidism. The typical appearance of a lingual thyroid is a focal or nodular accumulation at the base of the tongue and absence of tracer uptake in the expected cervical location (Fig. 8.22). However, ectopic thyroid tissue may occur in the mediastinum or even in the pelvis (struma ovarii). Lateral rests usually function poorly, but they can hyperfunction or be the focus of thyroid cancer. Ectopic thyroid tissue should be considered metastatic until proven otherwise.

Radioiodine I-131 Therapy of Thyrotoxicosis
Graves Disease

Patients with Graves disease are often initially treated with beta-blockers and antithyroid drugs (propylthiouracil [PTU] or methimazole [Tapazole]). These drugs block organification and reduce hormone production. They can "cool" the patient down and render the patient euthyroid, providing time to consider further therapeutic options. Often the drugs are prescribed for 6 to 12 months, sometimes longer. They have a reported high incidence of adverse effects (50%), the most serious being liver dysfunction and agranulocytosis. Thyroidectomy is an uncommon therapy except for concomitant cosmetic reasons and to relieve mass effect on the airway. Most patients with Graves ultimately receive radioiodine I-131 therapy.

Radioactive iodine is effective therapy for the majority of patients with Graves disease. Full effectiveness may take 3 to 6 months. A small minority of patients require repeat treatment (<10%) with a higher administered dose. Pregnancy must be excluded before I-131 therapy. Women should be counseled to avoid pregnancy for 3 to 6 months after therapy in the event that retreatment is necessary. The exophthalmos of Graves is not controlled by antithyroid drugs or I-131 therapy. In fact, exacerbation of exophthalmos may occur with I-131 therapy. Corticosteroids may be administered concomitantly to prevent this.

Many decades of experience have shown I-131 therapy to be safe and effective, even in children. The majority of these patients treated for Graves ultimately develop hypothyroidism and require replacement hormone therapy. This may occur as early as several months after therapy, particularly with higher doses. With lower administered doses, hypothyroidism is less common, but the likelihood of disease recurrence is higher.

Occasionally patients will develop radiation thyroiditis after I-131 therapy, causing neck tenderness, pain, or swelling that can be treated in most cases with acetaminophen. Rarely, thyroid storm occurs, potentially a life-threatening condition, and may require hospitalization and steroid therapy. Patients in a very toxic state and those treated with higher amounts of radioactivity are at greater risk. Beta-blockers and antithyroid drugs used before and after therapy can minimize the risk. Evidence over many decades of I-131 therapy for Graves disease has not shown a statistically significant increase in the frequency of secondary cancers, infertility, or congenital defects in the children of patients.

Iodine-131 Dose Selection for Graves. Various approaches have been used for selecting a specific I-131 therapy dose. One

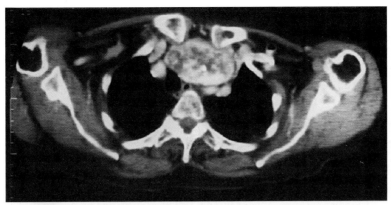

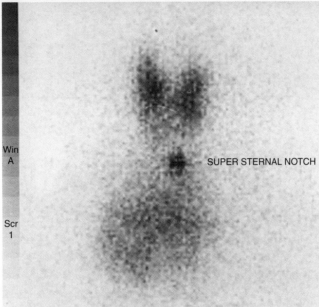

Win
A

SUPER STERNAL NOTCH

Scr
1

Fig. 8.19 Substernal goiter imaging with I-131. The contrast computed tomography (CT) image *(upper)* shows the presence of an anterior mediastinal mass. The thyroid scan *(below)* has uptake in a normal-appearing thyroid and a large substernal goiter that corresponds to the mediastinal mass seen on CT. A radioactive marker denotes the suprasternal notch. Similar images can be obtained with I-123.

method is to prescribe a standard empiric dose in the range of 10 to 15 mCi (370–555 MBq). This often works. However, factors such as the size of the gland and %RAIU may result in very different radiation doses to the thyroid between patients. Large glands require a relatively higher therapeutic dose, and patients with a high %RAIU may be effectively treated with a lower dose. Some physicians adjust this dose based on these factors.

A common individualized approach is to use a formula that takes into consideration gland size, the %RAIU, and the I-131 dose per gram of thyroid tissue (an example is shown Box 8.6):

$$\text{I-131 administered dose} = \frac{\text{gram size of thyroid gland} \times 100-180\mu\text{Ci/gram}}{24\text{ hour \% RAIU}}$$

Estimation of the gram weight of the gland is required. A normal gland weighs 15 to 20 g. Patients with Graves disease often have glands in the range of 40 to 80 g or larger. Although

experienced physicians may produce reproducible estimates, actual gland size is very difficult to estimate. This is especially true in large glands, which are often underestimated. Attempts to calculate volumes from ultrasound images are also generally inadequate.

Another important variable in this calculation is the microcurie per gram dose. In the past, referring physicians often preferred relatively low I-131 doses to minimize radiation to the patient, for example, 60 to 80 μCi (2.2–3.0 MBq)/g tissue. Today, referring physicians are more comfortable with the safety of higher doses, 120 to 180 μCi (4.4–6.6 MBq)/g tissue, and prefer the improved likelihood of success with a single therapeutic dose. With the higher dose, earlier-onset hypothyroidism is likely to occur, but this allows for prompt appropriate replacement therapy, which many endocrinologists prefer. Patients with rapid radioiodine turnover (high 4-hour but normal or significantly lower 24-hour %RAIU) have a shorter I-131 thyroid residence time. Thus, a higher I-131 dose than normally would be administered is indicated.

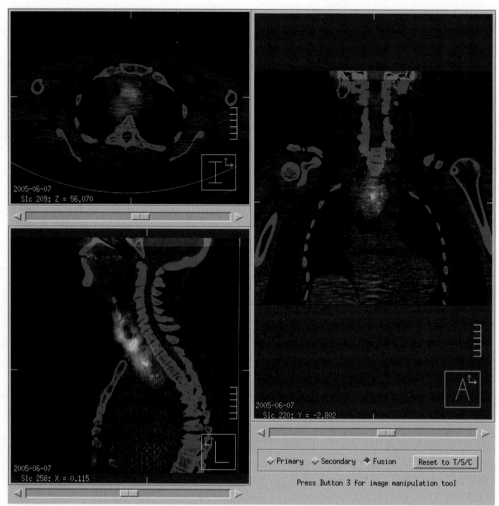

Fig. 8.20 Substernal goiter with I-123 hybrid single-photon emission computed tomography with computed tomography (SPECT/CT). I-123 thyroid scan is fused with the CT scan in selected transverse, sagittal, and coronal views. This patient had a clinically multinodular toxic goiter with substernal extension.

Toxic Nodular Disease

Toxic nodules are more resistant to therapy with radioiodine than Graves. The reason is uncertain, but it may be that I-131 thyroid residence time in the nodule(s) is reduced, leading to a lower retained dose. The administered I-131 therapeutic dose is often increased by 50% over what would be prescribed for Graves. An empirical dose of 20 to 30 mCi (740–1110 MBq) is often used. Because extranodular tissue is suppressed and relatively spared from radiation, normal function usually resumes after successful therapy.

Thyroid Cancer

Well-differentiated thyroid cancer originates from thyroid follicular epithelium. It retains biological characteristics of healthy thyroid tissue, including expression of the sodium iodide symporter, which is responsible for radioiodine uptake. Prognosis with appropriate treatment is generally good, with an estimated 10-year survival rate of greater than 85%. Even with distant metastases, the 10-year survival is 25% to 40%. The lifetime recurrence rate is 10% to 30%; therefore, long-term follow-up is required, and repeat therapy is necessary for some patients.

Papillary thyroid carcinoma is the most common histopathological type of well-differentiated thyroid malignancy (85%). Pure follicular cell carcinoma occurs less frequently (12%) and poorly differentiated tumors (3%). Papillary thyroid cancer spreads via regional lymphatic vessels; however, follicular thyroid carcinoma, a more aggressive tumor with worse prognosis, is likely to disseminate hematogenously and result in distant metastases. Hürthle cell, tall cell, and columnar variants of papillary cancer behave similar to follicular cell and have a similarly poorer prognosis. Medullary, anaplastic, and poorly differentiated carcinomas do not concentrate radioiodine, are not detected with radioiodine scintigraphy, and are not treated with I-131.

The American Thyroid Association (ATA) Initial Risk Stratification System is increasingly used to classify patients as having low, intermediate, or high risk of recurrence, rather than the traditional TNM system. This is important to estimate prognosis and provide appropriate therapy.

Low-risk patients have intrathyroidal cancer, usually small with no evidence of extrathyroidal extension, vascular invasion, or metastases.

Intermediate-risk patients have either microscopical extra-thyroidal extension, cervical lymph node metastases, vascular invasion, aggressive tumor histology, or radioactive iodine avid disease in the neck outside the thyroid bed.

High-risk patients have gross extrathyroidal extension, incomplete tumor resection, distant metastases, or inappropriately high postoperative serum thyroglobulin (Tg) values.

The primary treatment for newly diagnosed thyroid cancer is surgery. The presence of metastatic disease does not obviate the need for surgical excision of the primary tumor and accessible local/regional disease. In most cases, near-total thyroidectomy is the standard operation, with the removal of as much tumor, tumor-involved tissue, and lymph nodes as possible. Lesser surgery is at times performed for low-risk patients.

Postoperative radioactive iodine (RAI) therapy is administered either as *adjunctive* tumor therapy after total thyroidectomy or as *ablative* therapy for the remaining normal thyroid tissue. Effective RAI I-131 therapy requires eradication of the remaining thyroid cancer and ablation of the uninvolved normal thyroid. Ablation of normal thyroid tissue allows for clinical follow-up of the patient utilizing serum Tg and the whole-body RAI thyroid cancer scan. After total thyroidectomy, the serum thyroglobulin level should not be detectable. Thus, it becomes a specific thyroid cancer marker. The sensitivity of Tg for the detection of residual or recurrent cancer is enhanced when it is stimulated by serum TSH.

Lower RAI doses are being recommended today than in the past, especially for the therapy of low-risk patients. There is also less frequent use of the RAI scan for follow-up. Serum Tg and ultrasound are increasingly the primary methods for patient follow-up, although RAI is still recommended for some intermediate and many high-risk patients.

Initial therapy recommendations according to 2015 American Thyroid Association (ATA) management guidelines are as follows:

- *Low-risk* patients who have undergone total thyroidectomy: Routine postoperative evaluation of disease status with serum Tg. RAI scan and or ultrasound can be considered. RAI remnant ablation not routinely recommended. If performed, 30 mCi (1110 MBq) is generally favored.
- *Intermediate-risk* patients who have had a total thyroidectomy and therapeutic neck dissection: Routine postoperative evaluation of serum Tg. Postoperative diagnostic RAI scan and or ultrasound should be considered. For *remnant ablation*, 30 mCi is favored over a higher dose. Data suggest that the effectiveness of I-131 thyroid bed ablation plateaus at 30 to 50 mCi (740–1110 MBq), so higher amounts are not likely to be more effective. For *adjuvant therapy*, 30 mCi to 150 mCi (5550 MBq) is recommended in the absence of distant metastases.
- *High-risk* patients who have undergone total thyroidectomy, therapeutic neck dissection, and possibly central neck dissection: Postoperative RAI scan and or ultrasound should be considered. For adjuvant therapy, administered activities up to 150 mCi (5550 MBq). For known structural disease, 100 to 200 mCi

(370–740 MBq, 100–150 for patients > 70 years old). Evaluate response to therapy with serum Tg and neck ultrasound, and consider whole-body RAI scan, CT/magnetic resonance (MR), and or fluorodeoxyglucose (FDG) positron emission tomography (PET)/CT scan.

The ATA recommendations are guidelines. The nuclear medicine community, both in the United States and Europe, has raised concerns that the guidelines were written without sufficient nuclear medicine input and marginalized the role of nuclear medicine in the care of both nodular thyroid disease and thyroid cancer. One concern is that these guidelines are not always supported by strong data and are sometimes more conservative in the use of imaging and therapy dose than is in common practice at many centers.

Postoperative diagnostic radioiodine whole-body scans (RAI WBS) can help determine the extent of the thyroid remnant or residual disease when it cannot be accurately ascertained from the surgical report or neck ultrasonography alone and when the results may alter the decision to treat or the amount of RAI activity that is to be administered. This includes patients where serum thyroglobulin measurements are less accurate due to persistent antithyroglobulin antibodies. Unsuspected regional and distant metastases can also be identified. Localization of uptake may be enhanced by SPECT/CT, which can alter clinical management in up to 25% to 53% of patients.

All patients are prescribed thyroid hormone after surgery, not only as replacement therapy but also to suppress TSH, which could otherwise stimulate tumor growth. Serum Tg reaches its nadir 3 to 4 weeks postoperatively. Tg values of > 1 ng/mL or TSH-stimulated Tg values of > 10 ng/mL are evidence of biochemical incomplete response to therapy in patients treated with total thyroidectomy and RAI ablation. Serum Tg is often obtained 6 to 18 months after initial therapy. Risk assessment is then reclassified.

A *biochemical* incomplete response is seen in approximately 15% to 20% of patients. Many of these patients are eventually reclassified as having no evidence of disease at final follow-up, without any additional RAI or surgical treatment. A *structural* incomplete response to initial therapy is seen in 2% to 6% of ATA low-risk patients, 19% to 28% of intermediate-risk patients, and 67% to 75% of high-risk patients. Despite additional treatment, the majority of these patients will have persistent structural and/or biochemical evidence of persistent disease at final follow-up. Persistent/recurrent loco-regional structural disease may have a higher likelihood of responding to additional treatments and has significantly lower disease-specific mortality rates than persistent/recurrent distant metastases.

Whole-Body Thyroid Cancer Scintigraphy

Well-differentiated thyroid cancer cells are hypofunctional compared with normal thyroid tissue and so take up radioiodine to a lesser degree than adjacent normal thyroid. This is the reason thyroid cancer nodules appear cold on routine thyroid scans. However, after thyroidectomy with endogenous TSH stimulation by hormone withdrawal or by exogenous stimulation with recombinant TSH (Thyrogen), thyroid cancer imaging with radioiodine becomes feasible.

Postthyroidectomy Scan Preparation. Two methods are used for patient preparation. In one, the patient is not prescribed thyroid hormone replacement/suppression postoperatively; the serum TSH progressively rises as the patient becomes increasingly hypothyroid. The patient's serum TSH level should be

greater than 30 U/mL before radioiodine is administered, to ensure good uptake. This takes 4 to 6 weeks. Alternatively, the patient is placed on replacement/suppression thyroid hormone after surgery. Then Thyrogen, a recombinant form of TSH (rTSH), is administered on 2 consecutive days as an intramuscular injection of 0.9 mg. A serum TSH level is usually obtained. On the third day, radioiodine is administered. Imaging is performed on day 4 for I-123 and day 5 for I-131.

Subsequent Follow-Up Whole-Body Thyroid CANCER Scans. If the hormone withdrawal method is chosen, the patient discontinues the long-acting thyroid hormone T4 analog levothyroxine (Synthroid) for 4 to 6 weeks, until the TSH level is greater than 30 U/mL. To minimize hypothyroid symptoms, some patients are prescribed a shorter-half-life T_3 thyroid hormone analog, triiodothyronine (Cytomel). However, this must be discontinued 2 weeks before radioiodine administration to ensure an adequate rise in the serum TSH.

Because symptoms of hypothyroidism can be quite debilitating for some patients, particularly those with concomitant medical problems who cannot be taken off their thyroid hormone. Thyrogen is increasingly used as an alternative, as described previously.

Hypothyroidism causes a decrease in the glomerular filtration rate (GFR) and radioiodine clearance. Recombinant TSH does not affect GFR. Thus, to expose these thyroid cancer cells to similar extracellular RAI as the thyroid withdrawal method, a larger RAI dose is administered.

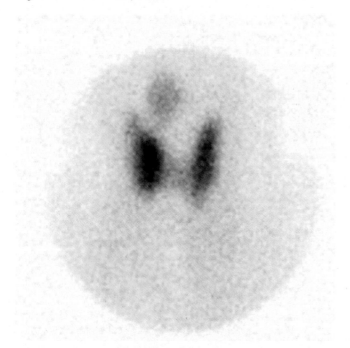

Fig. 8.21 Ectopic thyroid. The 40-year-old patient presented with an anterior midline neck mass. Ultrasonography described it as a solid, oval homogenous hypoechoic soft tissue mass measuring 11 cm, suggestive of thyroid tissue. The thyroid scan confirms that it is ectopic tissue thyroid superior to the normal right thyroid lobe.

Methodology for Whole-Body RAU Thyroid Cancer Scintigraphy.

Iodine-131 Whole-Body Scan. In the recent past, 5 mCi (185 MBq) or more of I-131 was a commonly administered dose for diagnostic thyroid cancer scans. However, because of reports of thyroid "stunning" after this dose (i.e., reduced uptake of the subsequent therapeutic dose), the recommended I-131 diagnostic dose was reduced to 2 to 3 mCi (74–111 MBq). Whole-body imaging is then acquired 48 hours after oral administration, which allows detection of thyroid metastases at distant sites, including the bones, liver, and brain. After I-131 therapy, a second whole-body scan is routinely acquired approximately 7 days posttherapy when the I-131 total-body RAI dose is low enough not to overwhelm the crystal of the gamma camera. This yields a high target-to-background ratio. A protocol summary is detailed (Box 8.7).

Iodine-123 Whole-Body Scan. I-123 is increasingly used as an alternative to I-131 for diagnostic thyroid cancer scans. Stunning is not an issue with I-123, image quality is superior, and the study is completed 24 hours after dose administration rather than 48 hours for I-131. I-123 might be expected to detect fewer tumors than I-131 because of the earlier imaging period, which allows less time for background clearance; however, investigations have shown similar sensitivity for detection of metastases, possibly because of the higher photon flux of I-123. The administered oral dose of I-123 is 1.5 to 3 mCi (55–111 MBq). Whole-body imaging and high-count spot images of the head, neck, and chest are obtained. SPECT/CT improves anatomical localization.

Interpretation of the Diagnostic Whole-Body Thyroid Cancer Scan. Diagnostic scans performed after near-total thyroidectomy but before therapy often show some residual focal thyroid uptake in the neck, often with a %RAIU uptake of less than 1% to 2%. Surgeons may not be able to remove all of the normal thyroid tissue, either because of the volume of tissue, tumor involvement of normal tissues, or care not to damage the parathyroid glands. If limited to the region of the thyroid bed with no known residual tumor, the neck uptake is often merely normal thyroid remnant. It is not uncommon to also see uptake

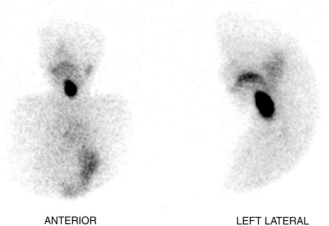

ANTERIOR   LEFT LATERAL

Fig. 8.22 Lingual thyroid. Hypothyroid infant with upper midline neck mass. Thyroid scan pinhole images (anterior view and left lateral views) show prominent uptake within the midline mass. There is no thyroid uptake lower in the region of the thyroid bed.

BOX 8.6 Calculation of Iodine-131 Therapeutic Dose for Graves Hyperthyroidism

Input Data
Gland weight: 60 g
24-hour uptake: 80%
Desired dose to be retained in thyroid (selected to deliver 8000–10,000 rads to thyroid): 100 μCi/g

Calculations

$$\text{Required dose (μCi)} = \frac{60g \times 100\mu Ci/g}{0.80} = 7500$$

$$\text{Dose (mCi)} = \frac{7500}{1000} = 7.5 mCi$$

BOX 8.7 Iodine-131 (or) Iodine-123 Whole-Body Imaging for Thyroid Cancer: Protocol Summary

Patient Preparation
Low-iodine diet for 10 days
Discontinue thyroid hormone for a sufficient period (T_4 for 6 wk, T_3 for 2 wk) to ensure maximum endogenous thyroid-stimulating hormone response (>30μU/mL) **(or)**
Administer Thyrogen (rTSH) 0.9 mg intramuscular × 2 days; on third day, administer radioiodine.

Radiopharmaceutical Dose: I-123
Withdrawal: 1.5 mCi (56 MBq), orally
Thyrogen: 2 to 4 mCi (74–148 MBq), orally

Radiopharmaceutical Dose: I-131
Withdrawal: 2 mCi (74 MBq), orally
Thyrogen: 4 mCi (148 MBq), orally

Imaging Time
24 hours after I-123 administration
48 hours after I-131 administration

Procedure—I-123
Wide field-of-view gamma camera with computer acquisition
Medium-energy parallel-hole collimator and a 20% window centered at 123 keV
Whole-body scan and a 10-minute spot views of the head, neck, and mediastinum
Single-photon emission computed tomography (SPECT) or SPECT with computed tomography (SPECT/CT) as indicated.
Calculate the percent radioactive iodine uptake.
SPECT/CT optional

Procedure—I-131
Wide field-of-view gamma camera with computer acquisition
High-energy parallel-hole collimator and a 20% window centered at 364 keV
Perform whole-body scan and 10-minute spot views to include head, neck, and mediastinum
Calculate the percent radioactive iodine uptake.
SPECT/CT optional

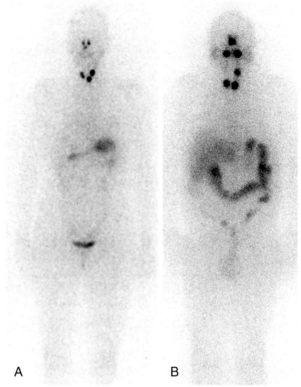

A   B

Fig. 8.23 Whole-body thyroid cancer scans before and after I-131 ablation. (A) Pretherapy (post-thyroidectomy) I-123 scan shows abnormal uptake limited to three focal areas in the region of the thyroid bed. No local or distant metastases are seen. Gastric and urinary clearance are normal. (B) Posttherapy I-131 scan. Six days after 30 mCi of I-131 therapy, the scan shows no significant change, with the exception of normal posttherapy liver uptake due to metabolism of I-131-labeled thyroid hormone, and some gastric and intestinal clearance.

Gastric and intestinal activity is also seen (Fig. 8.23). Normal uptake in the breasts should not be confused with lung uptake. It is only seen anteriorly. Thyroid cancer metastases have a predilection for the mediastinum and lung. Bone, brain, and liver metastases are less common and have a worse prognosis.

Approximately 7 days after RAI therapy, whole-body radioiodine I-131 scans are often obtained. Up to 10% of patients will have abnormal uptake on this posttherapy scan that was not seen on the pretherapy scan, potentially changing staging, risk assessment, and subsequent therapy (Fig. 8.24). SPECT/CT is increasingly used to improve localization of uptake (Fig. 8.25). There are some differences seen between the diagnostic pretherapy radioiodine scan and the 7-day posttherapy scan. Liver activity is almost always seen on the posttherapy scan because of the high administered dose, which allows for visualization of radiolabeled hormone metabolism in the liver, but almost never on the pretherapy scans. Considerably less intestinal or urinary activity is typically seen because most background radioiodine has cleared by 7 days, although this is variable. The high administered therapeutic dose may result in intense uptake in the thyroid bed ("star" artifact). The star has six points, caused by septal penetration of the hexagonal shaped collimator holes (Fig. 8.26).

Whole-Body Percent Radioactive Iodine Thyroid Uptake (%RAIU). Quantification of %RAIU after thyroidectomy is an

in the thyroglossal duct region superior to the thyroid bed. However, uptake lateral or inferior to the thyroid bed is suspicious for nodal tumor. Normal activity is seen in the nasal area, oropharynx and salivary glands, and genitourinary tract.

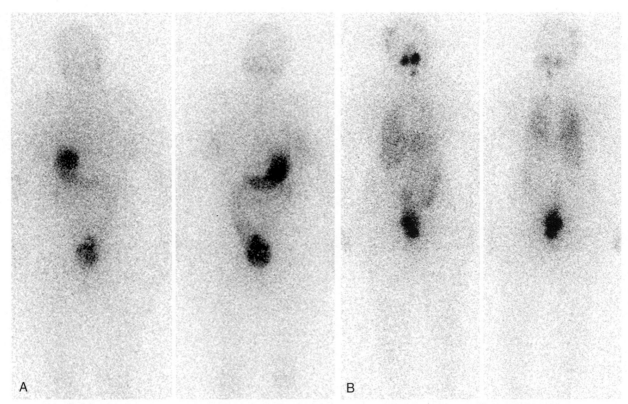

Fig. 8.24 Lung uptake due to miliary metastases seen only on the posttherapy scan. (A) Pretherapy I-123 scan in a patient with follicular cell thyroid cancer is negative, showing only normal gastric, intestinal, and bladder radiotracer. (B) Posttherapy I-131 scan shows diffuse lung uptake consistent with bilateral miliary pulmonary metastases.

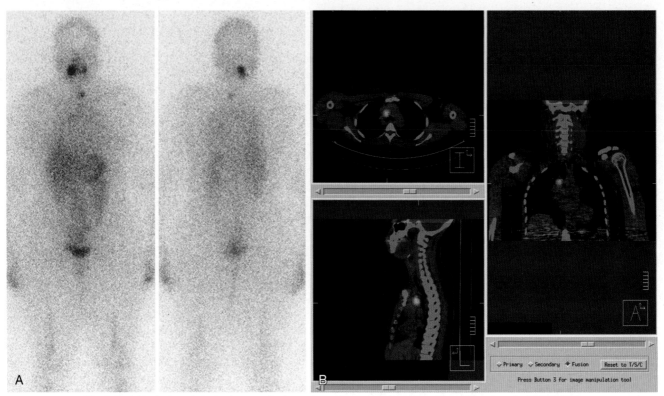

Fig. 8.25 Added value of single-photon emission computed tomography with computed tomography (SPECT/CT) for metastatic thyroid cancer. (A) A 48-year-old female whole-body posttherapy I-131 scan. Lymph node dissection of the neck had revealed tumor-positive nodes. The whole-body scan shows uptake in the lower neck versus upper mediastinum. (B) SPECT/CT three-view fused images precisely localize the uptake to pretracheal nodes.

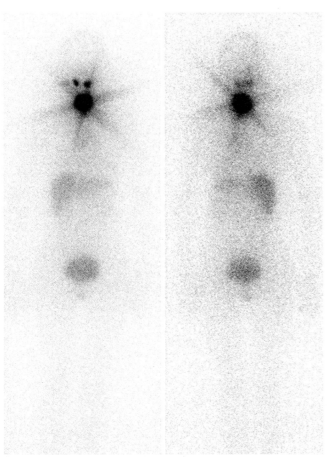

Fig. 8.26 Star artifact. Whole-body thyroid cancer scan (anterior and posterior views) obtained 7 days after high-dose I-131 therapy. The intense uptake in the thyroid bed results in a star artifact caused by septal penetration of the hexagonal-shaped collimator holes by the high-energy photons.

indicator of the adequacy of surgery and residual thyroid tissue. Subsequent follow-up scan uptake allows for evaluation of therapeutic effectiveness or recurrence. The %RAIU is determined from the scan itself, rather than using a probe detector generally used for routine thyroid scans. A radioiodine standard with calibrator-measured activity is also imaged. Regions of interest (ROIs) are drawn for the thyroid, background, and standard.

Dosimetry Calculation for Planning High-Dose I-131 Therapy. Patients at high risk requiring high-dose radioiodine therapy are often prescribed a standard dose of 150 to 200 mCi MBq. However, radioiodine uptake and clearance rate vary between patients; thus, patients ultimately receive different therapeutic doses to their thyroid cancer. One would like to administer as large a dose as possible while minimizing toxicity to the bone marrow and lungs. The accepted maximal allowable absorbed dose to the bone marrow is 200 rads at 48 hours, and the maximal accumulated activity to the lungs is 80 mCi (2960 MBq). Dosimetry calculations before therapy can produce an individualized dose based on the patient's radioiodine clearance. Thus, some patients may be able to receive considerably > 200 mCi (7400 MBq), whereas others should receive less.

For dosimetry calculation, a patient is administered a diagnostic dose of I-131 (1 mCi [37 MBq]). Blood clearance

sampling is acquired at 2, 4, 24, 48, 72, and 96 hours after tracer administration, and whole-body images are obtained daily for a week, usually with a probe detector. Blood serves as a surrogate for the red bone marrow. Total-body residence time and blood curve analysis are performed to evaluate the lung dose. The maximal I-131 dose to be administered is determined.

The Nuclear Regulatory Commission (NRC) patient release regulations (10 CFR 20 and 35) are based on likely radiation exposure to others. The regulations state that no one should receive more than 5 millisieverts (0.5 rem) from exposure to a released I-131 therapy patient. Agreement States generally follow NRC guidelines. Hospitals vary as to their own release requirements, which are never less stringent than the NRC regulations. At many centers, patients are treated primarily on an outpatient basis for doses < 200 mCi (7400 MBq). For > 200 mCi or for radiation safety for family members, patients are treated as inpatients. Posttherapy NRC patient release requirements are < 33 mCi (1121 MBq), or < 7 mrem/hour measured at 1 m. Radiation safety instructions should be discussed with the patient and family. Patient-specific information regarding limiting close contact and other measures to prevent exposure to others should be provided to the patient and family (Boxes 8.8 and 8.9).

Iodine-131 Therapy for Thyroid Cancer

Patient Preparation. A low-iodine diet is recommended for 7 to 14 days before the administration of therapy to increase radioiodine uptake and improve the likelihood of effectiveness.

Written Directive. Before administering greater than 30 microcuries (1.11 MBq) I-131 to a patient, a written directive must be dated and signed by an authorized user. A directive is also required for other therapeutic radiopharmaceuticals.

Adverse Effects of Therapy. Side effects soon after radioiodine I-131 therapy are usually mild but may include nausea and vomiting and sialoadenitis. The latter can be minimized with oral hydration and sour candy or lemon juice, although there is some disagreement about its utility. Late complications are usually related to the total I-131 dose received. Chronic sialadenitis and xerostomia may result. Infertility is quite uncommon, although sperm or egg harvesting is recommended by some physicians. Pulmonary fibrosis and bone marrow aplasia may be seen in patients with high tumor burden and repeated high-dose I-131 therapy. Concern for bone marrow suppression and leukemia increase as the total therapy dose increases above 500 mCi (18,500 MBq). There is some evidence, although inconclusive, for increased risk of secondary malignancies with RAI doses > 150 mCi (550 MBq). Physicians and technologists who administer the therapy dose are required by NRC regulations to have a thyroid "bioassay" (neck uptake counts) within a week of dose administration to determine whether they have received any internal dose during patient administration.

F-18 Fluorodeoxyglucose. 18 FDG PET is not useful for the initial detection of metastatic disease in well-differentiated thyroid cancer because F-18 FDG is generally more intense in aggressive cancers and has much lower sensitivity for disease detection compared with radioiodine. However, F-18 FDG PET/CT is indicated for high-risk patients with elevated serum thyroglobulin (Tg) and a negative radioiodine whole-body scan. The lack of radioiodine uptake signifies that the tumor has dedifferentiated into a higher-grade tumor, increasing the likelihood of FDG

uptake (Fig. 8.27). Localization of the tumor allows for possible surgical resection or other nonradioiodine therapy. FDG PET/CT in the setting of a rising serum Tg of > 10 ng/mL with a negative radioiodine scan has a sensitivity of about 83% and specificity of 84%, with particular increased sensitivity in the retropharyngeal and retroclavicular regions. Sensitivity is even higher in aggressive subtypes (e.g., tall cell, Hurthle cell, and poorly differentiated).

On whole-body FDG PET/CT performed for oncological staging or surveillance of nonthyroid tumors, uptake is sometimes seen in the thyroid. Diffuse gland uptake is usually caused by chronic thyroiditis (Hashimoto disease) and less frequently subacute thyroiditis, or Graves. Focal increased FDG uptake in a thyroid nodule, seen on the CT portion, has approximately a 30% likelihood of primary thyroid malignancy. Ultrasonography and biopsy are indicated.

PARATHYROID SCINTIGRAPHY

Parathyroid scintigraphy is a routine part of the preoperative workup of patients with the clinical diagnosis of hyperparathyroidism (elevated serum calcium and serum parathormone [PTH] level). Normally there is feedback between the serum calcium and serum PTH. Patients with hypercalcemia due to causes other than hyperparathyroidism (e.g., bone metastases) have low or suppressed PTH. PTH production is autonomous in hyperparathyroidism, and the serum PTH level is increased in spite of an increased serum calcium. The purpose of the parathyroid scan is to localize the hyperfunctioning parathyroid gland(s) before surgery, thus making minimally invasive surgery possible.

Anatomy and Embryology

There are usually four parathyroid glands, two superior and two inferior, measuring approximately 6 × 3 mm and weighing 35 to 40 mg each. A fifth supernumerary gland occurs in less than 10% of individuals. The inferior glands arise embryologically from the third brachial pouch and migrate caudally with the thymus. Their ultimate normal location is somewhat variable, with 60% located immediately posterior and lateral to the thyroid lower poles and 40% in the cervical portion of the thymus gland (Fig. 8.28). The superior glands arise from the fourth brachial pouch and migrate with the thyroid.

BOX 8.9 Patient Instructions After I-131 Therapy for Thyroid Cancer

Remain home from work for 2 to 3 days.

For 3 days after treatment:
Avoid prolonged sitting near others, including during travel.
Sleep in a separate bed.
Avoid close contact with children.
Drink at least 2 quarts of fluid daily.
Use sour candy to keep saliva flowing.
If you vomit, immediately contact Dr. _____ at (___) -___- ____.

For 3 to 7 days after treatment:
Men and women: Sit while urinating, and flush the toilet twice with the lid down after each use. If possible, use a separate bathroom. If not possible, clean the toilet seat after use.
Wash hands frequently. Shower or bathe daily, cleaning the tub or sink afterward.
Cover mouth when coughing or sneezing.
Do not engage in kissing or sexual relations.
Use separate towels and bed linens. Launder these items separately.
Do not share food or drink with others.
Place eating utensils in the dishwasher or wash them separately from others.
Maintain 1 to 2 arm's lengths from others when possible.
Dispose of toothbrush after using for 1 week.
For 6 months: Avoid pregnancy (use two forms of birth control for 3 months).

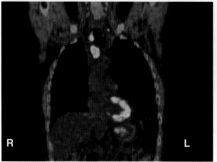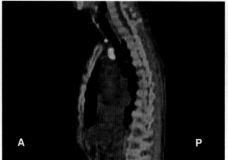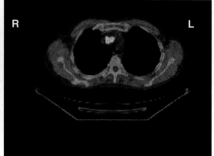

Fig. 8.27 F-18 fluorodeoxyglucose (FDG) positron emission tomography (PET) scan for thyroid cancer. Patient had elevated serum thyroglobulin but a negative I-123 whole-body scan. On the FDG PET study, multiple hypermetabolic lymph nodes from levels II to IV in the right neck and levels III to IV in the left neck, right paratracheal region, and left hilum consistent with thyroid cancer metastases.

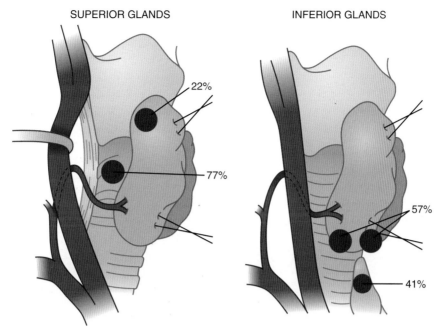

SUPERIOR GLANDS   INFERIOR GLANDS

Fig. 8.28 Normal parathyroid gland locations. The superior pair of glands *(purple circles on left image)* usually lie within the fascial covering of the posterior aspect of the thyroid gland outside the capsule. They are located just posterior to the superior pole or midpole of the thyroid. Intrathyroidal locations are rare. Most are adjacent to the thyroid or cricothyroid cartilage. Inferior glands *(purple circles on right image)* are located immediately posterior or lateral to the inferior pole of the thyroid or in the thyrothymic ligament *(right)*.

Approximately 75% are posterior to the midpoles of the thyroid and 25% posterior to the upper poles. The distinction between superior and inferior glands has surgical implications because the inferior glands are anterior to and the superior glands posterior to the recurrent laryngeal nerve. Resection of the superior glands poses a potential risk for nerve damage. The term *ectopic* refers to glands that have descended to an unusual location. Ectopic glands can be found as far cephalad as the carotid bifurcation, inferior to the mediastinum and pericardium, anterior to the thyroid, or posterior in the superior mediastinum into the tracheoesophageal groove and paraesophageal region (Fig. 8.29).

Physiology of the Parathyroid Gland

PTH is an 84-amino acid polypeptide hormone synthesized, stored, and secreted by the chief cells of the parathyroid glands. PTH regulates calcium and phosphorus homeostasis by its action on bone, the small intestine, and the kidneys.

Primary hyperparathyroidism is caused by autonomous hyperfunction of a parathyroid adenoma or, less frequently, four-gland hyperplasia. Adenomas are caused by somatic mutations with clonal expansion of the mutated cells; primary hyperplasia is a polyclonal proliferation. More than 85% of patients have a single adenoma, < 5% have two adenomas, and approximately 10% have four-gland hyperplasia (Table 8.7). Patients with multiple endocrine neoplasia syndrome may develop hyperparathyroidism as one of its manifestations due to multigland hyperplasia. Parathyroid carcinoma occurs in < 1% of patients with hyperparathyroidism. It typically presents with very elevated serum calcium, a palpable neck mass, bone pain, fractures, and renal colic.

Secondary hyperparathyroidism occurs in all patients with severe renal disease. It manifests as hypocalcemia, elevated serum phosphorus, and increased PTH. The cause is multifactorial due to vitamin D deficiency, phosphorus retention, and skeletal resistance to PTH. Despite an elevated serum PTH, the serum calcium remains below normal levels. Most patients are successfully managed medically. However, in symptomatic patients unresponsive to medical therapy with bone or joint pain, bone loss, muscle weakness, itching, irritability, anemia, or osteitis fibrosis, parathyroid surgery may be indicated.

Tertiary hyperparathyroidism presents as hypercalcemia in some patients with renal failure. One or more parathyroid glands becomes autonomous, and PTH is no longer responsive to the feedback of an elevated serum calcium. Surgical resection is indicated.

Primary Hyperparathyroidism
Clinical Presentation

In the past, patients presented with symptoms of nephrolithiasis, osteitis fibrosa cystica, osteoporosis, pathological fractures, gastrointestinal and neuropsychiatric symptoms, and brown tumors. Today, the majority of patients are asymptomatic at diagnosis, with hypercalcemia detected during routine blood screening.

Diagnosis

An elevated PTH level in a patient with hypercalcemia is diagnostic of hyperparathyroidism. Other causes for hypercalcemia without PTH elevation include malignancy, vitamin D intoxication, sarcoidosis, and thiazide diuretics. These patients have reduced serum PTH levels because of a normal physiological feedback mechanism.

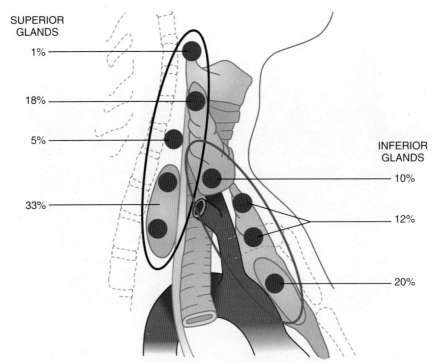

SUPERIOR
GLANDS

1%

18%

5%

33%

INFERIOR
GLANDS

10%

12%

20%

Fig. 8.29 Ectopic gland locations. Because of abnormal embryological descent, ectopic glands can be found as cephalad as the carotid bifurcation, as inferior as the pericardium, anterior to the thyroid, posterior in the tracheoesophageal groove, and in the superior mediastinum. In the anterior-posterior plane, inferior glands descend anteriorly and superior glands descend more posteriorly.

TABLE 8.7	**Hyperparathyroidism—Causes**
Cause	**Percentage**
Adenoma	85
Hyperplasia	10
Ectopic	<5
Carcinoma	<1

Treatment

Surgical resection is curative. In the past, the standard surgical operation was bilateral neck exploration with localization of each parathyroid gland by the surgeon and removal of the offending adenoma. Hyperplasia required removal of 3.5 glands, sometimes with placement of one gland elsewhere (e.g., in the arm) to ensure a functioning parathyroid gland. Preoperative imaging for hyperparathyroidism was controversial because all glands were localized at surgery, and some surgeons reported a > 90% detection/cure rate.

Today, the operation of choice is minimally invasive unilateral surgery using a small incision. This results in reduced operation time and fewer complications. However, this approach requires imaging for preoperative localization. The radionuclide method has proven to have superior detection accuracy compared with ultrasonography, CT, and magnetic resonance imaging (MRI) for the preoperative localization of a hyperfunctioning parathyroid adenoma. However, CT or sonography is often ordered for anatomical correlation and confirmation. The anatomical imaging methods are particularly insensitive for detecting ectopic and mediastinal glands.

During surgery, some surgeons use a specialized small gamma probe to help localize the hyperfunctioning gland or glands. Others do not feel it is necessary. An intraoperative reduction in the serum PTH level by 50% after surgical removal of the hyperfunctioning gland confirms successful surgery. Postoperative recurrence rates are approximately 5%. Common reasons for surgical failure include (1) an ectopic location of the tumor in the neck or in the mediastinum, (2) failure to recognize hyperplasia, or (3) the presence of an undiscovered fifth gland. Reexploration has increased morbidity and a poorer success rate than the primary procedure.

Radiopharmaceuticals

In the 1980s, Tl-201 was routinely used for parathyroid scintigraphy in conjunction with Tc-99m pertechnetate for imaging the thyroid. Detection and localization were subsequently shown to be superior for Tc-99m sestamibi compared with Tl-201, and Tc-99m sestamibi became the standard radiopharmaceutical used for hyperfunctioning parathyroid localization.

Tc-99m sestamibi (Cardiolite) is most commonly used as a myocardial perfusion imaging agent. Chemically, it is a lipophilic cation member of the isonitrile family (Hexakis 2-methoxyisobutyl isonitrile). Uptake is related to the parathyroid adenoma's high vascularity and cellularity. The radiotracer localizes and is retained in the region of mitochondria. The large number of mitochondria in oxyphil cells in parathyroid adenomas is thought responsible for its avid uptake and slow release. Normal functioning parathyroid glands are not visualized. Tc-99m tetrofosmin (Myoview) has a similar mechanism of uptake and localization and is reported useful for parathyroid imaging; however, published data are limited.

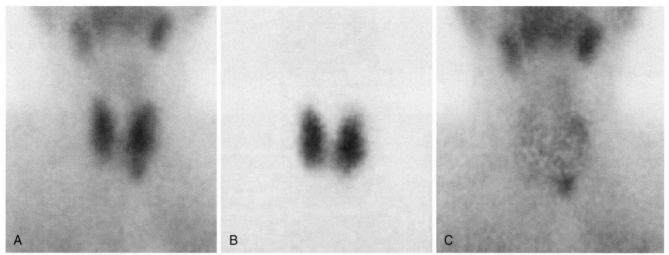

Fig. 8.30 Parathyroid subtraction scintigraphy. (A) Tc-99m sestamibi scan. (B) I-123 scan. (C) Computer subtraction of the I-123 scan from the Tc-99m sestamibi scan reveals uptake only in the parathyroid, consistent with an adenoma. In this case visual comparison would also suggest a left inferior parathyroid adenoma.

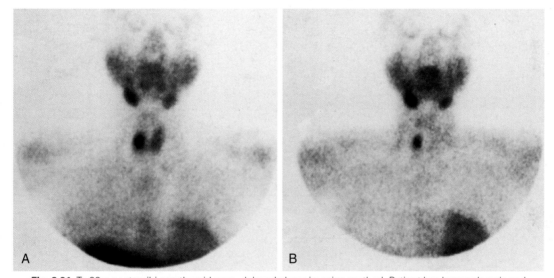

Fig. 8.31 Tc-99m sestamibi parathyroid scan, delayed planar imaging method. Patient has hypercalcemia and increased serum parathyroid hormone (PTH). (A) Early planar imaging at 15 minutes with Tc-99m sestamibi reveals somewhat asymmetrical activity with slightly more uptake in the region of the right thyroid gland, which appears larger. (B) Delayed imaging at 2 hours demonstrates washout of thyroid activity in both lobes; focal retained uptake on the right is retained, consistent with a parathyroid adenoma.

After intravenous injection, peak accumulation of Tc-99m sestamibi occurs in a hyperfunctioning parathyroid gland at 3 to 5 minutes, with a variable clearance half-time of approximately 60 minutes. Similar rapid uptake occurs in the thyroid; however, it usually washes out more rapidly than the parathyroid, thus the rationale for two-phase parathyroid scintigraphy.

Methodology

Tc-99m sestamibi, 20 to 25 mCi (740–925 MBq), is injected intravenously. Imaging begins 10 to 15 minutes later. Generally, two different acquisition methodologies have been used:

- Combined thyroid and parathyroid imaging—The rationale for a combined imaging protocol is to help differentiate a parathyroid adenoma from normal thyroid and thyroid nodules. The protocol is similar to that used in the past for Tl-201/Tc-99m pertechnetate, with the use of subtraction imaging.

Tc-99m sestamibi is injected, and images are acquired 10 minutes later. I-123 is then injected, and images are acquired 20 minutes later. Images are compared for different distribution. Digital subtraction of the I-123 thyroid image from the Tc-99m sestamibi image is performed, often resulting in an image only of the hyperfunctioning parathyroid gland (Fig. 8.30). This methodology works well, although technical errors may occur as a result of patient movement and image misalignment.

- Two-phase parathyroid imaging—This is the more commonly used methodology. Initial images are obtained 10 to 15 minutes after Tc-99m sestamibi injection. A second set of images is obtained at 2 hours. Because of more rapid washout of the thyroid, the delayed images often primarily show the hyperfunctioning parathyroid (Fig. 8.31). In up to a third of patients, this characteristic differential washout pattern is not seen. Either both the thyroid and the parathyroid wash

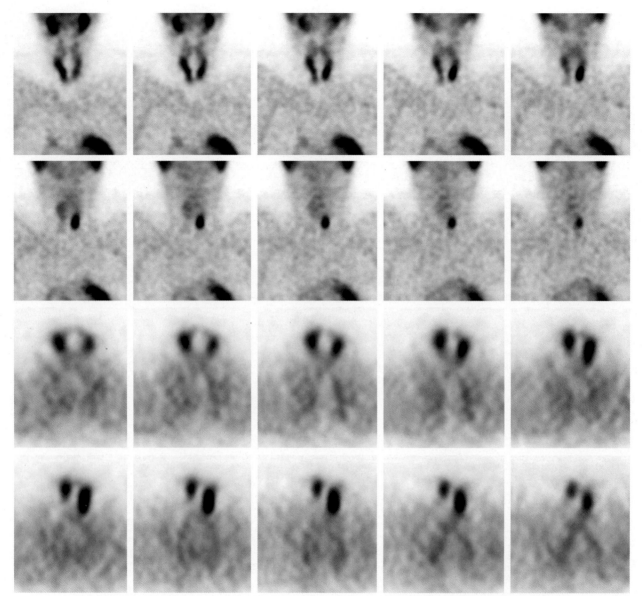

Fig. 8.32 Tc-99m sestamibi single-photon emission computed tomography (SPECT) parathyroid scan. Increased serum calcium and serum parathyroid hormone (PTH). Scan ordered for localization of hyperfunctioning parathyroid adenoma. Sequential coronal *(top two)* and transverse *(bottom two),* each with early images *(above)* and delayed images *(below).* The coronal images show that the adenoma is at the inferior and posterior aspect of the left thyroid lobe. The transverse images confirm that the parathyroid is quite posterior on the left side.

out at the same rate or both wash out so rapidly that little tracer remains on delayed images.

Many variations and combinations of these two methods are used at different imaging centers, which may include planar imaging, SPECT, or SPECT/CT:

- Planar imaging—Two-dimensional planar imaging has long been the standard methodology. The two options are a parallel-hole collimator that permits simultaneous imaging of the neck and mediastinum often with the addition of magnified pinhole imaging of the neck with oblique as images. The disadvantages of planar imaging are overlapping thyroid and parathyroid activity and limited two-dimensional information.

- Single-photon emission computed tomography (SPECT)—SPECT provides improved target-to-background compared

with planar imaging, minimizes overlapping activity, improves detectability, and localizes the hyperfunctioning gland(s) in three dimensions (Fig. 8.32).

- SPECT with computed tomography (SPECT/CT)—Hybrid SPECT/CT systems are increasingly used because they combine the functional information from SPECT and the anatomical information from CT (Figs. 8.33–8.35) and make possible attenuation correction.

Various combinations of these techniques are used at different imaging centers.

Image Interpretation

Initial images at 10 to 15 minutes after injection typically show prominent thyroid uptake, unless the patient has had a thyroidectomy or is on thyroid hormone, causing suppression. Focal

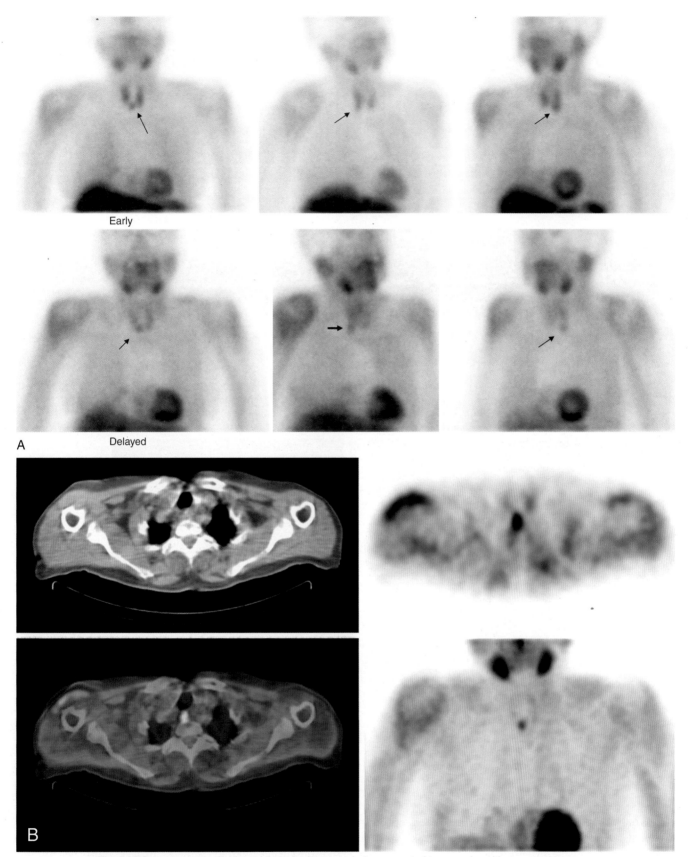

Fig. 8.33 Retrosternal localization with single-photon emission computed tomography with computed tomography (SPECT/CT). (A) Early and delayed planar images. Anterior *(left),* right anterior oblique (RAO; *middle*), left anterior oblique (LAO; *right*). In the anterior view, a suspicious adenoma is noted midline just below the two thyroid lobes. On the RAO and LAO views, the adenoma appears to be in the lower right lobe and lower left lobe, respectively. (B) The fused SPECT/CT images *(left lower)* show that the parathyroid adenoma is clearly retrotracheal.

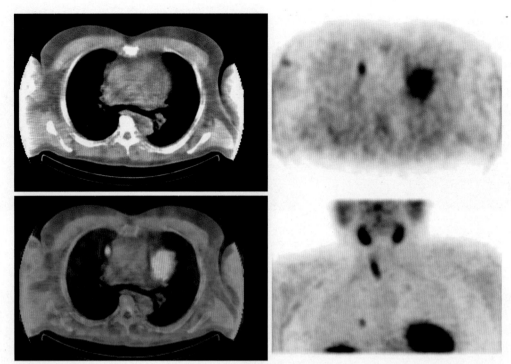

Fig. 8.34 Pericardial localization with single-photon emission computed tomography with computed tomography (SPECT/CT). Patient has had prior parathyroid surgery and left thyroidectomy and now has recurrent hypercalcemia. The maximal-intensity projection (MIP; *right lower*) view shows focal uptake in the right mediastinum. The fused SPECT/CT image shows localization in the region of the right pericardium.

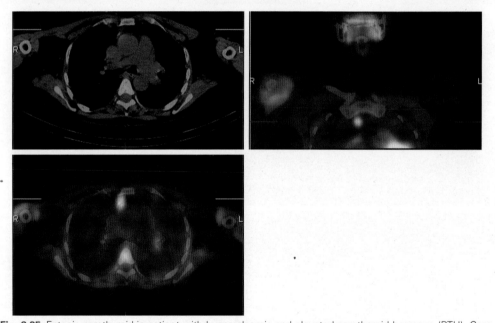

Fig. 8.35 Ectopic parathyroid in patient with hypercalcemia and elevated parathyroid hormone (PTH). Computed tomography (CT; *upper left*), fused single-photon emission computed tomography with computed tomography (SPECT/CT) transverse *(lower left),* and coronal *(right)* images. The parathyroid adenoma is localized anterior to the aorta, immediately behind the sternum.

parathyroid uptake greater than thyroid may be seen on occasion. On delayed imaging, much of the thyroid uptake has usually washed out, and the hyperfunctioning parathyroid gland persists and is a focus of increased activity. Occasionally there is rapid washout of the parathyroid adenoma as well as the thyroid, and a false-negative study may result. In both cases interpretation can sometimes be made on the initial image where the

focal parathyroid uptake is greater than the thyroid uptake. Ectopic glands are more easily detected because often there is no obscuring thyroid activity. Images must be routinely reviewed from the neck through the mediastinum, where adenomas may reside.

Although a parathyroid adenoma located in the region of the inferior thyroid lobe is often an inferior parathyroid adenoma,

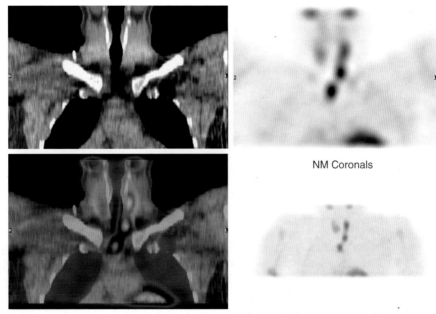

NM Coronals

Fig. 8.36 Tertiary hyperparathyroidism. Patient with renal failure and elevated serum calcium and parathyroid hormone (PTH). Three adenomas, two in the left neck and one in the anterior mediastinum.

superior glands may descend to that region. Inferior parathyroid glands are usually located immediately adjacent to the posterior aspect of the thyroid, while superior glands that have descended tend to be more posterior and clearly separated from the thyroid. This is sometimes distinguishable with oblique static images; however, SPECT and SPECT/CT can more easily allow differentiation.

Accuracy

The sensitivity for the detection of parathyroid adenomas larger than 300 mg approaches 90%. The most common cause of a false-negative study is small size. The sensitivity for detection of second adenomas or four-gland hyperplasia is lower than for single adenomas (50–60%). Localization of autonomous tertiary hyperfunctioning adenomas is also quite good (Fig. 8.36). The most common cause of a false-positive parathyroid study is a thyroid follicular adenoma. Thyroid cancer, benign neoplasms, and metastatic tumors may also show Tc-99m sestamibi uptake. Some drugs may cause rapid washout (e.g., calcium channel blockers, which activate p-glycoprotein). Although there few published data directly comparing the dual-isotope method combining thyroid and parathyroid imaging with the early and delayed image method, the reported accuracy of each suggests similar accuracy. There is some evidence suggesting that SPECT is superior to planar imaging and good evidence that SPECT/CT is superior to SPECT and planar imaging.

Other Radiopharmaceuticals

F-18 fluorodeoxyglucose has shown poor sensitivity for detecting parathyroid adenomas. It may have a role in the diagnosis of parathyroid carcinomas. C-11 methionine PET has shown good results in several publications, used most commonly for patients with negative Tc-99m sestamibi scans. However, C-11 has a very short half-life and requires on-site cyclotron production. Preliminary evidence suggests that F-18 fluorocholine provides very good localization accuracy.

SUGGESTED READING

Avram AM, Fig LM, Frey KA, Gross MD, Wong KK. Preablation 131-I scans with SPECT/CT in post-operative thyroid cancer patients: what is the impact on staging? *J Clin Endocrinol Metab*. 2013;98:1163–1171.

Bahn RS, Burch HB, Cooper DS, et al. Hyperthyroidism and other causes of thyrotoxicosis: management guidelines of the American Thyroid Association and the American Association of Clinical Endocrinologists. *Thyroid*. 2011;21:593–641.

Chapman EM. History of the discovery and early use of radioactive iodine. *JAMA*. 1983;250:2042–2044.

Haugen BR, Alexander EK, Bible KC, et al. American Thyroid Association management guidelines for adult patients with thyroid nodules and differentiated thyroid cancer. *Thyroid*. 2015;2016(26):1–133.

Lavely WC, Goetz S, Friedman KP, et al. Comparison of SPECT/CT, SPECT, and planar imaging with single-and dual-phase (99m) Tc-sestamibi parathyroid scintigraphy. *J Nucl Med*. 2007;48:1084–1089.

Nichols KJ, Tomas MB, Tronco GG, et al. Preoperative parathyroid scintigraphic lesion localization: accuracy of various types of readings. *Radiology*. 2008;248:221–232.

Shankar LK, Yamamoto AJ, Alavi A, Mandel SJ. Comparison of I-123 scintigraphy at 5 and 24 hours in patients with differentiated thyroid cancer. *J Nucl Med*. 2002;43:72–76.

Taillefer R, Boucher Y, Potvin C, Lambert R. Detection and localization of parathyroid adenomas in patients with hyperparathyroidism using a single radionuclide imaging procedure with technetium-99m sestamibi (double-phase study). *J Nucl Med*. 1992;33:1801–1807.

Van Nostrand D, Moreau S, Varalakshmi V, et al. 124I Positron emission tomography versus 131I planar imaging in the identification of residual thyroid tissue and/or metastasis in patients who have well-differentiated thyroid cancer. *Thyroid*. 2010;20:879–883.

Wong KK, Fig LM, Gross MD, Dwamena BA. Parathyroid adenoma localization with Tc-99m sestamibi SPECT/CT: a meta-analysis. *Nucl Med Commun*. 2015;36:363–375.

9

Hepatic, Biliary, and Splenic Scintigraphy

Liver, biliary, and splenic scintigraphy have played an important diagnostic imaging role in patient management since the 1960s. Today's radiopharmaceuticals have mechanisms of uptake and localization that take advantage of the complex anatomy and physiology of the liver (Table 9.1; Figs. 9.1 to 9.4). Although many of the radiopharmaceuticals, methodologies, and indications have changed, hepatobiliary and splenic scintigraphy continue to provide unique functional diagnostic information not available from anatomical imaging such as computed tomography (CT) or ultrasonography.

CHOLESCINTIGRAPHY

Cholescintigraphy is ordered by physicians and surgeons for the diagnosis of a variety of acute and chronic hepatobiliary diseases, including acute cholecystitis, biliary obstruction, biliary leak, and chronic acalculous gallbladder disease (Box 9.1).

Radiopharmaceuticals

Three Tc-99m-labeled hepatobiliary radiopharmaceuticals have been approved by the Food and Drug Administration (FDA) for clinical use (see Fig. 9.4). The first, Tc-99m dimethyl imino-diacetic acid (Lidofenin or hepatic iminodiacetic acid [HIDA]), is no longer used because of its poor uptake in patients with hepatic dysfunction. The term *HIDA* is now commonly used to describe all Tc-99m hepatobiliary radiopharmaceuticals. The two presently in clinical use in the United States are Tc-99m disofenin (Hepatolite) and Tc-99m mebrofenin (Choletec; Table 9.2).

For these hepatobiliary radiopharmaceuticals, Tc-99m serves as a bridging atom between two iminodiacetic acid (IDA) ligand molecules, both of which bind to a lidocaine analog that determines the radiopharmaceutical's biologic and pharmacokinetic properties (see Fig. 9.4). Minor structural changes in the phenyl ring (N substitutions) result in significant alterations in the pharmacokinetics of IDA radiopharmaceuticals (Table 9.3). Numerous Tc-99m HIDA analogs have been investigated; however, all had less uptake and slower clearance than the two currently approved radiopharmaceuticals (Fig. 9.5).

After intravenous injection, Tc-99m HIDA radiopharmaceuticals are tightly bound to protein in the blood, thus minimizing renal clearance. They are organic anions extracted and excreted by the liver in a manner similar to bilirubin and bile. Unlike bilirubin, Tc-99m HIDA radiopharmaceuticals are excreted in their original radiochemical form without conjugation or metabolism. Because Tc-99m HIDA travels the same pathway as bilirubin, it is subject to competitive inhibition by elevated serum bilirubin levels. The

radiotracer enters the gallbladder via the cystic duct and the second portion of the duodenum via the common bile duct (Fig. 9.6; see also Fig. 9.2). Distribution between the gallbladder and biliary ducts varies depending on the patency of the ducts, sphincter of Oddi tone, and intraluminal pressures. The gallbladder normally begins to fill before biliary-to-bowel transit.

Hepatic dysfunction results in altered HIDA pharmacokinetics—delayed uptake, secretion, and clearance (Figs. 9.7 and 9.8). Therefore, the normal time of gallbladder filling and biliary-to-bowel clearance may be delayed. The kidneys serve as the alternative route of excretion. Although only a small percentage of the dose is normally cleared by this path, urinary excretion increases with hepatic dysfunction. Because of high radiopharmaceutical extraction efficiency, diagnostic images can be obtained in patients with bilirubin levels of 20 to 30 mg/dL, although image quality lessens. Mebrofenin has greater hepatic extraction and resistance to displacement by bilirubin than disofenin does; thus, it is preferred in patients with poor liver function. Radiation dosimetry is detailed in the Appendix.

Patient Preparation

Patients must ingest nothing by mouth for 3 to 4 hours before the study because food stimulates the endogenous release of

TABLE 9.1 Liver and Spleen Radiopharmaceuticals, Mechanisms, and Clinical Indications

Radiopharmaceutical	Mechanism of Uptake	Indication
Tc-99m mebrofenin, disofenin	Hepatocyte	Cholescintigraphy
Tc-99m red blood cells	Blood-pool distribution	Hemangioma, splenosis
Tc-99m sulfur colloid	Kupffer cell	Focal nodular hyperplasia, splenosis, liver function
Tc-99m MAA	Blood flow, capillary occlusion	Hepatic arterial perfusion
Y-90 microspheres	Blood flow, capillary occlusion	Hepatic arterial tumor therapy
F-18 FDG	Glucose metabolism	Tumor/infection imaging
Gallium-67 citrate	Iron binding	Tumor/infection imaging

FDG, Fluorodeoxyglucose; *MAA,* macroaggregated albumin.

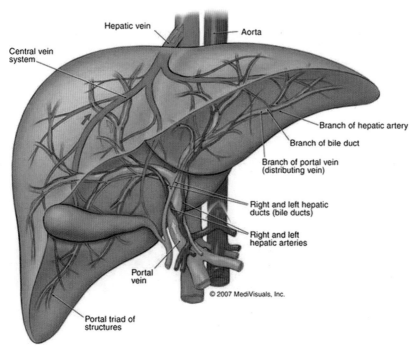

Fig. 9.1 Anatomy of the liver. Diagram of the internal anatomy of the liver, its biliary ducts, and arterial and venous vascularity.

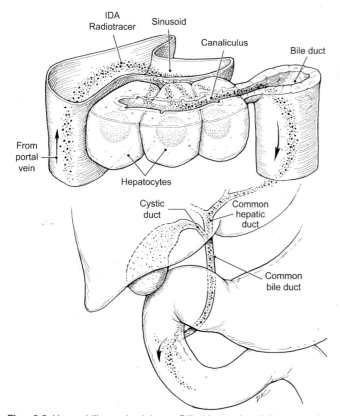

Fig. 9.2 Hepatobiliary physiology. Bilirubin, a breakdown product of hemoglobin, is extracted by hepatocytes in the liver, conjugated, secreted into the bile canaliculi, and cleared through the biliary tract into the bowel. Hepatic uptake and clearance of Tc-99m hepatic imino-diacetic acid (HIDA) radiopharmaceuticals is similar to that of bilirubin except that they are not conjugated or metabolized.

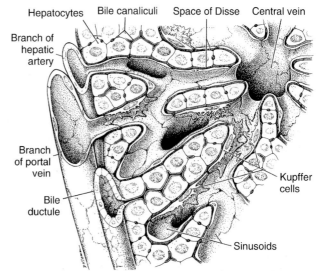

Fig. 9.3 Anatomy of a liver lobule. Plates of hepatocytes and Kupffer cells are distributed radially around the central vein. Branches of the portal vein and hepatic artery located at the periphery of the lobule deliver blood to the sinusoids. Blood leaves through the central vein (proximal branch of hepatic veins). Peripherally located bile ducts drain bile canaliculi that course between hepatocytes.

cholecystokinin (CCK) from the proximal small bowel, resulting in gallbladder contraction and thus potentially preventing radiotracer entry. On the other hand, if the patient has been fasting for > 24 hours, the gallbladder has no stimulus to contract and thus will likely contain viscous bile, which can also prevent radiotracer entry. In this situation, the patient should be administered sincalide (Kinevac, CCK) before the clinical study to empty the gallbladder. Tc-99m HIDA should be administered at least 30 minutes after the completion of sincalide infusion to allow sufficient time for gallbladder relaxation. All opiate drugs should be withheld for at least 6 hours or three half-lives before radiopharmaceutical injection. Opiates contract the sphincter of Oddi, potentially producing a picture of functional partial biliary obstruction, indistinguishable from a true obstruction.

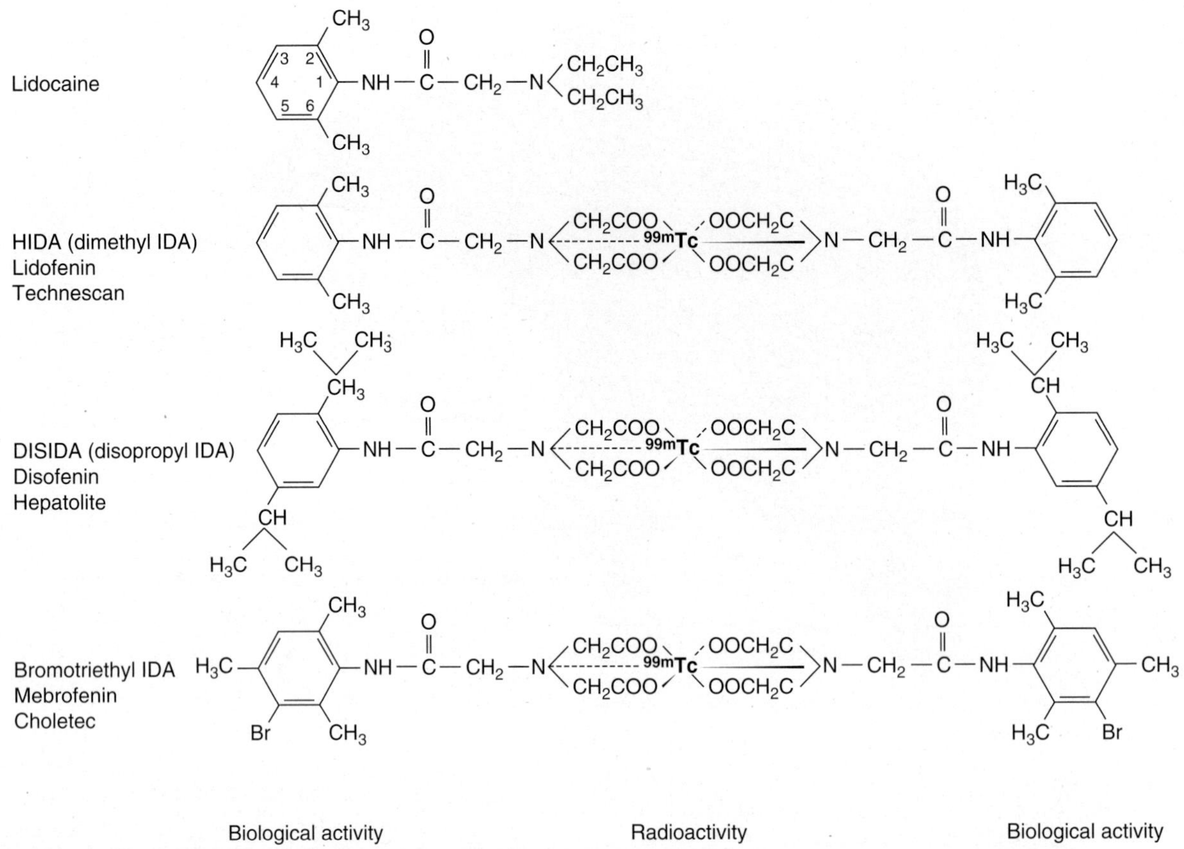

Fig. 9.4 Chemical structure of Tc-99m hepatic iminodiacetic acid (HIDA) radiopharmaceuticals. All are analogs of lidocaine *(top)*. Tc-99m is located centrally, bridging two ligand molecules of iminodiacetate (NCH₂COO; IDA), which bind to the lidocaine acetanilide analog. Substitutions on aromatic rings differentiate the various Tc-99m HIDAs and determine their pharmacokinetics. Tc-99m disofenin and mebrofenin are in clinical use.

BOX 9.1 Cholescintigraphy: Clinical Indications

Acute cholecystitis
Acute acalculous cholecystitis
Chronic cholecystitis
Chronic acalculous gallbladder disease
Biliary obstruction
Biliary atresia
Sphincter of Oddi dysfunction
Biliary leak
Biliary diversion assessment
Biliary stent function
Focal nodular hyperplasia
Enterogastric bile reflux

TABLE 9.2 Tc-99m Hepatobiliary Radiopharmaceuticals—Chemical, FDA, and Commercial Names

Chemical Name	FDA Name	Commercial Name
Tc-99m diisopropyl IDA (DISIDA)	Disofenin	Hepatolite
Tc-99m bromotriethyl IDA	Mebrofenin	Choletec

FDA, U.S. Food and Drug Administration. *IDA,* iminodiacetic acid.

TABLE 9.3 Uptake and Clearance of FDA-Approved Tc-99m Hepatic Iminodiacetic Acid (HIDA) Radiopharmaceuticals

Radiopharmaceutical	Hepatic Uptake (%)	Biliary Clearance Half-Time (min)	2-hr Renal Excretion
Tc-99m disofenin (Hepatolite)	88	19	<9%
Tc-99m mebrofenin (Choletec)	98	17	<1%

Pertinent patient history before starting the study includes the following: What is the clinical question being asked by the referring physician? Are the symptoms acute or chronic? Has sonography or other imaging been performed, and what were the results? Has the patient had biliary surgery? If the patient had a biliary diversion procedure, what is the anatomy? Are there intraabdominal tubes or drains? If so, where are they placed, and which tubing drains each? Should the drains be open or clamped to answer the clinical question? Did the patient's most recent meal contain sufficient fat (10 g) to contract the gallbladder?

Methodology

A protocol for cholescintigraphy is detailed (Box 9.2). Acquisition of 1-minute frames for 60 minutes is standard. An

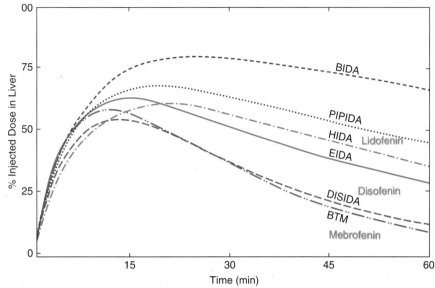

Fig. 9.5 Pharmacokinetics of many hepatobiliary radiopharmaceuticals that were investigated in the 1970s and 1980s (Tc-99m BIDA, PIPIDA, EIDA, etc.). Tc-99m Lidofenin (HIDA) was the first agent approved by the Food and Drug Administration (FDA) but was later withdrawn. Tc-99m disofenin (DISIDA) and Tc-99m mebrofenin (BTM) showed superior uptake and rapid clearance. They were subsequently FDA approved. (Adapted from Krishnamurthy GT. *Nuclear hepatology.* New York: Springer; 2000.)

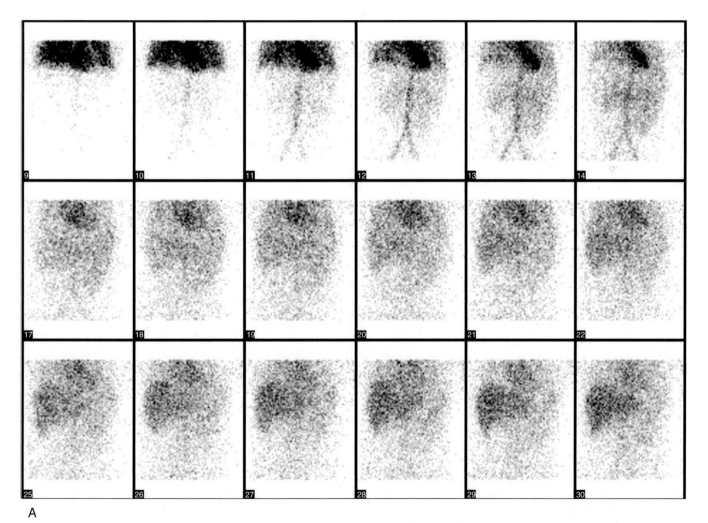

A

Fig. 9.6 Normal Tc-99m hepatic iminodiacetic acid (HIDA) study. (A) Normal blood flow to the liver (2-second frames). First visualized are the left ventricle and aorta. As the radiotracer transits, the kidneys are seen. The spleen is not well seen in the left upper quadrant (LUQ), being a posterior structure. The liver is perfused after the kidneys because the majority of its blood flow is from the portal vein.

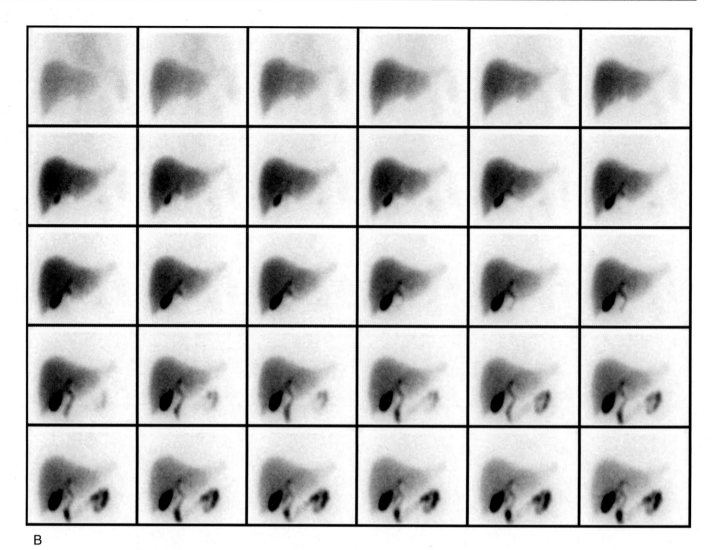

B

Fig. 9.6, cont'd (B) Normal Tc-99m HIDA 60-minute study (1-minute frames). Good hepatic uptake. Blood pool clears by 7 minutes, consistent with good hepatic function. Gallbladder fills early, then bile duct visualization and biliary-to-bowel transit.

initial 60-second flow study is optional (1–3 seconds/frame) but can occasionally add useful information. At 60 minutes, right lateral and left anterior oblique views should be performed to confirm or exclude gallbladder filling, which at times may be uncertain due to bile in the biliary ducts and duodenum overlapping the gallbladder fossa. Delayed imaging, morphine sulfate, and CCK are options for specific clinical indications.

Cholescintigraphic Diagnostic Patterns
Blood Flow
During the arterial flow phase, the spleen and kidneys are first seen (see Fig. 9.6). The liver appears during the venous phase because of its predominantly portal blood flow (75% portal vein, 25% hepatic artery). Early hepatic flow may be seen with arterialization of the liver's blood supply (e.g., in cirrhosis or generalized tumor involvement; see Fig. 9.7). With severe acute cholecystitis, there may be increased flow to the gallbladder fossa (Fig. 9.9). Focal increased flow may also be seen with intrahepatic abscess, malignant mass, and focal nodular hyperplasia.

Hepatic Uptake and Function
Liver function is best judged by noting how rapidly the cardiac blood pool clears. With good hepatic function, it clears within 5 to 10 minutes (see Fig. 9.6). With hepatic dysfunction, there is delayed clearance (see Figs. 9.7 and 9.8). During the early hepatic uptake phase, liver size can be approximated and intrahepatic lesions noted. Most intrahepatic masses will have decreased uptake compared with adjacent liver, except for focal nodular hyperplasia.

Gallbladder Filling
The normal gallbladder begins to fill by 10 minutes and is usually well seen by 30 to 40 minutes (see Fig. 9.6). Visualization beyond 60 minutes is considered delayed (Fig. 9.10). Right lateral and left anterior oblique views can help confirm or exclude gallbladder filling (Fig. 9.11). In the right lateral projection, the gallbladder is anterior and to the viewer's right. In the left anterior oblique view, the gallbladder, an anterior structure, moves toward the patient's right; the common duct and duodenum, more posterior structures, move to the patient's left. Upright imaging and ingestion of water can be used to clear duodenal activity when needed.

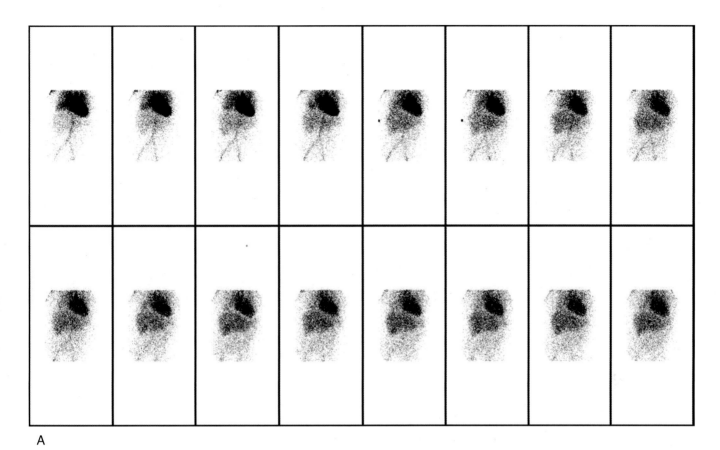

A

Fig. 9.7 (A to C) Hepatic dysfunction. Patient was referred with elevated bilirubin and abdominal discomfort, to rule out biliary obstruction. (A) Tc-99m hepatic iminodiacetic acid (HIDA) flow study (2-second frames). Blood flow to the liver is arterialized and early. The liver visualizes immediately after aorta flow.

Biliary Clearance

Duct size is not well assessed with cholescintigraphy. The smaller peripheral biliary ducts are seen. The larger left and right hepatic bile ducts, common hepatic duct, and common bile duct are typically seen. Prominent ducts do not necessarily signify obstruction. The left hepatic ducts sometimes appear more prominent than the right because of the anterior position of the left lobe and close proximity to the gamma camera. The strength of scintigraphy is to confirm or exclude duct patency, not to diagnose dilatation. The common bile duct is normally seen by 20 minutes. By 60 minutes, ductal activity decreases by > 50% of peak activity, and clearance into the small bowel is seen.

Pharmacological Interventions Before or During Cholescintigraphy
Morphine Sulfate

Morphine sulfate (MS) can be used as an alternative to 3- to 4-hour delayed imaging in patients with nonfilling of the gallbladder referred for suspected acute cholecystitis. If the gallbladder has not visualized by 60 minutes, low-dose morphine (0.04 mg/kg) is infused intravenously, producing contraction of the sphincter of Oddi, thus increasing intrabiliary pressure, resulting in preferential filling of the gallbladder, if the cystic duct is patent (Fig. 9.12). The answer to filling or nonfilling of

the gallbladder is known by 30 minutes. Some clinics give morphine at 30 minutes if bowel activity is seen. Be aware that morphine may inhibit the effect of subsequently administered cholecystokinin.

Cholecystokinin

CCK is a polypeptide hormone released by mucosal cells in the proximal small bowel in response to ingested fat and protein. The terminal octapeptide of CCK is the physiologically active portion of the hormone (Fig. 9.13). Binding of CCK with receptors in the gallbladder wall and sphincter of Oddi results in gallbladder contraction and sphincter relaxation. Bile is then discharged into the small intestines, where it facilitates intestinal fat absorption. Sincalide (Kinevac), an analog of the terminal octapeptide of CCK, is the commercial form of CCK. In patients who have not eaten within 24 hours, it should be administered before the study to empty the gallbladder. Tc-99m HIDA should not be injected until at least 30 minutes after the conclusion of sincalide infusion, to allow time for gallbladder relaxation so that the radiotracer can enter.

Imaging Gallbladder Contraction

Fatty meals and CCK have been used to evaluate gallbladder contraction. An underlying assumption is that gastric emptying is normal. Delayed gastric emptying results in delayed

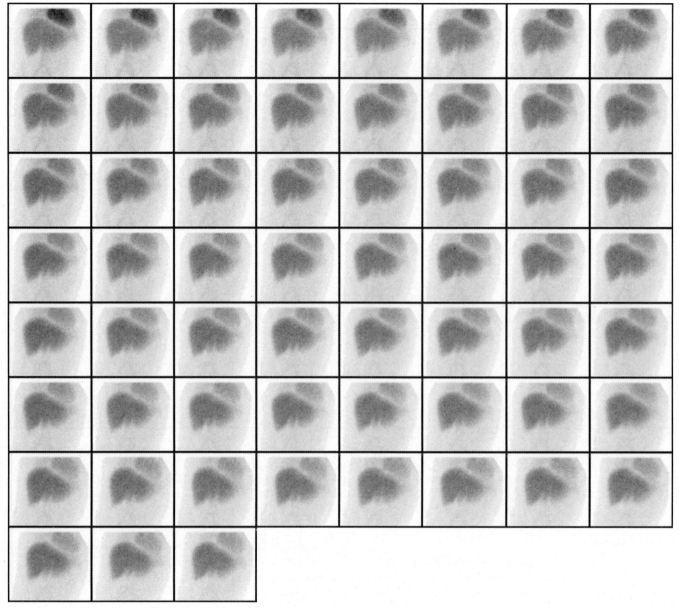

B

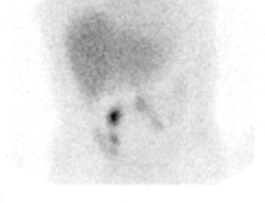

ANT DELAY
11:04:06.0

C

Fig. 9.7, cont'd (B) Very slow background and blood-pool clearance seen as prominent retained activity within the heart. This illustrates severe hepatic dysfunction. Obstruction has not been ruled out because biliary clearance and transit to the bowel has not occurred. (C) Delayed image at 4 hours. Background has further cleared, and there is now evidence of transit into the bowel without retention in biliary ducts. This rules out biliary obstruction. Acute cholecystitis has not been excluded. Further imaging up to 24 hours may be desirable (see Fig 9.8). The final diagnosis was cirrhosis.

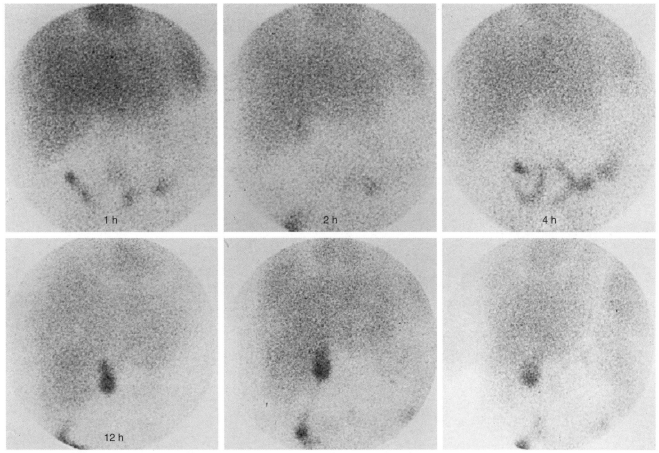

Fig. 9.8 Severe hepatic dysfunction with delayed gallbladder visualization. Slow blood-pool clearance and poor liver-to-background ratio. Gallbladder is not visualized until 12 hours. Last two images are right and left anterior oblique views, respectively.

BOX 9.2 Cholescintigraphy: Protocol Summary

Patient Preparation

Nothing by mouth for 4 hours before the study.

If the patient is fasting for >24 hours, infuse sincalide 0.02 μg/kg over 60 minutes. Wait at least 30 minutes after sincalide infusion is complete before infusing the radiopharmaceutical.

Hold all opiate drugs for at least 6 hours.

Radiopharmaceutical

Tc-99m Mebrofenin—Intravenous Injection

	Bilirubin	Dose
Adults		
	<2 mg/dL	5.0 mCi (185 MBq)
	2–10 mg/dL	7.5 mCi (278 MBq)
	>10 mg/dL	10.0 mCi (370 MBq)
Children		
	0.05 mCi/kg (1.85 MBq/kg)	Minimum dose 0.5 mCi (18.5 MBq)

Instrumentation

Camera: Large-field-of-view gamma camera
Collimator: Low-energy parallel hole—high resolution
Window: 15% to 20% over 140-keV photopeak

Patient Positioning

Supine; field of view should include upper abdomen.

Computer Setup

1-second frames × 60 for flow study, then 1-minute frames × 59

Imaging Protocol

1. Start computer, then inject Tc-99m mebrofenin intravenously.
2. At 60 minutes, acquire right lateral and left anterior oblique images.
3. If acute cholecystitis is suspected and the gallbladder has not filled, inject morphine sulfate (or) obtain delayed images up to 3 to 4 hours.
   A. If liver activity has washed out, reinject half-dose Tc-99m mebrofenin before morphine infusion.
   B. Morphine infusion: If good biliary duct clearance and biliary-to-bowel transit, inject intravenously 0.04 mg/kg over 1 minute. Acquire 1-minute frames for 30 minutes.
   C. As alternative to morphine for poor biliary duct clearance (<50%) and poor biliary-to-bowel transit, obtain delayed images at 2 and 4 hours.
4. If suspected partial biliary obstruction (delayed biliary duct clearance and biliary-to-bowel transit) at 60 minutes, administer sincalide over 60 minutes or obtain delayed 2- and 4-hour images.
5. Delayed imaging is also indicated in the setting of hepatic insufficiency or suspected slow leak.

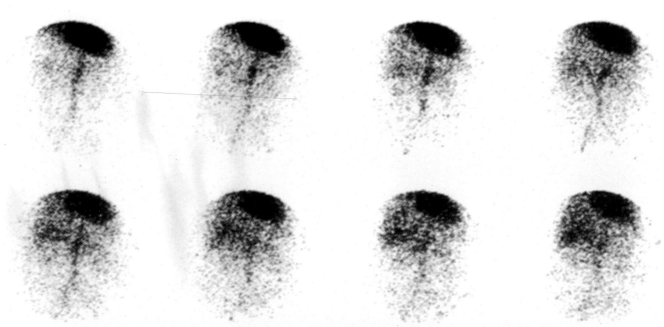

Fig. 9.9 Increased flow to the gallbladder fossa in a patient with acute cholecystitis. Increased focal flow to the region of the gallbladder fossa is seen beginning with the first several images. This is seen with severe inflammation of the gallbladder and adjacent liver with acute cholecystitis.

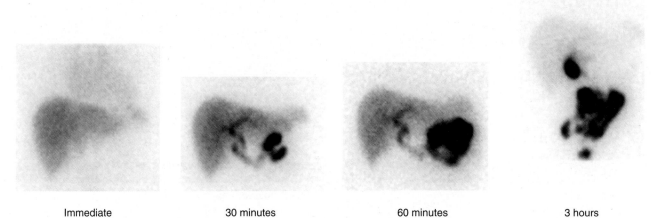

| Immediate | 30 minutes | 60 minutes | 3 hours |

Fig. 9.10 Delayed gallbladder visualization in a 50-year-old female with episodic abdominal pain. Immediate, 30-, and 60-minute images show good hepatic uptake and biliary-to-bowel clearance but no gallbladder visualization. Delayed image at 3 hours shows gallbladder filling. Delayed filling of the gallbladder rules out acute cholecystitis and is often seen with chronic cholecystitis.

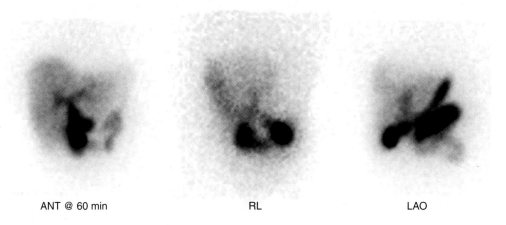

| ANT @ 60 min | RL | LAO |

Fig. 9.11 Overlapping duodenal and biliary activity in gallbladder fossa. On the anterior (ANT) 60-minute image, gallbladder filling is uncertain due to overlap. Right lateral (RL) and left anterior oblique (LAO) views confirm that the gallbladder has filled. In the RL, the gallbladder is anterior, and in the LAO view, it has moved to the left.

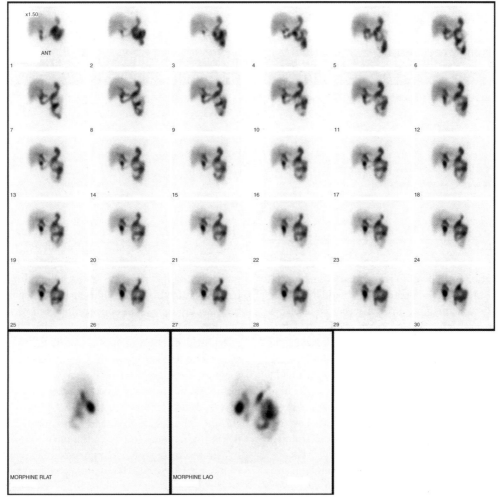

Fig. 9.12 Morphine-augmented cholescintigraphy. *(Above)* The gallbladder was not seen during the initial 60 minutes of the study (not shown). Bowel clearance was seen, and then morphine was administered intravenously. Over 30 minutes, the gallbladder visualizes, confirmed by right lateral (RL) and left anterior oblique (LAO) views, ruling out acute cholecystitis. *ANT,* Anterior.

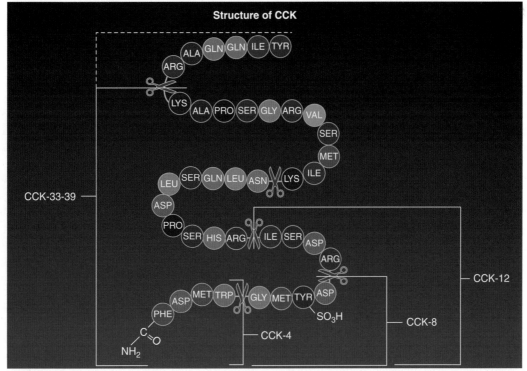

Fig. 9.13 Cholecystokinin (CCK) is a 33- to 39-polypeptide hormone endogenously released from the proximal small bowel in response to ingested fat. The terminal octapeptide is the physiologically active portion of the hormone (CCK-8), which binds to receptors in the gallbladder and sphincter of Oddi to produce gallbladder contraction and sphincter relaxation.

BOX 9.3   Clinical Indications for Sincalide Infusion

Before Tc-99m Hepatic Iminodiacetic Acid (HIDA) Examination
To empty gallbladder in patient fasting longer than 24 hours
To diagnose sphincter of Oddi dysfunction (see Box 9.15)

After Initial 60-Minute Tc-99m HIDA Examination
Differentiate common duct obstruction from functional causes.
Exclude acute acalculous cholecystitis if gallbladder fills (rule out a false-negative study).
Diagnose chronic acalculous gallbladder disease.

BOX 9.4   Acute Cholecystitis: Sequential Pathophysiology

1. Cystic duct obstruction
2. Venous and lymphatic outflow obstruction
3. Mucosal edema and congestion
4. Neutrophilic leukocyte infiltration
5. Hemorrhage and necrosis
6. Gangrene, abscess
7. Perforation

---

endogenous stimulation of CCK from the proximal small bowel and thus potentially delayed and reduced gallbladder contraction during the standard imaging time. Alternative cholecystogogues have been used and normal values established (e.g., whole milk, EnsurePlus, and corn oil emulsion). However, sincalide is preferable because it has been best standardized and gastric emptying is not an issue. Other uses for sincalide include the calculation of a gallbladder ejection fraction (GBEF) in patients to diagnose chronic acalculous gallbladder disease, diagnose acute acalculous cholecystitis, and differentiate biliary obstruction from functional delayed biliary clearance into the small bowel (Box 9.3).

The use of sincalide to empty the gallbladder in a fasting patient can result in delayed biliary-to-bowel transit. Because of its short half-life in serum, CCK can be infused a second time during a patient study (e.g., before the study in a patient who has been fasting > 24 hours and after the initial 60-minute study to calculate a GBEF). The sincalide infusion methodology should be identical for all indications, 0.02 µg/kg infused over 60 minutes.

Common Clinical Applications

Acute Cholecystitis

The most frequent indication for cholescintigraphy is to confirm or exclude the diagnosis of acute cholecystitis. Patients present with colicky right upper quadrant abdominal pain, nausea, and vomiting. Physical examination often detects right upper quadrant tenderness. Laboratory studies show leukocytosis. Liver function tests are usually normal. A confirmatory imaging study is required for the diagnosis before surgery. The cause is usually due to obstruction of the cystic duct secondary to cholelithiasis. Soon after obstruction, a series of sequential histopathological inflammatory changes occurs—first, venous and lymphatic obstruction, followed by edema of the gallbladder mucosa, then white blood cell infiltration, and, ultimately, hemorrhage, ulceration, necrosis, and if left untreated, gangrene, abscess, and perforation (Box 9.4).

Imaging for Acute Cholecystitis

Ultrasonography. Most patients with acute cholecystitis have gallstones noted on sonography; however, the presence of stones is not specific for acute cholecystitis. Asymptomatic gallstones are common and may be unrelated to the cause of the abdominal pain. Other sonographic findings seen with acute cholecystitis are also nonspecific. Thickening of the gallbladder wall and peri-cholecystic fluid occur with various acute and chronic diseases. A more specific indicator of acute inflammation is intramural lucency. The sonographic Murphy sign (localized tenderness in the region of the gallbladder) is reported to have high accuracy in experienced hands; however, this finding is operator dependent and not always reliable. The combination of gallstones, intramural lucency, and the sonographic Murphy sign makes the diagnosis of acute cholecystitis likely. However, many patients with acute cholecystitis do not have all of these findings, and the diagnosis is less certain. Ultrasonography may reveal other factors causing the patient's symptoms (e.g., common duct dilation due to biliary obstruction, pancreatic or liver tumors, renal stones, pulmonary consolidation).

Cholescintigraphy. A major advantage of HIDA scintigraphy is that it demonstrates the pathophysiology of acute cholecystitis (i.e., nonfilling of the gallbladder secondary to cystic duct obstruction). No filling by 60 minutes after Tc-99m HIDA injection is abnormal; however, it is not, by itself, diagnostic of acute cholecystitis. However, no filling on further delayed imaging at 3 to 4 hours or 30 minutes after morphine infusion is diagnostic of acute cholecystitis. Delayed filling of the gallbladder (i.e., after 60 minutes) rules out acute cholecystitis. Common reasons for delayed gallbladder filling are chronic cholecystitis and hepatic dysfunction (see Figs. 9.7–9.9).

Cholescintigraphy has high accuracy for the diagnosis of acute cholecystitis (Table 9.4). The sensitivity (nonfilling of the gallbladder in those with the disease) is 95% to 98%, and the specificity (filling of the gallbladder in patients who do not have the disease) is > 90%. Studies that have directly compared cholescintigraphy with ultrasonography have found cholescintigraphy superior for this diagnosis (see Table 9.4). However, in spite of its high specificity, false-positive studies may occur. These can be minimized by anticipating the potential situations where it can happen (Box 9.5) and using state-of-the-art methodology. Ensuring that patients have fasted for 3 to 4 hours before the study is critical. Those fasting > 24 hours or receiving hyperalimentation likely have a gallbladder full of viscous bile and should be administered sincalide before the study to empty the gallbladder. In these cases, false positives may still occur because of a poorly contracting gallbladder in response to CCK due to chronic cholecystitis. Patients with poor hepatic function have delayed uptake and clearance of the radiotracer and often delayed gallbladder filling. In these patients, delayed imaging for up to 24 hours may be necessary to confirm or exclude gallbladder filling; false positives may still occasionally occur.

TABLE 9.4 Accuracy for Diagnosis of Acute Cholecystitis: Cholescintigraphy and Ultrasonography

Study First Author, Date	Patients	SENSITIVITY/SPECIFICITY (%) Cholescintigraphy	Ultrasonography
Stadalnik, 1978	120	100/100	70/93
Weissmann, 1979	90	98/100	
Freitas, 1980	186	97/87	
Suarez, 1980	62	98/100	
Szalabick, 1980	271	100/98	
Weissmann, 1981	296	95/99	
Zeman, 1981	200	98/82	67/82
Worthen, 1981	113	95/100	67/100
Mauro, 1982	95	100/94	
Rails, 1982	59	86/84	86/90
Freitas 1982	195	98/90	60/81
Samuels, 1983	194	97/93	97/64
Chatziioannov, 2000	92	92/89	40/89
Overall	1988	97/94	77/84

BOX 9.5 Causes of False-Positive Cholescintigraphy for Acute Cholecystitis

Fasting <4 hours before hepatic iminodiacetic acid (HIDA) study
Fasting >24 hours before HIDA study
Parenteral alimentation
Concurrent severe illness
Chronic cholecystitis
Hepatic dysfunction

Patients with chronic cholecystitis may have false-positive findings for acute cholecystitis (nonfilling of the gallbladder) caused by a fibrotic obstruction of the cystic duct or a functional obstruction caused by a gallbladder filled with viscous bile. Even if a patient has received sincalide before the study, a diseased gallbladder, whether acute or chronic, may not contract. Very ill hospitalized patients with a concurrent serious illness may also have false-positive scintigraphic results for acute cholecystitis. The reason for this is uncertain.

False-negative results (gallbladder filling in a patient with acute cholecystitis) are rare. One important cause to be avoided is misinterpretation of the *cystic duct sign,* specifically cystic duct dilation proximal to its obstruction, which might be misinterpreted as a gallbladder. The focal activity is typically smaller than a gallbladder and in a more medial position (Fig. 9.14).

If the gallbladder does not fill by 1 hour, either delayed imaging for up to 4 hours or morphine administration is indicated to confirm or exclude gallbladder filling. The accuracy of morphine is similar to the delayed imaging method (Table 9.5) and is preferred whenever possible because it confirms or excludes the diagnosis by 30 minutes after administration. Morphine produces a functional partial common duct obstruction that cannot be differentiated by scintigraphy from a pathological partial common duct obstruction caused by stone or stricture. Thus, morphine should not be administered if scintigraphic findings show delayed clearance from the common duct and delayed transit into the small bowel. Delayed imaging is indicated for these patients. With cystic duct patency, the gallbladder begins to fill within 5 to 10 minutes after morphine infusion and is complete by 20 to 30 minutes. If no gallbladder filling is seen by the end of the 30-minute infusion, acute cholecystitis is confirmed.

Ancillary Scintigraphic Findings of Acute Cholecystitis. Increased blood flow to the gallbladder fossa secondary to severe inflammation is seen in some patients (see Fig. 9.9). Increased hepatic uptake of HIDA tracer adjacent to the gallbladder fossa in patients with acute cholecystitis is called the *rim sign* (Fig. 9.15) and is seen in approximately 25% of patients with acute cholecystitis. The rim sign is more common than increased flow to the gallbladder fossa. Sometimes they occur together. The rim sign can usually be seen throughout the duration of the study but is best seen as the radiotracer clears from the uninvolved liver. It is caused by inflammation of the liver adjacent to the gallbladder fossa. With severe acute cholecystitis, inflammation may spread to the adjacent normal liver, which can result in increased blood flow to that region, increased radiotracer delivery, and thus increased Tc-99m HIDA hepatic extraction.

The importance of the rim sign is twofold. First, it is a very specific scintigraphic finding of acute cholecystitis. It increases interpretive confidence that nonfilling of the gallbladder is caused by acute cholecystitis (true positive) in a patient at increased risk for a false-positive study (see Box 9.5), for example, a sick hospitalized patient with concurrent serious illness. Second, the rim sign identifies patients with acute cholecystitis who have more severe disease and are at increased risk for complications (e.g., gangrene and perforation). Even without these complications, patients with the rim sign tend to be sicker and at a later stage of the pathophysiological spectrum of disease, with hemorrhage and necrosis rather than edema and leukocyte infiltration (see Box 9.4).

Acute Acalculous Cholecystitis. The acalculous form of acute cholecystitis is not common; however, it can be life-threatening. It occurs in seriously ill hospitalized patients, often those in the intensive care unit (ICU; Box 9.6). Because of its high mortality (30%) and morbidity (55%), early diagnosis is imperative; however, because of concomitant serious illness, diagnosis is often delayed. In the majority of patients, acute acalculous cholecystitis is initiated by cystic duct obstruction but not by cholelithiasis, rather, by inflammatory debris, inspissated bile, and local edema, aggravated by dehydration. To complicate the diagnosis further, some of these patients do not have cystic duct obstruction but, rather, direct inflammation of the gallbladder wall caused by systemic infection, ischemia, or toxemia. This results in a lower diagnostic sensitivity for HIDA imaging.

The sensitivity of cholescintigraphy for diagnosis of acute acalculous cholescintigraphy is approximately 80%, compared with 95% to 98% for acute calculous cholecystitis (Table 9.6). The lower sensitivity is at least partially due to the fact that some of these patients do not have cystic duct obstruction. If a false-negative study result (filling of the gallbladder in acute acalculous cholecystitis) is suspected in a patient with a high

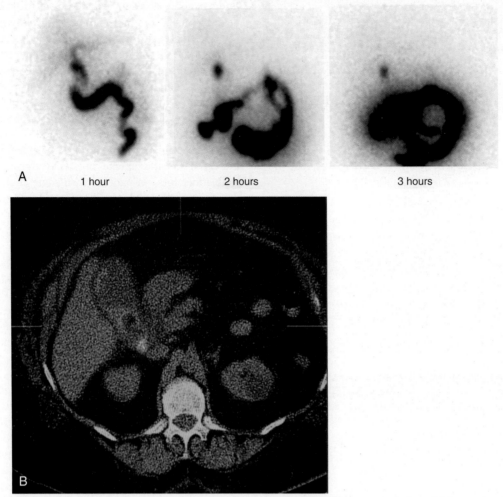

Fig. 9.14 Cystic duct sign. (A) Tc-99m hepatic iminodiacetic acid (HIDA) images at 1, 2, and 3 hours show focal accumulation of activity medial to the usual position of the gallbladder, which remains mostly unchanged over this time. (B) Single-photon emission computed tomography with computed tomography (SPECT/CT; 10-minute acquisition time) fused transverse images show that the focal activity is in the cystic duct, obstructed by a hypodense stone immediately proximal to it.

TABLE 9.5   Accuracy of Morphine-Augmented Cholescintigraphy

Study Author, Date	Patients	Sensitivity (%)	Specificity (%)
Choy, 1984	59	96	100
Keslar, 1987	31	100	83
Vasquez, 1987	40	100	85
Fig, 1990	51	94	69[a]
Flancbaum, 1994	75	99	91
Fink-Bennett, 1991	51	95	99
Kistler, 1991	32	93	78[a]
Overall	339	96	86

[a]High percentage of patients with concurrent illness and chronic cholecystitis.

clinical suspicion, sincalide infusion with a gallbladder ejection fraction can be helpful. An acutely inflamed gallbladder does not contract normally. Good contraction excludes the diagnosis of cholecystitis. Poor contraction is consistent with cholecystitis but not necessarily acute cholecystitis. It could be caused by chronic cholecystitis, medications that inhibit contraction, or concomitant acute or chronic illness (Boxes 9.7 and 9.8). In uncertain cases, a radiolabeled leukocyte study could confirm the diagnosis. Although it is urgent for these sick patients to have gallbladder surgery, the increased risk of surgery may call for more certainty and a willingness to wait for the leukocyte study. Indium-111 (In-111) leukocytes are preferable because they have no intraabdominal clearance. Tc-99m-labeled leukocytes are cleared through the biliary and urinary system. However, early-same-day Tc-99m HMPAO leukocyte imaging at 1 to 2 hours, before biliary clearance occurs, may avoid this problem. Although the standard imaging time for In-111 leukocytes is at 24 hours, imaging at 4 hours may be diagnostic if gallbladder uptake is seen.

Chronic Cholecystitis

Recurrent episodes of right upper quadrant pain, usually in a middle-aged female, although occasionally in men and children, are suggestive of chronic cholecystitis. The clinical diagnosis is often confirmed by detection of gallstones on sonography. The standard therapy is cholecystectomy; gallbladder histopathology

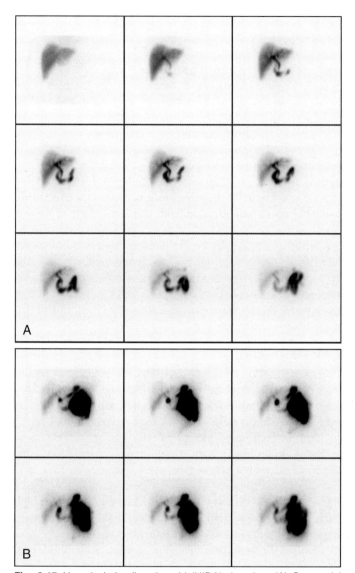

A

B

Fig. 9.15 Hepatic iminodiacetic acid (HIDA) rim sign. (A) Sequential anterior images over 60 minutes show no gallbladder filling but good biliary-to-bowel transit. Increased activity is seen in a curvilinear pattern along the inferior right hepatic lobe (rim sign), which persists from the beginning of the study through 60 minutes. (B) Sequential images for 30 minutes after morphine injection show no gallbladder filling but persistence of the rim sign. Surgery confirmed severe acute cholecystitis.

BOX 9.6 Clinical Settings Associated With Acute Acalculous Cholecystitis

Postoperative
Multiple trauma
Extensive burns
Shock
Acquired immunodeficiency syndrome
Mechanical ventilation
Multiple transfusions
Vasculitis

TABLE 9.6 Acute Acalculous Cholecystitis: Accuracy of Cholescintigraphy

Study Author, Date	Patients	Sensitivity (%)	Specificity (%)
Shuman, 1984	19	68	
Weissmann, 1983	15	93	
Mirvis, 1986	19	90	61
Swayne, 1986	49	93	
Ramanna, 1984	11	100	
Flancbaum, 1995	16	75	100
Prevot, 1999	14	64	100
Mariat, 2000	12	67	100
Overall	155	81	90

BOX 9.7 Drugs Known to Inhibit Gallbladder Contraction

Opiates
Atropine
Nifedipine (calcium channel blocking agents)
Indomethacin
Progesterone
Oral contraceptives
Octreotide
Theophylline
Isoproterenol
Benzodiazepine
Phentolamine (alpha-adrenergic blocking agent)
Nicotine
Alcohol

BOX 9.8 Diseases or Conditions Associated With Poor Gallbladder Contraction

Diabetes mellitus
Sickle cell disease
Irritable bowel syndrome
Truncal vagotomy
Pancreatic insufficiency
Crohn disease
Celiac disease
Achalasia
Dyspeptic syndrome
Obesity
Cirrhosis
Pregnancy

shows evidence of chronic inflammation. On occasion, a clinician suspecting that a patient's pain is not due to cholecystitis and that the gallstones seen are incidental may refer the patient for cholescintigraphy and a GBEF. Although chronic cholecystitis classically shows delayed filling after 60 minutes, some cases will show normal gallbladder filling. When CCK is administered after gallbladder filling, patients with asymptomatic cholelithiasis will have normal gallbladder contraction, whereas patients with chronic cholecystitis have a poor gallbladder response.

Chronic Acalculous Gallbladder Disease. The acalculous form of chronic cholecystitis occurs in approximately 10% of patients with symptomatic chronic gallbladder disease. It is clinically and histopathologically indistinguishable from chronic

BOX 9.9   Synonyms for Recurrent Pain Syndromes of Biliary Origin

Chronic Acalculous Gallbladder Disease
Chronic acalculous cholecystitis
Gallbladder dyskinesia
Gallbladder spasm
Cystic duct syndrome
Functional gallbladder disease

Sphincter of Oddi Dysfunction
Papillary stenosis
Biliary dyskinesia
Biliary spasm

calculous cholecystitis, except that there are no gallstones. This entity has been called by various names in the literature and by referring physicians, including gallbladder dyskinesia, gallbladder spasm, cystic duct syndrome, and functional gallbladder disease (Box 9.9). Patients present with recurrent right upper quadrant biliary colic, have poor gallbladder contraction, and are usually cured with cholecystectomy.

Many investigations have found that sincalide cholescintigraphy can confirm the suspected clinical diagnosis of chronic acalculous gallbladder disease. A poor GBEF predicts postcholecystectomy symptomatic relief and histopathological evidence of chronic gallbladder inflammation; a normal GBEF excludes the disease (Fig. 9.16). Publications report that a low GBEF has a positive predictive value of > 90%. However, most published studies were retrospective. There is only one small (21 patients) randomized prospective study. In that study, 92% were cured with surgery. Some gastroenterologists have stated that a larger, multicenter, well-controlled randomized prospective study is needed to confirm the utility of sincalide cholescintigraphy. Meanwhile, the GBEF study is commonly ordered by clinicians and surgeons in the United States, although less commonly outside the United States.

Sincalide cholescintigraphy should be performed on an outpatient basis after a clinical evaluation has excluded other diseases. It is best performed as an outpatient because acute illnesses and numerous therapeutic drugs can adversely affect gallbladder contraction and result in a false-positive study (see Boxes 9.7 and 9.8). If a clinician insists that a GBEF be performed on an inpatient, a normal study excludes gallbladder disease. However, a positive study (low GBEF) should be repeated as an outpatient when the patient is asymptomatic to confirm the disease.

Sincalide Infusion Methodology. The methodology used for sincalide infusion has varied in regard to the dose administered, infusion length, and normal values. A 3-minute infusion of 0.02 μg/kg was commonly used in the past. However, investigations have found that this results in a wide range of response in normal subjects and many false-positive studies (i.e., normal GBEFs in the same subjects when sincalide was infused for 30 or 60 minutes; Table 9.7). This raised concern that unnecessary surgeries might be performed as a result of this method. Furthermore, 50% of normal subjects have nausea and/or abdominal cramping with the 3-minute infusion but not with

slower infusions. The likely explanation is that rapid infusion of sincalide causes intestinal cramping, resulting cramping/pain, and nausea. A common misconception is that "reproduction of a patient's pain" with sincalide infusion is diagnostic of chronic acalculous gallbladder disease. This is not true. The pain is the result of rapid infusion. Pain almost never occurs with slow, more physiological infusions, regardless of whether the patient has chronic cholecystitis or not.

A prospective multicenter study of 60 normal subjects at four institutions, each given 0.02 μg/kg over 15 minutes, 30 minutes, and 60 minutes on different days, found the least variability (lowest coefficient of variation) and narrowest normal range using the 60-minute infusion, with the lower range of normal for the GBEF being 38% (see Table 9.7). Subsequently, a consensus report published by expert gastroenterologists, surgeons, and nuclear medicine physicians recommended that the 60-minute infusion method should become the standard methodology (Box 9.10). Society of Nuclear Medicine and Molecular Imaging (SNMMI) procedure guidelines also recommend this method of sincalide infusion.

Biliary Obstruction

Biliary obstruction is usually caused by cholelithiasis or malignancy (e.g., pancreatic or biliary duct cancer). Malignancy typically presents as painless obstructive jaundice, whereas choledocholithiasis causes acute or recurrent abdominal pain.

High-Grade Biliary Obstruction

Pathophysiology. With high-grade obstruction, the sequence of pathophysiological events progresses in a predictable manner (Box 9.11). Obstruction results in increased intraductal pressure and thus biliary ductal dilatation. The high back pressure from obstruction reduces bile flow. Ultimately, hepatocellular damage and biliary cirrhosis result.

Clinical Presentation. Patients present with abdominal pain, jaundice, and elevated alkaline phosphatase and direct serum bilirubin. With obstruction due to stones, the symptom of pain is dominant. With obstruction caused by tumor, jaundice is often the presenting finding.

Diagnosis. The diagnosis can often be made with anatomical imaging (e.g., ultrasonography or magnetic resonance cholangiopancreatography [MRCP]) demonstrating biliary duct dilation and either an obstructing mass or cholelithiasis. However, small obstructing biliary stones may be missed on anatomical imaging, and ductal dilation may not become evident until 24 to 72 hours after acute obstruction. Thus, a patient with an acute obstructing stone presenting in the emergency room may not have dilatation. In this situation, cholescintigraphy can diagnose the obstruction before dilation occurs because it depicts the underlying pathophysiology (i.e., reduced bile flow). A high-grade obstruction will show liver uptake but no biliary secretion (Fig. 9.17). If a patient has had prior obstruction, the biliary ducts may remain chronically dilated even after the obstruction has been relieved. In that case, cholescintigraphy can determine whether the dilated biliary ducts are patent or again obstructed.

Partial Biliary Obstruction. Patients with a partial biliary obstruction typically present with intermittent recurrent abdominal pain. Liver function tests and serum bilirubin are often

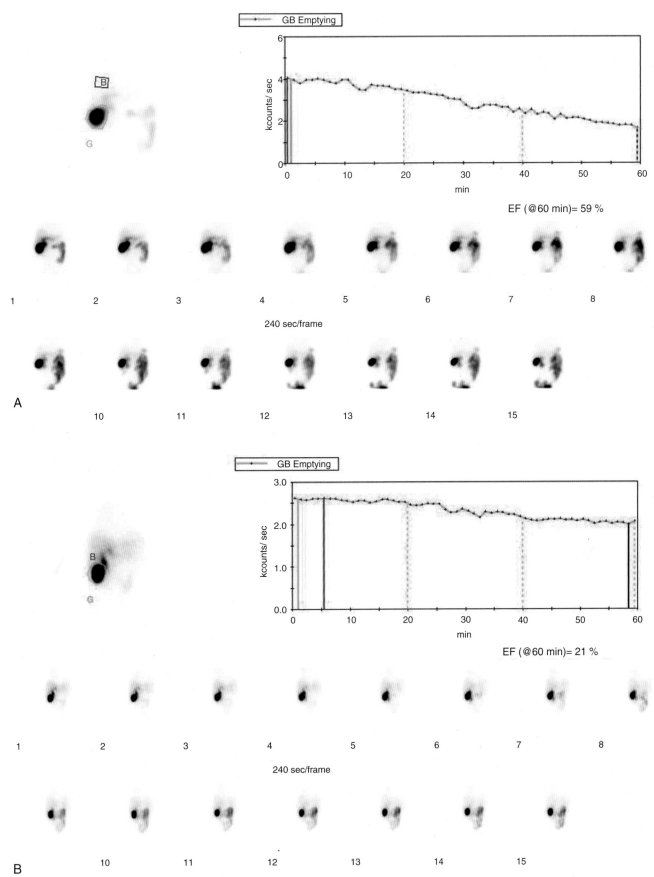

Fig. 9.16 Normal and abnormal gallbladder ejection fraction (GBEF). Both patients (A and B) were referred for suspected chronic acalculous gallbladder disease (gallbladder dyskinesia). Sincalide was infused over 60 minutes after gallbladder visualization. A region of interest (ROI) was drawn for the gallbladder and background. (A) Good gallbladder contraction, GBEF 59%. (B) Poor gallbladder contraction, GBEF 21% (abnormal <38%). The patient in B had a cholecystectomy with relief of his chronic recurrent biliary colic-like symptoms.

TABLE 9.7 Comparison of 3-, 15-, 30-, 60-Minute Sincalide Infusions (0.02 µg/kg) in Normal Subjects

Infusion Length	Subjects	CV[a] (%)	Range of GBEFs (%)	Calculated Abnormal GBEF (%)	Subjects With Abdominal Cramping (%)
3 minutes	43	48	0–100	<0	50
15 minutes	60	52	5–92	<17	5
30 minutes	60	35	20–95	<19	0
60 minutes	60	19[b]	50–96	<38	0

[a]Coefficient of variation (CV) as a measure of variability (standard deviation [SD]/mean).
[b]CV was statistically different (<0.0001) for 60 minutes versus 30 minutes and 30 minutes versus 15 minutes.

BOX 9.10 Consensus Methodology for Sincalide (Cholecystokinin [CCK]) Cholescintigraphy: Gallbladder Ejection Fraction (GBEF) Calculation

1. Ensure that the gallbladder has filled.
2. Position camera in left anterior oblique projection (35–40 degrees).
3. Draw 0.02 µg/kg sincalide into a 30- to 50-mL syringe and dilute with normal saline to the volume of the syringe.
4. Set up infusion pump so that the entire volume of the syringe will be infused slowly and continuously over 60 minutes.
5. Begin imaging at the start of sincalide infusion and stop imaging at the end of 60-minute infusion.

Computer-Processing GBEF

1. Select region of interest for the gallbladder and adjacent liver background.
2. Generate time–activity curve.
3. Calculate GBEF at 60 minutes = maximum counts − minimum counts divided by maximum counts, all corrected for background. (Abnormal GBEF is <38%.)

BOX 9.11 High-Grade Biliary Obstruction: Sequential Pathophysiology

1. Obstruction of hepatic or common bile duct
2. Increased intrabiliary pressure
3. Decreased bile flow
4. Ductal dilation
5. Biliary cirrhosis

normal. Biliary ducts are not usually dilated. Cholelithiasis is the usual cause. Ultrasonography is often the first imaging study ordered. If the ducts are dilated, this is diagnostic, unless the patient had prior obstruction. MRCP is superior to sonography for detecting stones that do not result in ductal dilation; however, small obstructing stones may not be detected, and MRCP does not evaluate bile flow.

Cholescintigraphy can determine whether the patient's symptoms are biliary in origin when anatomical imaging is uncertain, before a more invasive workup by percutaneous cholangiography or endoscopic retrograde cholangiopancreatography (ERCP). Discordance between anatomical and functional imaging is not uncommon. Functional abnormalities precede morphologically evident disease. When there is no anatomical evidence of biliary dilation, scintigraphy may show evidence of partial biliary obstruction as manifested by delayed bile flow (Fig. 9.18). In patients without obstruction but with dilated ducts from prior obstruction, cholescintigraphy can exclude recurrent obstruction by demonstrating normal bile flow.

Image Analysis for Obstruction With Cholescintigraphy

High-Grade Obstruction. With obstruction of recent onset, the liver will show good hepatic function, manifested by rapid blood-pool clearance and good Tc-99m HIDA uptake, but no excretion into the biliary tree. Images show a characteristic persistent hepatogram with no bile excretion, the result of the high back-pressure (see Fig. 9.17). Delayed imaging for up to 24 hours is often unchanged. On occasion, with a less severe but still high-grade obstruction, there may be some delayed excretion into the biliary ducts. In patients with good hepatic function, delayed imaging beyond 2 hours is not usually necessary for diagnosis. However, in patients with poor hepatic function, delayed imaging is required to differentiate obstruction from primary hepatic dysfunction (see Figs. 9.7 and 9.8). At times, differentiating chronic obstruction from severe hepatic insufficiency can be difficult. Lack of biliary clearance by 24 hours is suggestive of obstruction.

Partial Biliary Obstruction. Although there is prompt hepatic uptake and secretion into biliary ducts, clearance from the biliary ducts is delayed, with common duct activity often decreasing by less than 50% from peak over 60 minutes (see Fig. 9.18), accompanied by delayed transit into the small intestines (delayed biliary-to-bowel transit; Box 9.12). Some transit into the small bowel may be seen with a partial obstruction. The most important criteria should be whether or not there is good common duct clearance. Delayed images at 2 hours or sincalide infusion can help to confirm or exclude partial obstruction (Figs. 9.19–9.21).

Patients may have delayed biliary-to-bowel transit for reasons other than obstruction (Box 9.13; e.g., received sincalide to empty gallbladder before the study [see Fig. 9.18]). As the gallbladder relaxes, the resulting relatively negative intraluminal gallbladder pressure causes bile to flow preferentially toward the gallbladder rather than through the common duct and sphincter of Oddi. Delayed transit can also be seen in patients with chronic cholecystitis and in some normal patients ("hypertonic sphincter of Oddi"). Delayed imaging or sincalide can usually differentiate a functional cause (good clearance) from obstruction (poor biliary duct clearance). Sincalide provides a more

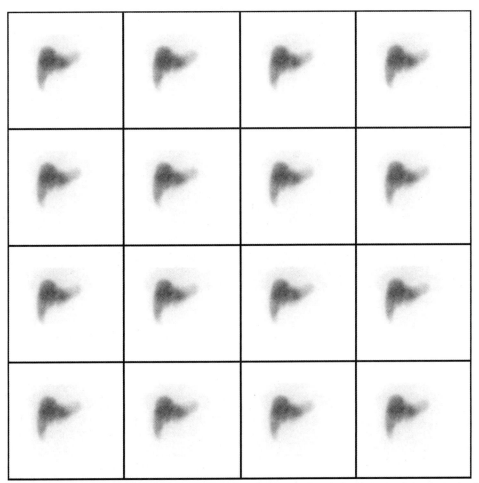

Fig. 9.17 High-grade biliary obstruction. Patient was admitted to the hospital with acute abdominal pain of 6 hours duration. Ultrasonography in the emergency room (ER) did not show biliary dilation. Cholescintigraphy sequential selected summed images over 2 hours show rapid clearance of cardiac blood pool consistent with good hepatic function. However, there is a hepatogram with no biliary duct activity or clearance. This is diagnostic of a high-grade biliary obstruction. A stone was found to be obstructing the common duct. With poor hepatic function, further delayed imaging is required.

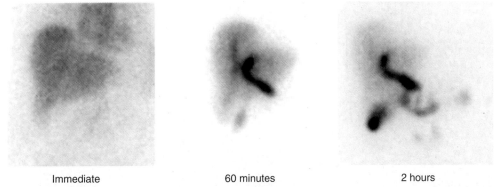

Immediate   60 minutes   2 hours

Fig. 9.18 Partial biliary obstruction. Patient had recurrent upper abdominal pain for 6 months. Normal ultrasonography. Cholescintigraphy immediately after injection *(left)*, at 60 minutes *(middle)*, and at 2 hours *(right)*. Cardiac blood pool cleared by 5 minutes (not shown). The common hepatic and common bile duct have retained activity at 1 hour, which increases at 2 hours, suggestive of partial biliary obstruction. Delayed gallbladder visualization (faint at 1 hour, filled by 2 hours) is suggestive of possible concomitant chronic cholecystitis. The gallbladder usually fills early with biliary partial obstruction in those without gallbladder disease.

rapid and standardized response. Opiate drugs may produce a functional partial biliary obstruction. Thus, they should be withheld for 6 hours before cholescintigraphy.

Accuracy of Cholescintigraphy for Biliary Obstruction. The sensitivity and specificity of cholescintigraphy for high-grade obstruction approach 100%. For low-grade, partial, or intermittent obstruction, the sensitivity and specificity of cholescintigraphy have been reported to be 95% and 85%, respectively, compared with ultrasonography with a sensitivity of 78% and specificity of 86%.

Choledochal Cyst

Choledochal cysts are not true cysts but, rather, congenital dilation of bile ducts. They usually involve the common hepatic duct or common bile duct but may occur anywhere in the biliary system, usually in an extrahepatic location but occasionally intrahepatic (Caroli disease), which may be multifocal (Fig. 9.22). The cysts may present in young children as biliary obstruction, pancreatitis, or cholangitis. Alternatively, they may be asymptomatic and detected incidentally and, rarely,

---

BOX 9.12 Scintigraphic Diagnosis of Partial Biliary Obstruction

Poor biliary duct clearance (<50% of peak common duct activity at 60 minutes)
Delayed or reduced biliary-to-bowel transit
No further biliary duct clearance on delayed imaging at 120 versus 60 minutes
No significant biliary duct clearance with sincalide infusion between 60 and 120 minutes

---

first detected in adulthood. Ultrasonography or CT may detect a saccular or fusiform cystic structure; however, it may be uncertain whether the cystic structure connects with the biliary tract. Cholescintigraphy can help confirm or exclude this. Nonobstructed choledochal cysts fill slowly, have prolonged retention, and show slow clearance of the HIDA radiotracer. Delayed imaging is often required (Fig. 9.23). However, with a high-grade obstruction, there will be no filling of the choledochal cyst because of the high back-pressure.

Biliary Atresia

Biliary atresia is characterized by progressive inflammatory sclerosis and obliteration of extrahepatic and intrahepatic biliary ducts. In the neonatal period, these infants present with cholestatic jaundice, acholic stools, and hepatomegaly. Without treatment, the disease leads to hepatic fibrosis, cirrhosis, liver failure, and death within 2 to 3 years. The cause is unknown. Early diagnosis is critical because surgery must be performed within the first 60 days of life to prevent irreversible liver failure. Surgery, hepatoportoenterostomy (Kasai procedure), is palliative. Ultimately, liver transplantation is required. Biliary atresia must be differentiated from neonatal hepatitis caused by various genetic, infectious, and metabolic causes, such as Alagille syndrome (arteriohepatic dysplasia), alpha-1-antitrypsin deficiency, and cystic fibrosis, to name a few. Importantly, a gallbladder seen on sonography does not rule out biliary atresia. Cholescintigraphy has been used successfully for decades to confirm or exclude biliary atresia.

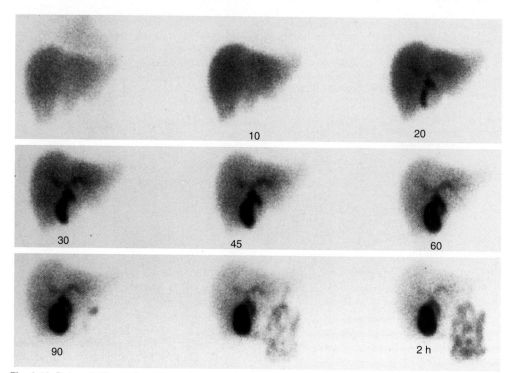

Fig. 9.19 Delayed biliary-to-bowel transit due to sincalide administered before the study because the patient had not eaten for more than 24 hours. The patient was referred with abdominal pain. The gallbladder fills by 30 minutes and the common duct is seen at 60 minutes, but there is no biliary-to-bowel clearance. Further imaging shows intestinal clearance first seen at 90 minutes and continued clearing of the common duct by 2 hours. This is a functional delay in biliary-to-bowel transit, in this case, due to the prestudy sincalide.

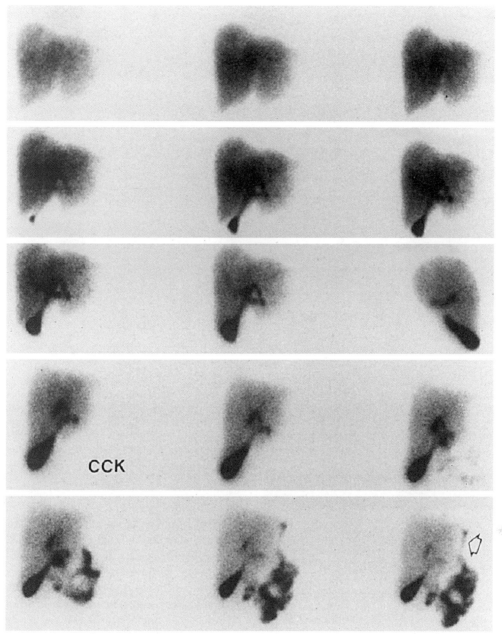

Fig. 9.20 Delayed biliary-to-bowel transit in normal subject. *(Top three rows)*, Sequential images acquired over 60 minutes. The gallbladder fills and the biliary ducts are visualized, but there is no biliary-to-bowel transit. *(Bottom two rows)* Sincalide infusion produces gallbladder contraction (gallbladder ejection fraction [GBEF], 51%) and biliary-to-bowel transit with relaxation of sphincter of Oddi. *(Arrowhead)* Mild enterogastric reflux. Interpreted as normal variation, "hypertonic sphincter of Oddi." *CCK,* Cholecystokinin.

Cholescintigraphy

Preparation. Patients should be pretreated with phenobarbital 5 mg/kg per day for 5 days before the study to activate liver excretory enzymes that increase bile flow. A serum phenobarbital level should be in the therapeutic range (10–30 mcg/mL) to maximize the specificity of the scintigraphy. Ideally, the patient should fast for 2 hours before the study. The recommended pediatric dose of Tc-99m HIDA is 0.05 mCi/kg (minimum dose, 0.5 mCi).

The atretic bile ducts of biliary atresia produce a picture of high-grade biliary obstruction, with good hepatic function as shown by rapid blood-pool clearance, but no biliary clearance, and a persistent hepatogram (Fig. 9.24). The obstructive pattern is caused by the high back-pressure, preventing secretion into biliary ducts or gallbladder. Neonatal hepatitis shows hepatic dysfunction, with delayed blood-pool clearance and delayed biliary-to-bowel transit, but transit is typically seen by 24 hours after Tc-99m HIDA injection (Fig. 9.25). Gallbladder filling excludes biliary atresia because the high back-pressure would prevent biliary secretion (Figs. 9.26 and 9.27).

The sensitivity for detection of biliary atresia with cholescintigraphy is very high, approaching 100%; however, the specificity reported in the older literature is considerably lower, averaging 75% to 80%, in some reports even less. However, a

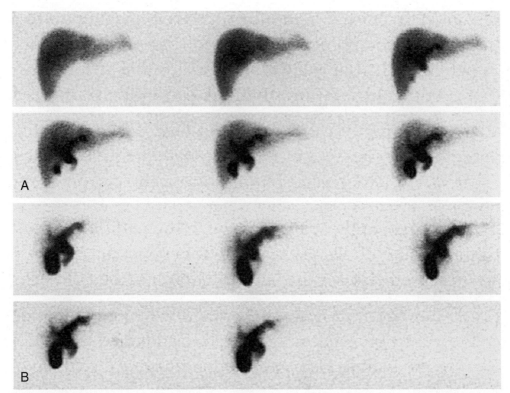

Fig. 9.21 Partial common bile duct obstruction with poor response to sincalide. (A) Increasing bile secretion over time. The gallbladder fills. The common duct is quite prominent. No biliary-to-bowel transit is seen at 60 minutes *(second line, last image)*. (B) Sincalide was infused over 60 minutes. No gallbladder contraction and no significant biliary-to-bowel transit is seen by the end of the study. This is consistent with a partial common bile duct obstruction. The high back-pressure likely prevented gallbladder contraction.

BOX 9.13   Causes of Delayed Biliary-to-Bowel Transit

Biliary obstruction
Sincalide administration before cholescintigraphy
Opiate drugs
Chronic cholecystitis
Normal variation ("hypertonic sphincter of Oddi")

---

recent publication of a 20-year experience at a children's hospital found that if phenobarbital is administered before the scan (5 mg/kg/day for 5 days in 2 divided doses) and the serum phenobarbital level is in the therapeutic range at the time of the scan, the specificity is 95%, with 100% sensitivity. When a false-positive study result is clinically suspected, a repeat study in several days to a week may be helpful for confirming a parenchymal cause. Single-photon emission computed tomography (SPECT) and SPECT with CT (SPECT/CT) may be occasionally helpful in specific cases (see Fig. 9.27).

Postcholecystectomy Pain Syndrome—Sphincter of Oddi Dysfunction. Approximately 10% to 20% of patients who have had a cholecystectomy for chronic cholecystitis subsequently develop recurrent abdominal pain. The most common biliary causes include retained or recurrent biliary duct stones, inflammatory stricture (Fig. 9.28), and, less commonly, sphincter of Oddi dysfunction (Figs. 9.29 and 9.30; Box 9.14). All can cause partial biliary obstruction. Cholescintigraphy will show evidence of this partial obstruction as delayed clearance from biliary ducts

and delayed biliary-to-bowel-transit. Delayed imaging at 2 hours usually reveals no reduction in common duct activity, and it is often increased (see Fig. 9.29). ERCP is ultimately used to make the final diagnosis of stone or stricture. Rarely, a cystic duct remnant acts like a small gallbladder, producing symptoms similar to those of acute or chronic cholecystitis.

Sphincter of Oddi dysfunction is the cause in approximately 10% of patients with postcholecystectomy pain syndrome. Symptoms are those of intermittent recurrent abdominal pain. Transient liver function abnormalities may be seen. It is caused by a partial biliary obstruction at the level of the sphincter of Oddi but not caused by stones, stricture, or tumor. The hypothesis for why the pain presents after cholecystectomy is that before surgery, the gallbladder acts as a pressure release valve that decompresses the biliary ducts when there are increases in intrabiliary pressure, thus preventing pain. There is no test that can reliably diagnose sphincter of Oddi dysfunction before cholecystectomy.

Sphincter of Oddi dysfunction may be a fixed obstruction (papillary stenosis) or a functional intermittent and reversible obstruction (biliary dyskinesia). The former is relatively straightforward to diagnose and treat with anatomical imaging and ERCP, whereas the latter can be more challenging. Therapy for sphincter dysfunction is usually sphincterotomy, particularly for a fixed obstruction, whereas a functional and reversible obstruction may sometimes respond to drugs (e.g., nifedipine, Botox), although ultimately, they usually require sphincterotomy.

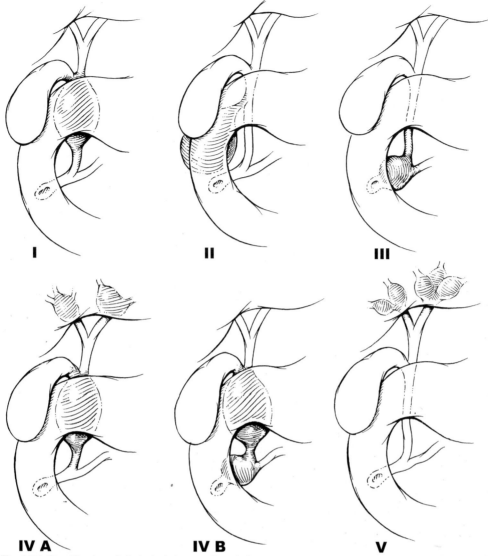

Fig. 9.22 Classification of choledochal cysts. Type I: Cystic dilation of an extrahepatic duct (most common). Type II: Sac or diverticulum opening from the common bile duct. Type III: choledochocele, located within the duodenal wall. Type IVA: Involving intrahepatic and extrahepatic biliary ducts. Type IVB: Dilation of multiple segments confined to extrahepatic biliary ducts. Type V: Multiple intrahepatic ducts (Caroli disease).

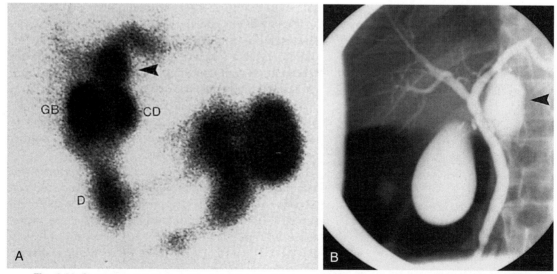

Fig. 9.23 Choledochal cyst in a 25-year-old patient being evaluated for abdominal pain. Ultrasonography detected a cystic structure adjacent to the common hepatic duct without definite connection to the biliary system. (A) Tc-99 hepatic iminodiacetic acid (HIDA) images acquired at 90 minutes after the liver had cleared show filling of choledochal cyst in the region of the common hepatic duct *(arrowhead),* confirming that the cystic structure was connected to the biliary system. *CD,* Common duct; *D,* duodenum; *GB,* gallbladder. (B) Cholangiogram confirmed the diagnosis.

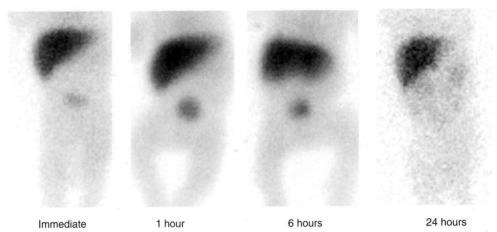

| | | | |
| Immediate | 1 hour | 6 hours | 24 hours |

Fig. 9.24 Biliary atresia in a 13-week-old child with jaundice, pretreated with phenobarbital for 5 days. Serum phenobarbital was in the therapeutic range. No biliary excretion occurred over 24 hours. Bladder clearance is seen. Biliary atresia was confirmed at cholangiography, and a Kasai procedure was performed.

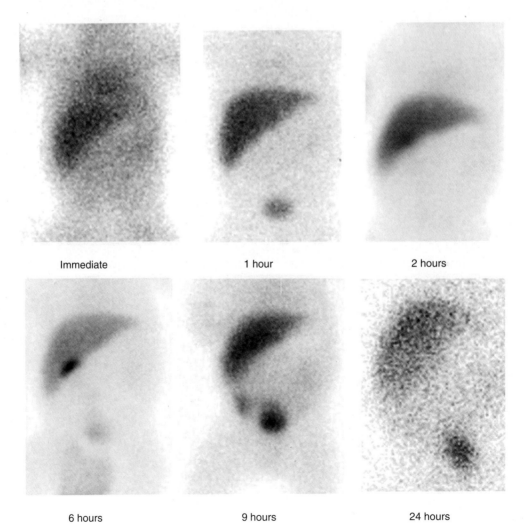

| | | |
| Immediate | 1 hour | 2 hours |

| | | |
| 6 hours | 9 hours | 24 hours |

Fig. 9.25 Neonatal hepatitis. Sequential Tc-99m hepatic iminodiacetic acid (HIDA) images. At 2 hours, gallbladder visualization is suggested. By 6 hours, good gallbladder filling is seen. At 9 hours, bowel clearance is noted, and the gallbladder has emptied. By 24 hours, image quality is reduced due to decay, with perhaps some mild bowel activity at the hepatic flexure. The patient was clinically followed, with progressive improvement in liver function tests. Imaging could have been discontinued at 6 hours because biliary atresia had been excluded with gallbladder filling. The high back-pressure of biliary obstruction in biliary atresia prevents any bile secretion.

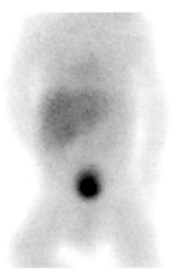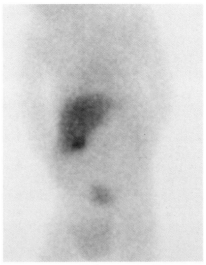

Fig. 9.26 Rule out biliary atresia. *(Left)* At 1 hour, there is no biliary clearance from the liver. *(Right),* At 4 hours, the gallbladder fills. The activity in the lower abdomen is bladder, and below that, diaper. Gallbladder filling rules out biliary atresia.

Sonography, CT, and MRCP may not be diagnostic. Sphincter of Oddi manometry was regarded as the diagnostic standard in the recent past, with a positive study revealing an elevated sphincter pressure (>40 mm Hg). However, this technique is invasive, not widely available, technically difficult, prone to interpretative errors, and associated with a significant incidence of adverse effects, the most serious of which is pancreatitis. It is rarely used today. ERCP ultimately excludes cholelithiasis or stricture; however, it is invasive and also associated with a relatively high incidence of postprocedure complications.

The potential utility of cholescintigraphy for the diagnosis of sphincter of Oddi dysfunction may seem obvious; however, its value is controversial among gastroenterologists and surgeons. Strong, evidence-based data are lacking. However, single-center studies have found cholescintigraphy to be diagnostically useful, and it is routinely performed at some biliary referral centers, although the quantitative methodology varies. Early studies suggested that image analysis could be diagnostic with findings of a partial biliary obstruction—delayed biliary duct clearance at 60 minutes and persistent or increased bile duct retention at 2 hours (see Fig. 9.29).

Various quantitative and semiquantitative methods have been used to improve on image analysis alone. One published method used routinely at Johns Hopkins University reported high sensitivity and specificity in 26 patients. The protocol requires the infusion of sincalide before the study, with the expectation that it will increase bile flow and stress the capacity of the biliary ducts, bringing out less severe abnormalities that might otherwise not be detected, similar to Lasix renography. This method incorporates image analysis and semiquantitative analysis (see Fig. 9.30). The methodology is detailed in Box 9.15. When the examination is negative, nonbiliary causes of pain are sought. If positive, the patient often proceeds to ERCP. If no stones or strictures are seen, a sphincterotomy is often performed for assumed sphincter dysfunction.

Postoperative Biliary Tract Complications

Cholescintigraphy can provide valuable diagnostic information for patients with suspected complications presenting after laparoscopic or open cholecystectomy, biliary duct surgery, gallstone lithotripsy, and biliary-enteric anastomoses.

Biliary Leaks. Bile leaks may occur after abdominal trauma, cholecystectomy, or other biliary tract surgery. The laparoscopic method has become the procedure of choice for elective cholecystectomy; however, it is associated with a higher incidence of bile duct injury than open cholecystectomy. Although ultrasonography and CT can detect fluid collections, cholescintigraphy is able to determine whether the fluid is of biliary origin and can estimate the rate of biliary leakage. Slow bile leaks usually resolve spontaneously with conservative therapy, whereas rapid leaks often require surgical correction. Only biliary scintigraphy can demonstrate communication between the biliary tree and space-occupying lesions that represent biloma formation after trauma.

Biliary leakage on cholescintigraphy is seen as a progressively increasing collection of radiotracer in the region of the gallbladder fossa or hepatic hilum. The activity may spread into the subdiaphragmatic space, over the dome of the liver, into the colonic gutters, or manifest as free bile within the abdomen (Fig. 9.31). Rapid leaks are detectable on early imaging, but slower leaks may require delayed imaging beyond 60 minutes. Positioning the patient in the right lateral decubitus position for several minutes may help demonstrate a fluid collection. Peritoneal tubing, drains, and collection bags may be the only evidence of a leak and should always be imaged.

Biliary Diversion Surgery. Biliary-enteric bypass procedures are performed for patients with biliary obstruction for both benign and malignant conditions and for liver transplantation. Ultrasonography has imaging limitations in the presence of gas in the anastomotic bowel segment or refluxed biliary air after surgery and thus may be reported as indeterminate. MRCP has become a standard diagnostic procedure because of its accuracy

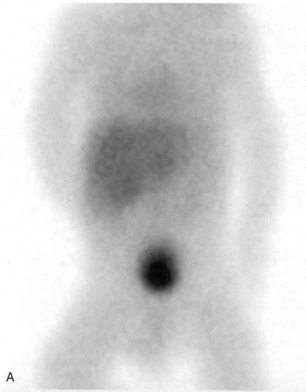

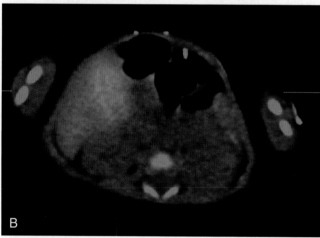

Fig. 9.27 Utility of single-photon emission computed tomography with computed tomography (SPECT/CT). (A) At 2 hours, *(left)* no definite biliary-to-bowel clearance. Mild increased uptake at the inferior border of the liver. The intensity is set high. (B) SPECT/CT confirms gallbladder filling. Biliary atresia is ruled out. With biliary atresia, bile cannot be excreted from the liver due to the high back-pressure.

in visualizing the postoperative stricture and detecting obstruction. Biliary dilation is present in > 20% of patients who have had these procedures, even though obstruction has been adequately relieved by surgery. Cholescintigraphy is well suited to diagnose bile leakage, patency of the anastomosis, or recurrent obstruction. It is important to know the postoperative anatomy of the patient being imaged. Cholescintigraphy also can be helpful if ERCP cannot reach the biliary tract when a long Roux-en-Y loop has been created (Figs. 9.32 and 9.33).

Cholescintigraphy is the only noninvasive method that can distinguish obstructed dilated ducts from chronically dilated but nonobstructed ducts. Biliary clearance into the bowel by 1 hour with or without ductal dilation is suggestive of functional patency. Intestinal activity seen after 1 hour suggests partial obstruction. Retention of activity in the biliary ducts is an even more reliable indicator. Persistent or worsening biliary duct retention between 1 and 2 hours is very suggestive of obstruction. Stasis with minimal intestinal excretion and pooling in the region of the biliary-enteric anastomosis may normally be seen at 1 hour. This may be positional and can be confirmed by imaging the patient upright. With complete biliary obstruction, there is persistent nonvisualization of the biliary system and intestine.

Cholescintigraphy can provide functional information about other surgical procedures involving the gastrointestinal tract (e.g., Billroth I and II and Whipple resection). In Billroth II anastomoses, afferent loop patency can be determined. The afferent loop should fill readily in an antegrade direction from the common duct. Normally, there is a progressive accumulation of activity within the loop. However, it should clear distally by 2 hours.

Primary Benign and Malignant Tumors of the Liver. Tumors that contain hepatocytes would be expected to take up Tc-99m HIDA. Thus, cholescintigraphy can be useful for the differential diagnosis of benign and malignant hepatic tumors, specifically focal nodular hyperplasia (FNH), hepatic adenoma, and hepatocellular carcinoma (Table 9.8).

Focal Nodular Hyperplasia and Hepatic Adenoma. The presentation and therapy of FNH and hepatic adenoma, both benign tumors, are quite different. FNH is usually asymptomatic, often discovered incidentally, and requires no specific therapy. Hepatic adenomas are often symptomatic and may cause serious hemorrhage that can be life threatening. They have a strong association with oral contraceptives; FNH has a weaker association.

FNH contains all hepatic cell types: hepatocytes, Kupffer cells, and bile canaliculi. The usual findings seen on cholescintigraphy are increased blood flow, prompt hepatic uptake, and delayed clearance (Fig. 9.34). Poor clearance may be due to abnormal biliary canaliculi. This characteristic pattern is reported to be seen in more than 90% of patients. Limited evidence suggests that the overall accuracy is higher than the traditional Tc-99m SC method to diagnose FNH. Tc-99m SC is taken up in only two-thirds of patients with FNH, one-third with increased uptake and one-third with uptake equal to other liver. Although hepatic adenomas consist exclusively of hepatocytes, it is surprising that they do not have uptake on cholescintigraphy and are hypofunctional.

Hepatocellular carcinoma (hepatoma) also demonstrates characteristic findings with cholescintigraphy. The malignant hepatocytes are hypofunctional compared with the normal liver. Thus, during the first hour of imaging, no uptake is usually seen within the lesion (cold defect). Delayed imaging at 2 to 4 hours often shows fill-in or continuing uptake within the tumor and concomitant clearing of the adjacent normal liver. This pattern is quite specific for hepatoma. However, poorly differentiated hepatomas may not fill in on delayed imaging. Tc-99m HIDA uptake may sometimes be seen at sites of hepatocellular metastases (e.g., in the lung).

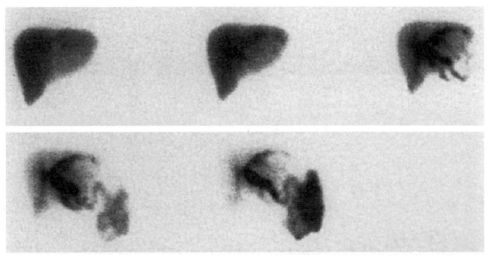

Fig. 9.28 Biliary stricture causing partial obstruction. Images at 5, 10, 20, 40, and 60 minutes. Common hepatic and common bile ducts are dilated proximal to the distal narrowing common duct, causing a partial obstruction. There is biliary-to-bowel transit.

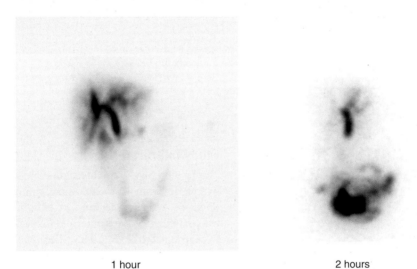

1 hour   2 hours

Fig. 9.29 Partial biliary obstruction postcholecystectomy—sphincter of Oddi dysfunction. Hepatic iminodiacetic acid (HIDA) images at 1 hour *(left)* and 2 hours *(right)*. At 1 hour, there is considerable retained activity in the common duct and more proximal ducts. At 2 hours, the liver has cleared; however, the common duct continues to retain activity and appears to be somewhat increased. The patient had a successful sphincterotomy.

Enterogastric Biliary Reflux. Cholescintigraphy can diagnose bile reflux into the stomach, which can result in an alkaline gastritis with symptoms often similar to those of acid-related disease (Fig. 9.35). It occurs most commonly after gastric resection surgery. Some reflux may be seen in normal subjects on routine cholescintigraphy, particularly if morphine or sincalide has been administered. Quantitative methods for estimating the amount of reflux have been described. The more reflux seen and the more persistent it is, the higher the likelihood that it is related to the patient's symptoms.

Tc-99M MACROAGGREGATED ALBUMIN (MAA) HEPATIC ARTERIAL PERFUSION SCINTIGRAPHY

Regional intraarterial therapy has been used to treat primary and metastatic cancer since the 1960s. The advantage of a

selective intraarterial approach is based on the dual blood supply to the liver. As a liver tumor grows, it derives most of its blood from the hepatic artery, whereas normal liver cells are supplied predominantly by the portal circulation. Intraarterial chemotherapy, chemoembolization, and therapeutic radiolabeled microspheres deliver therapy directly to the tumor, thus minimizing exposure to normal liver and to drug-sensitive dose-limiting tissues (e.g., gastrointestinal epithelium and bone marrow), which are often the source of side effects from conventional intravenous chemotherapy.

Contrast arteriography is used to position the therapeutic catheter. Incorrect positioning of the intraarterial catheter can result in inadequate delivery to the tumor and extrahepatic flow to the stomach, pancreas, spleen, or bowel. Collateral and anomalous arterial anatomy must be identified and the catheter repositioned or vessels occluded. Tc-99m MAA infused into the hepatic artery catheter can determine the adequacy of blood

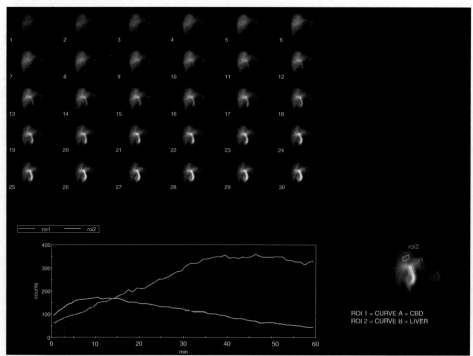

Fig. 9.30 Sphincter of Oddi dysfunction. *(Above),* The 2-minute sequential images demonstrate delayed clearance from the common duct. *(Below)* Regions of interest (ROIs) are drawn for the common duct and liver *(right).* Delayed clearance from the common hepatic and common bile duct is prominent. Time–activity curves for the common duct and liver are drawn *(left).* This patient had a scintigraphic score of 7 (see Box 9.15), positive for sphincter of Oddi dysfunction.

BOX 9.14 Causes of Postcholecystectomy Pain Syndrome

Retained or recurrent choledocholithiasis
Inflammatory biliary duct stricture
Sphincter of Oddi dysfunction
Cystic duct remnant (obstructed/inflamed)
Nonhepatobiliary origin

flow to the tumor; the presence or absence of extrahepatic perfusion, which can result in gastrointestinal toxicity; and right-to-left shunting within the tumor bed, which can result in pulmonary damage. Tumor arterial-venous shunting to the lung can be quantified before infusion of therapeutic Yttrium-90 radiolabeled microspheres (Therasphere, SIR-Sphere) to minimize pulmonary irradiation and toxicity.

Tc-99m MAA particles are larger than capillary size (range, 10–90 µm; mean 30–50 µm). When infused into the hepatic artery, they distribute according to blood flow and are trapped on first pass in the arteriolar-capillary bed of the liver. The particles partially occlude a small percentage of the liver capillary bed and cause no problem.

Methodology

After placement of the hepatic arterial catheter via contrast angiography, Tc-99m MAA is slowly infused. The procedure is summarized in Box 9.16. Liver and lung images are obtained to determine the extent of tumor and liver perfusion, extrahepatic perfusion in the abdomen, and the presence of left-to-right shunting.

Study Interpretation

The Tc-99m MAA ratio of tumor to nontumor uptake within the liver varies from 3:1 to 20:1. Small tumor nodules show uniform uptake, whereas larger tumors often have increased uptake at the periphery of the tumor and decreased uptake centrally due to central necrosis (Fig. 9.36). The hypervascular peripheral rim of the tumor is where active growth occurs (neovascularity). Extrahepatic intraabdominal perfusion to the stomach, spleen, pancreas, and so forth can result in adverse symptoms/complications (e.g., pain, hemorrhagic gastritis; see Fig. 9.36).

Although a small amount of arteriovenous shunting to the lungs is common (1% to <10%), abnormal shunting of 20% and higher can occur and is of concern for potential pulmonary toxicity by the therapeutic Y-90 microspheres (Fig. 9.37). Shunting to the lung of >20% usually results in cancellation of the planned intraarterial radioactive microsphere therapy, whereas a shunt of >10% but <20% usually results in dose reduction.

HEPATIC ARTERIAL RADIOLABELED MICROSPHERES FOR TUMOR THERAPY

Malignant tumors, primary and metastatic, commonly involve the liver. With hepatocellular cancer, surgical resection and liver transplantation are the only methods for cure, but the majority of patients present with unresectable disease. With liver metastases, palliative or adjuvant therapy is frequently needed in addition to chemotherapy to reduce tumor burden or symptoms. Thermal ablation (microwave and radiofrequency), cryoablation, and percutaneous injections can be effective but are not suitable for

CBD, Common bile duct.

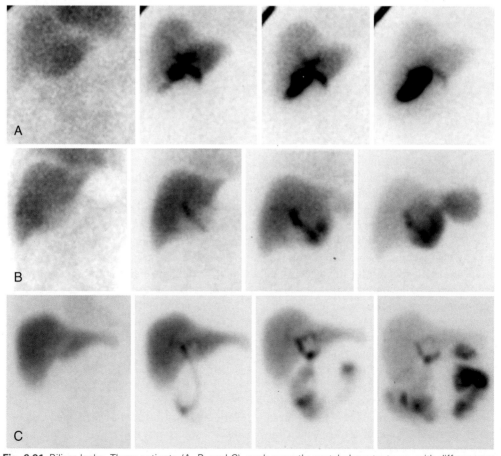

Fig. 9.31 Biliary leaks. Three patients (A, B, and C), each recently postcholecystectomy, with different patterns of biliary leakage. (A) Radiotracer extravasates along the inferior edge of the right lobe of the liver to the region of the gallbladder fossa. (B) Leak transits inferior to the left lobe, extending to the left upper quadrant. (C) Intraperitoneal extravasation.

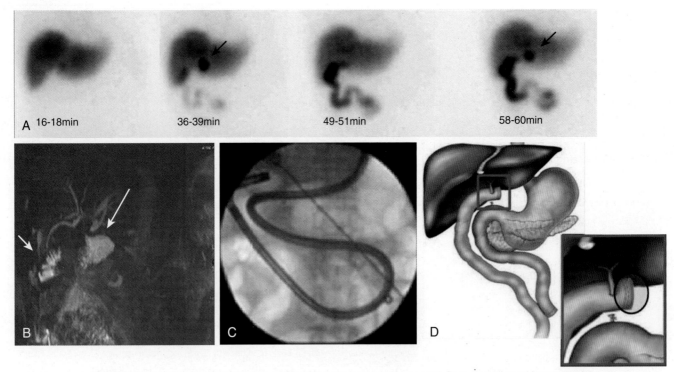

Fig. 9.32 Biliary-enteric anastomosis (hepatico-jejuno-anastomosis)—normal. Post–complicated laparoscopic cholecystectomy with injury of common hepatic duct. (A) Hepatic iminodiacetic acid (HIDA) images show biliary drainage initially toward the right flank through a retrocecal proximal jejunal limb (Roux limb). There is intermittent visualization of tracer at the blind end of the jejunum *(arrows)*. (B) Noncontrast coronal magnetic resonance (MR) T2 image shows the blind end of the mobilized jejunal loop *(long arrow)* and prominent intrahepatic right and left hepatic ducts. The jejunal loop descends toward the right flank *(short arrow)*. (C) Endoscopic retrograde cholangiopancreatography (ERCP) shows endoscopic tube passed through the duodenum and pushed retrograde into the Roux limb up to the site of hepatojejunal anastomosis. Anastomotic stricture was seen at the hepatico-jejuno-anastomosis, with no evidence of leak. (D) Illustration of Roux-en-Y hepatico-jejunostomy with end-to-side biliary enteric anastomosis and side-to side jejuno-jejunal anastomosis (proximal limb reanastomosed to the Roux limb. Magnified view of the end-to-side hepatico-jejuno-anastomosis and the blind end of the jejunal loop. (With permission from Matesan M, Bermo M, Cruite I, et al. Biliary leak in the postsurgical abdomen: A primer to HIDA scan interpretation. *Sem Nucl Med.* 2017;47:618–629, Elsevier Inc.)

patients with large or multiple lesions. Transarterial chemoembolization (TACE) has been recommended as a front-line therapy for patients with large or multifocal hepatocellular tumors. TACE involves a combination of chemotherapy and an embolic agent (steel coils, microspheres, particles, sponges) that induces ischemic necrosis and locally delivers chemotherapy. Newer drug-eluting microspheres provide sustained chemotherapy release.

Radiolabeled therapeutic microspheres can also be delivered via the hepatic artery, thereby offering the advantage of delivering a large dose of radiation directly to the region of the tumor (i.e., selective internal radiation therapy). These directed intraarterial therapy techniques take advantage of the primary blood supply to hepatic tumors that originates from the hepatic artery, whereas the majority of blood perfusing normal liver parenchyma is from the portal venous system. Therefore, tumors preferentially receive the therapy and do not need to be ablated individually, and flow to the normal liver is minimized. Two radioembolization microsphere agents are available clinically: Y-90 SIR-Sphere and Y-90 Therasphere. Y-90 SIR-Sphere has been FDA approved for use with adjuvant chemotherapy in

hepatic metastases from colon cancer, and Y-90 Therasphere was approved for unresectable hepatocellular carcinoma.

Radiopharmaceuticals

The physical characteristics of the two Y-90 microsphere agents are outlined (Table 9.9). The β-emissions from the Y-90 label have a mean penetration length of 2.5 mm and energy of 0.94 MeV, resulting in an intratumoral dose of 100 to 150 Gy. Nearby tumor cells are relatively spared. With a physical half-life of 2.7 days, approximately 94% of the Y-90 dose is delivered by 11 days. Dose calculation is based on the tumor burden within the liver and the amount of shunting from the liver to the lungs. The typical doses administered are in the range of 40 to 70 mCi (1.5–2.5 GBq); Table 9.10.

Methodology

Patients must be carefully screened before receiving radiolabeled microsphere therapy. The functional status of the patient, liver function, and estimated tumor burden are reviewed. Patency of the portal vein must be established because portal

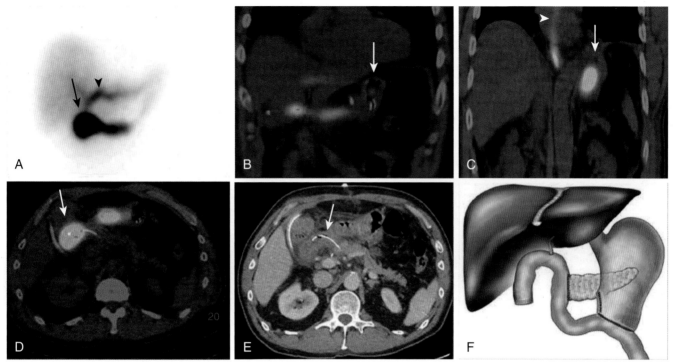

Fig. 9.33 Whipple procedure—hepatic iminodiacetic acid (HIDA) shows the jejunal loop brought to the right upper quadrant for gastrojejunal, cholecochojejunal, and pancreaticojejunal anastomosis. (A) HIDA at 60 minutes with radiotracer accumulation in the blind end of the mobilized jejunum in the right upper quadrant (RUQ; *arrow*) and normal progression of tracer distal in the afferent loop. Normal variant of more prominent visualization of the left hepatic duct *(arrowhead)* is also seen. (B and C) Fused coronal single-photon emission computed tomography with computed tomography (SPECT/CT) shows bile reflux into the stomach and esophagus. (D) Fused axial SPECT/CT image shows "blind-end sign" (arrow) at the end of the jejunum. (E) Contrast-enhanced CT shows pancreatic duct stent ending in the afferent jejunal loop. (F) Illustration of a variant of standard Whipple procedure (pancreatico-duodenectomy localized distal to the hepatico-jejuno-anastomosis as performed in this patient). (With permission from Matesan M, Bermo M, Cruite I, et al. Biliary leak in the postsurgical abdomen: A primer to HIDA scan interpretation. *Sem Nucl Med.* 2017;47:618–629, Elsevier Inc.)

TABLE 9.8 Differential Diagnosis of Primary Hepatic Tumors With Tc-99m Hepatic Iminodiacetic Acid (HIDA)

Lesion	Flow	Uptake	Clearance
Focal nodular hyperplasia	Increased	Immediate	Delayed
Hepatic adenoma	Normal	None	—
Hepatocellular carcinoma	Increased	Decreased and delayed	Delayed

vein thrombosis has been a contraindication, although some studies suggest it need not be absolute. Arteriography of hepatic vasculature is performed, and anomalous vessels that could result in accidental delivery into stomach, bowel, or other structures are embolized. With the catheter in position for therapy administration, tumor perfusion and arteriovenous shunting are assessed with Tc-99m MAA (Fig. 9.38). After administration, the catheter is removed and the groin stabilized. The patient is then scanned anteriorly and posteriorly. The shunt fraction is calculated. For Y-90 SIR-spheres, the dose is adjusted to help prevent radiation pneumonitis (Table 9.11). With Y-90 Theraspheres, the activity is higher on the glass beads, so a lower level of shunting (<10%) is acceptable.

After these procedures, the patient returns another day for the therapy itself. The catheter is placed in the same position under fluoroscopic guidance. The radioactive microsphere dose is administered with a slow push to prevent refluxing the dose into the systemic circulation. The patient can then be taken to nuclear medicine and imaged using the *bremsstrahlung* radiation emitted from the Y-90 to confirm proper localization (Fig. 9.39). Alternatively, positron emission tomography (PET) imaging can show posttherapy distribution because of a small amount of *positron decay* formed by pair production; however, imaging acquisition time is at least 30 minutes due to the low count rate. Patients can be discharged to home after the procedure. Some radiation safety precautions are needed because of some activity excreted via the kidneys and bladder.

Complications

The most frequent side effects are fatigue and loss of appetite, which typically resolve over 1 to 2 months. Potential serious side effects include gastric ulcers, radiation pneumonitis, and radiation hepatitis. Cholecystitis is a serious complication seen in patients when an accessory cystic artery has not been coil-embolized pretherapy. Thrombocytopenia can occur within 3 months of therapy. Transient intrahepatic bile duct obstruction due to edema occurs more frequently than cholecystitis, but is usually self-limiting.

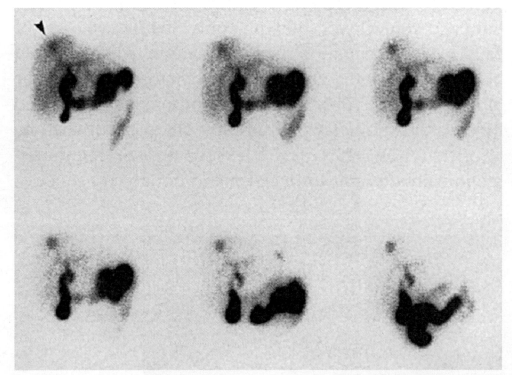

Fig. 9.34 Focal nodular hyperplasia. Sequential 5-minute images show early uptake by the benign tumor in the dome of the liver *(arrowhead)* that persists throughout the 60-minute study as the normal liver clears the tracer.

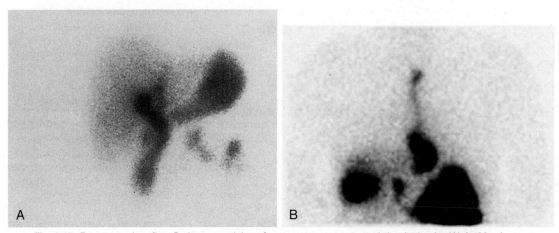

A

B

Fig. 9.35 Enterogastric reflux. Patient complains of recurrent vague upper abdominal pain. (A) At 60 minutes after Tc-99m hepatic iminodiacetic acid (HIDA) injection, reflux of a large amount of bile into the stomach can be seen. Bile gastritis was confirmed at endoscopy. (B) Entero-gastroesophageal reflux. This patient had a history of esophageal cancer and esophagectomy. Bile refluxes into the patient's gastric pull-up.

BOX 9.16 Tc-99m MAA Hepatic Arterial Perfusion Imaging With Lung Shunt Quantification: Protocol Summary

Patient Preparation

Intraarterial catheter must be positioned appropriately in the hepatic artery or its branches by interventional radiology.

Instrumentation

Gamma camera: Large field of view
Collimator: Low-energy parallel hole, high resolution
Energy window: 20% centered over 140-keV photopeak

Radiopharmaceutical

Tc-99m MAA, 4 mCi (148 MBq)
Infuse Tc-99m MAA in a small volume (0.5–1 mL) through the intraarterial catheter.

Imaging Protocol

Acquire anterior and posterior whole-body images.
Option: SPECT or SPECT/CT of abdomen to evaluate for adequacy of distribution and the presence and location of extrahepatic perfusion (e.g., stomach).

Calculation of Percent Shunt to Lung

1. Draw region of interest for the lung, for the liver, and for the thigh background (free Tc-99m pertechnetate is often present).
2. Percent shunt to lung = Lung (geometrical mean)/lung + liver (geometrical mean), all corrected for background.

CT, Computed tomography; *MAA,* macroaggregated albumin; *SPECT,* single-photon emission computed tomography.

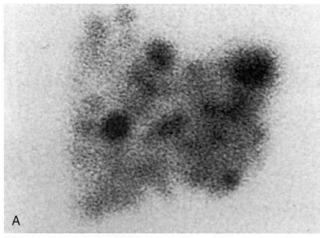

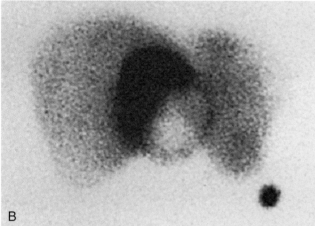

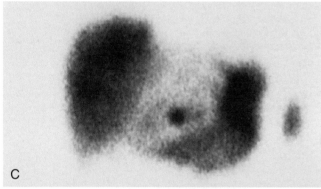

Fig. 9.36 Tc-99m macroaggregated albumin (MAA) hepatic arterial perfusion scintigraphy. (A) Patient with colon cancer metastatic to liver. Tc-99m MAA study shows multiple hyperperfused solid tumor nodules involving both lobes of liver. (B) Hyperperfusion of the periphery of the large tumor mass with a large cold necrotic center. (C) Perfusion of the right lobe, poor perfusion to the left lobe, and prominent extrahepatic perfusion to the stomach and spleen. The focal hot spot adjacent to the stomach is due to a thrombus at the chemotherapy infusion catheter tip.

Results

After Y-90 microsphere therapy, a significant response can be seen on CT in tumor appearance, with a decrease in size and development of necrosis within the lesion. F-18 fluorodeoxyglucose (FDG) PET/CT can be performed at 1 month and may help monitor response (Fig. 9.40). The majority of patients demonstrate at least partial response. Studies have shown responses in some patients with hepatocellular cancer who were not responding to chemotherapy and thus becoming resectable. Limited data suggest improvement in median survival, particularly with higher doses.

Tc-99M RED BLOOD CELL LIVER SCINTIGRAPHY

Cavernous hemangiomas are the most common benign tumor of the liver and the second most common hepatic tumor, behind liver metastases. They are usually asymptomatic and discovered incidentally on CT or ultrasonography during the workup or staging in a patient with a known primary malignancy or during evaluation of unrelated abdominal symptoms or disease. They require no specific therapy but must be differentiated from other, more serious liver tumors. The hemangiomas consist of dilated, endothelium-lined vascular channels of varying size separated by fibrous septa. Ten percent are multiple. Lesions larger than 4 cm are called giant cavernous hemangiomas. Non-invasive diagnosis of a cavernous hemangioma of the liver can obviate the need for biopsy, which could result in hemorrhage and morbidity.

Methodology

Radiolabeling RBCs with Tc-99m pertechnetate is performed using the methodology described for gastrointestinal bleeding (Chapter 10, Box X.11, Fig. X.24). After injection, Tc-99m-labeled red blood cells (RBCs) equilibrate within the relatively stagnant, nonlabeled blood pool of the hemangioma (Fig. 9.41). Equilibration time takes 30 to 120 minutes. With traditional planar imaging, a three-phase study is performed with flow images, blood-pool, and delayed multiple-view images (Box 9.17). SPECT and SPECT/CT are used for improved sensitivity and localization. Planar flow and early blood-pool images are no longer necessary for diagnosis, although they illustrate and teach the characteristic pathophysiology.

Image Interpretation

Radionuclide blood-flow imaging typically shows normal arterial flow to the cavernous hemangioma. Immediate blood-pool images show decreased activity within the hemangioma compared with adjacent liver. Early increased inhomogeneous uptake as a result of rapid equilibrium is sometimes seen (Fig. 9.42). On diagnostic 1- to 2-hour delayed imaging, hemangiomas show increased activity compared with that of the adjacent liver. Activity is equal to the blood pool of the heart and spleen. Giant cavernous hemangiomas show heterogeneity of uptake on delayed images, with areas of decreased and increased uptake. The cold regions are caused by thrombosis, necrosis, and fibrosis. Other benign and malignant liver tumors, abscesses, cirrhotic nodules, and cysts all have decreased activity compared with that of normal liver.

Accuracy

Tc-99m RBC scintigraphy has a positive predictive value approaching 100%. False-positive studies are rare. Sensitivity and false negatives depend primarily on lesion size and the methodology used. The sensitivity for planar imaging is 55% and SPECT 88%. Lesion

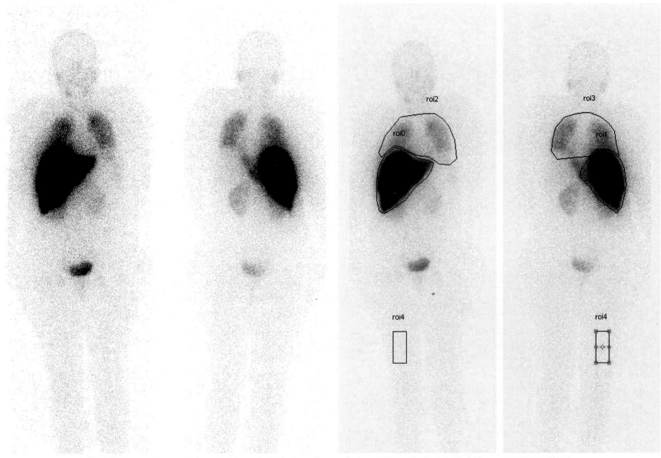

Fig. 9.37 Hepatic shunting to the lung. Calculation of percent lung shunt. Patient with colon cancer metastatic to the liver, unresponsive to chemotherapy, underwent this study before Theraspheres therapy. Tc-99m macroaggregated albumin (MAA) was injected via a hepatic artery catheter. Whole-body imaging was acquired. Regions of interest (ROIs) were selected for the lungs, liver, and background (thigh). The calculated shunting to the lung was 9%. Scatter from the liver can artificially elevate the shunt percent; thus, the lung ROI should not be immediately adjacent to the hot liver.

TABLE 9.9 Physical Characteristics of Therapeutic Radiolabeled Microspheres

Agent	Radiolabel	Particle Size (microns)	Particle Material	Activity (Bq/particle)
SIR-Sphere	Y-90	Mean 35 Range 20–60	Resin	50
Therasphere	Y-90	Mean 25 Range 20–30	Glass	2500

TABLE 9.10 Yttrium-90 Microsphere Therapy Calculations

Liver Involvement by Tumor (%)	Recommended Y-90 Dose (GBq)
>50	3
25–50	2.5
<25	2

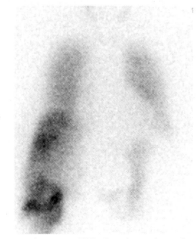

Fig. 9.38 Liver arteriovenous (AV) shunting to lung. Intraarterial administration of Tc-99m macroaggregated albumin (MAA) into the liver for quantification of shunting to the lung. The lung shunt was calculated to be 40%. Thus, therapy with the Ytrium-90-labeled microspheres was cancelled.

size is the main determinant of detectability (Table 9.12). SPECT can visualize most hemangiomas larger than 1.4 cm and may detect some as small as 0.5 cm. SPECT/CT can be helpful for the detection of smaller, centrally located, multiple hemangiomas and those adjacent to the heart, kidney, and spleen (Fig. 9.43). SPECT, contrast CT, and magnetic resonance (MR) have similar accuracy for the diagnosis of cavernous hemangioma (Fig. 9.44).

TABLE 9.11 Yttrium-90 SIR-Sphere Dose Correction Based on Lung Shunting[a]

Hepatopulmonary Shunting (%)	Dose Reduction (%)
<10	0
10–15	20
15–20	40
>20	100

[a]Maximum allowable shunting for Y-90 Therasphere = 10%.

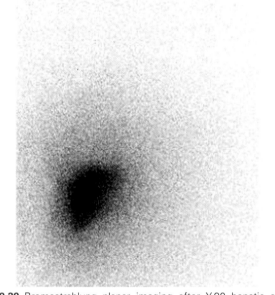

Fig. 9.39 Bremsstrahlung planar imaging after Y-90 hepatic arterial microsphere therapy. This confirmed that therapy was delivered to the whole liver. In some cases, single-photon emission computed tomography (SPECT) or SPECT with computed tomography (SPECT/CT) can be helpful in defining localization of the radiotracer.

Tc-99M SULFUR COLLOID LIVER AND SPLEEN IMAGING

Tc-99m sulfur colloid (SC) liver and spleen imaging was first introduced in 1963 and was the standard clinical method for liver and spleen imaging until the advent of CT in the 1970s. Although not a frequently requested study today, it still has a few important clinical indications.

Mechanism of Localization and Pharmacokinetics

After intravenous injection, the Tc-99m SC particles, 0.1 to 1.0 um in size, are extracted from the blood by Kupffer cells of the liver (85%), macrophages of the spleen (10%) and bone marrow (5%). Tc-99m SC has a blood clearance half-life of 2 to 3 minutes and single-pass liver extraction efficiency of 95%. Uptake is complete by 15 minutes. After phagocytosis, the Tc-99m SC particles are fixed intracellularly.

Kupffer cells line the walls of the liver sinusoids (see Fig. 9.3), make up less than 10% of liver cell mass, and are fixed phagocytic cells. Most liver diseases affect hepatocytes and Kupffer cells similarly, causing local, diffuse, or heterogeneously decreased uptake as a result of the destruction or displacement of normal liver. With severe diffuse liver disease, a generalized reduction in hepatic extraction and increased uptake by the spleen and bone marrow occur (colloid shift). Increased splenic uptake is also seen with immunologically active states.

Clinical Applications

Currently, the clinical role for Tc-99m SC liver and spleen imaging is limited to situations in which the study can provide functional diagnostic information, such as suspected focal nodular hyperplasia, splenosis, cirrhosis, and bone marrow imaging.

Methodology

No patient preparation is required. Four mCi (148 MBq) is the standard adult dose of Tc-99m SC; the pediatric dose is 0.05 mCi/kg (minimal dose 500 µCi). Imaging begins 20 minutes later. Planar static images are obtained in multiple views. SPECT or SPECT/CT is increasingly becoming standard.

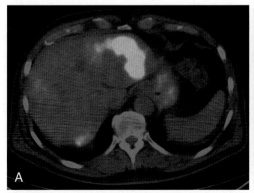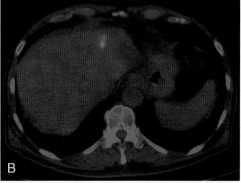

Fig. 9.40 Monitoring response to therapy. F-18 fluorodeoxyglucose (FDG) positron emission tomography (PET)/computed tomography (CT) images of the liver in a patient with unresectable hepatocellular carcinoma (A) before and (B) 1 month after Y-90 Therasphere administration. The patient shows marked improvement.

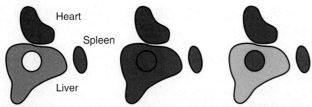

Fig. 9.41 Tc-99m red blood cell (RBC) diagram illustrating radiotracer pharmacokinetics seen with liver hemangioma. *(Left)* Immediately after injection, the hemangioma is "cold." Time is required for the radiolabeled RBCs to equilibrate with the unlabeled RBCs in the blood pool of the hemangioma. *(Middle)* As the Tc-99m-labeled RBCs increasingly enter the hemangioma and mix with the unlabeled cells, activity in the hemangioma equalizes with normal liver. *(Right)*, When fully equilibrated (60–120 minutes), activity within the hemangioma exceeds that in the surrounding liver and is equal to activity in the heart and spleen.

CT, Computed tomography; *RBC,* red blood cell; *SPECT,* single-photon emission computed tomography.

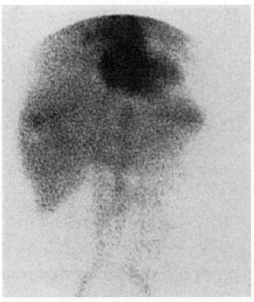 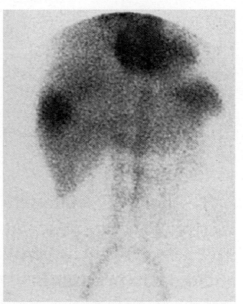

Fig. 9.42 Cavernous hemangioma. *(Left)* Static planar Tc-99m red blood cell (RBC) postflow immediate image. The lesion in the right lobe is partly cold but to a great extent showing early filling. *(Right)* Delayed image at 2 hours shows increased activity in the lesion compared with background liver, equal to heart blood pool.

Image Interpretation

Abnormal scintigraphic findings include hepatomegaly, heterogeneity of distribution, splenomegaly, colloid shift, focal defects, and focal increased uptake. Hepatomegaly suggests acute hepatic dysfunction or an infiltrating process. Splenic uptake on the posterior view is normally equal to or less than that of the liver. Colloid shift (increased splenic uptake compared with the liver) occurs in some hepatic diseases, particularly cirrhosis

(Fig. 9.45). A posterior spleen-to-liver count ratio > 1.5 is abnormal.

Liver Diseases
Decreased Uptake

Most benign and malignant lesions of the liver produce cold or "photopenic" defects on Tc-99m SC liver imaging (Fig. 9.46). Radiation therapy produces a characteristic rectangular

TABLE 9.12 Sensitivity for Hemangioma Detection by Lesion Size With Tc-99m RBC SPECT	
Lesion (cm)	Sensitivity (%)
>1.4	100
>1.3	91
1.0–2.0	65
0.9–1.3	33
0.5–0.9	20

RBC, Red blood cell; *SPECT,* single-photon emission computed tomography.

port-shaped hepatic defect. Diffusely decreased uptake is usually caused by hepatocellular disease or infiltrating tumor. With increasing severity and chronicity of cirrhotic liver disease, the right lobe of the liver shrinks; the left lobe and caudate compensates with hypertrophy, and colloid shift becomes marked due to portal hypertension.

Increased Uptake

Increased hepatic uptake on Tc-99m SC imaging is uncommon but quite characteristic for specific pathological conditions (Box 9.18).

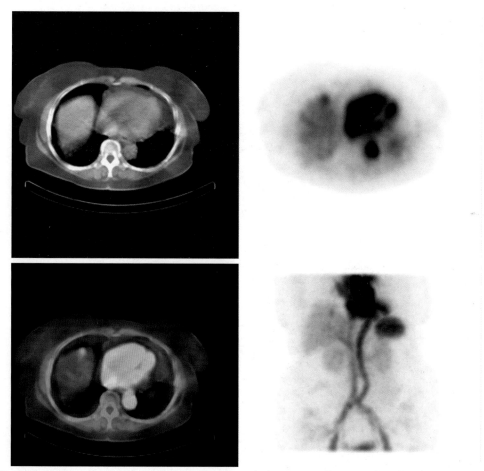

Fig. 9.43 Tc-99m red blood cell (RBC) single-photon emission computed tomography with computed tomography (SPECT/CT) of cavernous hemangioma. Small focus of mildly increased Tc-99m RBCs in the dome of the liver on the maximal-intensity projection (MIP) image *(bottom right).* Small hypodense lesion seen on CT *(left upper).* SPECT *(upper right)* shows increased focal uptake in anterior aspect of the dome of the liver. The fused SPECT/CT transverse image helps confirm the cavernous hemangioma.

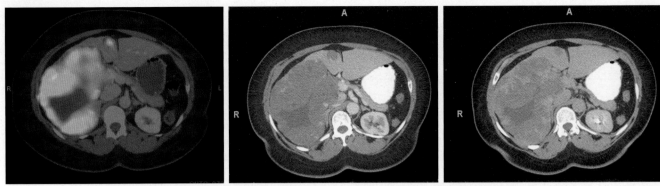

Fig. 9.44 Tc-99m red blood cell (RBC) single-photon emission computed tomography with computed tomography (SPECT/CT) study versus contrast CT. Both SPECT *(left)* and early and delayed contrast CT *(right)* confirm the diagnosis of cavernous hemangioma.

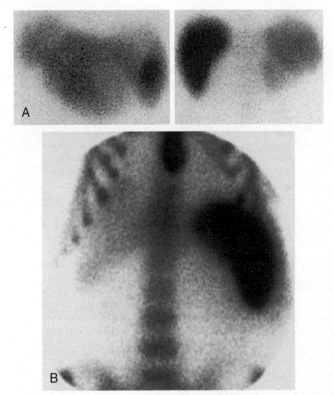

Fig. 9.45 Hepatic parenchymal disease with Tc-99m sulfur colloid. (A) A 52-year-old man with hyperpigmentation and biopsy-proved hemochromatosis. Anterior *(left)* and posterior *(right)* views show small right lobe, hypertrophied left lobe, large spleen, and colloid shift. (B) Severe cirrhotic liver disease. Anterior view shows very small liver with poor uptake, enlarged spleen, and prominent colloid shift to the marrow and spleen.

Superior Vena Cava Obstruction

Collateral thoracic and abdominal wall vessels communicate with the recanalized umbilical vein delivering Tc-99m SC via the left portal vein to the region of the quadrate lobe. Thus, relatively more concentrated Tc-99m SC is delivered to that region compared with the remainder of the liver, producing a hot spot (Fig. 9.47). This same phenomenon can be seen on FDG PET and Tc-99m MAA lung perfusion studies. Injection in the lower extremity rather than the upper extremity results in a normal scan (see Fig. 9.47).

Focal Nodular Hyperplasia

FNH results in increased Tc-99m SC uptake because of the vascular nature of the tumor and increased density of functioning Kupffer cells. This tumor has all three hepatic cell types. Tc-99m SC uptake occurs in two-thirds of patients with FNH (one-third with increased uptake and one-third with normal uptake; Fig. 9.48). Another third are cold, for unclear reasons. Hepatic adenoma is usually cold, comprising only hepatocytes.

BOX 9.18   Causes of Increased Focal Liver Uptake on Tc-99m SC Imaging

Superior vena cava syndrome (arm injection)
Inferior vena cava obstruction (leg injection)
Focal nodular hyperplasia
Budd–Chiari syndrome
Regenerating nodule in cirrhosis

SC, Sulfur colloid.

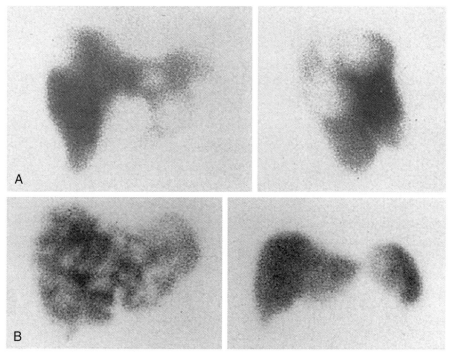

Fig. 9.46 Colon cancer metastases on Tc-99m sulfur colloid (SC) scan. (A) Anterior and right lateral views show large metastases in the right and left lobes. (B) In a different patient, extensive liver metastases are seen on initial Tc-99m SC study *(left),* but good response to therapy is seen on follow-up study 4 months later *(right).*

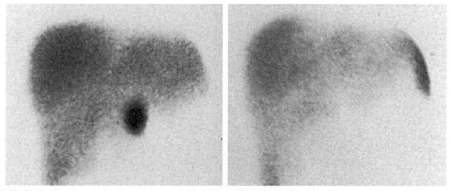

Fig. 9.47 Superior vena cava syndrome. *(Left)* Tc-99m sulfur colloid (SC) liver and spleen scan in a patient with lung cancer. Focal increased uptake in the region of the quadrate lobe. Radiotracer was injected in the arm. *(Right)* A repeat study with radiotracer injected in lower extremity shows no abnormal uptake.

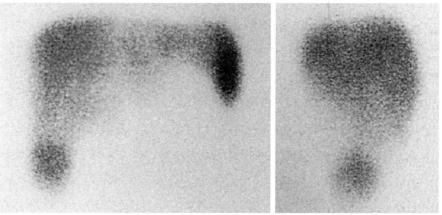

Fig. 9.48 Focal nodular hyperplasia. Tc-99m sulfur colloid (SC) study (anterior *[left]* and right lateral *[right]*) shows increased uptake in the inferior aspect of the right lobe of liver. Angiography confirmed the diagnosis of focal nodular hyperplasia (FNH).

Budd-Chiari Syndrome

Hepatic vein thrombosis is characterized by relatively more uptake in the caudate lobe than the remainder of the liver. The impaired venous drainage of most of the liver results in poor hepatic function. The caudate lobe retains good function because of its direct venous drainage into the inferior vena cava.

SPLENIC SCINTIGRAPHY

The spleen serves as a reservoir for formed blood elements, as a site for clearance of microorganisms and particle trapping, as a potential site of hematopoiesis during bone marrow failure, and as a source of humoral or cellular response to foreign antigens. It plays a role in leukocyte production, contributes to platelet processing, and has immunological functions.

Tc-99m SC can confirm splenic remnants, accessory spleens, splenosis, splenules, polysplenia-asplenia syndromes, and splenic infarction. Imaging with heat or chemically damaged Tc-99m RBCs is occasionally useful to detect accessory spleens or splenosis immediately adjacent to the liver (Fig. 9.49). However, with Tc-99m SC SPECT and SPECT/CT, damaged RBCs are rarely needed (Fig. 9.50). Nonvisualization of the spleen may result from congenital absence, from acquired functional asplenia caused by interruption of the blood supply (splenic artery occlusion), or secondary to reticuloendothelial system (RES) dysfunction (sickle cell crisis). Asplenia may be irreversible (Thorotrast irradiation, chemotherapy, amyloid) or functionally reversible (sickle cell crisis). With sickle cell, there is discordance between RES function and other splenic functions.

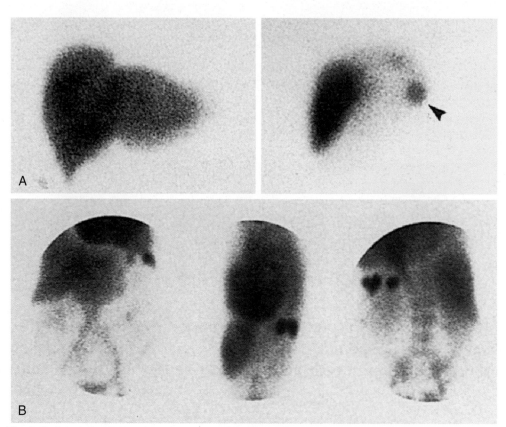

Fig. 9.49 Splenosis. (A) Tc-99m sulfur colloid (SC) with splenic remnant postsplenectomy, seen in the left lateral view *(arrowhead)*. (B) Chemically damaged Tc-99m red blood cells (RBCs). Auto-transplantation of splenic tissue after trauma and splenectomy. Multiple foci of uptake in the left upper quadrant consistent with splenosis (anterior, left lateral, posterior views).

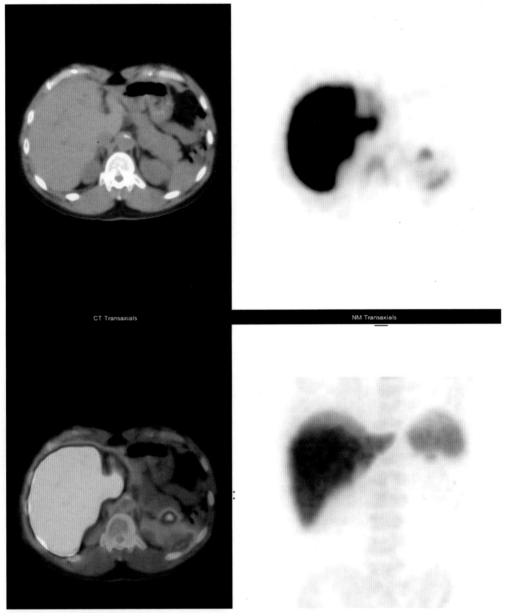

Fig. 9.50 Splenic tissue in tail of pancreas. Patient with prostate cancer and known metastases had a computed tomography (CT) scan that showed a soft tissue density mass in the tail of the pancreas with attenuation similar to that of the spleen. The Tc-99m sulfur colloid (SC) single-photon emission computed tomography with computed tomography (SPECT/CT) scan confirms that it is splenic tissue. This is best seen on the fused SPECT/CT image but can also be seen in the maximal-intensity projection (MIP) image just below the spleen.

SUGGESTED READING

Bozkurt MF, Salanci BV, Ugur O. Intra-arterial radionuclide therapies for liver tumors. *Semin Nucl Med*. 2016;46:324–339.

Choy D, Shi EC, McLean RG, et al. Cholescintigraphy in acute cholecystitis: use of intravenous morphine. *Radiology*. 1984;151:203–207.

DiBaise JK, Richmond BK, Ziessman HA, et al. Cholecystokinin-cholescintigraphy in adults: consensus recommendations of an interdisciplinary panel. *Clin Nucl Med*. 2012;37:63–70.

Fig LM, Stewart RE, Wahl RL. Morphine-augmented hepatobiliary scintigraphy in the severely ill: caution is in order. *Radiology*. 1990;175:473–476.

Kwatra N, Shalaby-Rana E, Narayanan S, et al. Phenobarbital-enhanced hepatobiliary scintigraphy in the diagnosis of biliary atresia: two decades of experience at a tertiary care center. *Pediatr Radiol*. 2013;43:1365–1375.

Sostre S, Kaloo AN, Spiegler EJ, et al. A noninvasive test of sphincter of Oddi dysfunction in post-cholecystectomy patients: the scintigraphic score. *J Nucl Med*. 1992;33:1216–1222.

Yap L, Wycherley AG, Morphett AD, Toouli J. Acalculous biliary pain: cholecystectomy alleviates symptoms in patients with abnormal cholescintigraphy. *Gastroenterology*. 1991;101:786–793.

Ziessman HA. Hepatobiliary scintigraphy—2014. *J Nucl Med*. 2014;55:967–975.

Ziessman HA. Sincalide Cholescintigraphy—32 years later: evidence-based data on its clinical utility and infusion methodology. *Semin Nucl Med*. 2012;42:79–83.

Ziessman HA, Tulchinsky M, Lavely WC, et al. Sincalide-stimulated cholescintigraphy: a multicenter investigation to determine optimal methodology and gallbladder ejection fraction normal values. *J Nucl Med*. 2010;51:229–236.

10

Gastrointestinal System

Janis M. O'Malley, Harvey Ziessman

The use of a radionuclide to measure gastric transit was first described in 1966. Radionuclide gastric emptying scintigraphy has long been the standard methodology for measuring gastric transit. In this section, the recommended standardized gastric emptying protocol is described in some detail, followed by a discussion of esophageal and intestinal transit (Fig. 10.1). Other topics include gastrointestinal bleeding, Meckel, peritoneal, and salivary gland scans.

GASTROINTESTINAL TRANSIT SCINTIGRAPHY

Gastric Emptying

The radionuclide gastric-emptying study is the accepted standard methodology used to measure gastric transit. It is physiological, quantitative, accurate, and reproducible. An upper gastrointestinal contrast study can detect a gross delay in gastric emptying, but it is not sensitive for the detection of less severe but symptomatic gastroparesis. Other methodologies have been proposed and investigated, most recently the wireless motility capsule; however, all have issues, and none has found routine clinical use. However, the radionuclide study cannot differentiate a severe functional delay from anatomical obstruction, such as a tumor or pyloric channel ulcer. Endoscopy or contrast barium radiography is required for that purpose.

Patients with delayed gastric emptying (gastroparesis) present clinically with symptoms of postprandial nausea, vomiting, and abdominal pain. Some of the clinical indications for the radionuclide gastric emptying study are listed (Box 10.1). Rapid gastric emptying is less common than delayed. Patients may present with similar symptoms, although more commonly postprandial abdominal cramps, diarrhea, flushing, and tachycardia (dumping syndrome).

Anatomy and Physiology

The regions are designated from proximal to distal as cardia, fundus, body, antrum, and pylorus (Fig. 10.2). Gastric mucosal glands secrete hydrochloric acid and digestive enzymes. Gastric motility is controlled by both neuromuscular gastric activity and small intestinal neuroendocrine feedback.

The gastric fundus and antrum have distinct functions. The more proximal fundus acts as a reservoir, accepting large meals with only a minimal increase in pressure (receptive relaxation and accommodation). Fundal tonic contractions produce a constant pressure gradient between the stomach and pylorus, resulting in liquid emptying. The more distal antrum has phasic contractions initiated by a neural pacemaker. Muscular contractions sweep down the antrum in a ring-like pattern,

squeezing food toward the pylorus. Larger food particles are not allowed to pass and are retropelled. The solid material is converted into chyme through contact with acid and peptic enzymes and mechanical grinding. Food particles must be broken down until they are small enough to pass through the pyloric sphincter (1–2 mm). The antrum is responsible for solid emptying. The pylorus, at the junction of the antrum and duodenal bulb, acts as a sieve, regulating gastric outflow (Fig. 10.3).

The pattern of emptying for solid and liquid meals is different. Solids have a delay before emptying begins (lag phase) lasting 5 to 25 minutes. This is the time required to grind the food into small enough particles so that they can pass through the pylorus. Following the lag phase, solids empty in a relatively linear pattern (Fig. 10.4). The rate of emptying depends on the size and contents of the meal. Meals with greater volume, weight, carbohydrates, protein, or fat empty slower (Box 10.2). Liquids have no delay before emptying begins.

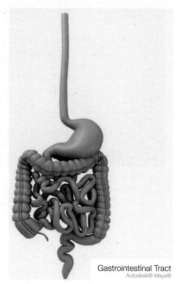

Gastrointestinal Tract
Autodesk® Maya®

Fig. 10.1 Diagram of gastrointestinal tract from esophagus through rectum.

BOX 10.1 Clinical Indications for Radionuclide Gastric-Emptying Study

Insulin-dependent diabetics with persistent postprandial symptoms
Diabetics with poor blood glucose control
Nonulcer dyspepsia
Unexplained postprandial nausea, vomiting, and abdominal pain
Severe reflux esophagitis
To assess response to a motility drug

Clear liquids empty in a monoexponential pattern (Fig. 10.5A and B). Full liquids and clear liquids ingested simultaneously with a solid meal empty in a slower multiexponential pattern.

Gastric Stasis Syndromes

The majority of patients with chronic gastroparesis have a functional cause; that is, there is no known pathological etiology. An exception is diabetic gastroenteropathy, which occurs in patients with long-standing insulin-dependent diabetes. Here gastroparesis is caused by vagal nerve damage as part of a generalized autonomic neuropathy. In addition to producing disagreeable postprandial symptoms, the delay in emptying may exacerbate the problem of diabetic glucose control because the timing of the insulin dose with food ingestion and absorption may be

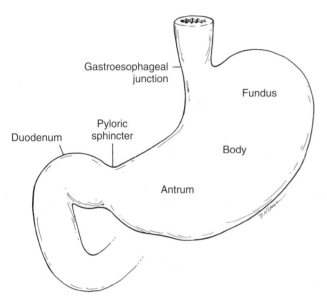

Fig. 10.2 Gastric anatomy. The proximal stomach (fundus) undergoes receptive relaxation and accommodation of ingested food. Its tonic contraction is responsible for liquid emptying. The distal stomach (antrum) is responsible for solid emptying. It has phasic contractions that mix and grind food into small enough particles to pass through the pylorus.

unpredictable. A common gastric disorder is nonulcer dyspepsia, characterized by ulcer-like or dyspeptic symptoms. It is reported that gastroparesis occurs in 20% to 40% of these patients.

Most patients with gastroparesis have a chronic problem with delayed emptying. However, some have acute and potentially reversible causes (e.g., due to viral gastroenteritis, trauma, metabolic derangements). Common causes of and associations with chronic and acute gastric stasis syndromes are listed in Box 10.3. Rapid gastric emptying is most commonly seen in patients who have had gastric surgery (e.g., pyloroplasty or gastrectomy), in patients with hyperthyroidism, or in those with a gastrinoma producing large amounts of the hormone gastrin (Zollinger–Ellison syndrome). A minority of patients with insulin-dependent diabetes have rapid gastric emptying (Box 10.4), with symptoms of palpitations, diaphoresis, weakness, and diarrhea.

Patient Preparation

Hyperglycemia per se, independent of diabetic gastroenteropathy, may cause a delay in gastric emptying. Thus, gastric-emptying studies should be performed when patients are under good diabetic control, with a fasting blood preferably <250 mg/dL. Also, many commonly used nongastric therapeutic drugs can delay gastric emptying (Table 10.1). In our clinic, we allow the referring physician to decide whether the patient should continue to take his or her medications before the study. This will depend on the study indication (e.g., whether to make the diagnosis of gastroparesis or to determine whether a specific therapeutic drug has been effective). When indicated, the drugs should be stopped 48 to 72 hours before the study. Medications taken should be considered when interpreting the study.

Therapy of Gastroparesis

Metoclopramide (Reglan) is the most common therapeutic drug prescribed for delayed gastric emptying. It is not effective in all patients, symptom relief is not always accompanied by an improvement in gastric emptying, and serious side effects may occur in some patients (e.g., tardive dyskinesia seen in 10% of

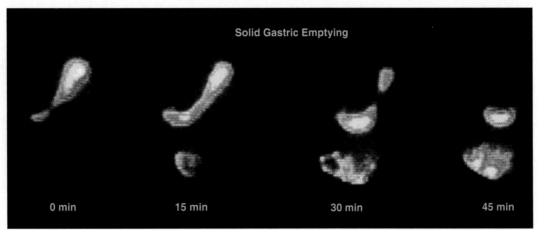

Fig. 10.3 Solid gastric emptying. Four selected images, from left to right, at time 0, 15 minutes, 30 minutes, and 60 minutes. Initially, the solid meal resides in the fundus; then it moves into the antrum, where it is ground up to a small enough size to pass through the pylorus into the small intestines.

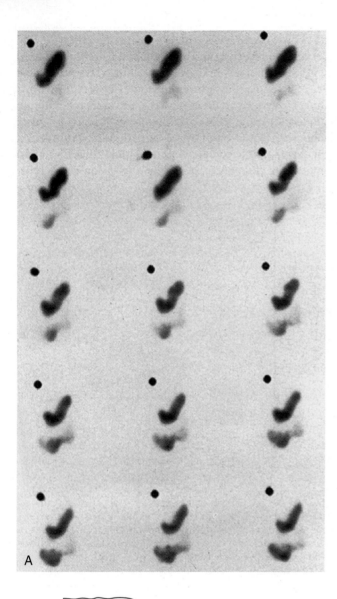

A

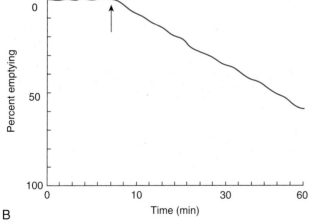

B

Fig. 10.4 Biphasic pattern of solid emptying. (A) Sequential solid gastric-emptying images over initial 60 minutes. The ingested meal moves normally from the gastric fundus to the antrum and then begins to clear into the small intestines. (B) Time–activity curve for the patient generated by a region of interest (ROI) around the stomach shows a biphasic pattern of solid gastric emptying. An initial delay (lag phase) of 9 minutes is seen before emptying begins. Emptying clears the stomach in a linear pattern for the remainder of the 60-minute study.

patients taking the drug for longer than 3 months). Domperidone (Motilium), used in Europe, is not approved for clinical use in the United States. Cisapride (Propulsid) was removed from the U.S. market due to serious arrhythmias. Erythromycin, a motilin agonist, improves gastric motility; however, it has a high incidence of nausea and vomiting. Analogs of erythromycin as well as other potential therapeutic drugs are in development. Surgical intervention is sometimes used to treat refractory gastroparesis. One approach is implantation of an electrical gastric stimulator. In patients who are not responsive to standard therapies, gastric resection may be indicated.

Radiopharmaceuticals

For accurate and reproducible quantification of solid gastric emptying, the radionuclide must be tightly bound to the solid component of the meal. Elution of the radiolabel results in a part-solid, part-liquid labeled mixture and may be quantitatively unreliable. Radiolabeled eggs are most commonly used for solid gastric-emptying studies. Tc-99m sulfur colloid (Tc-99m SC) binds to albumen in egg white during cooking. Although whole eggs work well for gastric emptying, egg whites have higher percent binding. Tc-99m SC remains stable in the acidic stomach and is not absorbed by the gastrointestinal (GI) tract.

For liquid meals, the radiotracer must equilibrate rapidly within the liquid and be nonabsorbable in the gastrointestinal tract. Tc-99m- or In-111-labeled diethylenetriaminepentaacetic acid (DTPA) and Tc-99m SC meet these criteria. Dual-phase solid-liquid studies use one radiotracer for the solid meal and another for the liquid phase, for example, In-111 DTPA as the liquid marker (171, 247 keV) and Tc-99m SC (140 keV) as the solid marker (Fig. 10.6). They are differentiated by their separate photopeaks.

Standardization of Solid Gastric-Emptying Scintigraphy

Various methodologies have been used over the years for solid gastric-emptying studies, including different meals, patient positioning, instrumentation, framing rate, and study length as well as quantitative methods. All of these factors may affect normal values. Thus, normal values must be well

---

BOX 10.2   Factors Other Than Medications That Affect the Rate of Gastric Emptying

Meal content
Fat, protein, acid, osmolality
    Volume
    Weight
    Caloric density
    Particle size
Time of day
Patient position (standing, sitting, supine)
Gender
Metabolic state
Stress
Exercise

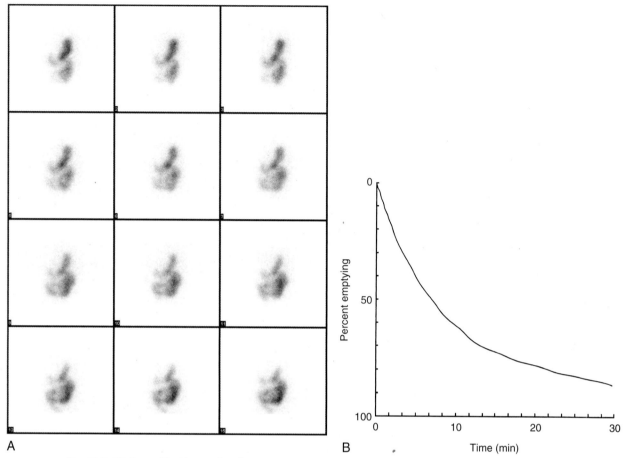

A

B

Fig. 10.5 (A) Normal liquid emptying. Sequential 1-minute images of a 30-minute study after ingestion of 300 mL water with 100 μCi Tc-99m diethylenetriaminepentaacetic acid (DTPA). Distribution is uniform in the stomach throughout the study. Hot spot in lower portion of the stomach in second row of images is due to overlap with small bowel activity. (B) Time–activity curve was generated by drawing a whole-stomach region of interest (ROI). Emptying begins immediately. The clearance pattern is monoexponential, with a half-emptying time of 15 minutes (normal <25).

validated for the specific meal and methodology used. In the past, gastroenterologists have expressed concern about the different methodologies and different normal values. They advocated for a standardized gastric emptying protocol.

Standardized Solid Gastric-Emptying Study

In 2008, an expert panel of gastroenterologists and nuclear medicine physicians published Consensus Recommendations for Radionuclide Gastric Emptying. The recommendations were based on a protocol published by Tougas and colleagues in 2000 and are described in detail in Box 10.5. The protocol was selected because it simplified the procedure and because the normal values were considered valid based on the large number of normal subjects studied (123). The meal consists of an egg-substitute sandwich (4 oz egg white, equivalent to 2 whole eggs, 2 slices of bread), strawberry jam (30 g), and water (120 mL). The study requires 1-minute anterior and posterior images acquired at four time points (immediately after meal ingestion and at 1, 2, and 4 hours) and calculation of the percent gastric retention at each time point (Figs. 10.7–10.9).

The Tougas and colleagues publication found that infrequent imaging (each hour) was as accurate as more frequent imaging (e.g., every 10 minutes). The rationale for a 4-hour study length was based on several publications reporting a higher rate of detection of gastroparesis at 4 hours compared with 2 hours. One investigation reported that by extending the study from 2 to 4 hours, the number of patients diagnosed with gastroparesis increased by 30%. Widespread use of this protocol ensures that results are comparable between institutions. Although a 4-hour study length might at first seem demanding of clinic logistics, the standardized protocol can actually improve patient flow. Multiple patients can be studied on one camera in a single morning because total imaging time per patient is short.

Interpretation of Solid Gastric-Emptying Studies

A standardized gastric-emptying study is considered normal if the 2-hour retention value is <60% retention (>40% emptying) and the 4-hour value is <10% retention (>90% emptying; see Fig. 10.7). The Tougas protocol used "percent retention" for the normal values. This textbook prefers "gastric emptying." Normal values are based on ingestion of the entire meal. Ingestion of a smaller volume or less eggs, bread, jam, or water will likely result in more rapid emptying than if the entire meal was ingested. Normal values have not been published for partial

BOX 10.3   Gastric Stasis Syndromes—Causes and Associations

Acute Gastroparesis—Potentially Reversible
Trauma
Postoperative ileus
Acute viral infections (e.g., gastroenteritis)
Hyperalimentation
Metabolic: Hyperglycemia, acidosis, uremia, hypokalemia, hypercalcemia, hepatic coma, myxedema
Physiological: Labyrinth stimulation, physical and mental stress, gastric distention, increased intragastric pressure
Hormone increases: Gastrin, secretin, glucagon, cholecystokinin, somatostatin, estrogen, progesterone

Chronic Gastroparesis
Anatomical
Gastric ulcer
Surgery, vagotomy
Pyloric hypertrophy
Postradiotherapy
Tumors
Diabetic gastroenteropathy
Functional
 Nonulcer dyspepsia
 Dermatomyositis
 Systemic lupus erythematosus
 Amyloidosis
 Hypothyroidism
 Familial dysautonomia
 Pernicious anemia
 Tumor-associated gastroparesis
 Progressive systemic sclerosis
 Fabry disease

BOX 10.4   Rapid Gastric Emptying—Causes

Prior surgery
Pyloroplasty
Hemigastrectomy (Billroth I, II)
Diseases
 Duodenal ulcer
 Gastrinoma (Zollinger–Ellison syndrome)
 Hyperthyroidism
 Diabetics (subgroup)
Hormones
 Thyroxine
 Motilin
 Enterogastrone

TABLE 10.1   Drugs That Delay Gastric Emptying

Drug Type	Specific Drugs
Cardiovascular	Calcium channel blockers (e.g., nifedipine) Beta-adrenergic antagonists (e.g., propanolol)
Respiratory	Isoproterenol, theophylline
Gastrointestinal	Sucralfate, anticholinergics, tegaserod
Reproductive	Progesterone, oral contraceptives
Neuropsychiatric	Valium, Librium, Librax, Ativan, tricyclic antidepressants, levodopa Phenothiazines (e.g., Thorazine)
Opiates	OxyContin, Percodan, Percocet
Alcohol and nicotine	

>90% emptying. Rapid emptying has been defined as >70% emptying at 1 hour (see Fig. 10.9).

Two published large investigations have now reported that the solid gastric-emptying study can be stopped at 2 hours in >50% of patients because the 2-hour emptying value can predict 4-hour emptying in those patients. If 2-hour gastric emptying is <35%, the study can be interpreted as delayed emptying and stopped. If there is >55% emptying, it can be interpreted as normal with high accuracy and the study discontinued. If emptying is between those two values, the study must be continued to 4 hours. The disadvantage of stopping early is that it may be more difficult to compare subsequent follow-up studies.

Alternative Solid Meals

Some patients cannot eat eggs for dietary or allergic reasons. Limited data exist regarding normal values for alternative meals. One small published study found that EnsurePlus (8 oz) had normal values that did not differ significantly from the standardized meal, in spite of the fact that it is a full liquid meal. A few other meals have been reported with established normal values, but their contents and use are often unique to their country of origin. One alternative meal with well-established published normal values is a clear liquid-meal, described in the following section. It can be used when the patient cannot ingest the standard meal or EnsurePlus.

Liquid Gastric Emptying

Accepted teaching had long been that liquid gastric-emptying studies were less sensitive for the detection of gastroparesis than solid studies, that liquids become abnormal only in late stages of gastroparesis, and that only a solid gastric-emptying study is necessary for clinical purposes. However, no data had been published to support this, and it has recently proven to be incorrect.

Two publications of 140 patients have compared clear-liquid (water)-only emptying with the standardized solid gastric-emptying meal in patients referred for suspected gastroparesis. More patients had abnormal liquid than solid emptying. The most important finding was that 25% of patients who had a normal solid study had delayed liquid emptying. The pathophysiologic explanation for these findings is unclear; however, it may help explain the patient's symptoms. Many of our patients are referred for both studies.

meal ingestion. Thus, if a patient cannot ingest the whole meal, a statement should be added to the interpretation (e.g., "Because the patient did not ingest the entire meal, the study likely overestimates the rate of gastric emptying").

Delayed emptying may occur at both 2 and 4 hours, only at 2 hours, or only at 4 hours. All these patterns are abnormal and may be causing the patient's symptoms. The study can be discontinued early (e.g., 2 hours) if the 4-hour normal values have been achieved. Some clinics obtain a 3-hour image for this same reason, potentially stopping the study early if there has been

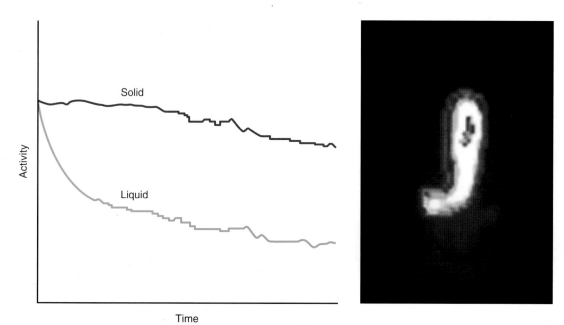

Fig. 10.6 Dual-isotope, dual-phase solid–liquid emptying. Simultaneously ingested solid and liquid meals. The solid egg meal is labeled with Tc-99m sulfur colloid (SC), and the liquid (water) meal is mixed with In-111 diethylenetriaminepentaacetic acid (DTPA). One-minute images were acquired. Time–activity curves were generated by drawing regions of interest (ROIs) around the stomach. The solid and liquid meals are distinguished by their different photopeaks. This study shows very delayed solid emptying but normal liquid emptying.

BOX 10.5   Standardized Gastric-Emptying Scintigraphy: Summary Protocol

Patient Preparation

The referring physician should decide which medications are to be continued/discontinued before the study.

For diabetics, a fasting blood sugar (FBS) is recommended before the study. The study should not be performed if the FBS is >250 mg/dL.

Begin the study in the morning after an overnight fast. The patient should be NPO for at least 6 hours before study.

Radiopharmaceutical and Meal

Tc-99m SC 1 mCi (37 MBq) bound to 4 oz egg substitute (Egg-Beaters or generic egg-white equivalent) by microwaving or scrambling after mixing egg with Tc-99m SC. Stir once or twice while cooking until mixture reaches consistency of omelet. Meal also consists of two slices of white bread, strawberry jam (30 g), and water (120 mL).

Meal should be ingested within 10 to 15 minutes.

Instrumentation

Gamma camera: Large-field-of-view, dual-detector camera

Collimator: Low energy, parallel hole, high resolution or general purpose

Tc-99m photopeak with a 20% window around 140 keV photopeak

Computer setup: 1-minute frames (128 × 128 word mode matrix)

Patient Position

Position patient either standing upright or lying supine, with camera heads anterior and posterior. A single-head camera can be used, acquiring an image first anteriorly, then posteriorly.

Imaging Procedure

Acquire 1-minute frames at time 0 (immediately after ingestion) and 1, 2, and 4 hours; 3-hour images are optional.

Processing

Draw region of interest for anterior and posterior stomach views.

The geometrical mean of the anterior and posterior views is determined at each time point. The percent retention or gastric emptying is calculated at each imaging time point.

Decay correction is mandatory.

Interpretation

Delayed gastric emptying:

    1 hour <10% emptying (>90% retention)

    2 hours <40% emptying (>60% retention)

    4 hours <90% emptying (>10% retention)

Rapid gastric emptying:

    >70% emptying at 1 hour

    >90% emptying at 2 hours

    These values apply to the entire meal and are not valid for different meals or incomplete ingestion of the standard meal.

NPO, Nil per os; *SC,* sulfur colloid.

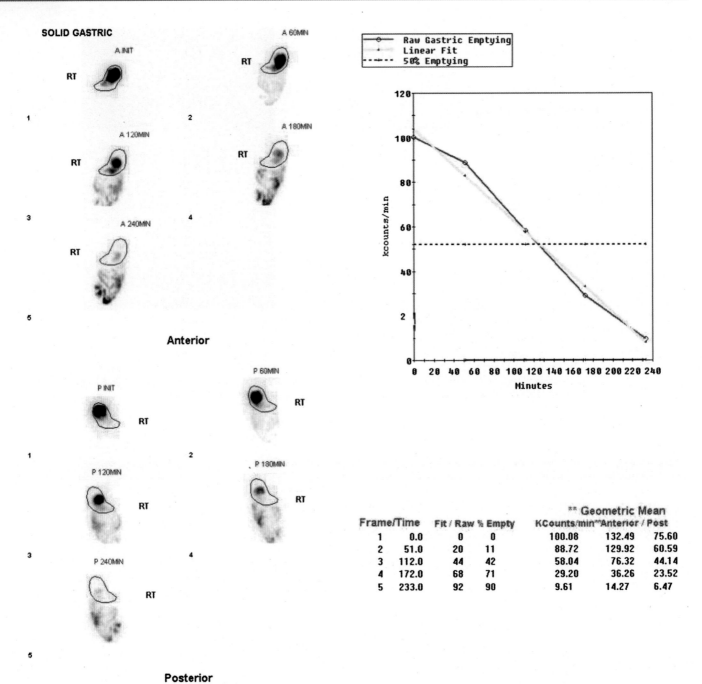

Fig. 10.7 Normal solid gastric emptying using the standardized Tougas and colleagues protocol. *(Left)* Anterior *(above)* and posterior *(lower)* images acquired simultaneously at time 0, 1, 2, 3, and 4 hours. Three-hour images are not required. Regions of interest are drawn around the stomach. *(Right)* Time–activity curve and results *(below)*. The percent geometrical-mean-corrected gastric emptying result at 2 hours (112 minutes) is 44% (normal >40%), and at 4 hours (233 minutes), it is 90% (normal >90%).

The methodology for clear-liquid-only studies is detailed in Box 10.6. Because water empties rapidly, only a 30-minute study is required (1-minute framing rate). Imaging begins immediately after ingestion of the 300 mL water containing 1 mCi Tc-99m DTPA or Tc-99m SC. Alternatively, the liquid and solid studies can be performed sequentially on the same day, the clear liquid first with In-111 DTPA, followed by the solid study labeled with Tc-99m SC. Simultaneous evaluation of liquid and solid gastric emptying is possible and done at some institutions using a dual-isotope acquisition technique (Fig. 10.10). Liquids radiolabeled with In-111 and ingested simultaneously with the standardized Tc-99m-labeled solid meal empty slower than liquid-only meals. The results of liquid-only and simultaneously ingested liquids and solids correlate poorly and likely provide different pathophysiologic information, although at present the reason is uncertain. However, if abnormal, either may explain the patient's symptoms.

Quantification of Gastric Emptying

Various methods have been used over the years to quantify gastric-emptying studies. However, investigations have found no clinical advantage to more frequent imaging, other

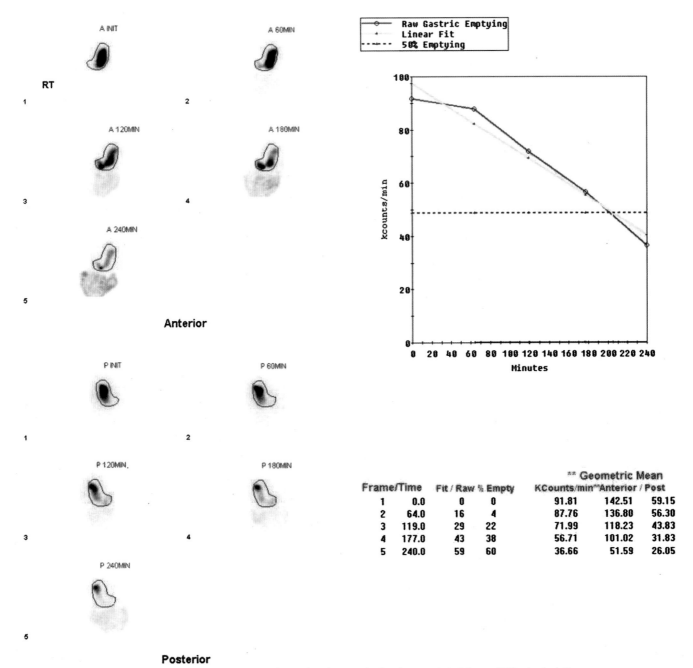

Frame/Time		Fit / Raw % Empty		KCounts/min	** Geometric Mean Anterior / Post	
1	0.0	0	0	91.81	142.51	59.15
2	64.0	16	4	87.76	136.80	56.30
3	119.0	29	22	71.99	118.23	43.83
4	177.0	43	38	56.71	101.02	31.83
5	240.0	59	60	36.66	51.59	26.05

Fig. 10.8 Delayed solid gastric emptying, using the standardized protocol. At 2 hours (119 minutes), the percent gastric emptying is 22% (normal >40%), and it is 60% at 4 hours (240 minutes; normal >90%).

methods of quantification, or calculation of the lag phase. Percent emptying is more accurate than a rate of emptying ($T_{1/2}$) with the standardized methodology because there are only 4 to 5 data points. For the standardized solid gastric-emptying study, a gastric region of interest (ROI) is drawn for all anterior and posterior views at each time point (see Figs. 10.7–10.9). Decay and attenuation correction is required for accurate quantification. The percent emptying is calculated at each time point.

Percent emptying = initial meal counts minus meal counts at 1, 2, and 4 hours, each divided by initial meal counts, and all corrected for attenuation and decay.

Attenuation Correction

Attenuation on gastric-emptying studies varies as the ingested meal transits the stomach because stomach contents move from the relatively posterior fundus to the more anterior antrum. With a single gamma camera detector positioned anteriorly, the counts increase during the early portion of the study in spite of the fact that all the food is already in the stomach from time zero. This results in a quantitative error. Attenuation correction is mandatory for correct results (see Fig. 10.10). Otherwise, there may be an underestimation of emptying, by as much as 10% to 30%. This is most pronounced in obese patients; however, it also occurs in

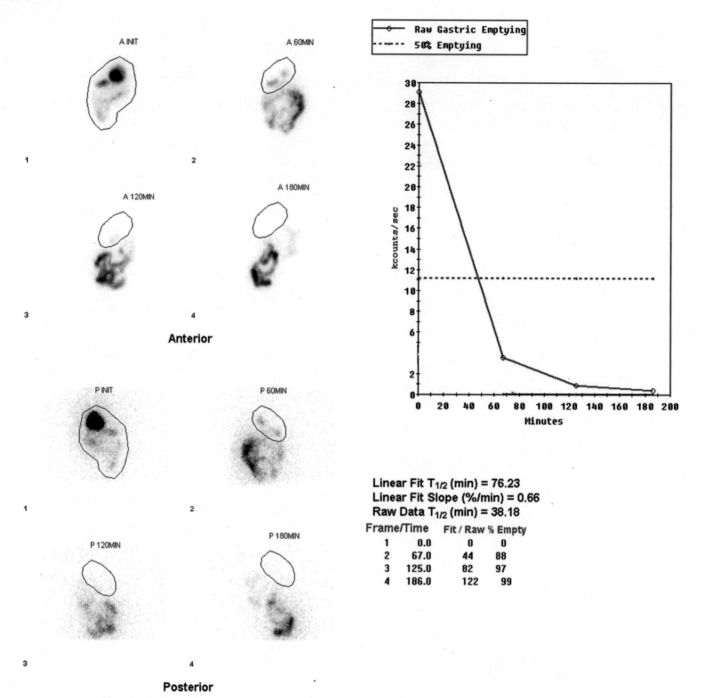

Linear Fit T$_{1/2}$ (min) = 76.23
Linear Fit Slope (%/min) = 0.66
Raw Data T$_{1/2}$ (min) = 38.18

Frame/Time		Fit / Raw % Empty	
1	0.0	0	0
2	67.0	44	88
3	125.0	82	97
4	186.0	122	99

Fig. 10.9 Rapid solid gastric emptying. At 1 hour (67 minutes), solid gastric emptying is 88% (abnormal >70%). We also consider >90% emptying at 2 hours to be rapid. The initial (time 0) region of interest (ROI) includes abdominal activity. Because of the rapid emptying, there was transit to the small bowel by the first image after ingestion. Thus, for accurate calculation of the total ingested radiolabeled meal, the large ROI is required for the initial image.

nonobese patients and is not predictable between patients. The commonly used method for attenuation correction is mathematical and involves calculating the geometrical mean (square result of the product of the anterior and posterior counts) at each time point.

The left anterior oblique projection acquisition method is an alternative approach that minimizes the effect of attenuation. The study is acquired in this one projection. It compensates for attenuation because the head of the gamma camera is roughly parallel to the movement of the stomach contents, and thus the effect of attenuation is minimized (Fig. 10.11). The advantages of this method are that it requires only a single-headed camera, and no mathematical correction is needed. Results correlate well with those of the geometrical mean method, although the geometrical mean is more accurate and preferable whenever possible (Fig. 10.12).

Correction for radioactive decay is mandatory for solid-meal studies because of the short half-life of Tc-99m (6 hours) and

BOX 10.6 Liquid (Water) Gastric Emptying: Summary Protocol

Patient Preparation
Patient must fast for 4 to 6 hours before study.

Radiopharmaceutical and Meal
Tc-99m DTPA or Tc-99m SC, 1 mCi (37 MBq) in 300 mL water

Instrumentation
Gamma camera: Large field of view, dual detector
Collimator: Low energy, parallel hole, high resolution or general purpose
Tc-99m photopeak with a 20% window around 140 keV
Computer setup: 1-minute frames (128 × 128 word mode matrix) × 30

Patient Position
Semiupright (30–45 degrees) on a hospital gurney with the gamma camera placed in the left anterior oblique (LAO) projection (makes it convenient for patient to ingest meal and imaging be started promptly with the camera in the LAO projection)

Imaging Procedure
Have patient swallow radiolabeled water. Immediately after ingestion of the water, acquire 1-minute images for 30 minutes.

Processing
Draw region of interest (ROI) to outline stomach on all images. Correct for decay.
Observe for ROI overlap of the stomach with small intestines. If there is overlap, redraw ROI to exclude overlap.
Calculate a half-time of emptying and exponential $T_{1/2}$.

Interpretation
Normal values: Less than 25 minutes
Use the half-time of emptying and/or exponential fit depending on which best represents the apparent emptying.
DTPA, diethylenetriaminepentaacetic acid; *NPO*, nil per os; *SC*, sulfur colloid.

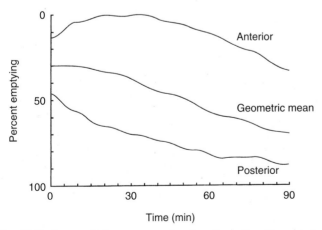

Fig. 10.10 Geometrical mean correction for attenuation. The anterior detector time–activity curve (TAC) shows a rising curve before emptying begins; however, all the food is in the stomach at time 0. The posterior detector curve shows decreasing counts from time 0. The geometrical-mean-corrected curve has a normal pattern with an initial lag phase, then linear emptying.

the relatively long duration of the study (4 hours). Down-scatter (In-111 into the Tc-99m window) and up-scatter (Tc-99m into the In-111 171 keV window) have been shown to be inconsequential if the administered dose ratio of Tc-99m to In-111 is at least 4:1. Therefore, with standard doses of 1 mCi Tc-99m and 100 to 200 μCi In-111, no correction is necessary.

Liquid Gastric Emptying Quantification

Attenuation correction is not necessary for liquid gastric emptying because of its rapid transit. A gastric ROI is drawn, and a half-time of emptying (time in minutes when counts become half of peak counts) and/or an exponential mathematical fit $T_{1/2}$ is calculated (Figs. 10.13 and 10.14). If small bowel activity moves into the ROI, it should be excluded to correct for potential artificial delay. Normal values for a clear-liquid (water) study alone have been well validated, with a half-emptying time of <25 minutes. Adding salt, sugar, and so forth to the clear liquid meal slows the rate of emptying.

Gastric Accommodation

Some patients with symptoms suggestive of gastroparesis are found to have normal emptying. Some of these patients have a problem with gastric accommodation, the ability of the gastric fundus to relax with ingestion of a meal. Direct methods are insufficient and unpleasant for clinical diagnosis. The radionuclide approach is straightforward and simple for the patient. Tc-99m pertechnetate is injected intravenously. Single-photon emission computed tomography (SPECT) of the stomach is acquired. The patient ingests a meal, and then a second SPECT is obtained. The stomach volume is calculated before and after the meal. When ratios are compared with normal values, a diagnosis can be made. This has been a diagnostic test at only a limited number of centers around the world, but interest is increasing at other centers.

ESOPHAGEAL TRANSIT SCINTIGRAPHY

Abnormal esophageal transit usually presents with dysphagia or chest pain and occurs in patients with achalasia, scleroderma, systemic lupus, muscular dystrophy, polymyositis, diffuse esophageal spasm, and so forth. Barium swallow esophagrams can detect mucosal changes and anatomical lesions but provide only a rough qualitative assessment of motility. Manometry measures esophageal pressure, peristalsis, and sphincter contraction/relaxation but not transit (Fig. 10.15). Esophageal transit scintigraphy is a time-proven test with good accuracy, particularly for achalasia and scleroderma. It is most commonly ordered today to screen patients who have a low suspicion of a motility disorder, to avoid invasive manometry, or to evaluate patient response to therapy. Sensitivity is reported to be 92% and specificity 88% for abnormal transit. However, it is not particularly useful in differentiating the underlying cause.

Methodology for Esophageal Transit Scintigraphy

Tc-99m SC or Tc-99m DTPA, 100 to 250 μCi, in 5 mL water is swallowed as a bolus. A clear-liquid protocol is described (Box 10.7). Acquisition in the posterior view allows for

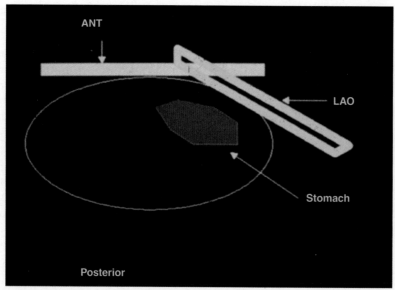

Fig. 10.11 Left anterior oblique (LAO) acquisition—diagram of transverse view. When the camera is placed in the LAO projection, rather than the anterior view, the stomach contents move roughly parallel to the head of the gamma camera, compensating for the effect of varying attenuation. No mathematical correction for attenuation is required. *ANT,* Anterior.

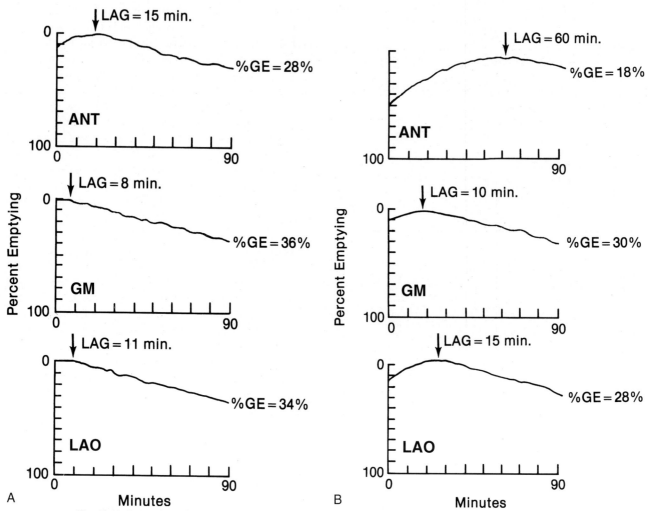

Fig. 10.12 Comparison of lag phase (LAG) and percent emptying (%GE) in two patients (A *[left]* and B *[right]*) using anterior (ANT)-only camera head, geometrical mean (GM), and left anterior oblique (LAO) attenuation correction, from top to bottom. (A) ANT-acquisition time–activity curve (TAC) shows a modest rise in counts over 15 minutes before declining. GM correction of anterior and posterior views *(middle)* results in a shortened lag phase of 8 minutes and greater %GE than the ANT view. LAO uncorrected method *(bottom)* results are very similar to GM method. (B) Different patient. ANT acquisition shows very long lag phase of 60 minutes and slowly rising TAC. GM correction shortens the lag phase considerably, although there is still some initial rise, suggesting incomplete correction *(middle)*. The %GE is improved greatly. The LAO results are similar, although not identical, to the GM.

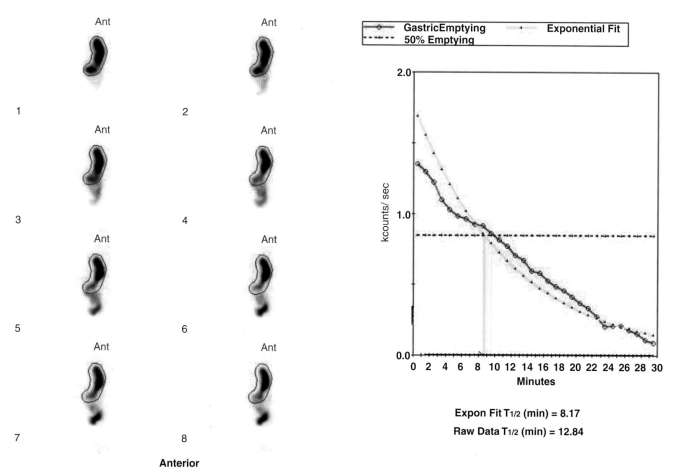

Fig. 10.13 Normal liquid-only (water) gastric emptying. Only the first 8 of 30 1-minute images are shown. A region of interest (ROI) was drawn for the stomach, and a time–activity curve was generated. The half-time of emptying was 12.84 min (normal <25 minutes). The exponential $T_{1/2}$ fit *(yellow line)* was 8.17 minutes. *Expon,* Exponential

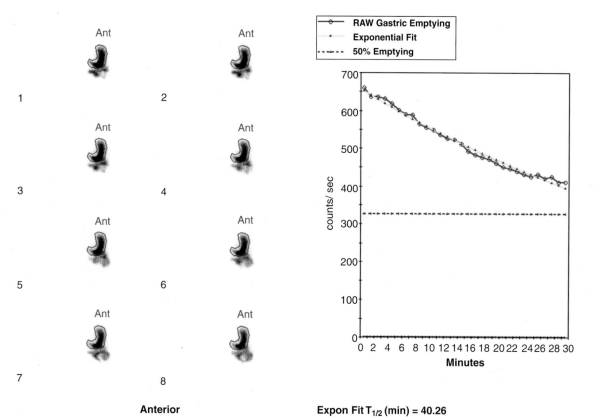

Fig. 10.14 Delayed liquid-only (water) gastric emptying. Only the first 8 of 30 1-minute images are shown. $T_{1/2}$ of >40 minutes is delayed emptying (normal <25). *Expon,* Exponential.

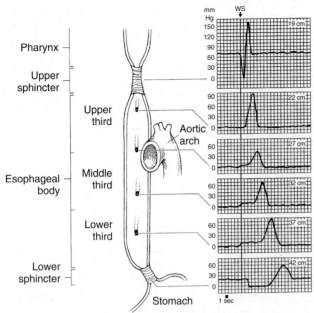

Fig. 10.15 Esophageal motility. Swallowing initiates a coordinated peristaltic contraction that propagates down the esophagus. The esophagus has three regions: the upper esophageal sphincter (UES), which allows food to pass from the mouth to the esophagus and prevents tracheobronchial aspiration; the esophageal body, with striated muscle proximally and smooth muscle distally; and the lower esophageal sphincter (LES), a high-pressure smooth muscle region that prevents gastric reflux but relaxes during swallowing to allow passage of food into the stomach. Shown are manometric pressure changes with a bolus water swallow (WS). After WS, UES pressure falls transiently, then LES pressure falls and remains low until the peristaltic contraction passes aborally through the UES and esophageal body, closing the LES.

BOX 10.7 **Esophageal Transit (Clear Liquid) Scintigraphy: Summary Protocol**

Patient Preparation
Patient should fast overnight.
Place radioactive marker next to cricoid cartilage.
Position the camera posteriorly.
Patient should be standing or supine (must be upright for achalasia).
Practice swallow(s) with nonradioactive bolus.

Radiopharmaceutical
Tc-99m SC or DTPA, 100 to 250 µCi (11 MBq) in 10 mL of water

Instrumentation
Camera setup: Tc-99m 140 keV photopeak with 20% window
Computer setup: 0.5-second frame × 120; byte mode, 64 × 64

Swallowing Procedure
Practice swallow with nonlabeled bolus.
Swallow radiolabeled liquid as a bolus.

Processing and Quantification
Time–activity curves, condensed dynamic images
Calculate
Transit time:
Time of initial esophageal entry until all but 10% of peak clears (abnormal >15 sec)
Percent emptying:
Maximal counts—counts 10 seconds after maximal counts divided by maximal counts before swallow (normal >83%)
DTPA, diethylenetriaminepentaacetic acid; *SC*, sulfur colloid.

---

easier administration of the liquid bolus and closer observation of the patient. The supine position eliminates the effect of gravity on esophageal clearance and thus is thought to be more sensitive for detection. However, in achalasia, gravity is the only emptying mechanism, and thus upright positioning is required for serial studies. Multiple swallows are suggested for complete esophageal emptying and to increase the sensitivity for abnormal transit in mild disease. Limited data suggest that semisolid meals may be more sensitive for detecting esophageal dysmotility; however, data are limited.

Analysis and Quantification

Viewing the individual sequential esophageal swallow images as well as the cinematic display may be adequate for diagnosis of serious transit abnormalities. Quantification, however, is helpful for diagnosis of less severe abnormalities and for comparison of serial studies over time to determine therapeutic effectiveness. Time–activity curves are typically derived for the entire esophagus and for selected regions (e.g., upper, middle, lower; Figs. 10.16–10.18). Esophageal transit has been quantified by calculating either a transit time, percent emptying, or residual in the esophagus at a defined time point. Transit time has been defined as the time from the initial entry of the bolus into the esophagus until all but 10% of peak activity clears (abnormal >15 seconds). Percent emptying has been quantified as maximal counts minus counts 10 sec after maximal counts/maximal counts before swallow (normal >83%).

GASTROESOPHAGEAL REFLUX DISEASE

Gastroesophageal reflux disease (GERD) is a common and sometimes serious medical disorder. In adults, heartburn is the major symptom. Complications include esophagitis, bleeding, perforation, stricture, Barrett esophagus, and cancer. In children, reflux often presents differently, with respiratory symptoms, iron-deficiency anemia, and failure to thrive. Reflux is normal in infants and usually resolves spontaneously by 18 months of age. However, a minority will have persistent symptoms with serious sequelae. Symptomatic disease is more common in patients with an associated esophageal motility disorder, which increases the duration of mucosal exposure to refluxate. Delayed gastric emptying may exacerbate symptoms and inhibit effective therapy.

Diagnosis of GERD

Various tests are used to confirm the diagnosis. Barium esophagography can detect mucosal damage, stricture, and tumor but has low sensitivity for reflux. Endoscopy allows direct visualization of esophageal mucosa and permits biopsy of ulcerations and areas suspicious for malignancy. With the Bernstein acid infusion test, hydrochloric acid (0.1 N) is infused

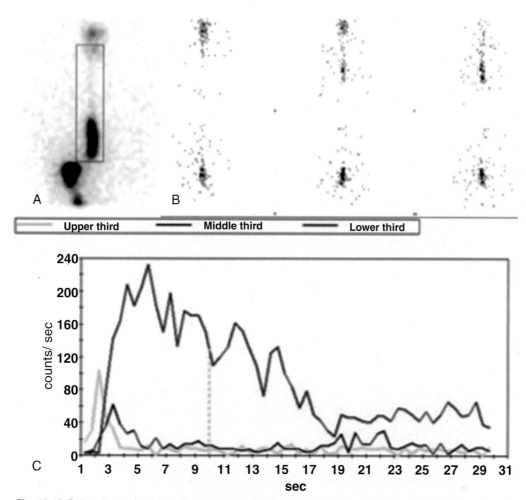

Fig. 10.16 Delayed esophageal swallow and quantification. (A) Summed image demonstrates delayed transit through the lower third of the esophagus. (B) Selected sequential dynamic 0.5 images show normal transit through the upper two-thirds of the esophagus but slow transit in the distal third. (C) Time–activity curves for upper, mid-, and lower regions. The red curve (lower third of esophagus) confirms delayed transit. The esophageal transit time was not reached by 30 seconds. Percent esophageal emptying at 10 seconds was 54% (normal >83%).

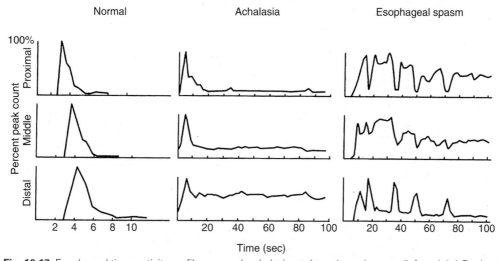

Fig. 10.17 Esophageal time–activity profiles: normal, achalasia, and esophageal spasm *(left to right)*. Regions of interest (ROIs) were drawn for the proximal, middle, and distal esophagus, and time–activity curves were generated. *(Left)* Normal subject. Bolus proceeds promptly sequentially from proximal to distal esophagus. *(Middle)* Achalasia. Delayed transit most prominent in the lower esophagus. *(Right)* Spasm, uncoordinated contraction. Bolus has poor esophageal progression.

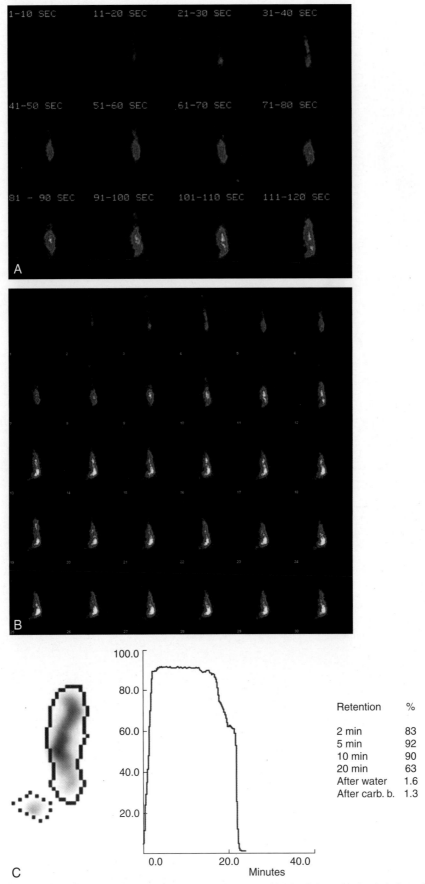

Fig. 10.18 Achalasia: semisolid meal. This methodology is most useful for follow-up of achalasia patients. (A) Ten-second frames. Retention of activity in the esophagus, most prominently in the distal esophagus. (B) Two-minute frames. Persistent distal esophageal retention with minimal clearance into the stomach over 30 minutes. (C) Quantification of esophageal emptying. Time–activity curve shows very delayed transit until ingestion of carbonated beverage, when rapid emptying occurs. Calculated retention at 20 minutes: 63% (<5% is normal).

into the distal esophagus to reproduce reflux symptoms and confirm its esophageal origin. Monitoring of pH can be diagnostic. A pH electrode is placed in the distal esophagus for 24-hour monitoring. An abrupt drop in pH to less than 4.0 is diagnostic of reflux; however, the study is invasive and technically demanding.

Scintigraphy

The radionuclide gastroesophageal reflux study is quantitative, noninvasive, and technically easy to perform. Although most commonly requested for neonates, with simple modifications it can also be quite useful for adults. In the past, the study was performed in a manner similar to the barium contrast study, using Valsalva maneuvers and an abdominal binder to progressively increase intraabdominal pressure during each sequential static 30-second image. However, this is not physiological, had poor sensitivity, and is no longer recommended. Known as the "milk study," the infant or child ingests this or her normal formula or milk feeding mixed with Tc-99m SC. With older children and adults, the radiotracer is typically mixed in orange juice.

After ingestion, the study is acquired on a computer at a framing rate of 5- to 10-second frames for 60 minutes. This rapid temporal acquisition rate provides high sensitivity for the detection of reflux events. Gastric emptying can also be determined by acquiring static images immediately after ingestion and at 1 and 2 hours. See the protocol in Box 10.8.

Image Interpretation

All frames should be reviewed. The window should be adjusted to maximize esophageal detection sensitivity. Cinematic display may also be helpful. The reflux events are seen as distinct spikes of activity into the esophagus (Fig. 10.19). Normal values for neonates or young children have not been established. Neonates normally have some reflux. The greater the number of high reflux events and the longer they last, the more likely and severe is the problem. Reflux events that occur with small gastric volumes have more clinical significance because reflux is occurring without the effect of the increased pressure of a full meal volume. Detection of reflux events is affected by the volume of the ingested meal and the rate of gastric emptying. Sensitivity for the detection of reflux events is highest with a full stomach and decreases as the stomach empties.

Image Interpretation and Quantification

All images should be reviewed for evidence of reflux events. A marker noting the mouth is useful for estimating the degree of reflux. One approach to quantification is a simple semiquantitative method that grades each reflux event as high- or low-level ($\geq$ or < midesophagus), by its duration (<10 secs or $\geq$10 secs), and by the temporal relationship to meal ingestion (reflux events at low gastric volume carry greater significance). The total number and level of reflux events can be summed into four categories:
1. Low level, <10 seconds
2. Low level, $\geq$10 seconds

3. High level, <10 seconds
4. High level, $\geq$10 seconds

Other quantitative parameters have been used (e.g., ROIs can be drawn for the esophagus and time–activity curves [TACs] generated. Peaks >5% have been reported to be diagnostic of gastroesophageal reflux.

Accuracy

With current protocols using rapid framing rates, the sensitivity for the detection of reflux is reported to be 75% to 100%, superior to barium studies. The standard technique of pH monitoring has limitations (i.e., 24-hour monitoring and poor temporal resolution [detecting recurrent events]) because since clears slowly from the pH monitors. The highest sensitivity is achieved using both scintigraphy and pH monitoring. Normal gastric-emptying values for formula or milk are not well established, but the consensus is that 1-hour emptying should be 40% to 50% and 2-hour emptying, 60% to 75%. The 2-hour value is considered more reliable.

Salivagram

Although aspiration should always be looked for on gastroesophageal reflux studies, the sensitivity for the detection of aspiration on radionuclide milk studies is reported to be poor,

---

BOX 10.8 Gastroesophageal Reflux ("Milk Study") Scintigraphy: Summary Protocol

Patient Preparation
NPO 3 hours

Computer Setup
Framing rate of 5 to 10 seconds per frame for 60 minutes

Radiopharmaceutical
Tc-99m SC, 0.1 mCi mixed with formula or milk

Feeding Meal
Infants: Normal feeding meal (formula or milk). Mix radionuclide with half of the meal and feed to the child. The second "cold" half of the meal is then fed to the child. Orange juice is used for older children and adults.

Imaging Procedure
After mother burps infant, place patient supine with gamma camera positioned posteriorly and the chest and upper abdomen in the field of view. Place radioactive marker at the mouth for several frames.
Obtain 1-minute anterior/posterior image immediately after ingestion of feeding and at 1 hour and 2 hours.
Acquire 5- to 10-second frames for 60 minutes starting after first 1-minute static image.
Acquire image of the chest at 2 hours. Review for aspiration with computer enhancement.
Quantify gastroesophageal reflux events and gastric emptying:
  Short reflux events ≤ 10 seconds
  Long reflux events >10 seconds
  Low reflux events < half distance up esophagus
  High reflux events ≥ half distance up esophagus
Sum events for each category.
  Normal gastric emptying >50% at 1 hour and 75% at 2 hours
NPO, nil per os; *SC*, sulfur colloid.

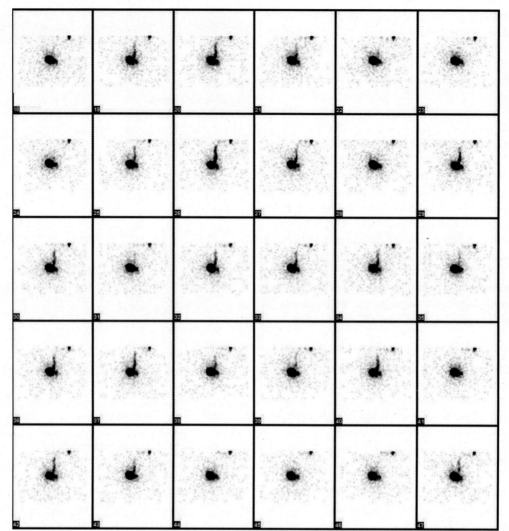

Fig. 10.19 Gastroesophageal reflux. Sequential 5-second frames show multiple episodes of long-lasting (>15 seconds) high-grade (above midesophagus) reflux events.

1% to 25%. However, a "salivagram" can often demonstrate clinically suspected aspiration when the gastroesophageal reflux study is negative. The salivagram is a variation of an esophageal transit study. A drop of radiotracer is placed in the back of the infant's mouth or tongue. Acquisition uses a framing rate similar to the reflux study, followed by static images (Fig. 10.20).

Intestinal Transit Scintigraphy

Intestinal transit scintigraphy is not yet a routine study in many nuclear medicine imaging clinics. However, this seems to be changing. Gastroenterologists are finding intestinal transit scintigraphy useful for evaluating patients with various symptoms related to the gastrointestinal (GI) tract. Small intestinal dysmotility may present with a wide range of clinical manifestations and symptoms, including some that overlap with those of gastric dysmotility, including postprandial epigastric or periumbilical abdominal pain, bloating, nausea, dyspepsia, vomiting, and diarrhea. Large intestinal dysmotility symptoms may include constipation, diarrhea, fecal incontinence, lower abdominal pain, and upper abdominal symptoms. Abnormal intestinal

transit may involve the entire colon or may be regional (e.g., limited to the right colon, descending colon, or rectosigmoid), and differentiating these is important for appropriate therapy.

Nonscintigraphic Methodologies

Oral contrast ingested with radiopaque markers and obtaining abdominal radiographs to plot its movement has been used as an index of intestinal transit; however, it is not physiological (i.e., it is not food and is likely treated differently than food by the intestines). The radiation dose from repeated abdominal films can be high. The hydrogen or lactose breath test sometimes used to estimate small bowel intestinal transit measures H_2 produced when a carbohydrate is fermented by colonic bacteria. However, fermentative bacteria are absent in the colon in a quarter of the population. The test only measures the transit time of the meal's leading edge from the mouth to the cecum, not bulk transit. The wireless motility capsule (Smartpill) measures pH and pressure within the intestines, but it must be swallowed and requires multiple-day monitoring; however, it is costly, published data are limited, and it is not truly physiological.

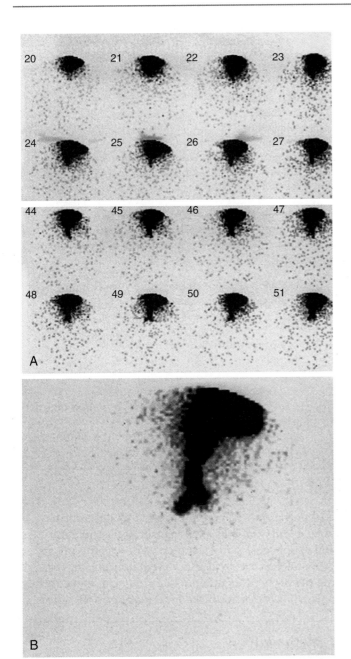

Fig. 10.20 "Salivagram" (esophageal swallow): aspiration. Neonate with swallowing and neurological problems. A prior gastroesophageal reflux study showed numerous reflux events but no aspiration. Tc-99m pertechnetate was placed on the posterior tongue so that the child would swallow it. (A) Sequential 5-second frames show transit into the tracheal bifurcation. (B) High-count anterior image at 1 hour shows persistent retention at the tracheal bifurcation.

Scintigraphy for Small Intestinal Transit

Scintigraphic quantification of intestinal transit is not as straightforward as gastric emptying. With gastric emptying, all of the meal resides within the stomach at the start of acquisition, and quantification depends on how much of or how fast the meal empties. With small intestinal transit, there is continual movement of food into the small intestine from the stomach as well as from the small bowel into the large bowel, making quantification challenging. Various scintigraphic quantitative methods have been published.

A common approach has been the use of an orally ingested liquid marker (e.g., In-111 DTPA), with or without a solid meal. In-111 DTPA is not reabsorbed and has a sufficiently long half-life. Images are typically acquired for 5 to 6 hours. The radiolabel spreads out as it moves through the small bowel. Identification of the first accumulation of radiotracer or the percent reaching the ileocecal valve or cecum at specific time intervals has been used to estimate the small bowel transit (Figs. 10.21–10.23). Limited data using Tc-99m HIDA radiotracers have been reported.

Large Bowel Transit Scintigraphy

Various radiopharmaceuticals that do not break down before reaching the large bowel have been used, such as I-131-radiolabeled cellulose fiber. There are some limited data on the use of Ga-67 citrate to measure transit. The most commonly used method has been the oral ingestion of In-111 DTPA, with or without a concomitant meal. One approach to quantification has been to calculate a geometrical center of activity, that is, the weighted average of the counts in five to seven sequential regions of the large bowel at specific time intervals over several days (Fig. 10.24). This provides a semiquantitative assessment of transit. However, it is demanding to draw all these regions and not always reproducible. Alternatively, a method that calculates the percent transit, similar to percent gastric emptying, at 24, 48, and 72 hours has been published and correlates well with the geometrical center method (Figs. 10.25 and 10.26). The diffuse or regional nature of delayed transit is then assessed by image analysis.

Whole-Gut Transit or Comprehensive Gastrointestinal Transit Scintigraphy

Studies at several institutions now have protocols that assess the upper and lower gastrointestinal tract transit as a single combined sequential study. Solid and liquid gastric emptying and small and large bowel transit are combined into a several-day study, using the standardized solid egg meal for solid emptying with In-111 DTPA for liquid emptying, and small and large intestinal transit. Esophageal transit is also an easy add-on at the beginning of the study. Different approaches have been used. A sample summarized protocol is described in Box 10.9. Because the symptoms of upper and lower tract disease may overlap, these studies allow for evaluation of the entire gastrointestinal tract in one study over 72 hours (Fig. 10.27). Furthermore, many of these patients have transit abnormalities in more than one region of the gastrointestinal tract.

GASTROINTESTINAL BLEEDING

Because acute gastrointestinal bleeding is potentially life threatening, effective therapy requires prompt localization of the site of hemorrhage. The history and physical examination can often distinguish upper from lower tract bleeding (above or below the ligament of Treitz). Upper-tract bleeding typically presents with melena; bright red blood suggests a lower-tract origin. Hemorrhage from the upper tract is often confirmed with gastric intu-

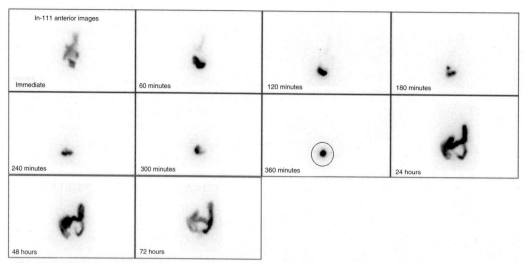

Fig. 10.21 Small and large bowel transit—normal small bowel transit; delayed large bowel transit. Images start immediately after ingestion of In-111-labeled water *(left upper)*. Radiotracer can be seen in the stomach. It promptly moves distally to the small bowel and then to the region of the ileo-cecal valve, best demonstrated at 360 minutes, where the region of interest (ROI) is drawn. At 24 hours, the radiotracer has moved to the transverse colon and, to a lesser extent, the descending colon. However, there is poor progression of transit at 48 and 72 hours, which is delayed.

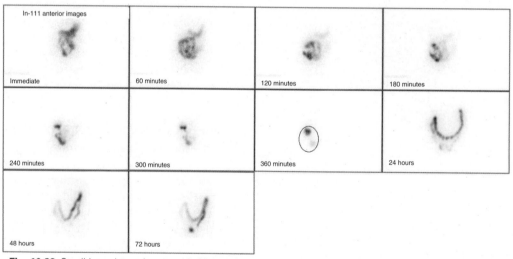

Fig. 10.22 Small bowel transit—normal. All anterior In-111 images beginning with ingestion of radiolabeled water (immediate). The stomach is seen as well as transit to the proximal small bowel. Then images every 60 minutes until 6 hours (360 minutes). Finally, images for colonic transit at 24, 48, and 72 hours. On sequential images, the small bowel activity moves distally, localizing in the region of the ileocecal valve and cecum. On the 360-minute image, a region of interest (ROI) is drawn to include the distal ileum and cecum in both the anterior and posterior views (posterior not shown). In this case it is assumed that the inferior activity is the ileocecal valve and the superior activity is the cecum. If activity had progressed further along the large bowel, it would have been included. The amount of radiotracer that reaches this region is an index of small intestinal transit. In this case it was 69% or normal (>49% is normal). At 24 hours, the activity has reached the transverse colon.

bation and treated with flexible fiberoptic endoscopy. Lower-tract bleeding is more challenging. Colonoscopy is difficult and of limited value during active hemorrhage.

The radionuclide gastrointestinal bleeding study has been a standard imaging test to detect gastrointestinal bleeding for decades, first described in 1977. Only 2 to 3 mL of extravasated blood is required for detection. Contrast computed tomography (CTA) is being used at some centers as an alternative to the scintigraphic study because of its ready availability

and superior anatomical visualization of the bleeding site. However, because gastrointestinal bleeding is intermittent, the radionuclide study has the distinct advantage of being able to image patients over time for up to 24 hours, not just immediately after injection. Other disadvantages of CTA include the need for intravenous contrast and a higher radiation dose to the patient. The radionuclide study can detect bleeding rates of 0.1 mL/min, versus 0.3 mL/min for CTA or 1.0 mL/min for visceral contrast angiography. An important reason for

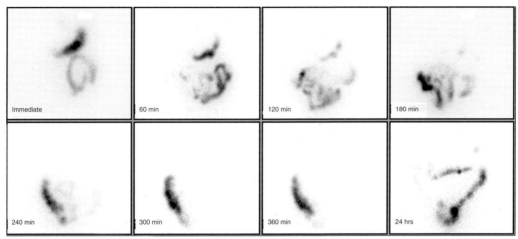

Fig. 10.23 Small bowel transit—rapid. Anterior In-111 images after ingestion of water with In-111 diethylen-etriaminepentaacetic acid (DTPA) and solid meal. In the top row, the stomach is almost completely emptied by 180 minutes *(first row, top right)*. There is rapid transit through the small bowel so that by 240 minutes *(second row, far left)*, the activity is almost all in the ascending colon. The ileocecal valve can be seen at its inferior aspect. By 24 hours *(second row, far right)*, the activity has almost all transited from ascending colon, with some in the transverse colon, but most is in the descending colon and rectosigmoid. The region of interest (ROI) was drawn at 360 minutes to include all activity that has reached the ileocecal value or that which is distal to it. In this case the entire image is included because it is beyond the ileocecal valve. Small bowel transit was 100%. The 24-hour image shows rapid large bowel transit, with most activity in the descending colon and rectosigmoid.

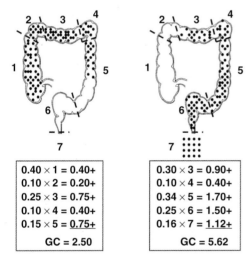

Fig. 10.24 Geometrical center of colonic activity. The geometrical center is a weighted average of the radioactivity counted over specific segments of the colon, the ascending, transverse, descending, and rectosigmoid colon. The geometrical center is calculated as the sum of a weighted fraction represented by the counts in each region multiplied by the region number divided by the total counts. (From Maurer AH, Camilleri M, Donohoe K, et al. The SNMMI and EANM practice guideline for small-bowel and colon transit 1.0. *J Nucl Med.* 2013;54:2004–2013.)

performing scintigraphy or CTA is to determine whether bleeding is active so that invasive mesenteric angiography can be performed for therapeutic intervention. Which approach is used depends on the local situation. Lack of availability of nuclear studies in some hospitals on weekends and or at night may give preference there to CTA.

Gastrointestinal Bleeding Scintigraphy

A method using Tc-99m SC was first described. After intravenous injection, it is rapidly extracted by the liver, spleen, and marrow, resulting in a high target-to-background ratio. The diagnosis was made by observing intraabdominal extravasation at the site of bleeding. The study was complete in 20 to 30 minutes. The disadvantage of this method was that intermittent bleeding could be missed during the short duration of the examination, similar to CTA. Tc-99m serum albumen, a blood-pool agent, was subsequently used, permitting a longer imaging time. In 1979, radiolabeling of the patient's red blood cells (RBCs) with Tc-99m pertechnetate was introduced, and this continues to be the standard methodology used today. Image quality is superior to Tc-99m serum albumen, and imaging is possible for up to 24 hours. Advances and modifications in instrumentation and methodology have enhanced detection.

Image quality is best when Tc-99m pertechnetate binds tightly to the RBCs, with minimal residual free Tc-99m. Free Tc-99m is taken up by the salivary glands and gastric mucosa and secreted into the stomach, which then transits the gastrointestinal tract, potentially complicating study interpretation (i.e., differentiating free Tc-99m from active bleeding).

Before initiating a radionuclide GI bleeding study, it is helpful to have a discussion with the referring clinician, angiographer, and/or surgeon regarding the specific plan should the bleeding study be positive. Contrast angiography should be performed promptly after a positive radionuclide study to maximize the likelihood of detection and treatment of the bleeding site.

RBC Radiolabeling

Tc-99m must be reduced before it can bind to the beta chain of hemoglobin. Stannous ion (tin) in the form of stannous chloride or stannous pyrophosphate is used for this purpose. Several methodologies have been utilized over the years for labeling of RBCs with Tc-99m and are briefly described in Box 10.10.

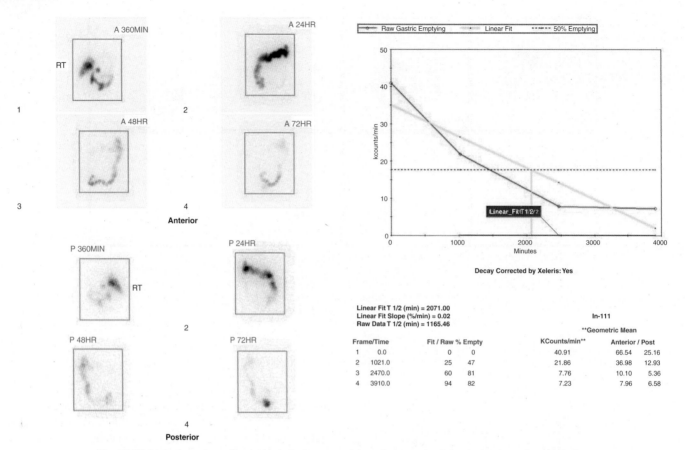

Fig. 10.25 Large bowel transit—normal. Patient complains of recurrent abdominal pain and constipation. Format and software are similar to the gastric-emptying program. At 360 minutes *(left upper corner of anterior and posterior images)*, there is predominantly small bowel activity. At 24 hours *(right upper corner)*, activity has transited to the ascending and, even more so, the transverse colon. By 48 hours, activity is in the descending colon and rectosigmoid, but with much-reduced overall activity from 24 hours. At 72 hours, most activity has exited, with a small residual in the descending colon and rectosigmoid *(bottom right anterior and posterior images)*. Quantification is 47% at 24 hours, 81% at 48 hours, and 82% at 72 hours—all normal (see % emptying column; normal is >14% at 24 hours, >41% at 48 hours, >67% at 72 hours).

In Vivo Method. This was the original method described. Stannous pyrophosphate is injected intravenously (IV), followed 15 minutes later by IV Tc-99m pertechnetate. Both diffuse across the RBC membrane. The stannous ion reduces the Tc-99m intracellularly, which then binds to hemoglobin. Although a simple method, the labeling yield is at best 75%. Poor labeling can be exacerbated by various drugs and other interactions (Table 10.2). This method is suboptimal by today's standards and used only for patients who cannot receive blood products for religious reasons.

Modified In Vivo (In Vitro) Method. Stannous pyrophosphate is injected into the IV line. After 15 minutes, 3 to 5 mL of blood is withdrawn through the IV line into a lead-shielded syringe that contains Tc-99m pertechnetate and a small amount of anticoagulant. The syringe is left attached to the IV line during the procedure so that it is a closed procedure. The syringe is agitated gently for 10 minutes, and then its contents are reinjected into the patient. Labeling efficiency is approximately 85%. Although it is clearly superior to the in vivo method and acceptable for GI bleeding studies, some drugs and other factors may still interfere with labeling (see Table 10.2).

In Vitro Method. Originally, the in vitro method required drawing the patient's blood, centrifuging it to separate the RBCs

from serum, radiolabeling the RBCs, resuspending it in plasma, and then infusing it back into the patient. Binding was excellent. However, today, a simple commercial kit method (UltraTag) is available for this purpose. Labeling efficiency is >97%. The method uses whole blood and does not require centrifugation (Fig. 10.28). The patient's blood is withdrawn and added to a reaction vial contacting stannous chloride. The stannous ion diffuses across the RBC membrane. After adding Tc-99m pertechnetate, which also crosses the RBC membrane, it is reduced by the stannous ion within the cell, allowing for binding to the RBC. The mixture is allowed to incubate for 20 minutes before reinjection into the patient. This approach is much less subject to drug-labeling interference than the other methods. Although the in vivo and modified in vivo methods both depend on biological clearance of undesirable extracellular reduced stannous ion, the in vitro method adds sodium hypochlorite to oxidize any extracellular stannous ion and thus prevent extracellular reduction of Tc-99m pertechnetate, ensuring only RBC cellular radiolabeling.

Image Acquisition

An imaging protocol is described (Box 10.11). Images are acquired in the supine position, and the camera is placed

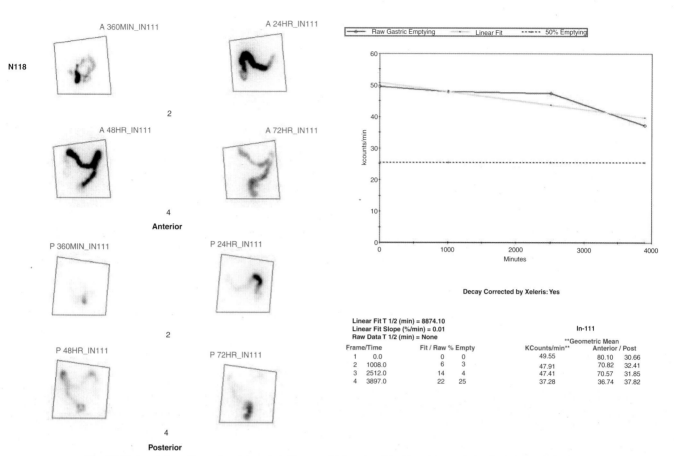

Fig. 10.26 Large bowel transit—delayed. A 50-year-old female with scleroderma, abdominal discomfort, and constipation. Esophageal study showed delayed transit (not shown here). Gastric emptying was normal. At 360 minutes *(anterior image, upper left)*, activity is predominantly in the small bowel, most prominently at the ileocecal valve and cecum. By 24 hours *(upper right)*, activity is in the ascending and transverse colon. By 48 hours *(lower left)*, activity is in the transverse and descending colon. At 72 hours *(lower right)*, the distribution is mostly unchanged, although the activity has decreased somewhat, and some has reached the rectosigmoid area *(posterior image, bottom right)*. However, quantification shows diffusely delayed transit. This patient had minimal transit or percent emptying, even at 72 hours, 25% (frame/time 4). Normal transit (emptying) values are 14% at 24 hours, 41% by 48 hours, and 67% by 72 hours.

BOX 10.9   Comprehensive Gastrointestinal Transit—Protocol Summary

Esophageal transit:
Posterior view, standing
  Computer setup: 0.5-second frames × 60
  Practice 2 dry swallows initially; then swallow 15-cc water bolus with 100 µCi.
Normal values: Percent transit (>83%), transit time (<15 seconds)
  Liquid-only gastric emptying:
In-111 100 µCi in 300 cc water
Left anterior oblique (LAO) projection
1-minute frames × 30
Normal values: <25 minutes half-time ($T_{1/2}$)
  Liquid emptying simultaneous with solid gastric emptying:
In-111 100 µCi in 120 mL water
Tc-99m SC standardized egg-white sandwich, jam
Anterior/posterior imaging at 0, 1, 2, 3, 4 hours
Normal values: 39% at 1 hour
  Small intestinal transit:

In-111 window: 1-minute anterior/posterior images at 5 and 6 hours
Calculation: Percent of activity that reaches ileal-cecal valve or beyond at 360 minutes
Normal values: >50 at 6 hours
  Large intestinal transit:
In-111 window: 5-minute anterior/posterior images at 24, 48, 72 hours
Calculation: % activity transited (gastric-emptying program) from 360-minute baseline
Interpretation: Include image analysis to determine whether regional or diffuse delay.
  Normal values: 14% at 24 hours, 41% at 48 hours, 67% at 72 hours; rapid emptying >40% at 24 hours.
For further details of methodology, processing, and normal values, refer to Antoniou AJ, Ziessman HA, et al. Comprehensive radionuclide esophago-gastrointestinal transit: methodology, normal values, and initial clinical experience. *J Nucl Med.* 2015;56:721–727.
  SC, Sulfur colloid.

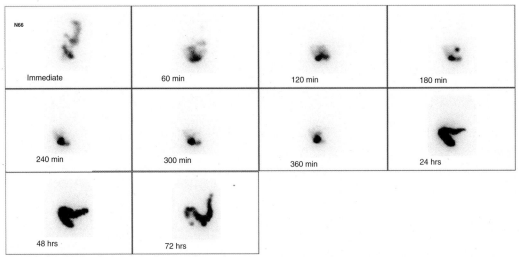

Fig. 10.27 Comprehensive gastrointestinal (GI) transit. A 35-year-old female with symptoms of postprandial nausea, abdominal discomfort, and constipation. Anterior In-111 images after ingestion of combined soli–liquid meal. The esophageal and liquid and solid gastric-emptying portions of the study are not shown. *(Upper row)* In-111 activity in the stomach *(first image)* transits normally to the small bowel over 180 minutes. *(Second row)* The majority of tracer is at the ileocecal valve by 240 minutes *(second row, left),* which is normal small bowel transit. By 24 hours, activity is in the ascending and transverse colon. No change is seen at 48 hours, and there is very delayed transit at 72 hours, never reaching the descending colon.

BOX 10.10 Methods of Tc-99m Red Blood Cell (RBC) Labeling

In Vivo Method (Labeling Efficiency, 75–80%)
1. Inject stannous pyrophosphate.
2. Wait 10 to 20 minutes.
3. Inject Tc-99m sodium pertechnetate.

Modified In Vivo (In Vitro) Method (Labeling Efficiency, 85–90%)
1. Inject stannous pyrophosphate.
2. Wait 10 to 20 minutes.
3. Withdraw 5 to 8 mL of blood into shielded syringe with Tc-99m.
4. Gently agitate syringe contents for 10 minutes at room temperature.

In Vitro Commercial Kit (UltraTag; Labeling Efficiency, >97%)
1. Add 1 to 3 mL of blood (heparin or acid citrate dextrose as anticoagulant) to reagent vial (50–100 μg stannous chloride, 3.67 mg Na citrate) and mix. Allow 5 minutes to react.
2. Add syringe 1 contents (0.6 mg sodium hypochlorite) and mix by inverting 4 to 5 times.
3. Add contents of syringe 2 (8.7 mg citric acid, 32.5 mg Na citrate, dextrose) and mix.
4. Add Tc-99m 10 to 100 mCi (370–3700 MBq) to reaction vial.
5. Mix and allow to react for 20 minutes, with occasional mixing.

TABLE 10.2 Causes of Poor Tc-99m Red Blood Cell Labeling

Drug–drug interactions	Heparin, doxorubicin, methyldopa, hydralazine, contrast media, quinidine
Circulating antibodies	Prior transfusion, transplantation, some antibiotics
Too little stannous ion	Insufficient to reduce Tc (VII)
Too much stannous ion	Reduction of Tc (VII) outside of red blood cell before cell labeling
Carrier Tc-99	Buildup of Tc-99m in the Mo-99/Tc-99m generator due to long interval between elutions
Too short an interval for "tinning"	Not enough time for stannous ion to penetrate the red blood cells before addition of Tc-99m
Too short an incubation time	Not enough time for reduction of Tc (VII)

Image Interpretation

The purpose of the radionuclide bleeding study is (1) to determine whether hemorrhage is active, (2) to estimate the approximate rate of bleeding, and (3) to determinate the site of bleeding. If the study is negative, angiography is also likely to be negative because of the greater sensitivity of the radionuclide study. If scintigraphy is positive, it should be promptly followed by angiography. Because intestinal anatomy is complex due to its embryological development (Fig. 10.29) and because scintigraphic image resolution is limited, all sequential 1-minute frames should be carefully reviewed to observe the path of intestinal blood flow to determine with certainty the site of bleeding. Prematurely stopping the study before that is a mistake, unless the patient is unstable and needs to be sent immediately to angiography. Displaying the frames dynamically can help pinpoint the vascular origin of the bleed.

anteriorly. Following IV injection, a flow study may be acquired (1- to 3-second frames), then 1-minute dynamic images for up to 90 minutes. A static left lateral or left anterior oblique view of the pelvis is obtained to help differentiate activity in the bladder and genital area from blood in the rectum. If the study is not diagnostic, delayed imaging can be acquired as needed for up to 24 hours. Delayed images should always be acquired at the same framing rate and for approximately 30 minutes in duration.

Excessive gastric, thyroid, and soft tissue background activity suggests poor labeling. A routine anterior image of the neck and abdomen can confirm free Tc-99m pertechnetate by noting uptake in the thyroid, salivary glands, and stomach. The iodine from a recent contrast study can block thyroid uptake, but salivary uptake is usually seen. Bladder filling with Tc-99m pertechnetate or other reduced Tc-99m compound may make it difficult to see a rectal bleed in the anterior view. The left lateral or left anterior oblique (LAO) view can help to confirm or exclude blood in the rectum.

Flow Phase

Rapid hemorrhage may rarely be seen during this phase. However, it is probably most helpful when bleeding is not active, such as for detection of a vascular blush, which at times can be seen with angiodysplasia, arteriovenous (AV) malformations, or tumor, at a time when there is no active bleeding (Fig. 10.30). The flow study on occasion may also help with image interpretation (e.g., defining a vascular lesion, aneurysmal vessels, kidneys, or uterus).

Dynamic Phase

Approximately 80% of bleeding sites are detected during the initial 90-minute study (0.5- to 1.0-minute frames; Figs. 10.31–10.36). Because bleeding is intermittent, further delayed imaging may be necessary to confirm the site and/or detect the other 20% of bleeding sites. On occasion, SPECT with computed tomography (SPECT/CT) can sometimes be helpful in confirming the site of bleeding.

Delayed Imaging

Further imaging can be obtained as needed for up to 24 hours. Images should always be dynamic over 20 to 30 minutes.

Interpretative Criteria

Specific diagnostic criteria should be used to diagnose active bleeding and its site of origin (Box 10.12). The radiotracer activity must (1) first appear where there was none before, (2) then increase over time, and (3) move in a pattern consistent with intestinal anatomy, antegrade and/or retrograde. Fixed nonmoving activity should not be diagnosed as an active bleeding site and is likely due to a vascular structure (e.g., hemangioma, accessory spleen, ectopic kidney; Box 10.13). Large intestinal bleeds typically appear as curvilinear activity moving along the periphery of the abdomen in the expected anatomical pattern.

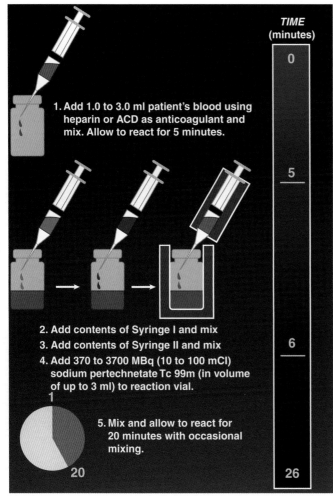

Fig. 10.28 In vitro red blood cell (RBC) labeling with Tc-99m (UltraTag). The kit consists of three nonradioactive components: a 10-mL vial of stannous chloride; syringe 1 containing sodium hypochlorite (to oxidize the extracellular stannous ion to prevent extracellular reduction of Tc-99m pertechnetate); and syringe 2 containing citric acid, sodium citrate, and dextrose (ACD). Labeling efficiency is >97%.

BOX 10.11 Gastrointestinal Bleeding—Tc-99m Red Blood Cell (RBC) Scintigraphy: Summary Protocol

Patient Preparation
None

Radiopharmaceutical
Tc-99m-labeled RBCs; in vitro kit labeling method (UltraTag)

Instrumentation
Gamma camera: Large field of view
Collimator: High resolution, parallel hole
Computer setup: 1-second frames for 60 seconds; 1-minute frames for 90 minutes
As needed up to 24 hours: Delayed image sequence should be acquired as 1-minute frames for 30 minutes.

Patient Position
Supine; anterior imaging, with abdomen and pelvis in field of view

Imaging Procedure
Inject patient's Tc-99m-labeled erythrocytes intravenously.
Acquire 1-second flow images × 60, followed by 1-minute images for 90 minutes.
Acquire image of neck for thyroid and salivary uptake and left lateral/left anterior oblique (LAO) view of pelvis.
If study is negative or bleeding is recurrent, may repeat with 30-minute acquisitions (1-minute frame × 30).

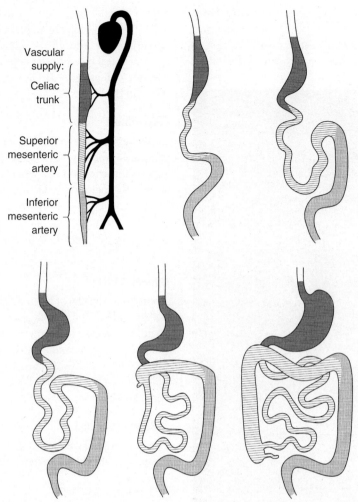

Vascular
supply:

Celiac
trunk

Superior
mesenteric
artery

Inferior
mesenteric
artery

Fig. 10.29 The embryological development of the gastrointestinal tract explains its ultimate anatomical configuration. The diagram relates this anatomy to its arterial supply (celiac, superior mesenteric, and inferior mesenteric arteries).

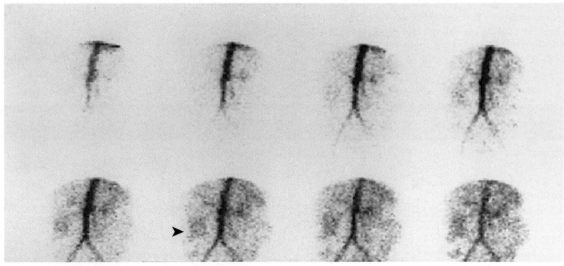

Fig. 10.30 Utility of blood flow on a gastrointestinal (GI) bleeding study. Increased blood flow (3-second frames) to the region of the right upper quadrant *(arrowhead)*. The subsequent 90-minute Tc-99m red blood cell (RBC) study (1-minute frames) was negative, as was a second acquisition for 30 minutes at 3 hours. Colonoscopy diagnosed angiodysplasia in the ascending colon.

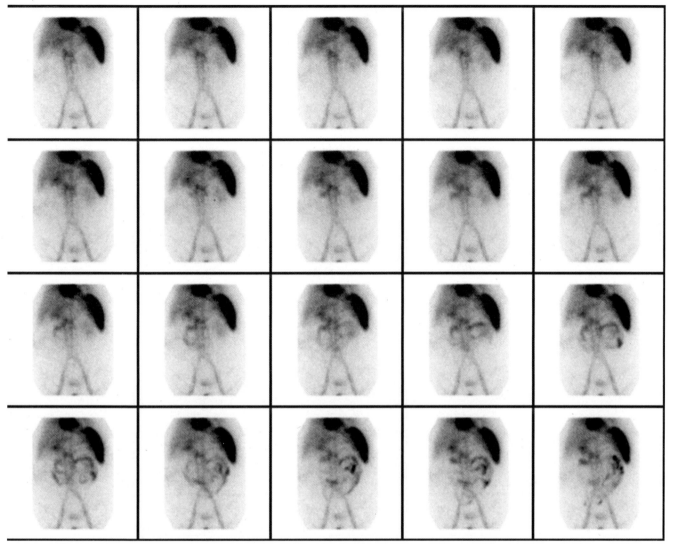

Fig. 10.31 Tc-99m red blood cell (RBC): Small bowel bleed. Sequential 1-minute images. *(Second row, left image)* New focal activity just below the liver, likely proximal small bowel. With time, the activity transverses the proximal and ultimately more distal small intestines. This was determined to be a duodenal ulcer bleed on endoscopy.

The small bowel is more centrally located, and blood moves rapidly through its looping (serpiginous) segments.

Scintigraphy has limitations in precise anatomical localization; however, a bleeding site can usually be localized to the proximal or distal small bowel, cecum, ascending colon, hepatic flexure, transverse colon, splenic flexure, descending colon, sigmoid colon, or rectum. This information can assist the angiographer in deciding which vessel (celiac, superior mesenteric, or inferior mesenteric artery) to inject first with contrast.

Although the radionuclide bleeding study is rarely requested for upper gastrointestinal bleeding because endoscopy is usually diagnostic, occasionally upper-tract bleeding will be seen on a study ordered for a suspected lower GI bleed. Gastric hemorrhage must be differentiated from free Tc-99m pertechnetate. With both, gastric activity will transit to the small bowel and eventually the large bowel. An image of the neck can help confirm free Tc-99m pertechnetate by the presence of salivary and thyroid gland uptake. A recent intravenous contrast study may prevent thyroid uptake.

Interpretive Pitfalls

Interpretive pitfalls are normal, technical, or pathological findings that might be misinterpreted as active hemorrhage (see Box 10.13). The presence of free Tc-99m pertechnetate caused by poor radiolabeling or dissociation of the label in vivo is a technical pitfall. A not uncommon imaging interpretive pitfall is activity in the genitourinary tract. Urinary renal pelvic or ureteral activity resulting from free pertechnetate or another Tc-99m labeled reduced compound might be wrongly thought to be active bleeding because of its movement. Upright positioning and oblique or posterior views can be helpful to clarify the source of activity.

Intraluminal intestinal radioactivity first detected on delayed static images can pose a diagnostic dilemma. Blood in the colon or rectum may have originated from anywhere in the gastrointestinal tract, and one should be cautious in diagnosing its site of origin on a single image. Misinterpretation can best be avoided by acquiring dynamic 1-minute images for at least 30 minutes whenever delayed imaging is required. An active bleeding site should only be

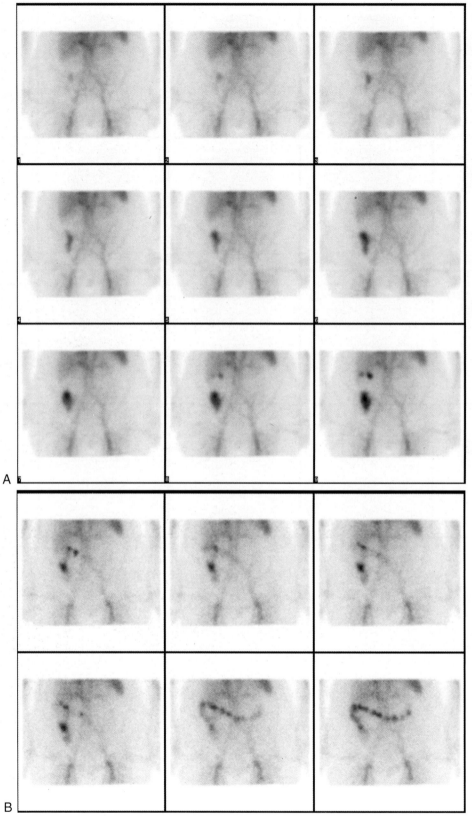

Fig. 10.32 Tc-99m red blood cell (RBC): Bleeding from cecum. (A) Focal low-intensity uptake is first seen on the first image, which increases over time and appears to be in the region of the cecum. The third row of images shows transit to the hepatic flexure. (B) Further imaging shows transit to the transverse colon.

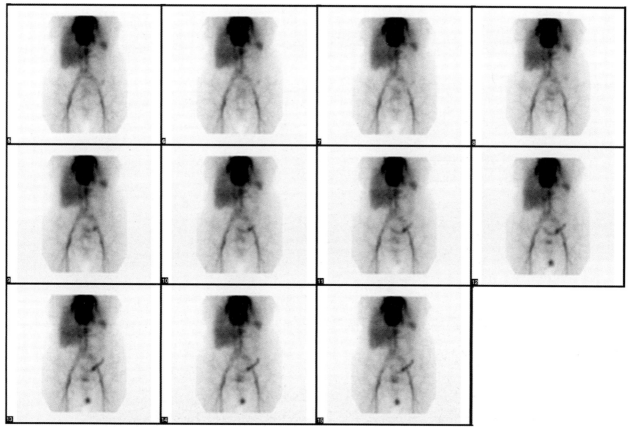

Fig. 10.33 Tc-99m red blood cell (RBC): Sigmoid bleed. *(First row):* No active bleeding. *(Second row)* Increasing activity is seen in the region of the sigmoid colon. *(Third row)* Activity is seen in the rectum just below the medial aspect of sigmoid activity. The bladder would be higher.

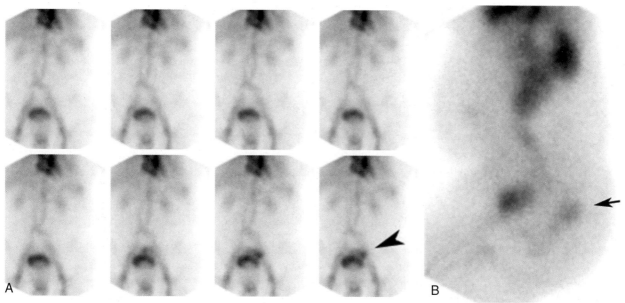

Fig. 10.34 Tc-99m red blood cell (RBC): Rectal bleed. (A) The last three 1-minute images show increasing activity just superior and to the left of the bladder *(arrowhead),* very suggestive of rectosigmoid colon bleed. (B) Left lateral view confirms that blood is in the rectum *(arrow).*

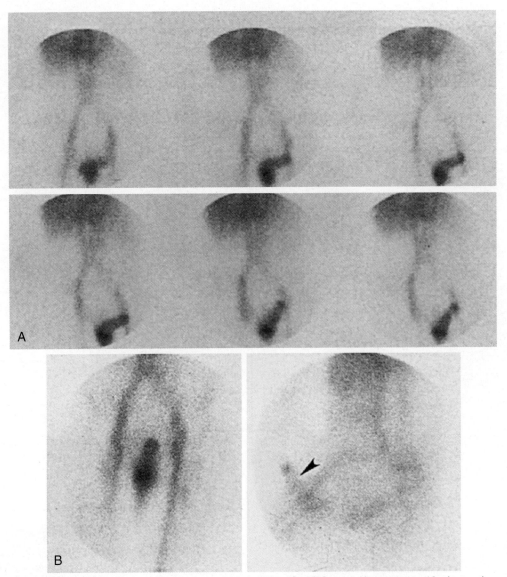

Fig. 10.35 Potential false positive for active gastrointestinal bleeding. (A) Summed images every 10 minutes show activity in the lower middle and left pelvic region that moves over time. (B) Anterior *(left)* and left anterior oblique (LAO; *right*) images acquired at 90 minutes show the activity to be penile blood pool *(arrowhead)*. Left lateral or LAO views should be obtained when pelvic activity is seen, to separate rectal, bladder, and penile activity.

diagnosed by using the criteria already described (i.e., new and increasing activity moving in a pattern consistent with intestinal transit; see Box 10.12). Background subtraction may be helpful.

Other potential pitfalls include abdominal varices, hemangiomas, accessory spleen, arterial grafts, aneurysms, ectopic kidneys, and renal transplants, all of which show fixed and nonmoving activity (see Fig. 10.35). Activity clearing through the hepatobiliary system and gallbladder can be caused by hemobilia; however, patients with renal failure may have gallbladder visualization as a result of radiolabeled fragmented heme breakdown products (porphyrins).

Accuracy

Many investigations have reported very good accuracy for the radionuclide GI bleeding study; however, some have not found it so helpful (Table 10.3), and thus controversy exists regarding its clinical utility. Reasons for the discrepancy are likely several.

Misinterpretation, especially in the older literature, may have been due to now-outdated methodology (e.g., infrequent image acquisition, static rather than dynamic imaging, pitfalls in interpretation already described, and incorrect localization based on single delayed images). An additional issue is whether the bleeding studies were performed early in the course of a workup or only after extended hospitalization and negative clinical workup. The radionuclide study has the highest yield when performed as soon as possible after arrival in the emergency room or on hospital admission.

The gold standard used in some published investigations is a potential problem for determining accuracy. Of patients who have visceral angiography, only the positive studies are diagnostic. False negatives may occur because the patient is not actively bleeding at the time of the study, which is not uncommon if not performed promptly after the scintigraphic study. Bleeding is intermittent. Colonoscopy is often not possible during active bleeding, but commonly patients are put to rest and prepped for

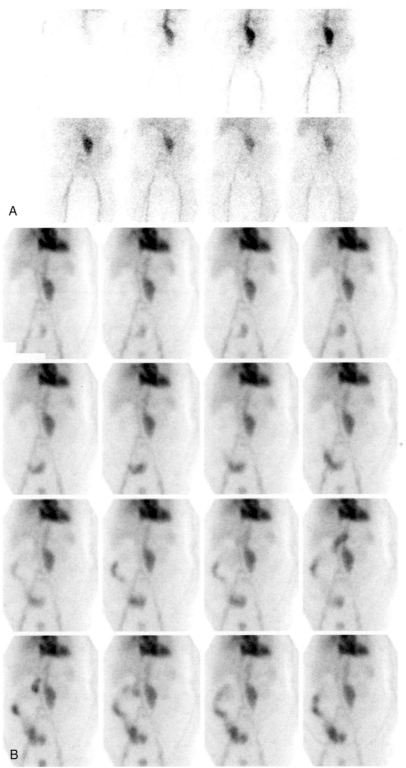

Fig. 10.36 Aortic aneurysm and acute bleed. (A) Blood-flow study demonstrates aortic flow and distal aorta fusiform configuration. (B) In 1-minute dynamic summed images over 90 minutes, an acute bleed originates in the midpelvic region, moving with time to the ascending and transverse colon, consistent with cecal bleeding. The abdominal aortic aneurysm shows persistent activity throughout the study. This fixed activity of an aortic aneurysm is unrelated to the active bleed.

BOX 10.12 Diagnostic Criteria for Diagnosis of Active Bleeding Site With Tc-99m Red Blood Cells (RBCs)

Focal activity appears where none was initially.
Radioactivity increases over time.
Movement of activity conforms to intestinal anatomy.
Movement may be antegrade and/or retrograde.

BOX 10.13 Pitfalls in Interpretation of Tc-99m Red Blood Cell (RBC) Scintigraphy for Gastrointestinal (GI) Bleeding

Common

Gastrointestinal (free Tc-99m pertechnetate): stomach, small and large intestine
Genitourinary
Pelvic kidney
Ectopic kidney
Renal pelvic activity
Ureter
Bladder
Uterine blush
Penis

Uncommon

Accessory spleen
Hepatic hemangioma
Varices, esophageal and gastric
Vascular
Abdominal aortic aneurysm
Gastroduodenal artery aneurysm
Abdominal varices
Caput medusae and dilated mesenteric veins
Gallbladder varices
Pseudoaneurysm
Arterial grafts
Cutaneous hemangioma
Duodenal telangiectasia
Angiodysplasia
Gallbladder (heme products in uremia)

TABLE 10.3 Correct Localization of Tc-99m Red Blood Cell (RBC) Gastrointestinal Bleeding

First Author	Year	Number of Scans	% Positive	% Correct
Suzman	1996	224	51	96
Orechhia	1985	76	34	94
O'Neill	2000	26	96	88
Emslie	1996	75	28	88
Leitman	1989	28	43	86
Bearn	1992	23	78	82
Dusold	1984	74	59	75
Rantis	1995	80	47	73
Van Geelen	1994	42	57	69
Nicholson	1989	43	72	67
Hunter	1990	203	26	58
Bentley	1991	182	60	52
Garofalo	1997	161	49	19
Voeller	1991	111	22	0

colonoscopy the next day. This is time lost for the GI bleeding study. Detection of pathological abnormalities on radiographic studies or colonoscopy after bleeding has ceased does not necessarily indicate that they were the source of bleeding.

Overall, many investigators, clinicians, and angiographers have found the gastrointestinal bleeding study to be clinically valuable and accurate in bleeding-site localization. A telling point is that at many institutions, angiographers are often the ones to request RBC scintigraphy before an invasive procedure. Being readily available when needed and having good communication with referring physicians is critical for success.

MECKEL SCAN

Meckel diverticulum is the most common and clinically important form of heterotopic gastric mucosa. Although *ectopic gastric mucosa* is the terminology frequently used, this is not really

correct. *Ectopic* refers to an organ that has migrated—for example, an ectopic kidney. *Heterotopic* refers to a tissue at its site of origin. Other causes of heterotopic gastric mucosa besides Meckel diverticulum are gastrointestinal duplications, postoperative retained gastric antrum, and Barrett esophagus.

Radiopharmaceutical

Tc-99m pertechnetate has been used since the 1970s to image and diagnose Meckel diverticulum as the cause of gastrointestinal bleeding.

Mechanism of Uptake

The mucosa of the gastric fundus contains multiple cell types, including parietal cells that secrete hydrochloric acid and chief cells that secrete pepsinogen and intrinsic factor. The gastric antrum and pylorus contain G cells that secrete the hormone gastrin. Columnar mucin-secreting epithelial cells are found throughout the stomach and excrete alkaline secretions that protect the mucosa from the highly acidic gastric fluid. Parietal cells were originally thought to be solely responsible for gastric uptake and secretion of Tc-99m pertechnetate. However, evidence points to the mucin-secreting cells being as important. Uptake has been found in gastric tissue with no parietal cells, and autoradiographic studies have shown mucin cell uptake.

Meckel diverticulum is the most common congenital anomaly of the gastrointestinal tract, occurring in 1% to 3% of the population. It is due to failure of closure of the omphalomesenteric duct in the embryo. The duct connects the yolk sac to the primitive foregut through the umbilical cord. This is a true diverticulum that arises on the antimesenteric side of the small bowel, approximately 80 to 90 cm proximal to the ileocecal valve. It is usually 2 to 3 cm in size but may be larger. Gastric mucosa is present in 10% to 30% of patients with Meckel diverticulum, in 60% of symptomatic patients with the diverticulum,

---

BOX 10.14 Meckel Diverticulum

1% to 3% incidence in the general population
50% occur by age 2 years
10% to 30% have ectopic gastric mucosa
25% to 40% are symptomatic; 50% to 67% of these have ectopic gastric mucosa
95% to 98% of patients with bleeding have ectopic gastric mucosa

---

and in 98% of those with bleeding (Box 10.14). More than 60% percent of patients with complications of Meckel diverticulum are under age 2. Bleeding after age 40 is uncommon.

Clinical Manifestations

Gastric mucosal secretions can cause peptic ulceration of the Meckel diverticulum or adjacent ileum, producing pain, perforation, or bleeding.

Diagnosis

Meckel diverticulum can be missed on small bowel radiography because of its narrow or stenotic ostium, which fills poorly and empties rapidly. Angiography is diagnostic only with brisk active bleeding and rarely used. The Meckel scan with Tc-99m pertechnetate is considered the standard method for preoperative diagnosis of a Meckel diverticulum.

Methodology

A Meckel scan protocol is described (Box 10.15). For patient preparation, barium studies should not be performed for several days before scintigraphy because attenuation by the contrast material may prevent lesion detection. Procedures such as colonoscopy or laxatives that irritate the intestinal mucosa can result in Tc-99m pertechnetate uptake and should be avoided. Ethosuximide (Zarontin), an anticonvulsant, is reported to cause uptake.

A full stomach or urinary bladder may obscure a Meckel diverticulum; thus, fasting for 2 to 4 hours before the study or continuous nasogastric aspiration to decrease stomach size is recommended. Patients should void before the study and at the end before imaging. A urinary catheter should be considered. Potassium perchlorate should not be used to block thyroid uptake because it will also block gastric uptake. It may be administered after the study to wash out the radiotracer from the thyroid and thus minimize radiation exposure.

Pharmacological Augmentation

Patient preparation with drugs to improve the detection of Meckel diverticulum has been used. Cimetidine, a histamine H2-receptor antagonist, is reported to increase Tc-99m pertechnetate uptake by inhibiting its release from gastric mucosa. The dose is 20 mg/kg orally in divided doses for 2 days before the study. It can also be given intravenously. Other related drugs, such as ranitidine and famotidine, have been used both orally and intravenously (see Box 10.15). No large or controlled studies have been reported to validate the diagnostic utility of cimetidine; however, its use has been recommended based on animal studies and case reports suggesting its effectiveness and

---

BOX 10.15 Meckel Scan: Summary Protocol

Patient Preparation
Fasting 4 to 6 hours before study to reduce size of stomach
No pretreatment with sodium perchlorate; may be given after completion of study
No barium studies should be performed within 3 to 4 days of scintigraphy.
Void before, during if possible, and after study.

Premedication
Cimetidine: 20 mg/kg/day orally for 48 hours in divided doses (or)
Intravenous: 300 mg in 100 mL 5% dextrose over 20 minutes; imaging begins 1 hour later
(or) Ranitidine: 2 mg/kg twice daily (or)
Intravenous: 1 mg/kg (maximum 50 mg) intravenously over 20 minutes; imaging begins 1 hour later
(or) Famotidine: 0.5 mg/kg once daily × 48 hours
Intravenous: 0.25 mg/kg intravenously 1 hour before procedure

Radiopharmaceutical
Tc-99m pertechnetate
    Children: 0.05 mCi/kg (1.85 MBq/kg)—minimum 1 mCi (37 MBq)
    Adults: 5 to 10 mCi (185–370 MBq) intravenously

Instrumentation
Gamma camera: Large field of view
Collimator: Low energy, all purpose or high resolution

Patient Position
Position patient supine under camera with xiphoid to symphysis pubis in field of view.

Imaging Procedure
Obtain flow images: 60 1-second frames.
Obtain static images: 500k-counts for first image, others for same time every 5 to 10 minutes for 1 hour.
Erect, right lateral, posterior, or oblique views may be helpful at 30 to 60 minutes.
Obtain postvoid image.

---

its low risk for side effects with short-term use. Pentagastrin was used in the past to stimulate uptake; however, it was removed from the U.S. market because of reported serious side effects.

Image Interpretation

On the scan, a Meckel diverticulum appears as a focal area of increased activity, usually in the right lower quadrant (see Fig. 10.37). Tc-99m pertechnetate uptake is seen within 5 to 10 minutes after injection and increases over time, typically at a rate similar to that of gastric uptake. Lateral or oblique views can help confirm the anterior position of the diverticulum versus the posterior location of renal or ureteral activity. Upright views may distinguish fixed activity (e.g., duodenum) from ectopic gastric mucosa, which moves inferiorly, and also renal pelvic activity. The intensity of activity may fluctuate because of intestinal secretions, hemorrhage, or increased motility washing out radiotracer. Postvoid images can empty the renal collecting system and aid in better visualization of areas adjacent to the bladder.

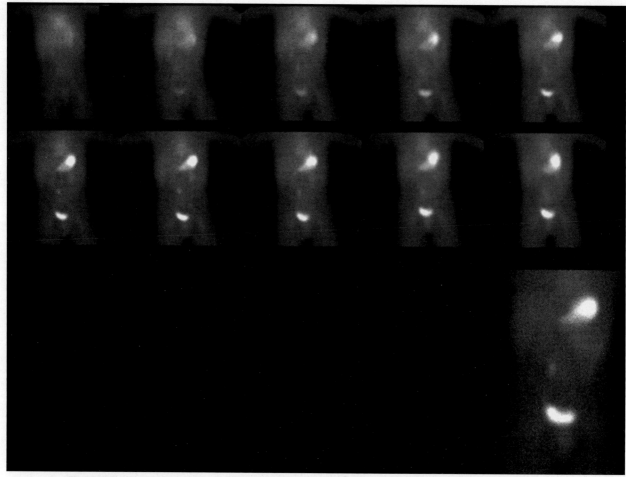

Fig. 10.37 Meckel diverticulum. Child referred with rectal bleeding. Sequential dynamic images *(top two rows)* and then static image *(below right)* show focal accumulation in the right lower quadrant. Note the simultaneous progressive uptake in the stomach and the Meckel diverticulum. Surgery confirmed the diagnosis.

Accuracy. The reported accuracy of Meckel scintigraphy is high. One large study reported results in 954 patients who had undergone scintigraphy for suspected Meckel diverticulum using modern imaging methods and found an overall sensitivity of 85% and specificity of 95%. Detection in adults is said to be lower, but data are quite limited.

False-negative studies may result from poor technique, rapid washout of the secreted Tc-99m pertechnetate, lack of sufficient gastric mucosa; a small diverticulum; and impaired diverticular blood supply from intussusception, volvulus, or infarction. Reported causes for false-positive study results are listed (Box 10.16). Activity in the genitourinary tract is the most common cause (see Fig. 10.38). Gastrointestinal duplications are potential false positives. These are cystic or tubular congenital abnormalities that have a mucosa, smooth muscle, and alimentary epithelial lining attached to any part of the gastrointestinal tract, often the ileum. Gastric mucosa occurs in 30% to 50% of duplications. Duplications often appear on scintigraphy as large, multilobulated areas of increased activity. Other false-positive causes include inflammatory and/or obstructive lesions of the intestines, as well as tumors. The final diagnosis of a duplication is made at surgery.

Retained Gastric Antrum

Retained gastric antrum may be left behind in the afferent loop after a Billroth II gastrojejunostomy. The antrum continues to produce gastrin, no longer inhibited by acid in the stomach because it is diverted through the gastrojejunostomy. The high acid production leads to marginal ulcers. Endoscopy or barium radiography may demonstrate the retained gastric antrum. A Tc-99m pertechnetate scan can be confirmatory. Uptake in the gastric remnant is seen as a collar of radioactivity in the duodenal stump of the afferent loop. The retained antrum usually lies to the right of the gastric remnant. In one series, uptake was detected in 16/22 patients.

Barrett Esophagus

Chronic gastroesophageal reflux can cause the distal esophagus to become lined by gastric columnar epithelium rather than the usual esophageal squamous epithelium. This condition is associated with complications of ulcers, strictures, and an 8.5% incidence of esophageal adenocarcinoma. Tc-99m pertechnetate scans show intrathoracic uptake contiguous with that of the stomach but conforming to the shape and posterior location of the esophagus. Today, the diagnosis is usually made with endoscopy and mucosal biopsy.

BOX 10.16 False-Positive Meckel Scan—Potential Causes

Urinary Tract
Ectopic kidney
Extrarenal pelvis
Hydronephrosis
Vesicoureteral reflux
Horseshoe kidney
Bladder diverticulum

Vascular
Arteriovenous malformation
Hemangioma
Aneurysm of intraabdominal vessel
Angiodysplasia

Hyperemia and Inflammatory
Peptic ulcer
Crohn disease
Ulcerative colitis
Abscess
Appendicitis
Colitis

Neoplasm
Carcinoma of sigmoid colon
Carcinoid
Lymphoma
Leiomyosarcoma

Small Bowel Obstruction
Intussusception
Volvulus

Other Sites of Ectopic Gastric Mucosa
Gastrogenic cyst
Enteric duplication
Duplication cysts
Barrett esophagus
Retained gastric antrum
Pancreas
Duodenum
Colon

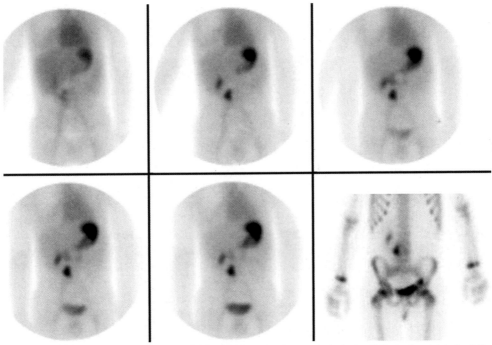

Fig. 10.38 Meckel scan: False positive. Sequential images show two foci of activity to the right of midline that progressively increase with time. A bone scan performed 6 months before this study showed a similar pattern, consistent with renal collecting-system clearance. The patient had crossed-fused ectopia.

PROTEIN-LOSING ENTEROPATHY

Excessive protein loss through the gastrointestinal tract is associated with a variety of diseases, including intestinal lymphangiectasia, Crohn, Ménétrier, amyloidosis, and intestinal fistula. Tc-99m human serum albumin, In-111 transferrin, and Tc-99m dextran have all been reported useful for confirming protein-losing enteropathy. However, these radiopharmaceuticals have not been approved for clinical use in the United States.

Case reports suggest that Tc-99m methylene diphosphonate bone scans can also be confirmatory.

PERITONEAL SCINTIGRAPHY

Peritoneal scintigraphy has been used for many years to evaluate intraabdominal distribution for planned intraperitoneal chemotherapy, to detect pleural-peritoneal communications (e.g., as the cause for a pleural effusion), to assess peritoneal

BOX 10.17 Peritoneal Scintigraphy: Summary Protocol

Patient Preparation

Place peritoneal catheter access.

Patients with minimal ascites may benefit from 500 mL of saline or other fluid infused into the peritoneal cavity before the study.

Patients on peritoneal dialysis should have 500 mL dialysate infused before study. They should have 100 mL dialysate with them for infusion after intraperitoneal injection of radiotracer.

Radiopharmaceutical

Tc-99m SC or Tc-99m MAA, 3 mCi (111 MBq)

Instrumentation

Gamma camera: Large field of view

Energy window: 20% window centered at 140 keV

Collimator: Low energy, parallel hole, high resolution or general purpose

Patient Position

Position patient supine under gamma camera.

Procedure

Check catheter patency before radiopharmaceutical injection.

Inject the radiopharmaceutical slowly 10 mL saline, followed by fluid flush.

Imaging

Obtain anterior and lateral static images for 5 minutes (128 × 128) or 500k counts.

Have patient ambulate if possible; alternatively, turn from side to side.

Repeat imaging 1 hour after injection.

Interpretation

Radiopharmaceutical should normally distribute throughout the peritoneal cavity, although often inhomogeneously.

MAA, Macroaggregated albumin; *SC*, sulfur colloid.

shunt patency, and to evaluate complications of peritoneal dialysis. Scintigraphy can diagnose pleural-peritoneal and scrotal-peritoneal communications, hepatic hydrothorax, traumatic diaphragmatic rupture, loculation of chemotherapy, peritoneal dialysis catheter flow, and obstructed LeVeen or Denver peritoneal venous shunts. A protocol is described in Box 10.17.

Methodology

Both Tc-99m SC and Tc-99m macroaggregated albumin (MAA) have been used because they do not diffuse through peritoneal surfaces. Both radiopharmaceuticals will stay below the diaphragm unless a pleural-peritoneal connection or a patent shunt is present (see Fig. 10.39). For purposes of chemotherapy, it can confirm good distribution throughout the peritoneum. SPECT may be helpful. To judge peritoneal venous shunt patency, Tc-99m MAA has the advantage of being taken up by the lungs, confirming patency.

Salivary Gland Scintigraphy

Xerostomia or dry mouth is due to salivary gland hypofunction resulting in reduced saliva production. This causes problems in tasting, chewing, and swallowing and can lead to tooth decay,

demineralization of teeth, tooth sensitivity, and oral infections. Etiologies include radiation therapy, chemotherapy, medications, radioactive iodine therapy, and Sjogren' syndrome, an autoimmune disorder in patients with rheumatoid arthritis and lupus.

Studies have shown that salivary gland dysfunction can be confirmed by scintigraphy, using Tc-99m pertechnetate, which can dynamically demonstrate abnormal or normal trapping and uptake and discharge of saliva after stimulation with sour candy or lemon juice.

Methodology

The fasting patient's head is placed in the Waters projection (anterior view with head tilted back 45 degrees), Tc-99m pertechnetate is injected intravenously, and dynamic images are obtained (15-second frames × 240; uptake phase). At frame 180 (end of uptake phase), lemon juice is administered to stimulate saliva (discharge phase). Normal quantitative values for uptake and discharge have been published for the parotid and submandibular glands.

Dacryoscintigraphy

Dacryoscintigraphy is an old nuclear medicine procedure that is still occasionally performed today to evaluate the drainage of nasolacrimal ducts, most commonly for epiphora, an overflow of tears that can be caused obstruction due to a variety of anatomical abnormalities. It is a noninvasive alternative to the contrast study. A droplet of normal saline with 100 µCi Tc-99m pertechnetate is instilled into the conjunctiva near the lateral canthus, and serial images are obtained every 15 to 30 seconds for 5 to 8 min. It can confirm subjective patient complaints. The contrast study is required for precise anatomical information as to the etiology of the obstruction.

HELICOBACTER PYLORI INFECTION

The 2005 Nobel Prize in Medicine was awarded for the discovery that ulcer disease is caused by *H. pylori*, a gram-negative bacterium. Antibiotic treatment often cures or greatly reduces the recurrence of duodenal and gastric ulcer disease. This was a major advance in therapy from the prior chronic medical symptomatic treatment and, in many cases, gastric surgery.

Urea Breath Test for *H. pylori*

In the presence of the bacterial enzyme urease, orally administered urea is hydrolyzed to carbon dioxide (CO_2) and ammonia. If the urea carbon is labeled with either the stable isotope carbon-13 or radioactive beta-emitter C-14, it can be detected in breath analysis as CO_2. *H. pylori* is the most common urease-containing gastric pathogen; thus, a positive breath test is equated with infection. Increasingly, the stable isotope breath test is being used clinically.

The initial diagnosis is usually made by gastric biopsy. The urea breath test is mostly used to determine the effectiveness of therapy against *H. pylori*. Serological tests cannot determine the effectiveness of therapy because the antibody titer falls too slowly to be diagnostically useful.

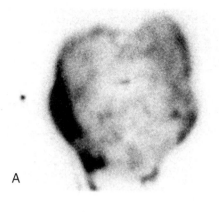
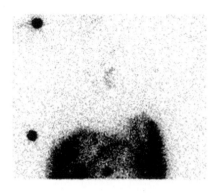
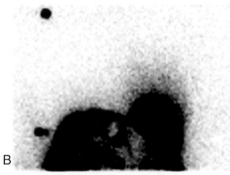
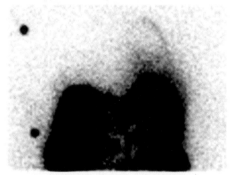

Fig. 10.39 Peritoneal perfusion studies. Two patients, A and B. Both patients are on peritoneal dialysis and had persistent pleural effusions. Tc-99m sulfur colloid (SC) was injected into the peritoneum. (A) Upper study; normal intraperitoneal distribution *(left);* only activity above the diaphragm is assumed to be thoracic duct *(right).* (B) Lower study; activity seen in left chest, suggestive of pleural distribution at 1 hour *(left);* definite uptake in pleural effusion at 2 hours *(right).*

The breath test is simple to perform, noninvasive, accurate, and inexpensive. An on-site analyzer is not needed because an expired air-filled balloon can be mailed for breath gas analysis. Overall accuracy is high. False-negative results may occur with recent use of antibiotics or bismuth-containing medications. False-positive results occur in patients with achlorhydria, contamination with oral urease-containing bacteria, and colonization with another *Helicobacter* species, such as *H. felis.* Increasingly today, the nonradioactive C-13 is more commonly used.

SUGGESTED READING

Abell TL, Camilleri M, Donohoe K, et al. Consensus recommendations for gastric emptying scintigraphy: a joint report of the American Neurogastroenterology and Motility Society and the Society of Nuclear Medicine. *J Nucl Med Technol.* 2008;36:44–54.

Antoniou AJ, Raja S, El-Khouli R, et al. Comprehensive radionuclide esophago-gastro-intestinal transit: methodology, normal values, and initial clinical experience. *J Nucl Med.* 2015;56:721–727.

Bonta DV, Lee HY, Ziessman HA. Shortening the four-hour gastric emptying protocol. *Clin Nucl Med.* 2011;36:283–285.

Diamond RH, Rothstein RD, Alavi A. The role of cimetidine-enhanced Tc-99m pertechnetate imaging for visualizing Meckel's diverticulum. *J Nucl Med.* 1991;32:1422–1424.

Grady E. Gastrointestinal bleeding scintigraphy in the early 21st century. *J Nucl Med.* 2016;57:252–259.

Klein HA. Improving esophageal transit scintigraphy. *J Nucl Med.* 1991;3:1372–1373.

Mariani G, Boni G, Barreca M, et al. Radionuclide gastroesophageal motor studies. *J Nucl Med.* 2004;45:1004–1026.

Maurer AH. Gastrointestinal motility, part 1: esophageal transit and gastric emptying. *J Nucl Med.* 2015;56:1229–1238.

Maurer AH. Gastrointestinal motility. Part 2: small-bowel and colon transit. *J Nucl Med.* 2015;56:1395–1400.

Parkman HP, Miller MA, Fisher RS. Role of nuclear medicine in evaluating patients with suspected gastrointestinal motility disorders. *Semin Nucl Med.* 1995;25:289–305.

Sachdeva P, Kantor S, Knight LC, et al. Use of a high caloric liquid meal as an alternative to a solid meal for gastric emptying scintigraphy. *Dig Dis Sci.* 2013;58:2001–2006.

Tougas G, Eaker EY, Abell TL, et al. Assessment of gastric emptying using a low fat meal: establishment of international control values. *Am J Gastroenterol.* 2000;95:1456–1462.

Ziessman HA, Chander A, Ramos A, Wahl RL, Clark JO. The added value of liquid gastric emptying compared to solid emptying alone. *J Nucl Med.* 2009;50:726–731.

Ziessman HA, Fahey FH, Atkins FB, Tall J. Standardization and quantification of radionuclide solid gastric-emptying studies. *J Nucl Med.* 2004;45:760–764.

11

Urinary Tract

Over the years, radiopharmaceuticals and scintigraphic techniques have been developed to assess different aspects of renal function. Using a variety of radiopharmaceuticals, these techniques can answer clinical questions not possible with ultrasound, computed tomography (CT), or magnetic resonance imaging (MRI). Some indications for nuclear scintigraphy are listed in Box 11.1. These include problem-solving and quantification applications that break down roughly into issues related to function and excretion and those related to cortical abnormalities.

RENAL ANATOMY AND PHYSIOLOGY

It is useful to know the anatomy and physiology of the kidney and urinary tract in order to best understand and interpret the functions and disease processes that affect various parts of the kidney (Fig. 11.1). The outer renal cortex contains the proximal convoluted tubules as well as the basic functional unit of the kidney, the nephron. Nephrons consist of glomeruli, the terminal capillary tufts from the renal arterial system, surrounded by the Bowman's capsule formed by the proximal end of the renal tubule. The more central medullary portion of the kidney contains the renal pyramids, collecting tubules, and the loops of Henle. At the apex of the pyramids, papillae drain into the renal calyces of the collecting system.

Normally, the kidneys receive 20% of cardiac output, with renal plasma flow (RPF) averaging 600 mL/min. The kidneys clear waste products from the plasma, which can be calculated as follows:

$$\text{Clearance (mL/min)} = \frac{\left[\text{Urine concentration}\left(\frac{mg}{mL}\right) \times \text{Urine flow}\left(\frac{mL}{min}\right)\right]}{\text{Plasma concentration}\left(\frac{mg}{mL}\right)}$$

Plasma clearance occurs by both glomerular filtration and tubular secretion (Fig. 11.2). If a substance undergoes 100% first-pass extraction, it could measure the total RPF. However, the actual extraction possible clinically is less than 100%, so the term *effective renal plasma flow* (ERPF) is generally a better description. The glomerular filtrate rate (GFR) is normally around 125 mL/min (approximately 20% of RPF delivered to the kidney) as water, polar molecules, and small crystalloids from the intravascular space pass through the semipermeable membrane into the ultrafiltrate. Larger material, such as cells, colloids, and protein-bound compounds, will not be filtered. The remaining plasma moves from the glomerulus into the efferent arteriole, where some molecules that could not be filtered are actively secreted by the tubular epithelial cells.

Paraaminohippurate (PAH) is the classic molecule used for ERPF measurement; its high clearance mirrors RPF distribution, with 20% of PAH cleared by glomerular filtration and 80% secreted into the proximal convoluted renal tubules by anionic transporters. The molecule inulin, on the other hand, is the historical gold standard for GFR measurement, with 100% of its clearance the result of filtration. These molecules help form the basis for some radiopharmaceuticals.

DYNAMIC RENAL IMAGING

Radiopharmaceuticals: Excretion and Washout

Renal radiopharmaceuticals are classified by their uptake and clearance mechanisms as agents for glomerular filtration, tubular secretion, or cortical binding. A list of important renal imaging agents is found in Table 11.1. The distribution and clearance rates vary considerably among these radiopharmaceuticals. Their uptake and clearance occur in different areas of the kidney (Fig. 11.3). Imaging characteristics and patterns vary considerably (Fig. 11.4), as do the clinical protocols used.

Of the various types of agents, those undergoing both filtration and secretion have greater clearance rates, allowing adequate visualization even in cases of fairly significant renal failure. The radiolabeled analog of PAH, I-131 Hippuran, with its high extraction of roughly 85%, could provide diagnostic

---

BOX 11.1 Clinical Indications for Urinary Tract Scintigraphy

Differential function quantification
Glomerular filtration rate (GFR) calculation
Hydronephrosis versus obstruction (ureteropelvic junction [UPJ], ureteral)
Renal artery stenosis
Monitoring partial UPJ obstruction
Assessing effects of corrective surgeries
Renal transplant rejection
Acute renal failure
Surgical and trauma complications: leak, vascular occlusion, etc.
Renal vein thrombosis
Renal artery occlusion
Pyelonephritis
Renal mass
Vesicoureteral reflux
Bladder residual volume (postvoid retention) calculation

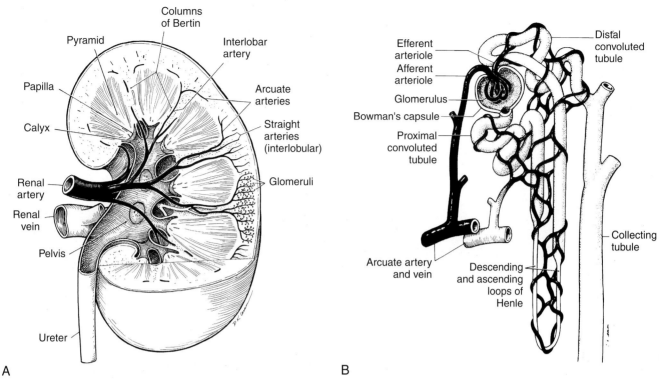

Fig. 11.1 Renal anatomy. (A) The outer cortex is made up of glomeruli and proximal collecting tubules. The columns of Bertin separate the pyramids in the cortex, extending into the medulla. The inner layer, or medulla, contains pyramids made up of distal tubules and loops of Henle. The tubules converge at the papillae, which empty into the calyces. The renal artery and vein enter at the hilum and divide and become arcuate arteries that give rise to the straight arteries, from which afferent arterioles feed the glomerular tuft. (B) The nephron consists of the glomerulus and the afferent vessels leading to the tuft of capillaries in the glomerulus and the efferent vessels leaving the glomerulus. Bowman's capsule surrounds the glomerulus and connects the proximal and distal renal tubules and loops of Henle.

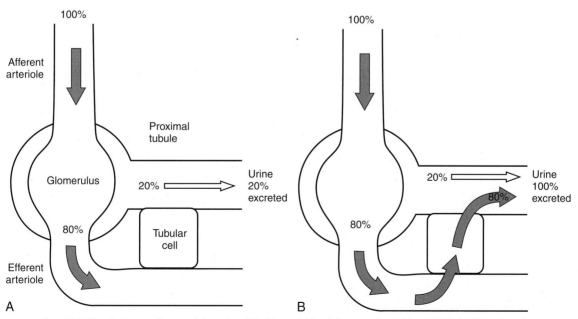

Fig. 11.2 Renal plasma flow and function. (A) Of renal blood flow to the kidneys, 20% is filtered at the glomerulus. (B) The remaining renal plasma flow moves on, with tubular secretion occurring into the proximal tubules, accounting for 80% of the output.

TABLE 11.1 Mechanism of Renal Radiopharmaceutical Clearance Agent

Clearance Agent	Glomerular Filtration (%)	Tubular Secretion (%)
Tc-99m DTPA	100	
Cr-51 EDTA[a]	100	
I-125 Iothalamate[b]	100	
Tc-99m MAG3		100
I-131 Hippuran[a]	20	80

[a]Currently not available in the United States for clinical use.
[b]Laboratory use without imaging.

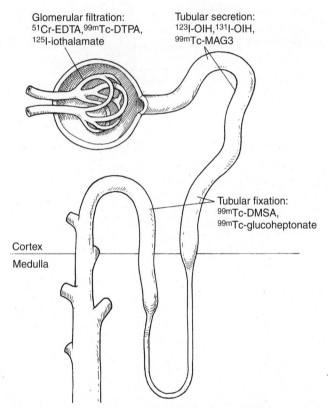

Glomerular filtration:
^{51}Cr-EDTA, ^{99m}Tc-DTPA, ^{125}I-iothalamate

Tubular secretion:
^{123}I-OIH, ^{131}I-OIH, ^{99m}Tc-MAG3

Tubular fixation:
^{99m}Tc-DMSA, ^{99m}Tc-glucoheptonate

Cortex
Medulla

Fig. 11.3 Different mechanisms of renal radiopharmaceutical uptake and excretion include glomerular filtration, tubular secretion, and cortical tubular binding.

studies as the creatinine rises, whereas radiopharmaceuticals dependent solely on glomerular filtration rapidly become nondiagnostic in the same situation. Although it was utilized in the past, the limited resolution of its images compared with Technetium-99m–based agents led to its replacement with another tubular agent, Tc-99m MAG3.

Tc-99m Diethylenetriaminepentaacetic acid

Diethylenetriaminepentaacetic acid (DTPA) is a heavy metal chelator used for the treatment of poisoning. When small, nontoxic amounts are labeled with Tc-99m, it is cleared via glomerular filtration with no tubular secretion or reabsorption, similar to other chelators. Different pharmaceutical preparation techniques result in variable impurities and, subsequently, different

levels of protein binding, which affects clearance because protein-bound DTPA cannot be filtered. In practice, normal first-pass Tc-99m DTPA extraction is less than the 20% of RPF because of binding, resulting in an underestimation of the GFR. However, if properly prepared, Tc-99m DTPA is generally adequate to measure GFR clinically. It should be noted that the alternative GFR agent, Cr-51 ethylene diamine tetraacetic acid (EDTA), does not suffer from such significant variable binding but is not available for clinical use in the United States. In addition to estimating GFR, Tc-99m DTPA imaging can assess flow and function in a variety of scenarios where Tc-99m MAG3 is also an option.

Technetium-99m Mercaptoacetyltriglycine

Currently, Technetium-99m mercaptoacetyltriglycine (Tc-99m MAG3) is the most commonly used renal radiopharmaceutical (Fig. 11.5). It is highly protein bound (97%), and because of this, it is essentially cleared entirely by tubular secretion. This also results in high target-to-background ratios because it cannot diffuse into the extravascular spaces. Although its clearance is only about 60% of that of I-131 Hippuran, the extraction efficiency is considerably higher than that of filtration agents, such as Tc-99m DTPA. This leads to excellent performance and less radiation exposure when function is compromised. However, when renal failure is significant, the alternative pathway of excretion through the hepatobiliary tract may be detected.

Tc-99m MAG3 images show significant anatomical detail while assessing function (Figs. 11.6 and 11.7). Later in the course of the examination, significant details can also be seen involving the collecting system (Fig. 11.8). Flow and plasma clearance can be evaluated in numerous clinical situations, often interchangeably with Tc-99m DTPA, but only Tc-99m MAG3 can be used to reproducibly measure ERPF. Tc-99m DTPA can be used to measure GFR.

Although the radiation dose to the patient from renal radiopharmaceuticals is low when renal function is normal, the absorbed dose rises significantly in the obstructed kidney or when renal function is poor. Dosimetry is listed in **Appendix 1**.

DYNAMIC RENOGRAPHY IMAGING PROTOCOLS

Preparation

Patients must also be properly hydrated to ensure prompt radiotracer clearance, avoiding any appearance of obstruction or decreased function. Because neurogenic bladder or bladder outlet obstruction can create the appearance of diminished renal function or obstruction, maneuvers including bladder catheterization, voiding, and upright positioning may be utilized. Finally, a clear understanding of the clinical question being posed and the patient's history is needed as protocols are tailored to each situation.

Acquisition and Processing

For both Tc-99m DTPA and Tc-99m MAG3, images are acquired in two phases utilizing similar protocols. An initial dynamic perfusion imaging sequence consists of images acquired every 1 to 4

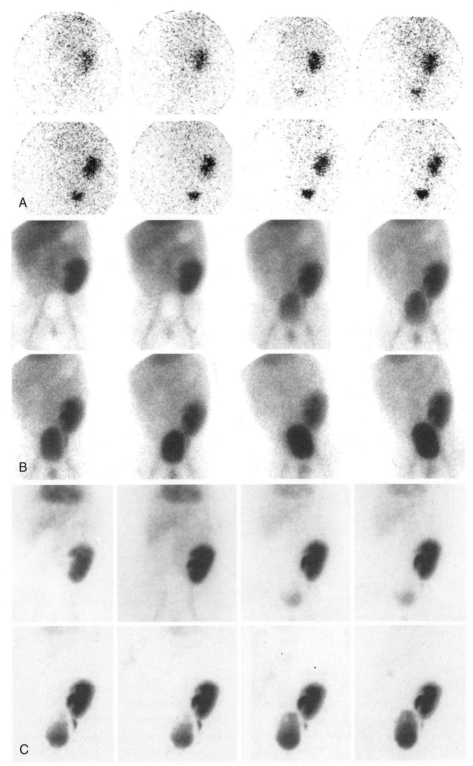

Fig. 11.4 Radiopharmaceutical comparison in a renal transplant patient. (A) I-131 Hippuran provides excellent functional information but has poor image quality compared with technetium agents. (B) Tc-99m DTPA image from the same day shows higher resolution. (C) Tc-99m MAG3 done 30 hours later reveals the highest level of detail as well as an improved target-to-background ratio compared with DTPA.

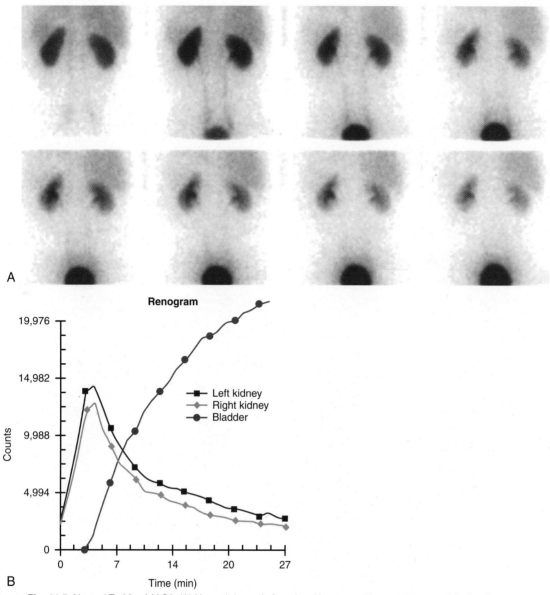

Fig. 11.5 Normal Tc-99m MAG3. (A) Normal dynamic functional images with prompt symmetrical radiotracer uptake and rapid clearance over the study. The liver is usually visible in the right upper corner of the images, which are usually acquired posteriorly. (B) Normal time–activity curves with a steep uptake slope, distinct peak, and rapid clearance confirming the visual analysis of the images.

seconds after radiotracer injection for 60 seconds. Then, over the next 25 to 30 minutes, images are acquired to assess renal uptake and clearance. An example protocol is provided in Box 11.2.

A time–activity curve (TAC) can be generated for both phases, placing a region of interest (ROI) on the aorta (or iliac artery for transplants), around the kidneys, and on a background near each kidney (Fig. 11.9). In cases of severe hydronephrosis, it may be desirable to draw the kidney ROI as a thin cortical crescent, excluding elevated counts from the central collecting system. Different types of background ROIs have been used, from small boxes to a 1- to 2-pixel rim around the kidney, but all are generally successful. The counts detected in the ROIs are then translated into a graph, a TAC, or a renogram (Fig. 11.10).

The differential or split function, the amount that each kidney contributes to overall function, is determined at the peak cortical

activity, before excreted activity is accumulating in the collecting system, usually about 2 to 3 minutes after injection. Children normally have more rapid transit, so a 1- to 2-minute interval may be more accurate. This measurement may be particularly useful when unilateral abnormalities have not been identified when global function and serum creatinine remain in the normal range (Fig. 11.11). Normally, each kidney contributes 50% of function, and each should normally contribute at least 45%. This information can be combined with measurements, such as GFR, to best indicate how the kidneys are functioning.

Interpretation

If the radiopharmaceutical dose is given as a rapid bolus, then perfusion to the kidneys should be seen immediately as the adjacent aorta (or iliac artery for transplants) and at a similar

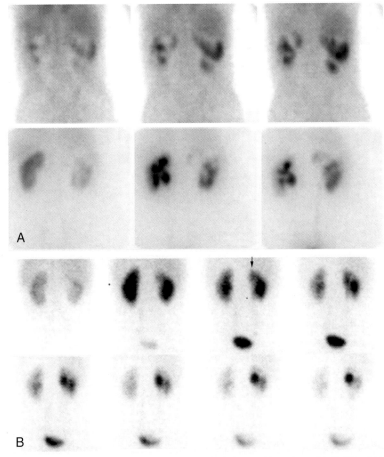

Fig. 11.6 Many abnormalities can be detected in the cortical phase of imaging with Tc-99m MAG3 examples revealing cortical abnormalities. (A) Multiple cortical defects from polycystic kidney disease are seen throughout the examination in poorly functioning kidneys. (B) Asymmetrical cortical uptake, decreased on the right, with a right upper pole scar *(arrow)* in a patient with a duplicated collecting system. The upper pole moiety collecting system fills without response to furosemide due to obstruction.

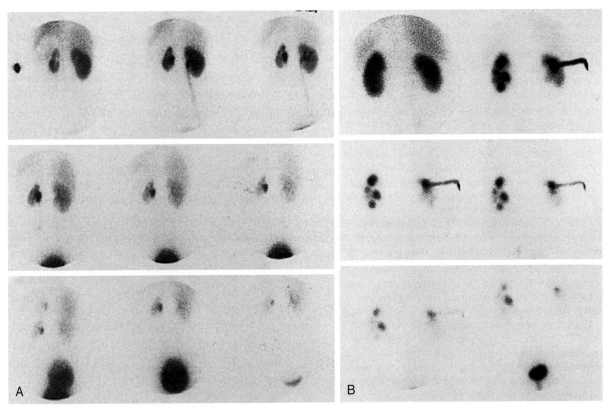

Fig. 11.7 Cortical function is readily assessed during the dynamic function portion of Tc-99m MAG3 imaging. The left kidney in (A) is small and scarred secondary to vesicoureteral reflux, contributing only 15% to overall function. (B) Obstructed right kidney secondary to cervical carcinoma is draining well through a nephrostomy tube, and function is relatively preserved, with good bilateral function. Prominent left pelvis and calyces are mostly cleared by the end of the study. The last image was taken with the bladder in view.

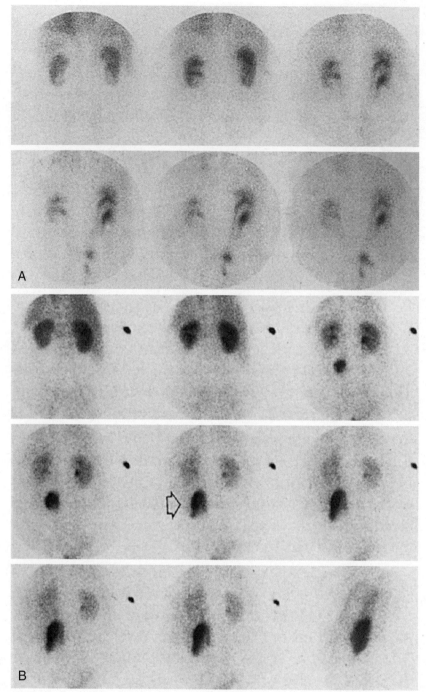

Fig. 11.8 After the peak cortical phase, many abnormalities can be detected during radiopharmaceutical excretion. (A) Duplicated right collecting system, a congenital abnormality sometimes associated with lower pole reflux and upper pole obstruction. (B) Postoperative ureteral leak on left *(arrow)* detected on sequential images.

BOX 11.2 Dynamic Renal Scintigraphy Protocol Summary

Preparation

Hydrate patient for 30 to 60 minutes.

    Adult: 300 to 500 mL

    Young children may require intravenous (IV) 10 to 15 mL/kg normal saline (with 5% dextrose for < 1 year).

Void bladder before injection.

Radiopharmaceuticals

Tc-99m MAG3

Adult: 78 to 111 MBq (2–3 mCi) if no flow, 111 to 185 MBq (3–5 mCi) if flow performed

Child: 3.7 MBq/kg (0.1 mCi/kg), minimum dose 37 MBq (1 mCi)

Tc-99m DTPA

Adult: 185 to 370 MBq (5–10 mCi) IV

Child: 1.9 MBq/kg (0.05 mCi/kg) IV, minimum dose 37 MBq (1 mCi)

Instrumentation

Large-field-of-view camera, positioned posteriorly for native kidneys (anterior for horseshoe or transplant)

Low-energy, high-resolution collimation; photopeak 15% to 20% window centered at 140 keV

Acquisition

Blood flow: 1 to 2 seconds/frame for 60 seconds

Dynamic: 30-second frames for 25 to 30 seconds

Prevoid image 500,000 counts; postvoid image for same time length

Processing

Draw region of interest around kidneys; draw background regions next to each.

Generate time–activity curves and differential function.

level within a couple seconds. Any asymmetry, delayed, or diminished flow on the images or TAC may represent decreased tissue volume from scarring or an active disease (Fig. 11.12).

During the initial cortical or nephrogram phase, the kidneys accumulate activity for the first 1 to 3 minutes, and the collecting system is either not seen or slightly photopenic. Peak overall

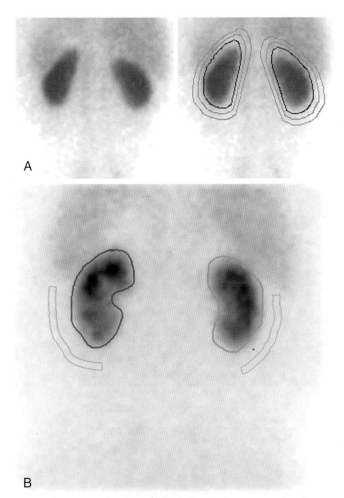

A

B

Fig. 11.9 Regions of interest (ROI) for time–activity curves. (A) *Left,* An image at 3 minutes with peak cortical activity is chosen for the ROIs. *Right,* Regions of interest are drawn for the kidney *(dark lines)* and for background correction *(gray lines)*. (B) Regions to assess background activity can also be drawn as smaller crescents below or laterally along the cortex.

activity on the TAC should normally occur by 4 to 6 minutes. The kidneys should be symmetrical in size. Chronic scarring causes an abnormal kidney to become smaller and less intense. Acutely, kidneys can appear enlarged, such as in high-grade obstruction.

During the clearance phase, activity moves from the cortex into the collecting system and is excreted into the bladder, with the TAC showing an exponential decline nearly to baseline by the end of the acquisition. In addition to slow uptake, when function is poor, the kidney may gradually accumulate activity over time with poor cortical washout, so-called cortical retention (Fig. 11.13). Cortical retention is a nonspecific finding that can be seen from multiple causes of acute and chronic renal failure (Box 11.3).

Normally, the calyces and pelvis usually begin filling by 3 minutes and ureters or bladder by 5 to 6 minutes, with the collecting-system activity decreasing through the final clearance phase. In some healthy subjects, pooling of activity in the dependent calyces can result in focal hot spots that usually clear at least partially over time. Hydronephrosis shows delayed or absent clearance, and the collecting system may appear enlarged, although areas with increased activity appear larger than they actually are, so caution must be taken when trying to gauge size.

Given the variability of peristalsis and other factors, the normal ureter may or may not be seen and may appear as a thin column of transient activity. Dilated ureters may visibly accumulate activity. Care must be taken in diagnosing reflux into the ureters. Indirect determination of reflux can be done when ureteral activity persists or recurs after the kidneys have cleared. However, reflux is best detected on a direct vesicoureterogram (VCUG) with activity introduced directly into the bladder via a catheter.

The prevoid and postvoid bladder images help evaluate emptying and postvoid residual. In infants and small children, the bladder may appear quite large and higher in position than might be expected when looking at the outline of the child's body on the image.

CLINICAL APPLICATIONS OF RENAL SCINTIGRAPHY

Urinary Tract Obstruction
Background
Obstruction can lead to recurrent infection, diminished function, progressive loss of nephrons, and parenchymal atrophy.

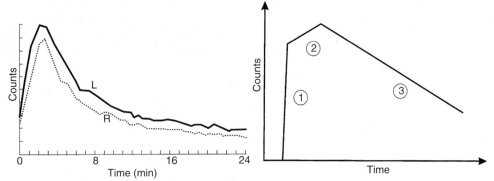

Fig. 11.10 Normal renogram time activity curve *(left)* can be divided into phases. *Right,* Initial blood flow (30–60 seconds). *2,* Cortical uptake phase (normally 1–3 minutes). *3,* Clearance phase representing cortical excretion and collecting-system clearance.

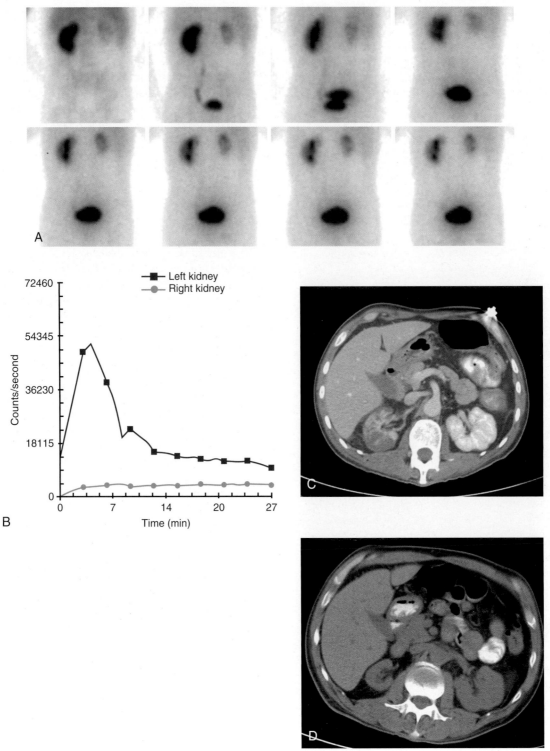

Fig. 11.11 Differential function and viability. (A) Tc-99m MAG3 images and time–activity curve (B) acquired shortly after injury from a car accident show little function in the right kidney (calculated at 6%). (C) Postcontrast computed tomography (CT) on admission revealed flow to the kidney but severe cortical injury. (D) 3 months later, a noncontrast CT shows chronic effects with the right kidney, now small and scarred.

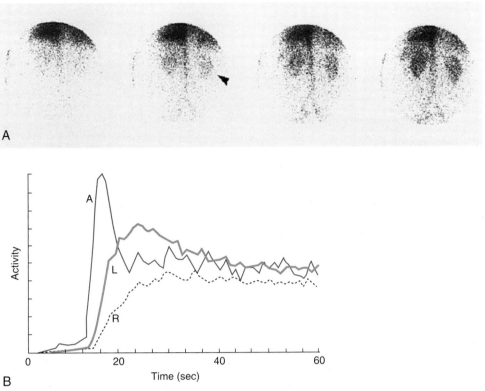

Fig. 11.12 Renal blood-flow analysis. (A) Sequential 2-second frames show moderately delayed and decreased blood flow to the right kidney *(arrowhead)*. (B) Sixty-second time–activity curves confirm the imaging findings. Initial upslope of the right kidney *(R)* is delayed compared with the aorta *(A)* and left kidney *(L)*.

Patients may present with pain, hematuria, or decreased function, or signs of obstruction may be discovered in the asymptomatic patient or neonate by ultrasound. Box 11.4 lists potential causes of hydronephrosis and obstruction—conditions for which furosemide (Lasix) renography is indicated. Within hours of onset, renal blood flow, glomerular filtration, and renal output are decreased. If a high-grade obstruction is corrected promptly, function can recover fully; however, if it is left uncorrected for more than a week, only partial recovery is expected.

Ultrasound is a sensitive method of identifying hydronephrosis but may not reliably indicate whether the dilation is due to mechanical obstruction or merely nonobstructive hydronephrosis (such as from reflux, primary megaureter, or a previous obstruction that has been relieved). CT and more invasive tests such as retrograde pyelography can often identify the cause of an obstructed system. However, the etiology of the hydronephrosis may not be evident.

The loop diuretic furosemide inhibits sodium and chloride reabsorption, markedly increasing dilute urine flow and renal washout. If mechanical obstruction is present, the narrowed lumen prevents augmented washout; prolonged retention of tracer is seen and can be measured with a Tc-99m MAG3 or Tc-99m DTPA nuclear medicine scan. This can help differentiate if dilation is the result of ongoing obstruction or prior obstruction, quantitate function to determine whether the kidney is salvageable were the obstruction corrected, and assess effects of therapy, helping plan safe stent removal or additional procedures. Additionally, some cases of partial ureteropelvic junction (UPJ) obstruction benefit from periodic

monitoring to determine whether critical obstruction is developing, requiring intervention.

Methods

Numerous diuretic renography protocols exist, although many areas have been agreed on. An example protocol is listed in Box 11.5. The 40-mg furosemide dose (80 mg or more when function is decreased) is injected slowly over 1 to 2 minutes, with an onset of action within 30 to 60 seconds and a maximal effect at 15 minutes. The time of diuretic administration varies at different centers. A commonly used method is the F + 20 furosemide protocol, giving furosemide 20 minutes after the radiotracer, allowing an identifiable of washout of pooled activity. However, earlier administration, giving furosemide at the same time (F + 0) as or 15 minutes before (F-15) the radiopharmaceutical may be useful in cases with diminished renal function because this gives additional time for the diuretic effect to occur, allowing radiotracer washout. Additionally, one study has shown that giving a diuretic at 10 minutes and imaging the patient in an upright position provides similarly accurate results. Alternatively, some centers still follow older methods and divide the examination into two parts, the first 30 minutes as described previously, then an additional 30-minute acquisition after Lasix injection.

Interpretation

Diuretic renography interpretation can be complex (Box 11.6). A dilated nonobstructed system responds to furosemide infusion and causes prompt clearance, in a linear or exponential manner, as a result of increased dilute urine flow (Fig. 11.14).

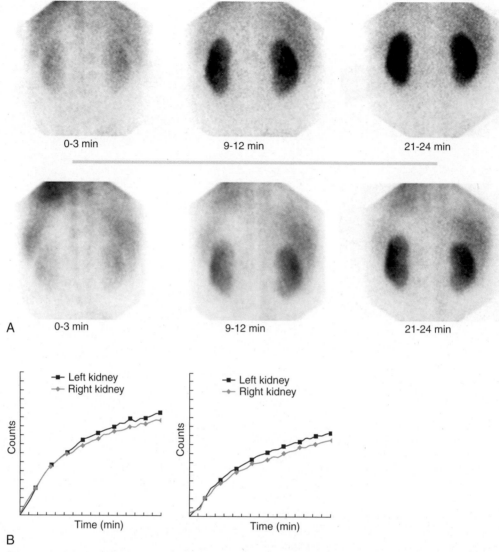

Fig. 11.13 Acute and chronic renal failure. (A) Tc-99m MAG3 images in a patient with newly elevated creatinine initially showed slow uptake and clearance with bilateral cortical retention *(top row)*. It is not possible to predict whether any improvement can be expected. No improvement occurred 6 months later, and uptake slightly diminished as function gradually worsened *(bottom row)*. (B) The time–activity curves show poor uptake and clearance with a slight worsening between the two studies, with a more gradually rising slope on the right. In long-standing renal failure, uptake tends to diminish over time, with kidneys appearing small, scarred, and less intense.

BOX 11.3   Causes of Cortical Retention

Native Kidneys
Severe obstruction
Chronic medical renal disease
Ischemia
Venous thrombosis
Acute tubular necrosis (ATN)
Dehydration

Renal Transplants
Posttransplant delayed graft function/ATN
Acute rejection
Immunosuppressive drug toxicity
Drug toxicity
Chronic rejection

BOX 11.4   Indications for Diuretic Renography

Hydronephrosis
Unexplained
Obstructing pelvic mass
Obstructing calculi: current, prior
Ureteropelvic junction (UPJ) obstruction
Ileal loop diversion
Megaureter: obstructive, nonobstructive, refluxing
Horseshoe kidney
Polycystic kidney

Prune-belly syndrome
Ectopic ureterocele
Urethral valves
Postoperative states
Pyeloplasty
Ureteral reimplantation
Urinary diversion
Renal transplant ureteral obstruction

BOX 11.5 Diuretic Renography Protocol Summary

Patient Preparation

Hydration should be as described in dynamic renography protocol.

Place Foley catheter in children; consider in adults with bladder outlet issues.

If not catheterized, complete bladder emptying before diuretic injection.

Furosemide (Lasix)

Children: 1 mg/kg to maximum 40 mg (may require more in severe azotemia)

Adults: 40 mg intravenous (IV) normal creatinine level, 80 to 100 mg for elevated creatinine

Timing: 20 minutes after injection; consider 15 minutes before (F-15) or with Tc-99m MAG3 (F + 0) in azotemia

Imaging Procedure

Inject Tc-99m MAG 3 to 5 mCi (111–185 MBq).

Acquire study for 20 minutes as per the renal scan protocol.

Slowly infuse furosemide intravenously over 60 seconds.

Continue imaging 10 to 30 minutes.

Obtain prevoid and postvoid images.

Image Processing

On computer, draw region of interest around entire kidney and pelvis.

Generate time–activity curves.

Calculate a half-emptying time or fitted half-time.

BOX 11.6 Factors Affecting Diuretic Renography Interpretation

Causes of diminished response to furosemide:
  Dehydration
  Pressure from distended bladder
  Massive hydronephrosis
  Azotemia
  In infants: insufficient time for diuretic action
Diuretic given at T0 or before Tc-99m MAG3
  Acts steadily, does not give visible drop in curve
  $T_{\frac{1}{2}}$ values not applicable
  Administration at T(0) or T(-15) useful with azotemia
Ureteropelvic junction may present with partial obstruction, but critical blockage is often detected on serial examinations.
Use of diuretics in patients with spinal cord injury can result in dangerous hypotension.
Postoperative obstruction in renal transplants can be best assessed with diuretic scans.
  External fluid collections
  Anastomotic swelling or stricture follow-up
  Hydronephrosis

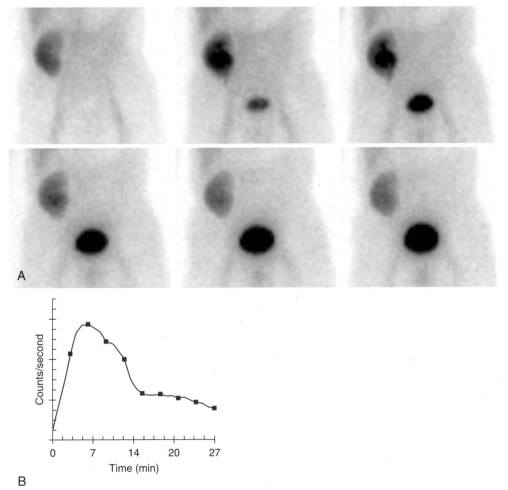

Fig. 11.14 Diuretic renography with no obstruction. A right pelvic renal transplant was noted to have new hydronephrosis on ultrasound. The Tc-99m MAG3 diuretic examination (A) and time–activity curves (B) with furosemide given at 10 minutes shows the prominent collecting system clearing promptly without evidence of obstruction.

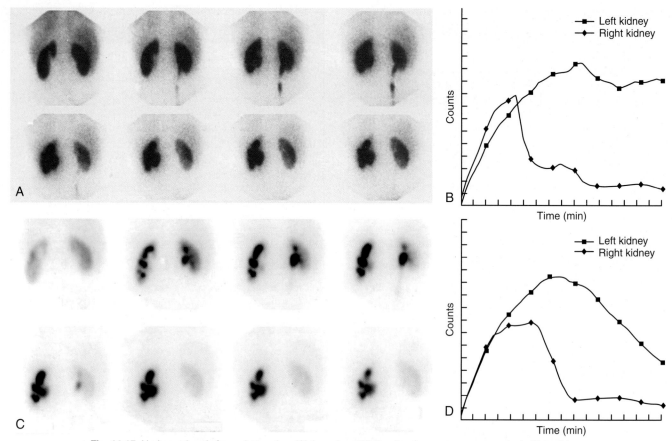

Fig. 11.15 Hydronephrosis from obstruction. (A) An enlarged left collecting system progressively fills, with no clearance in response to Lasix given at 10 minutes, unlike the normal right kidney. The visual impression of obstruction is confirmed by the time–activity curve (B). After left ureteropelvic junction obstruction correction in the same patient, Tc-99m MAGs Lasix images (C) and TAC (D) show residual hydronephrosis but correction of the obstruction.

An obstructed system, on the other hand, will not respond to the diuretic challenge; activity will continue to accumulate or sometimes stay at a plateau (Fig. 11.15). Acute high-grade obstruction often shows uptake but no excretion, which can look similar to severe cortical retention. Different patterns can be seen in response to furosemide (Fig. 11.16). In very distended systems, delayed washout may be seen regardless of whether obstruction is present. An "indeterminate" clearance pattern is seen with little change on the images or TAC (see Fig. 11.16D).

Diuretic response may also be diminished with azotemia, so an increased furosemide dose or early diuretic infusion (F-15) may be used. However, even with additional modifications, it may not be possible to induce sufficient diuresis to exclude obstruction in a poorly functioning kidney (Figs. 11.17 and 11.18). Although elevated serum creatinine may indicate severe renal dysfunction, GFR or ERPF may be more accurate, especially if the lesion is unilateral. If the GFR on the affected side is less than 15 mL/min, diuretic renography is unreliable.

At times, it is useful to quantitate collecting-system clearance half-time or washout half-time ($T_{1/2}$), the length of time it takes to reach half-peak after the diuretic. Generally, a $T_{1/2}$ less than 10 minutes indicates there is no significant obstruction present, whereas values greater than 20 minutes are considered obstructed. Values between 10 and 20 minutes fall in a gray zone or indeterminate range. When a collecting system is very large, it may clear abnormally slowly even if not obstructed.

RENOVASCULAR HYPERTENSION

Significant renal artery stenosis (RAS) causes glomerular perfusion pressure to drop, and as the GFR falls, renin secretion from the renal juxtaglomerular apparatus is stimulated, leading to angiotensin-converting enzyme (ACE) activation of the powerful vasoconstrictor angiotensin II. The resulting constriction raises blood pressure peripherally, including the efferent arterioles of the glomerulus, raising filtration pressure and thus maintaining GFR (Fig. 11.19).

Although more than 90% of patients with hypertension have essential hypertension, renovascular hypertension (RVH) from RAS is common among patients who have a correctable cause. Early intervention decreases arteriolar damage and glomerulosclerosis, increasing the chance for cure. However, in many cases, treating the stenosis does not cure the patient. ACE inhibitor (ACEI) renography (or "captopril scan") is an accurate method to diagnosis reversible RVH. ACEIs block conversion of angiotensin I to angiotensin II (Fig. 11.20). This causes patients with RVH who rely on the compensatory mechanism to show a

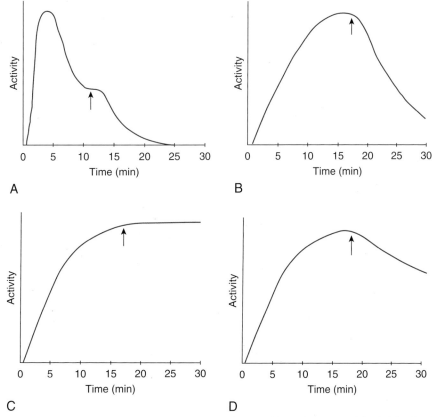

Fig. 11.16 Diuresis time–activity curve (TAC) examples of Lasix effects. Arrows mark Lasix injection. (A) Normal kidney response to diuretic. The short plateau before further emptying represents diuretic-induced flow just before rapid clearance. (B) Dilated nonobstructed kidney. The slowly rising curve represents progressive pelvocaliceal filling. With a diuretic, rapid clearance occurs. (C) Obstructed kidney. The diuretic has no effect on the abnormal TAC. (D) Indeterminate response. After the diuretic, very slow partial clearance is seen. This can be the result of an extremely distended system, but obstruction is not excluded.

drop in GFR and renal clearance, which can be imaged. The ACEI renal scan should be considered in scenarios such as those listed in Box 11.7.

Imaging Protocol

Patient preparation involves discontinuation of all ACEIs before the study or sensitivity for the diagnosis of RVH is reduced by approximately 15%. Stopping angiotensin receptor blockers and halting calcium channel blockers also should be considered. Care must be taken with other diuretics to prevent dehydration. Otherwise, most antihypertensive agents have little or no effect on the results.

A decision must be made as to which imaging protocol to use. Oral captopril requires an hour delay for absorption but does not require intravenous (IV) access and is usually cheaper than enalapril. A 1-day protocol can be performed by first doing a baseline examination using a low dose of 1 mCi (37 MBq) of Tc-99m MAG3 radiopharmaceutical followed by a post-ACEI study using 5 mCi (185 MBq) of Tc-99m MAG3. However, doing the pre- and post-examinations on separate days, at least 24 hours apart, makes interpretation easier, with the baseline examination performed only on those with an abnormal ACEI test. An example protocol is listed in Box 11.8.

Although a drop in blood pressure is expected after ACEI administration, blood pressure should be monitored, making sure the patient is stable.

Image Interpretation

In patients with renin-dependent RVH, decreased blood flow to the affected kidney is *not* seen, even after giving an ACEI. If decreased perfusion is seen, it is usually related to decreased tissue volume. Instead, effects from stenotic lesions are primarily manifested on the scan as cortical retention (cortical staining) from delayed Tc-99m MAG3 washout (Fig. 11.21). If the radiopharmaceutical used is Tc-99m DTPA, a positive scan will show a dramatic decrease in uptake and overall function instead (Fig. 11.22). Other signs have been reported but are less common or specific. Comparison to a baseline scan is needed to be sure the abnormal scan is an acute result of ACEI effects rather than chronic change from some other condition.

If the protocol has been properly followed, the sensitivity and specificity of ACEI renography are reportedly 90% and 95%, respectively. In general, ACEI renography is accurate when the serum creatinine is normal or only mildly elevated (creatinine < 1.7 mg/dL). False-positive results are rare but have been reported in patients on calcium channel blockers. If bilateral cortical

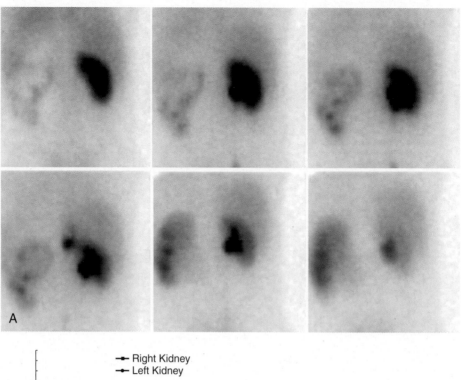

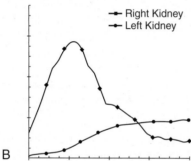

Fig. 11.17 Decreased function resulting from high-grade obstruction. (A) Dynamic sequential Tc-99m MAG3 images performed 15 minutes after giving Lasix reveal normal function on the right. The left kidney shows only a thin rim of cortex with delayed uptake, a photopenic hydronephrotic collecting system, and continual collecting-system filling without washout consistent with obstruction. (B) Findings are confirmed on the time–activity curve.

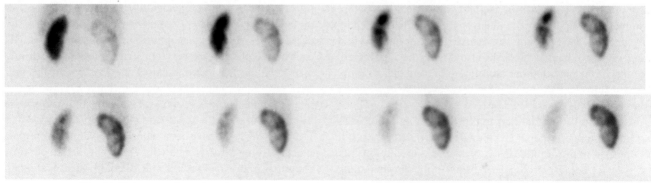

Fig. 11.18 Impact of ongoing obstruction. Untreated high-grade right-sided vesicoureteral junction obstruction secondary to tumor results in dilation of the central collecting system and a thin cortex functioning poorly, with slow uptake.

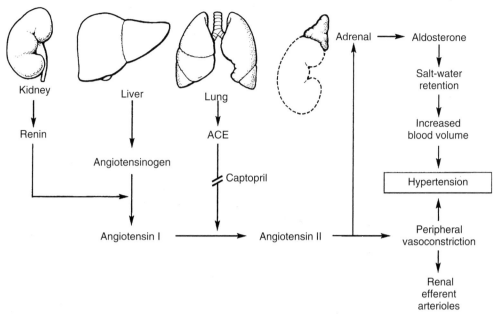

Fig. 11.19 Renin–angiotensin–aldosterone pathways and site of angiotensin-converting enzyme (ACE) inhibitor captopril action.

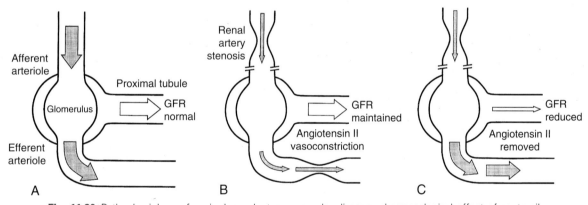

Fig. 11.20 Pathophysiology of renin-dependent renovascular disease: pharmacological effect of captopril. (A) Normal glomerular filtration rate (GFR). (B) Renovascular hypertension. Because of reduced renal plasma flow, filtration pressure and GFR fall. Increased renin and resulting angiotensin II produce vasoconstriction of the efferent glomerular arterioles, raising glomerular pressure and maintaining GFR. (C) Captopril blocks the normal compensatory mechanism, and GFR falls.

BOX 11.7 Indications for Angiotensin-Converting Enzyme Inhibitor (ACEI) Renography (Captopril Scan)

Severe hypertension
Hypertension resistant to medical therapy
Abrupt or recent onset of hypertension
Onset of hypertension < 30 years or over 55 years of age
Abdominal or flank bruits
Unexplained azotemia
Worsening renal function during ACEI therapy
Occlusive arterial disease in other beds
Known renal artery lesion to assess potential reversibility of renovascular hypertension (RVH)
Assess effects of therapy, also allowing differential function calculation.

---

retention is seen, it is likely artifact from dehydration or hypotension and not bilateral renal artery stenosis. Among patients with bilateral cortical retention undergoing arteriogram, roughly two-thirds had no significant stenosis (Fig. 11.23).

RENAL TRANSPLANT EVALUATION

Kidneys for transplantation come from one of three sources: a deceased donor (cadaveric kidney), a living related donor, or a living unrelated donor. Although cadaveric kidneys are carefully screened and transported, allografts from living donors generally have the best prognosis. Allograft 1-year survival rates are 90% to 94% for living-related-donor kidneys and 88% to 90% for cadaveric transplants. Having an understanding of common complications can help in correctly recommending

BOX 11.8   Angiotensin-Converting Enzyme Inhibitor (ACEI) (Captopril) Protocol Summary

Preparation

Discontinue ACEIs 2 to 3 days for short acting, 5 to 7 days for long acting.
  Consider stopping calcium channel blockers.
No food for 4 hours before examination; drink fluids to hydrate during this time.
Before injection, use hydration protocol as per the general renal protocol.

Medications and Dose

ACEI
  Captopril 50 mg PO, monitor blood pressure for 1 hour -OR-
  Enalapril 40 μCi/kg (minimum 2.5 mg) intravenous (IV) over 3 to 5 minutes,
    leave IV line in place, monitor for 5 minutes
  Lasix 40 mg IV
  Inject Tc-99m MAG3

Acquisition

  2-day protocol: day 1 Tc-99m MAG3 111 to 185 MBq (3–5 mCi); day 2 perform
    baseline if phase 1 is abnormal
  1-day protocol: 37 to 74 MBq (1–2 mCi) IV baseline before Captopril; then 185
    to 296 MBq (5–8 mCi) phase 2 after ACEI

Imaging

Use methods for dynamic imaging protocol (see Box 11.2).

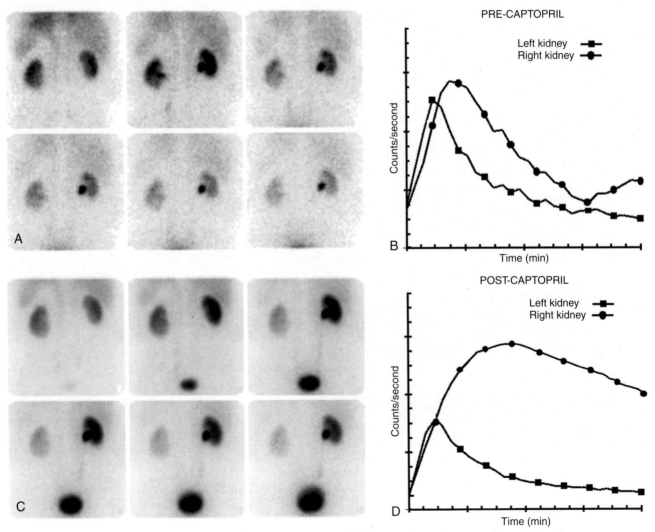

Fig. 11.21 Positive Tc-99m MAG3 captopril study. (A and B) The baseline study was performed first. Note prompt, fairly symmetrical initial uptake and good washout over time. (C and D) A follow-up examination performed later the same day with captopril shows marked cortical retention on the right, considered "high probability" for renal artery stenosis as a cause for renovascular hypertension.

Baseline

Captopril

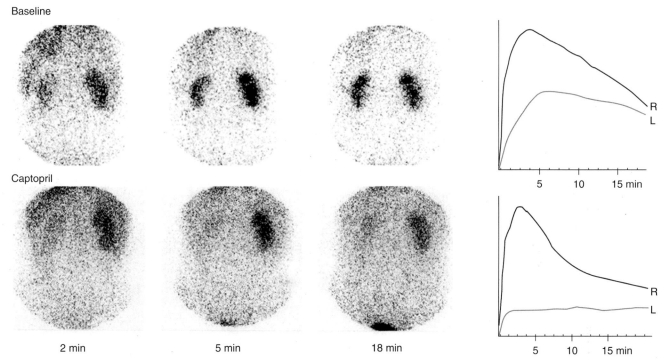

2 min   5 min   18 min

Fig. 11.22 Effects of captopril on renovascular hypertension with Tc-99m DTPA. *Top,* The baseline study shows mildly decreased function on the left. *Bottom,* Examination after captopril reveals severe deterioration on the left kidney with diminished peak and overall function.

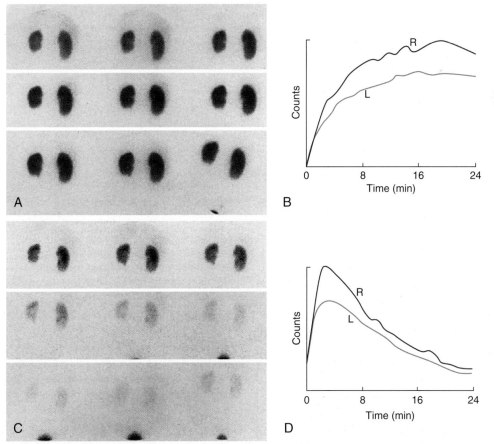

Fig. 11.23 Captopril-stimulated Tc-99m MAG3 study (A) and the captopril time–activity curve (TAC) (B) show marked bilateral cortical retention and minimal urinary bladder clearance over 30 minutes. The patient had abstained from food and drink for nearly 12 hours before the examination. Repeat captopril images (C) and TAC (D) after hydration are normal. Bilateral positive captopril findings are most commonly a false positive from dehydration.

testing and correctly interpreting scan findings. Table 11.2 lists common complications.

Transplant Complications
Delayed Graft Function (ATN)
Poor function in the immediate posttransplant period can be caused by ischemia, volume depletion, and nephrotoxic drugs in the pretransplant period. The terms *delayed graft function* and *acute tubular necrosis* (ATN) have been used interchangeably to describe this process, although ATN is just one of the possible causes. It is more common in cadaveric transplants, seen in up to 50%, but it can also occur in a small fraction of kidneys from living related donors (5%). Delayed graft function presents immediately or in the first few days as decreased urine output. This typically resolves from a few days to up to 4 to 6 weeks.

Acute Rejection
Hyperacute rejection is seen immediately from major incompatibilities, and the prognosis for survival is grim. Accelerated acute rejection develops in the first few days after transplantation, caused by preformed antibodies, likely from prior sensitization. Cellular-mediated acute rejection (AR) is not seen until after a week or so, commonly presenting with decreasing urine output, although the patient may have fever and painful swelling of the kidney. AR becomes less common after several

months or a year if the patient is taking his or her medication because the patient becomes relatively desensitized.

Chronic rejection is a common term for an autoimmune, cumulative, and irreversible process typically not seen for weeks to months. Vascular constriction, chronic fibrosis, tubular atrophy, and glomerulosclerosis from immunological and nonhumoral causes occur. Over months to years, this fibrosis causes cortical loss and decreased function. Relative dilation of the collecting system may be seen as the cortex thins. Risk factors for early development (<1 year) and allograft loss include damage from early ischemic injury (severe ATN), prior severe AR episodes, and subclinical rejection. Calcineurin-inhibitor therapy (cyclosporine and tacrolimus) is thought to play a role in thrombotic microangiopathy.

Immunosuppressive Drug Toxicity
Another important cause of allograft dysfunction is nephrotoxicity of therapeutic drugs. In the past, this was often due to high levels of cyclosporine. Cyclosporine toxicity is less commonly seen because it has been largely replaced with other agents or is prescribed at lower, safer levels. Similar changes can be seen with other antirejection agents.

Surgical Complications and Renal Diseases
Major vascular abnormalities can occur, including arterial thrombosis and renal vein thrombosis. Issues can also arise at the ureteral anastomosis: obstruction, leak, or lymphoceles. These issues generally present in the first few days after surgery. Transplanted kidneys may also develop problems like renal artery stenosis with renovascular hypertension as well as ureteral obstruction.

Transplanted kidneys are usually evaluated by ultrasound and biopsy when complications occur. However, radionuclide scintigraphy has been widely used to evaluate not only renal function but also complications in renal allografts.

Methods
Renal allograft evaluation is performed using the dynamic scintigraphy protocol with Tc-99m MAG3 listed in Box 11.2, except the camera is anterior, centered over the allograft in the lower pelvis. It is useful to include at least some of the native kidneys in the field of view because they may contribute to overall function. Some portion of the bladder should be seen, and the entire bladder is included on prevoid and postvoid images. Delayed images for up to 1 to 2 hours or single-photon emission computed tomography (SPECT)/CT may be helpful to assess fluid collections. Lasix or captopril studies can be performed when needed.

Interpretation
Renal transplant scans must be interpreted with the age of the transplant in mind as well as the type of allograft. The two most common issues to consider in the early posttransplant period are ATN/delayed graft function and AR (Table 11.3). Because both manifest clinically with decreased function, the scan typically shows slower uptake initially, progressively increasing cortical activity over time, and a delay in the appearance of collecting-system and bladder activity from the expected 3- to 6-minute time frame. Unlike ATN, AR affects the small renal

TABLE 11.2	Renal Allograft Complications	
Complications	**Timeline**	**Comments**
Delayed graft function/ acute tubular necrosis (ATN)	Minutes to hours	Presurgical damage Cadaveric transplants may take days or weeks to recover
Autoimmune Rejection and Functional Damage		
Hyperacute rejection	Minutes	Preformed antibodies, irreversible
Accelerated acute rejection	1–5 days	History of transfusion or prior transplant
Acute rejection	7 days on	Most common first 3 months Cell-mediated humoral
Chronic rejection	Months to years	Humoral, irreversible
Cyclosporine toxicity	months	Reversible with drug withdrawal
Surgical		
Urine leak/urinoma	Days or weeks	
Hematoma	First few days	
Infection	First week	
Lymphocele	2–4 months	
Vascular		
Renal artery stenosis	After first month	
Vascular occlusion	Days to weeks	
Infarcts		
Renal obstruction	Days to months	Pelvic mass, stricture, calculi

parenchymal vessels. The classic dynamic imaging pattern of AR is decreased perfusion and then marked cortical retention with Tc-99m MAG3 (Fig. 11.24). ATN, on the other hand, shows normal perfusion but poor function with delayed cortical clearance and decreased urine excretion immediately after surgery (Fig. 11.25).

ATN is the result of damage occurring before transplant insertion and so is present from the start. Although function usually improves in the first couple of weeks (Fig. 11.26), it often persists in severe cases, overlapping with the time frame expected of acute rejection. In these cases, worsening function suggests that another process is developing (Fig. 11.27).

The degree of renal dysfunction can vary widely. Severe cortical retention or function that does not rapidly improve on serial studies has strong negative prognostic implications, with increased transplant loss in the first 6 months. Multiple episodes of AR, especially if severe, also have a negative effect on transplant survival.

Nephrotoxicity from immunosuppressive drugs causes delayed clearance similar to that of delayed graft function/ATN.

The time frame of the examination usually allows these two processes to be differentiated. In some cases, the history will point to a cause for ATN occurring long after transplant surgery, such as from cardiovascular collapse or medication issues.

When renal function is initially normal, it is simpler to differentiate AR from delayed graft function. However, it may be difficult to differentiate AR from the toxicity effects of immunosuppressive therapy.

In chronic rejection, the blood flow and function images may initially appear normal. As it worsens, serial examinations show mild to moderate parenchymal retention. Over time, nephron loss causes cortical thinning and the associated "ex-vacuo" central collecting-system prominence. Uptake appears patchy, the allograft appears small or scarred, and clearance is delayed (Figs. 11.28 and 11.29).

The rare acute renal artery occlusion leads to absent perfusion and a photopenic defect on the functional portion of scintigraphy, often with a surrounding rim of activity. Renal vein thrombosis can have the same appearance. Because there are no collaterals or lymphatics, the kidney is rapidly destroyed and

TABLE 11.3 Comparison of Acute Rejection and Postoperative Acute Tubular Necrosis (ATN)

Disease	Baseline Scan	Early Follow-Up Scan	Perfusion	Renal Transit Time
Acute rejection	Normal	Worsens	Decreased	Delayed
ATN	Abnormal	Improves	Normal	Delated

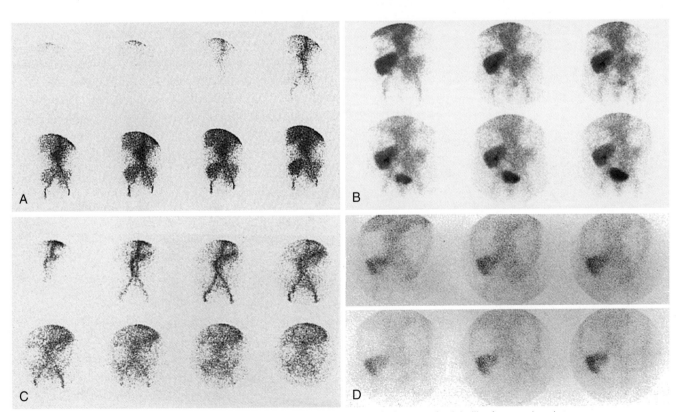

Fig. 11.24 Acute allograft rejection. Postoperative Tc-99m MAG3 images of a right iliac fossa cadaveric transplant show good baseline blood flow (A) and reasonably good function (B). Six days later, the patient developed fever, allograft tenderness, and elevated serum creatinine. Repeat blood flow is diminished (C), and functional images show cortical retention (D). These findings are consistent with acute rejection.

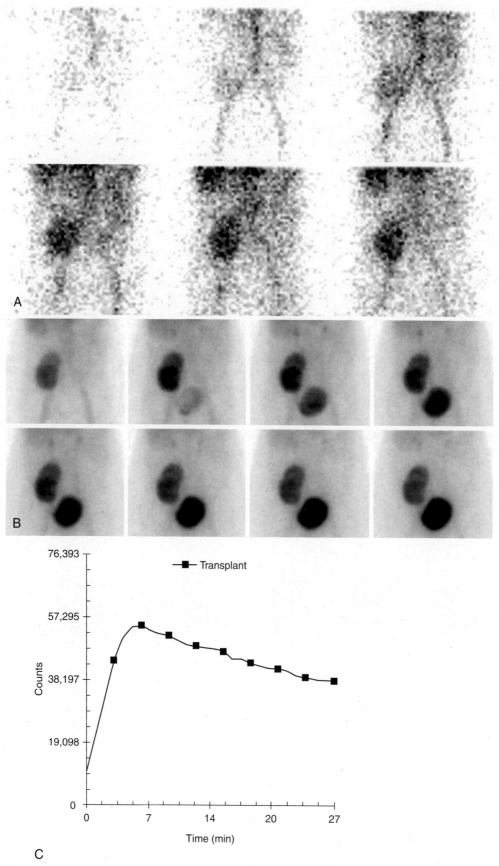

Fig. 11.25 Postoperative function in a cadaveric transplant. Imaging at 72 hours after surgery reveals normal perfusion (A) with decreased function (B) with slightly slower uptake, mildly delayed transit to bladder, and significant cortical retention. The time–activity curve (C) confirms the impression of postoperative acute tubular necrosis (ATN). If flow images are inadequate to differentiate delayed graft function from acute rejection, the time course of the functional changes or biopsy and follow-up may be needed.

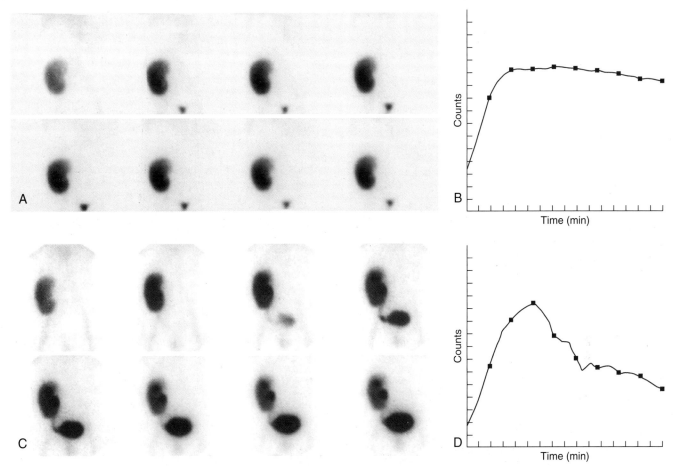

Fig. 11.26 Delayed graft function/acute tubular necrosis (ATN). *Top row,* Baseline blood-flow images (A) and time–activity curve (B) obtained 24 hours after transplantation reveal significant cortical retention, confirming the diagnosis of delayed graft function, often called acute tubular necrosis. *Bottom row,* A follow-up examination shows improving function (C), with more rapid transit into bladder and decreased cortical retention, confirmed on the time-activity curve (D).

does not look enlarged and hot like acute renal vein thrombosis in native kidneys (Fig. 11.30).

Other problems seen on CT or ultrasound can be characterized. Perinephric fluid collections from a leak can show radiotracer accumulation, sometimes not visible until delayed images at 1 to 2 hours (Fig. 11.31). An obstructed allograft may present with hydronephrosis or diminished urine output. Diuretic renography can be useful in suspected obstruction, as in native kidneys (Fig. 11.32). It is important that acute rejection is not present and that there is adequate function to respond to the diuretic.

MEASURING RENAL FUNCTION: GLOMERULAR FILTRATION RATE

The normal GFR varies according to age, sex, and body size. The estimated GFR can be fairly reliably calculated using these factors and the serum creatinine. However, these estimations may not be reliable when function is very abnormal, and changes from a unilateral abnormality may be difficult to detect. It should be noted that any method for measuring function may not be "precise," but the methods are generally reproducible and

generally superior to creatinine-based methods in the very young and the elderly or when function is poor.

Nuclear medicine techniques using different combinations of plasma sampling and imaging techniques have evolved. Although these are the most accurate, few institutions have the wet laboratory setup for the more accurate blood sample methods; therefore, camera-based techniques are more practical. Camera-based methods require no blood sampling and only a few minutes of imaging time (Fig. 11.33). Precise adherence to protocol is necessary, however, because they are more prone to error than the blood-sampling methods.

For camera-based GFR calculation, a small known dose of Tc-99m DTPA is counted at a set distance from the camera face. The actual administered dose is then corrected for the postinjection residual in the syringe and serves as a standard. If the dose is too large, it may overwhelm the counting capabilities of the system, and lost counts would affect accuracy, causing overestimation of GFR. Some camera systems no longer have software to easily perform these studies, but manual calculations are possible.

After injection, images are acquired for 6 minutes. ROIs are drawn around the kidneys, and the background is subtracted.

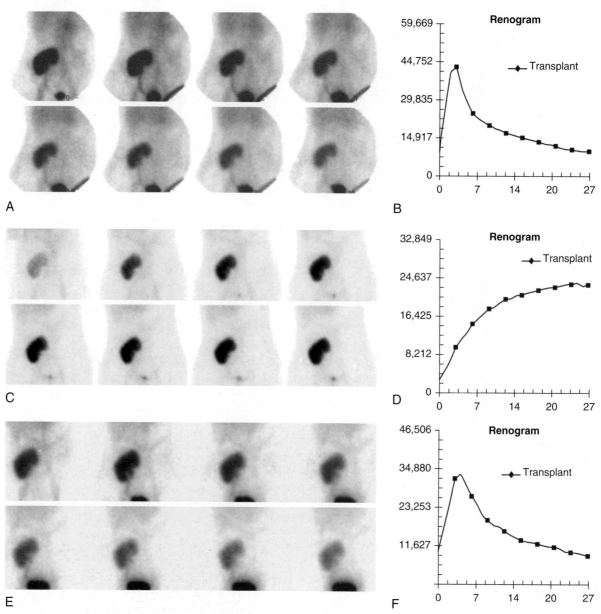

Fig. 11.27 Time course of acute rejection. Baseline Tc-99m MAG3 images (A) and curves (B) show prompt uptake and transit into ureter and bladder. Two months later, function deteriorated, and the scan (C) and time–activity curve (D) reveal marked cortical retention with delayed and decreased clearance into bladder. Function improved a week later with immunosuppressive therapy, as seen in (E) and (F).

Photon attenuation caused by varying renal depth is corrected using a formula based on patient weight and height. The fraction of the standard taken up by the kidneys in the 1- to 2.5-minute or 2- to 3-minute frames can be correlated with GFR measured by other methods (e.g., multiple blood sample, single blood sample, or, less accurately, by creatinine clearance). A similar camera-based approach can be used for a modified ERPF calculation using Tc-99m MAG3 but is less frequently performed.

RENAL CORTICAL IMAGING

It is often difficult to clinically distinguish upper urinary tract infections from lower tract infections. However, pyelonephritis can lead to cortical scarring, renal failure, and hypertension.

In specific instances, nuclear medicine cortical imaging can show changes over time that are difficult to see with anatomical imaging modalities. Tc-99m DMSA offers superior cortical resolution over Tc-99m MAG3 and can be used to evaluate suspected pyelonephritis or scarring in a patient with reflux. Differentiating benign oncocytoma from renal cell cancer has recently become an area of interest.

Technetium-99m Dimercaptosuccinic Acid

Although agents such as Tc-99m MAG3 and Tc-99m DTPA can provide significant information about the renal cortex, their dynamic clearance through the region does not allow optimal resolution. A significant fraction, roughly 40% to 50%, of Technetium-99m dimercaptosuccinic acid (Tc-99m DMSA),

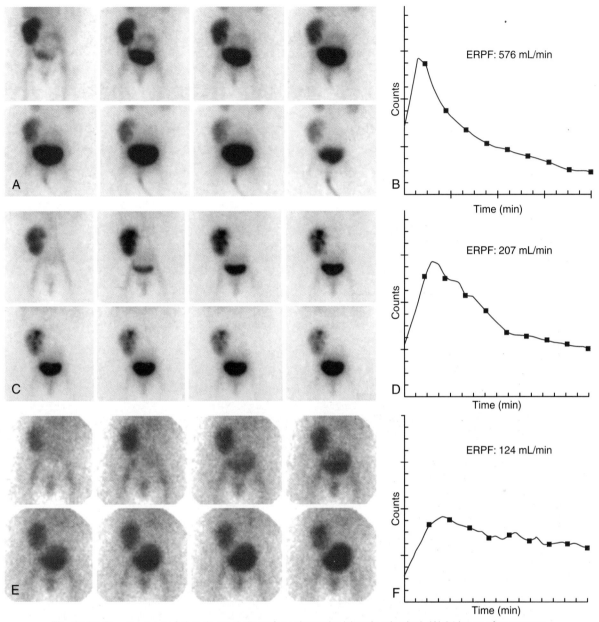

Fig. 11.28 Development of chronic renal allograft nephropathy (chronic rejection). (A) 24 hours after surgery, a baseline Tc-99m MAG3 study and (B) time–activity curve (TAC) are normal. A year later, the images and TAC show continued good function. Three years later, the patient presented with decreased urine output and rising creatinine. Images (E) and TAC show poor function, with decreased target to background, peak activity, and clearance rate in a patient found to have chronic rejection. Cortical retention is usually less significant than with acute rejection.

however, binds to the renal cortical proximal tubules, providing a stable target for high-quality, detailed pinhole or SPECT imaging (Fig. 11.34). Renal cortical imaging with Tc-99m DMSA is most commonly used to detect areas of pyelonephritis and differentiate areas of scarring. Pyelonephritis causes tubular dysfunction and thus reduced uptake. Although other radiopharmaceuticals were available in the past with cortical binding, only Tc-99m DMSA remains available.

Method

Pinhole images, SPECT, or SPECT-CT can be utilized; all provide improved resolution. The preference as to which

usually depends on the level of comfort or expertise at the individual center. A sample protocol is outlined in Box 11.9. Pinhole imaging requires precise positioning, with the patient at the same distance and angle on each oblique view. Children frequently require anesthesia for SPECT in order to keep them still.

Imaging is generally done after a 2- to 3-hour delay to allow for the relatively slow background clearance, and in cases of diminished renal function, further delay may be needed. The properties of the radiopharmaceutical make it unsuitable for the assessment of the collecting system and lower urinary tract given a low level of urinary excretion.

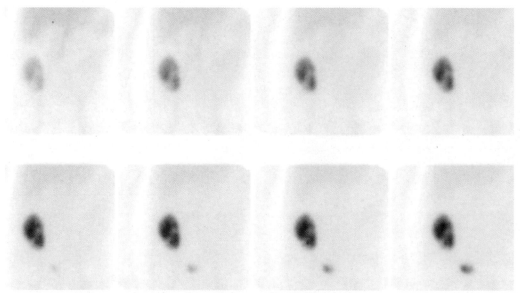

Fig. 11.29 Effects of long-standing chronic rejection. A Tc-99m MAG3 scan in a patient with an old transplanted kidney shows cortical scarring, delayed transit into collecting system, and slow washout. The prominent collecting system is often present at this stage but is not well seen in this particular case.

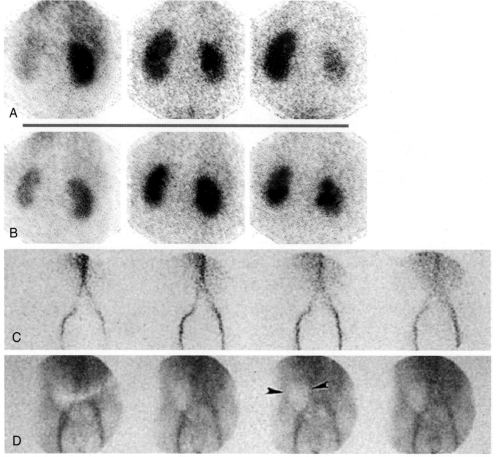

Fig. 11.30 Renal vein thrombosis. (A) Renal vein thrombosis in a native kidney. The Tc-99m DTPA scan reveals poor uptake and delayed clearance in the left native kidney. (B) Function improves on a follow-up scan 4 months later. Tc-99m MAG3 in another patient with a renal allograft and renal vein thrombosis shows no perfusion on the radionuclide angiogram (C) and a photopenic defect *(arrowheads)* resulting from nonviable allograft causing attenuation but having no uptake (D).

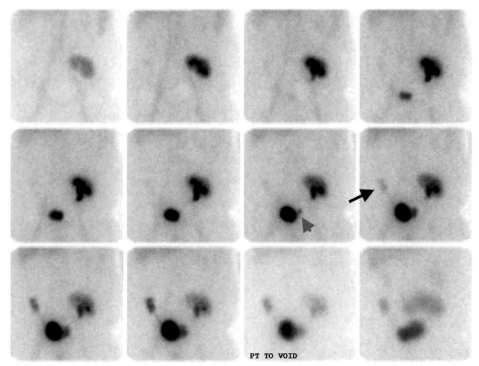

Fig. 11.31 Postoperative urinary leak.

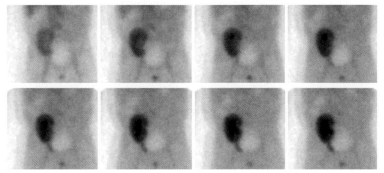

Fig. 11.32 Postoperative obstruction. Images from a recent transplant reveal a photopenic area in the pelvis from a postoperative fluid collection pressing on the ureter and causing obstruction. Delayed images (not shown) failed to show active urine leak in the region.

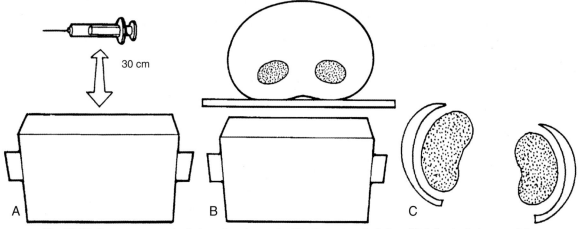

Fig. 11.33 Gamma camera technique for glomerular filtration rate calculation. (A) A 1-minute image of the Tc-99m DTPA syringe before and after injection is taken at a 30-cm distance from the center of the collimator. (B) After injection, 15-seconds-per-frame images are acquired for a total of 6 minutes. (C) Kidney and background regions are selected on images to obtain counts. After correcting for background and attenuation, the net renal cortical uptake as a percentage of the total injected dose is calculated.

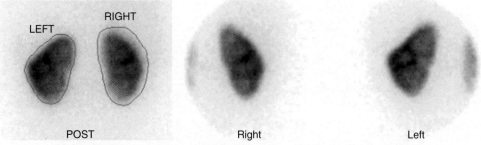

Fig. 11.34 Normal appearance of the kidneys in a child using Tc-99m DMSA.

BOX 11.9   Renal Cortical Imaging Protocol Summary

Radiopharmaceutical: Tc-99m DMSA
Child: 1.85 MBq/kg (50 µCi/kg) minimum dose: 22 MBq (600 µCi)
Adult: 185 MBq (5 mCi)

Instrumentation

Single-photon emission computed tomography (SPECT): dual-head camera; low-energy, high-resolution collimator
Planar: pinhole collimator for small children; converging may be used for adults
Differential calculation: parallel-hole collimator

Imaging Procedure

Patient should void before beginning.
After intravenous (IV) injection, delay imaging for 2 to 3 hours.

Planar Technique

Low-energy, high- or ultrahigh-resolution collimator
Acquire anterior and posterior 300,00 to 500,00 counts (or 10 minutes) for differential function:

$$\text{Differential function} = \sqrt{\text{anterior ROI counts} \times \text{posterior ROI counts}}$$

Pinhole: kidneys centered in field of view (FOV), equidistant from camera on each view,
posterior and posterior oblique images 100,000 to 150,000 counts/view (or 10 minutes)
SPECT
128 × 128 or 256 × 256 matrix, zoomed as needed for infants
Orbit: noncircular body contour, rotate 180 degrees; 40 views/head, 3 degrees/step, 40 sec/step
Reconstruction
Prefilter: Hann cutoff frequency 0.9/cm, order 0
Postfilter: Butterworth cutoff frequency 0.5/cm, order 10; 2 iterations, 10 subsets

Image Interpretation

The shape of the kidney is variable, as is the thickness of the cortex. The upper poles often may appear less intense because of splenic impression, fetal lobulation, and attenuation from the liver and spleen. The central collecting system and medullary regions are photon deficient because Tc-99m DMSA tubular binding occurs in the cortex. The columns of Bertin will show radiopharmaceutical uptake and may appear quite prominent.

When assessing the cortex, areas of abnormally decreased activity can be seen from infection or evolving scar not always obvious on anatomical imaging modalities like CT. Areas of cortical tubular dysfunction from infection or scarring present as cortical defects (Figs. 11.35 and 11.36). Scars would be expected to have localized, sharp margins and may occur in a small kidney with associated cortical loss. However, it is often difficult to tell an area of acute inflammation from a scar without serial images to show resolution, particularly in patients with clinically silent infections (Fig. 11.37).

Diseases affecting the renal tubules, such as renal tubular acidosis and Fanconi syndrome, inhibit Tc-99m DMSA uptake. Nephrotoxic drugs, including gentamicin and cisplatinum, also may inhibit uptake. When renal function is poor, uptake may be so poor that no useful diagnostic information can be gained.

A tumor will present as a defect because cortical scanning is not specific. Therefore, comparison with ultrasound is advisable. However, if increased activity is present, the area represents a prominent column of Bertin. Renal tumor imaging is discussed in the F-18 FDG oncology chapter (Chapter 12). Differentiating oncocytoma from renal cell carcinoma is covered in the section on Tc-99m sestamibi in oncology imaging beyond FDG (Chapter 12).

RADIONUCLIDE CYSTOGRAPHY

Untreated vesicoureteral reflux (VUR) and infection are associated with subsequent renal damage, scarring, hypertension, and chronic renal failure. If the intramural ureter does not normally traverse the bladder wall and submucosa to its opening at the trigone, the ureterovesical valve may fail to passively close as the bladder fills, resulting in reflux. As children grow, this spontaneously resolves in many cases; 40% to 60% of cases resolve by 2 to 3 years of age.

Renal damage that occurs from reflux of infected urine is more likely in patients with severe rather than mild or moderate grades of reflux. Antibiotic therapy has helped decrease scaring from 35% to 60% in untreated patients down to 10%. The goal of therapy is to prevent infection of the kidney until reflux resolves spontaneously. However, antibiotics do not completely protect the kidney from infection and scar. Therefore patients must be carefully monitored, and serial Tc-99m DMSA scans may be helpful.

Radionuclide voiding cystography (nuclear VCU) is more sensitive than contrast-enhanced cystography for detecting

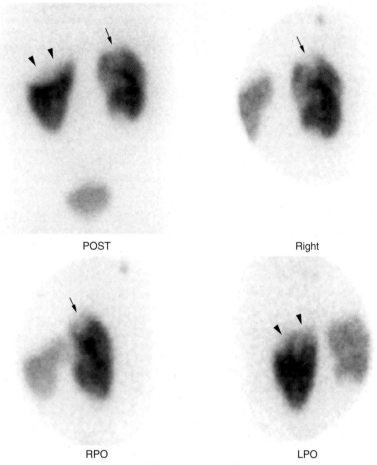

POST

Right

RPO

LPO

Fig. 11.35 Cortical scar. Anterior pinhole DMSA images reveal focal defects bilaterally. The sharp margins on the left *(arrowheads)* suggest scar. Smaller defects on the right *(small arrow)* are also present. When uncertain, serial studies can confirm lack of change in scar.

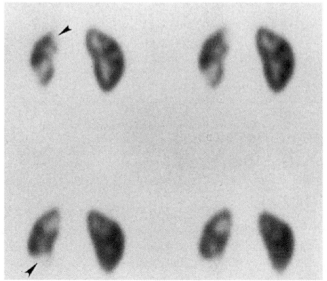

Fig. 11.36 Tc-99m DMSA single-photon emission computed tomography (SPECT). Sequential 3.5-mm coronal sections show great detail, such as cortical and medullary separation. Cortical defects in the upper pole and lower pole *(arrowheads)* are present in the slightly smaller right kidney from scarring.

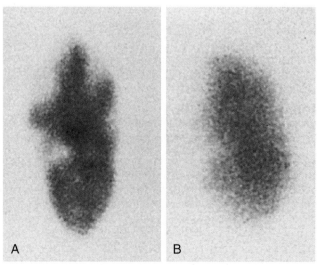

A

B

Fig. 11.37 Acute pyelonephritis. Tc-99m DMSA pinhole images study in an 11-year-old child show (A) multiple cortical defects, particularly in the upper pole, that nearly completely resolve on a follow-up study obtained 6 months later, after appropriate antibiotic therapy (B).

BOX 11.10   Radionuclide Retrograde Cystography Protocol Summary

Radiopharmaceutical: Tc-99m Sulfur colloid (Tc-99m DTPA alternative) 18.5 to 37 MBq (0.5–1.0 mCi)

Patient Preparation
Insert Foley using aseptic technique, inflate balloon, and tape to secure.
Use clean diaper that has been weighed for infants.

Position
Supine with camera under table
Bladder and kidneys in field of view

Instrumentation
Camera, large field of view
Collimator: converging for newborns < 1 year, low energy, high resolution
Computer 128 × 128 matrix (64 × 64 minimum)

Frame Rate
5 to 10 seconds/frame filling for 60 seconds
Prevoid 30 seconds
Voiding 2 seconds/frame 120 seconds
Postvoid 30 seconds

Imaging Procedure
Hang 500-mL bag saline 25 cm above table.
Inject radiotracer into tubing connecting bag to bladder.

Filling
Fill bladder no fuller than capacity: [Age (years) + 1] × 30 cc = volume.
Fill until drip slows or voiding begins around catheter.

Voiding
Place camera perpendicular to table; place patient on bedpan, back against camera.
Infants remain supine and void in the clean weighed diaper.
Measure voided urine volume or weigh diaper for output volume.

Interpretation
Calculate postvoid residual volume (RV):

$$RV\ (mL) = \frac{voided\ volume\ (mL) \times postvoid\ bladder\ counts}{initial\ bladder\ counts - postvoid\ bladder\ counts}$$

Or

$$RV\ (mL) = \frac{postvoid\ bladder\ counts \times infused\ volume\ (mL)}{prevoid\ bladder\ counts}$$

Place region of interest (ROI) over bladder.
Assess reflux (see Table 11.4).

---

reflux because of its continuous acquisition. It also results in considerably less radiation exposure to the patient, although it provides limited anatomical data. In many centers, contrast-voiding urethrocystography (VCUG) is reserved for the initial workup of male patients to exclude an anatomical cause for reflux, abnormal posterior urethral valves. VCUG screening is recommended for patients with reflux. Because pyelonephritis may be clinically silent and siblings are at an increased risk of approximately 40% for VUR, screening is also recommended for siblings.

Methodology

Indirect radionuclide cystography can be performed as part of routine dynamic renal scintigraphy done with Tc-99m MAG3. The child is asked to not void until the bladder is maximally distended, and then imaging is obtained. Although this test has an advantage because the bladder is not catheterized, upper-tract stasis often poses a problem for interpretation, and indirect VCUG cannot reliably detect the 20% of reflux that occurs during bladder filling.

Direct radionuclide cystography is the most commonly used, performed as a three-phase process with continuous imaging during bladder filling, during micturition, and after voiding. Besides diagnosing reflux, this procedure can quantitate postvoid bladder residuals.

The protocol for radionuclide retrograde cystography and residual bladder volume calculation is listed in Box 11.10. Tc-99m pertechnetate may be absorbed through the bladder, particularly if the bladder is inflamed. So, Tc-99m sulfur colloid and Tc-99m DTPA are the radiopharmaceuticals most commonly used. A solution of 37 MBq (1 mCi) of radiotracer in

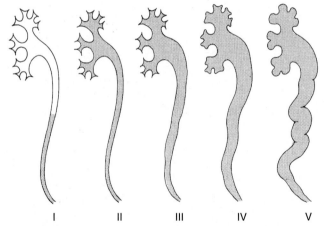

Fig. 11.38 Vesicoureteral contrast grading system (International Reflux Study Committee). *I*, Ureteral reflux only. *II*, Reflux into ureter, pelvis, and calyces without dilation. *III*, Mild to moderate dilation/tortuosity of ureter and calyceal dilatation. *IV*, Moderate dilation and tortuosity of ureter and moderate dilation of the renal pelvis. The angles of the fornices obliterated, but the papillary impressions maintained. *V*, Gross dilation and tortuosity of the ureter and gross dilation of the renal pelvis and calyces. Papillary impressions no longer visible in most calyces.

500 mL normal saline provides sufficient concentration. The absorbed radiation dose is quite low. From 50 to 200 times less radiation is delivered to the gonads from the radionuclide method than with contrast cystography.

Interpretation

Any reflux into the ureters is abnormal. Reflux grades have been described for radiographic contrast studies (Fig. 11.38). In this

TABLE 11.4

Vesicoureteral Reflux Characterization Reflux Level	DRC Grade	Radiological Grade
Ureter	A	I
Renal pelvis	B	II and III
Pelvis dilated/ureter appears dilated	C	IV and V

DRC, Direct radionuclide cystogram.

system, the level the reflux reaches, the dilation of the renal pelvis, and ureteral dilation and tortuosity are considered. However, anatomical resolution is much lower with scintigraphic methods, and calyceal morphology is not well defined (see outline in Table 11.4). A radionuclide grading system would report activity confined to the ureter grade I reflux, similar to the radiographic grade I. A scintigraphic grade II would include reflux to the renal pelvis and corresponds to x-ray cystography grades II and III (Fig. 11.39). If a diffusely dilated system is seen

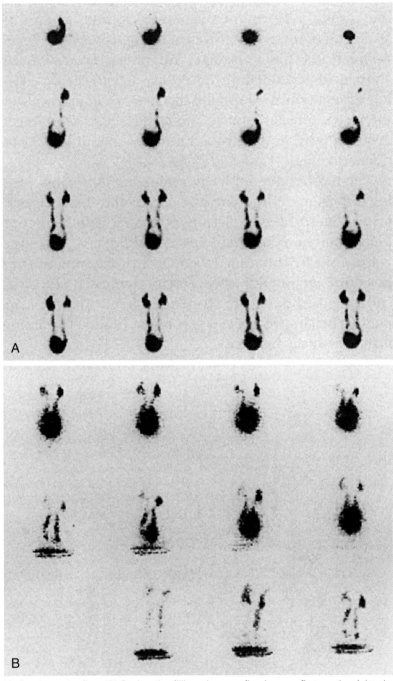

Fig. 11.39 Vesicoureteral reflux. (A) During the filling phase, reflux is seen first on the right, then bilaterally in (B). On voiding, the left side clears better than the right. Reflux is seen in the renal pelvic region bilaterally from grade II to III reflux.

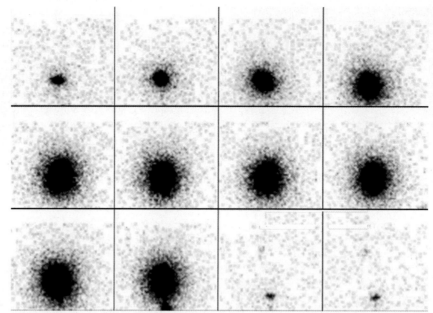

Fig. 11.40 Reflux can be limited to any phase on radionuclide voiding cystography (VCU). In some instances, it may only be brought on by voiding.

scintigraphically, it corresponds to grades IV and V seen with contrast cystography.

The radionuclide technique permits detection of reflux volumes on the order of 1 mL. In one study comparing the RVCUG and x-ray VCU techniques, 17% of reflux events were seen only on the RVCUG examination. Although radionuclide voiding cystography can miss low level I reflux because of the adjacent bladder activity, it is generally accepted that level I reflux is of little consequence. The act of voiding or rolling the patient with a full bladder into posterior oblique positions may reveal reflux not otherwise evident (Fig. 11.40). If a study is negative but clinical suspicion is high, refilling the bladder will improve sensitivity. This is not routinely done, however.

SUGGESTED READING

General Topics

Dubovsky EV, Russell CD, Bischof-Delaloye A, Bubeck B, et al. Report of the radionuclides in nephrourology committee for the evaluation of the transplanted kidney (review of techniques). *Semin Nucl Med*. 1999;29:175–188. https://doi.org/10.1016/S0001-2998(99)80007-5.

Prigent A, Cosgriff P, Gates GF, et al. Consensus report on quality control of quantitative measurements of renal function obtained from the renogram. international committee from the scientific committee of radionuclides in nephrology. *Semin Nucl Med*. 1999;29(2):146–159.

Taylor AT. Radionuclides in nephrourology, part 1: radiopharmaceuticals, quality control, and quantitative indices. *J Nucl Med*. 2014;55(4):608–615. https://doi.org/10.2967/jnumed.113.133447.

Taylor AT. Radionuclides in nephrourology, part 2: pitfalls and diagnostic applications. *J Nucl Med*. 2014;55(5):786–798. https://doi: 10.2967/jnumed.113.133454.

ACE Inhibitors and Renal Artery Stenosis

Taylor A, Nally J, Aurell M, et al. Consensus report on ACE inhibitor renography for detecting renovascular hypertension. *J Nucl Med*. 1996;37(11):1876–1882.

Lasix

Girolamo T, Alessandro D, De Waure C, et al. Tc-99m MAG3 diuretic renography in diagnosis of obstructive nephropathy in adults. A comparison between F-15 and as new procedure F+10 (sp) in seated position. *Clin Nucl Med*. 2013;38:432–436.

Gordon I, Piepsz A, Sixt R. Guidelines for standard and diuretic renogram in children. *Eur J Nucl Med and Mol Imaging*. 2011;38(6):1175–1188. https://doi.org/10.1007/s00259-011-1811-3.

Perez-Brayfield MR, Kirsch AJ, Jones RA. A prospective study comparing ultrasound, nuclear scintigraphy and dynamic contrast enhanced magnetic resonance imaging in the evaluation of hydronephrosis. *J Urol*. 2003;170(4 Pt 1):1330–1334.

Sfakianakis GN, Sfakianakis E, Georgiou M, et al. A renal protocol for all ages and indications: mercapto-acetyl-triglycine (MAG3) with simultaneous injection of furosemide (MAG3-F0)—a 17-year experience. *Semin Nucl Med*. 2009;39(3):156–173.

Turkolmez S, Atasever T, Turkolmez K, Gogus O. Comparison of three different diuretic renal scintigraphy protocol in patients with dilated urinary tracts. *Clin Nucl Med*. 2004;29:154–160. https://doi.org/10.1097/01.rlu.0000113852.57445.23.

Transplants

Ayse Aktas. Transplanted kidney function evaluation. *Semin Nucl Med*. 2014;44:129–145. https://doi.org/10.1053/j.semnuclmed.2013.10.005.

ERPF and GFR Calculations

Gates GF. Glomerular filtration rate: estimation from fractional renal accumulation of Tc-99m DTPA (stannous). *AJR Am J Roentgenol*. 1982;138:565–570.

Russell CD, Bischoff PG, Kontzen F, et al. Measurement of glomerular filtration rate using Tc-99m-DTPA and the gamma camera method. *Eur J Nucl Med*. 1985;10(11-12):519–521.

Taylor A, Manatunga A, Morton K, et al. Multicenter trial of a camera-based method to measure Tc-99m mecaptoacetyltriglycine, or Tc-99m MAG3, clearance. *Radiology*. 1997;204(1):47–54.

Tc-99m DMSA

Fouzas S, Krikelli E, Vassilakos P, et al. DMSA scan for revealing vesicoureteral reflux in children with urinary tract infections. *Pediatrics.* 2010;126(3):e513–e519.

Tc-99m Sestamibi

Campbell SP, Tzortzakakis A, Javadi MS, et al. Tc-99m sestamibi SPECT/CT for the characterization of renal masses: a pictorial guide. *Br J Radiol.* 2018;91(1084):20170526. https://doi.org/10.1259/bjr.20170526.

Gorin MA, Rowe SP, Baras AS, et al. Prospective evaluation of Tc-99m sestamibi SPECT/CT for the diagnosis of renal oncocytomas and hybrid oncocytic chromophobes tumors. *European Urology.* 2016;69:413–416. https://doi.org/10.1016/j.eururo.2015.08.056.

Reynolds AM, Porter KK. Characterizing indeterminate renal masses with molecular imaging: the role of Tc-99m MIBI SPECT/CT. *Curr Urol Rep.* 2017;18(11):86. https://doi.org/10.1007/s11934-017-0737-0.

12

Oncology: F-18 Fluorodeoxyglucose Positron Emission Tomography

BACKGROUND

For decades, positron emission tomography (PET) imaging was largely limited to use in research. The development of dedicated PET cameras, the widespread expansion of cyclotron production facilities, and the approval of new radiopharmaceuticals have all contributed to the dramatic growth of clinical PET in recent years. PET agents often incorporate radioactive isotopes of atoms normally present in organic substances (e.g., oxygen-15, nitrogen-13, carbon-11, and the hydroxyl analog, fluorine-18) and thus can image cellular or molecular processes that are otherwise difficult to image. Several different PET applications are clinically available (Box 12.1). However, most clinical PET imaging is currently done with the glucose analog F-18 fluorodeoxyglucose (F-18 FDG) for the evaluation of cancer. Malignant cells are usually more metabolically active than normal tissues and tend to accumulate higher levels of glucose, which is reflected in increased radiopharmaceutical uptake.

Functional imaging with PET can provide substantially different information than conventional modalities, such as computed tomography (CT). Because CT relies on changes in size and architecture to diagnose malignancy, sensitivity and specificity are limited. For example, in patients with cancer, enlarged lymph nodes are assumed to harbor malignancy, whereas nodes of normal size are characterized as benign. This can result in errors when adenopathy occurs from infection or when early metastases are present in small lymph nodes. In addition, the results of therapy can be difficult to determine because masses may change in size slowly or not at all, and residual or recurrent disease can be obscured by radiation or postsurgical scar distortion of normal tissues. Use of F-18 FDG, on the other hand, permits metabolic activity to be monitored serially, with quantitative and semiquantitative analysis helping to better characterize lesions and predict therapy outcome.

One limitation of PET is the lack of anatomical detail in the images. Normal uptake in structures such as the bowel, muscles, and ureters can be mistaken for tumor. Therefore, correlation with CT or magnetic resonance (MR) is critical for proper image interpretation. Differences in positioning between the two scans are minimized when studies are performed on a dedicated PET camera combining the CT or magnetic resonance imaging (MRI) scanner in a single hybrid PET/CT or PET/MR device.

F-18 FDG PET/CT has become a key component in tumor evaluation and significantly affects patient care. This was shown by data obtained during the National Oncologic PET Registry (NOPR) established by the U.S. Centers for Medicare and Medicaid Services (CMS) to gather evidence to help determine when payment would be authorized. Findings from the NOPR trial were impressive, with PET found to alter patient management in 36.5% of cases. Changes included redirecting biopsy, avoiding surgery (after upstaging a patient), changing the overall treatment goal or causing a major change in therapy, and detecting additional primary malignancies (Coleman et al. 2010; Hilner et al. 2008). Based on the success of the NOPR trial, F-18 FDG PET/CT reimbursement was approved for most solid tumors.

Radiopharmaceuticals
Physical Properties

In positron radioactive decay, a positron (β^+) ejected from the atom travels a short distance before meeting a negative particle (electron) and undergoing annihilation. The resulting two 511-keV photons travel at 180 degrees from each other. These high-energy photons do not interact well with routine gamma cameras but are optimally detected by the specialized ring of detectors in a PET camera. Photons received within a short enough time interval at opposing detectors are registered as "coincidence photons," or those originating from the same decay event. The result is a superior image to those achieved with gamma camera single-photon studies (e.g., with technetium-99m–labeled agents).

BOX 12.1 Common Clinical Applications of PET Imaging

F-18 Fluorine Deoxyglucose (F-18 FDG)
Cancer: Staging, restaging, therapy monitoring
Lung nodule diagnosis/characterization, localization of cancer of unknown primary
Dementia imaging
Seizures (interictal)
Cardiac: Viability, sarcoidosis

F-18 Florbetaben/F-18 Florbetapir/F-18 Flutemetamol: Detection of Amyloid
Rubidium-82 (Rb-82): Cardiac perfusion
Ammonia N-13: Cardiac perfusion
F-18 fluciclovine: Prostate cancer recurrence, metastasis
Gallium-68 prostate-specific membrane antigen (Ga-68 PMSA): Prostate cancer recurrence
Ga-68 DOTATE or DOTATOC: Neuroendocrine/somatostatin-receptor tumor imaging
F-18 sodium fluoride: Bone metastases and tumors

PET, Positron emission tomography.

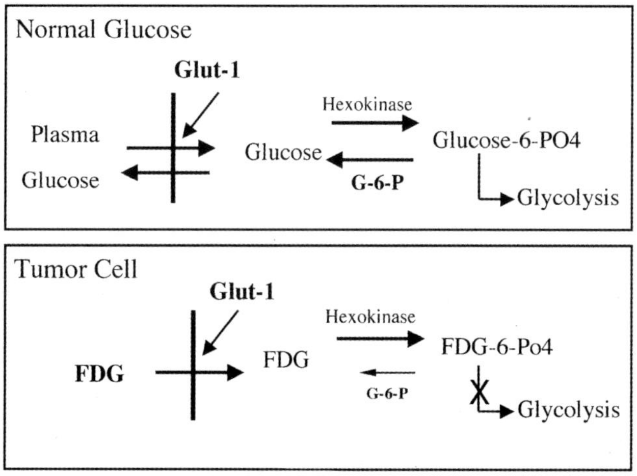

Normal Glucose

Glut-1

Plasma Glucose

Hexokinase

Glucose → Glucose-6-PO4

G-6-P

→ Glycolysis

Tumor Cell

Glut-1

FDG

Hexokinase

FDG → FDG-6-Po4

G-6-P

✗ → Glycolysis

*G-6-P: Glucose-6-Phosphatase

Fig. 12.1 Glucose and F-18 fluorodeoxyglucose (FDG) intracellular kinetics. F-18 FDG uses the same uptake and phosphorylation pathways as glucose, although it cannot be metabolized further through glycolysis. In cancer cells, radiotracer accumulation is increased because of different levels of enzymatic activity. *G-6-P*, Glucose-6-phosphatase.

Many PET-emitting isotopes have very short half-lives ($T_{1/2}$), requiring a cyclotron to be in extremely close proximity. The 109.7-minute $T_{1/2}$ of F-18 means it can be shipped from local and even regional production facilities. On the other hand, the $T_{1/2}$ is not excessively long, and radiation exposure is lower than many agents with longer-lived radiolabels. Dosimetry information is outlined in Appendix 1.

Kinetics and Distribution

In malignant cells, increased expression of membrane glucose transporters (e.g., glut-1) results in higher levels of intracellular glucose. Within these cells, the levels of hexokinase (hexokinase II) activity are also increased, phosphorylating glucose, which then moves through the glycolysis pathway. F-18 FDG is taken into the cell and phosphorylated by the same mechanisms as glucose, but F-18 FDG cannot be metabolized further (Fig. 12.1). In addition, due to the lower levels of glucose-6-phosphatase in cancer cells, FDG remains effectively trapped because phosphorylated FDG cannot diffuse back across the membrane. The normal distribution of F-18 FDG is shown in Figs. 12.2 and 12.3.

F-18 FDG ONCOLOGY PROTOCOL

PET/CT Imaging

Many factors affect F-18 FDG uptake, distribution, and clearance. Table 12.1 outlines different causes for altered F-18 FDG distribution in tissues. Measures are required to optimize tumor-to-background radiotracer uptake, making patient preparation and scheduling complex. An example protocol is listed in Box 12.2. PET/CT scheduling is often complicated by factors that alter F-18 FDG distribution, and some recommendations on PET scheduling modifications are outlined in Table 12.2.

Patient Preparation

Because glucose competes with F-18 FDG for uptake, the patient's glucose level should be checked before injection. The

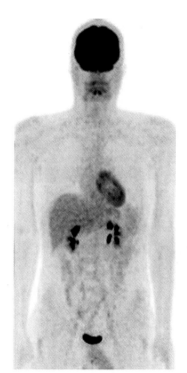

Fig. 12.2 Normal distribution of F-18 fluorodeoxyglucose (FDG). Uptake is normally intense in the brain and urinary tract, moderately intense in the liver, and variable in muscles (especially of the oropharynx), heart, and bowel.

upper-limit cutoff varies among institutions, but a value under 200 mg/dL is generally considered acceptable.

Insulin, whether endogenously released in response to a meal or following administration to diabetics, stimulates the glucose transporters (e.g., glut-1), which are highly expressed in muscle cell membranes. This dramatically increases muscle uptake (Fig. 12.4), thereby potentially decreasing uptake in tumor. To minimize the impact, patients fast overnight or for at least 4 to 6 hours before injection and avoid carbohydrates in the meal (or even the day) before injection. Patients with diabetes should not be given short-acting insulin within 2 hours of radiotracer injection, and long-acting insulin should be held overnight. The scan must be carefully scheduled because it may be difficult to coordinate with the diabetic patient's serum glucose levels, which can fluctuate widely over the course of the day. When this is the case, optimal times often include early morning, before eating or taking insulin, and early afternoon, with the patient fasting after eating a light early breakfast and taking the morning short-acting insulin dose. For non–insulin-dependent diabetics taking the medication metformin, consideration should be given to withholding it for 1 to 2 days because metformin has been shown to dramatically increase uptake in the bowel.

Muscle activity is also minimized by limiting vigorous exercise for 1 to 2 days before the examination, and sedatives (e.g., alprazolam oral 0.5 mg) are routinely administered for patients with head and neck cancer who have undergone surgery in the past, helping to prevent frequently problematic increased background muscle activity.

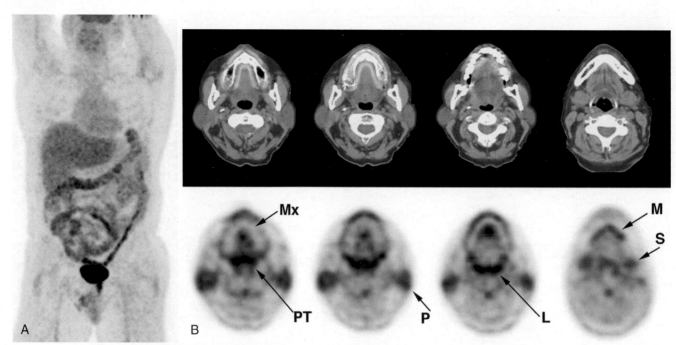

Fig. 12.3 Normal variants. (A) Marked uptake can be seen normally in the small and large bowel. In some cases, the increased bowel activity is related to metformin use. (B) Axial positron emission tomography (PET) and corresponding computed tomography (CT) images show uptake in the oropharynx. Normal activity is typically symmetrical and may be intense when patients swallow or talk. *L,* Lingual tonsil; *M,* mandible; *Mx,* maxilla; *P,* parotid gland; *PT,* palatine tonsils; *S,* submandibular gland.

TABLE 12.1 Lesion Characterization: F-18 Fluorodeoxyglucose (FDG) Activity Levels

Increased Uptake	Decreased Uptake
High-grade malignancy	Benign lesion
	Indolent or low-grade tumor
Highly cellular lesion	Low cellularity: mucinous, cystic/fluid filled
Increased patient body mass/weight	Lesion:
	• Size too small
	• In area of motion
Infection, abscess	Scar, chronic fibrosis
Increased vascularity, inflammation	Prior chemotherapy
Trauma, surgery	Attenuation: breast implant or metal
Radiation (acute)	Radiation (delayed)

Dose Administration and Uptake

Administered doses of F-18 FDG have been steadily decreased over the years. With the introduction of improved camera technology, such as time-of-flight (TOF) detection, typical doses are on the order of 7 to 8 mCi (259–296 MBq), up to half that used with the previous-generation scanners.

Patients should remain completely still and quiet for the uptake period, which is usually 50 to 65 minutes to achieve the optimum target-to-background ratio balanced with the physical decay $T_{1/2}$. Some studies have suggested that additional delayed images at 90 to 120 minutes may improve sensitivity and specificity because tumors tend to continue accumulating F-18 FDG while activity continues to decrease from other tissues and benign processes. In the case of astrocytomas, which are especially difficult to image with F-18 FDG, an even greater interval

BOX 12.2 Patient Protocol for Fluorine-18 Fluorodeoxyglucose (F-18 FDG) PET/CT Imaging in Oncology

Patient Preparation

Avoid exercise for 1 to 2 days.

Diabetes: Serum glucose controlled

Insulin: Stop long-acting insulin 8 to 12 hours before scan; no short-acting insulin within 2 hours of injection.

 Oral metformin (Glucophage): May continue

 If colon is area of concern, consider holding 48 hours if serum glucose can be controlled otherwise.

Hydrate patient orally.

NPO except water for 4 to 6 hours; avoid carbohydrates 6 to 24 hours prior; no caffeine.

Check serum glucose before dosing (<200 mg/dL).

Patient kept warm, quiet, and relaxed for 30 to 60 minutes before injection.

Consider sedation (diazepam, benzodiazepine) for claustrophobia, anxiety or tense muscles, or prior head and neck surgery.

 Prior brown-fat uptake: Warming the patient is best.

 Alternative: 5 mg intravenous (IV) diazepam 10 minutes prior or 80 mg oral propranolol 2 hours prior

Radiopharmaceutical

Adult: 8 mCi F-18 FDG IV [5–12 mCi (185–444 MBq)]

0.09 mCi/kg (3.2 MBq/kg) to 0.14 mCi/kg (5.3 MBq/kg)

Child: 0.10 mCi/kg (3.7 MBq/kg), minimum 1.0 mCi (37 MBq)

Wait (quiet, inactive) 50 to 65 minutes.

Void bladder immediately before imaging.

Image Acquisition

Patient supine

Field of view: 80 to 90 cm (varies by patient size and camera manufacturer, 50–90 cm for PET/CT)

CT transmission scan (varies):
  Scout: Determine bed/slice positioning and automatic CT exposure settings 5 mAs.
  Localizing (PET/CT): mAs automatic tube modulation (max 125 mAs), 100 kVp (70–120 kVp)
    CTDI: 3 to 7 mGy (arms down slightly higher)
  Diagnostic: 80 to 300 mAs; 100 to 140 kVp (e.g., 100 kVp in chest)
    CTDI: 10 to 15 mGy
PET emission scan: TOF scanner 1 to 4 minutes/bed position; non-TOF 5 to 10 minutes/position
Processing: Iterative reconstruction, 128 × 128 or 256 × 256 matrix, pixel size typically 2 to 4 mm

CT, Computed tomography; *CTDI,* computed tomography dose index; *PET/CT,* positron emission tomography with computed tomography; *TOF,* time of flight.

TABLE 12.2 Alterations in Scheduling Due to Clinical Factors

History	Course of Action
Prior surgery	Delay scan 4 weeks (2–6 weeks).
Chemotherapy	Delay scan 6–8 weeks posttherapy (minimum 3 weeks) or schedule just before next cycle.
Radiation therapy	Delay scan ≥ 3 months.
Colony-stimulating drugs	Consider scan delay of 1 week for short-acting drugs or several weeks for long-acting drugs.
Serum glucose	Reschedule until controlled (<200 mg/dL).
Insulin administration	Wait 2 hours for short-acting insulin or 8–12 hours for long-acting insulin. Turn off insulin pump for 4–6 hours.
Breastfeeding	Discontinue for at least 6 hours postexamination.
Prior brown-fat activity	Warm patient for 30–60 minutes before injection; consider medication if ineffective.

(on the order of hours) may increase the accuracy. However, prolonged waiting periods are not generally practical in the clinic. Whatever delay is used, subsequent studies should be performed in a consistent manner to be certain that the changes seen are not artificially created.

PET/CT Scan Acquisition

Patients are usually imaged in the supine position after bladder voiding. Because CT artifact occurs when the arms are in the field of view, they are most often placed above the head when the pathology is in the chest, abdomen, and pelvis but left at the patient's side when the tumor is in the head and neck.

The study is acquired in two phases. First, a transmission scan is performed using an external radiation source for attenuation correction. Originally, radiation sources (e.g., germanium-68 or cesium-137 rods) rotated around the patient, requiring several minutes. CT radiography, on the other hand, requires only seconds to cover the entire body. Based on the interactions of the x-ray photons with tissues, an attenuation-correction map is built and applied to the photons detected from the patient during the second phase of imaging, the emission PET scan. Attenuation correction allows PET data to be displayed with the proper intensity and is necessary for quantification of activity. The emission scan is acquired as a series of partially overlapping blocks of data, or bed positions, as the patient is moved through the camera. The scan time for each bed position can be modified depending on the patient's body habitus but is typically a couple of minutes on modern TOF scanners, nearly half that of previous-generation scanners. Traditionally, a whole-body PET/CT refers to a scan extending from skull base to midthigh, although studies can include the extremities and brain, depending on the situation.

Although most PET/CT studies are performed without intravenous CT contrast, its use has been increasing because it helps identify normal structures and makes pathology more conspicuous. Water can be used to distend the stomach and duodenum. Dilute oral or water-equivalent negative oral contrast are also acceptable. Attenuation correction can help overcome any questions or artifacts if dense contrast builds up, causing artificially elevated counts.

Displays include a three-dimensional maximum-intensity projection (MIP) image and sagittal, coronal, and axial fused and unfused slices. Software can fuse PET images to CT scans performed at other times or to an MR image if desired. If the examination was performed on a dedicated PET/MR camera, it is still advisable to compare the study to a recent CT in order to visualize some abnormalities, such as small lung nodules.

DEDICATED PET/MR

Although dedicated PET/MR scanners are still primarily a research tool, they are increasingly being utilized clinically. By eliminating the CT component, patient radiation exposure may be decreased by 50% to 70%, with the benefit of superior soft tissue characterization (Fig. 12.5). However, hybrid PET/MR scanners have a relatively small central bore, and examinations are much longer than PET/CT; thus, some patients may not tolerate the examination due to claustrophobia and positioning difficulties (Box 12.3). Before scheduling an examination, the patient should be prescreened for MR contraindications, the most important being metallic foreign bodies, implants, or devices.

Because the MR signal is based on proton density and not beam attenuation, attenuation correction needed for standardized uptake value (SUV) calculations is challenging. MR attenuation correction (MRAC) is only possible with a limited number of sequences. Most often, a two-point three-dimensional (3D) isotropic Dixon T1-weighted (T1W) sequence is used for a process called segmentation attenuation correction. Four components are identified: fat, soft tissue, lung, and air. MRAC maps built from this are then applied. This process does not fully compensate for cortical bone, and artifacts can result, especially in the skull base. Methods such as an atlas-based attenuation-correction algorithm are likely a better option when imaging the brain. The SUV measurements generated from the

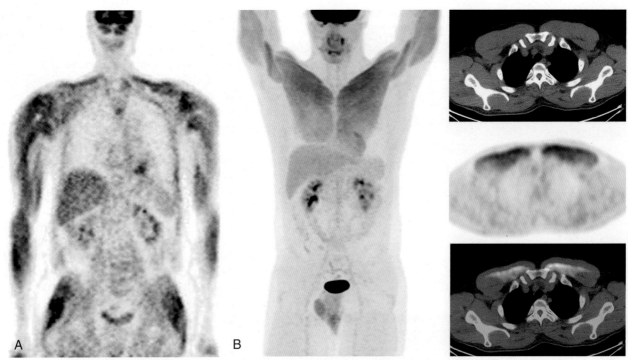

Fig. 12.4 (A) Elevated muscle activity can occur from increased insulin levels (i.e., injected insulin in a diabetic and postprandial secretion in nondiabetics) activating membrane glut-transporters. (B) Strenuous exercise can also alter distribution. When muscle activity is extensive, scans may need to be repeated after adequate preparation because it can result in diminished activity in lesions.

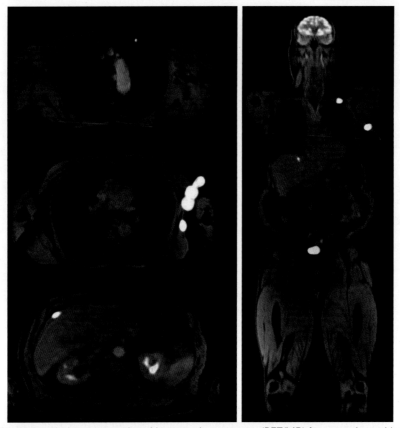

Fig. 12.5 Positron emission tomography with magnetic resonance (PET/MR) from a patient with metastatic recurrent melanoma of the left arm demonstrates intense F-18 fluorodeoxyglucose (FDG) activity in lesions in the axilla, chest wall, and liver capsule on axial *(left)* and coronal *(right)* projections. Whole-body images can be obtained from the top of the head through the toes when needed.

BOX 12.3   Example Protocol Items for Hybrid PET/MR Acquisition

Patient Preparation

Follow preparation guidelines for PET/CT.

Before arrival, screen for:

    Metal implants/implantable devices, fragments, or foreign bodies

    Assess the safety of the specific device model and serial number (resources include http://www.mrisafety.com).

    Claustrophobia, difficulty caused by body habitus given smaller scanner bore size

Radiopharmaceuticals

Follow guidelines for PET/CT.

Acquisition

Whole-body localizing scan

MR sequences for whole-body simultaneous PET and MR acquisition:

1. MR attenuation correction (MRAC):
   - Coronal isotropic fast T1-weighted three-dimensional (3D) 2-point Dixon sequence
   - For segmentation: spoiled 3D GRE (e.g., VIBE, LAVA)
   - Display in fat-only, water-only, in-phase, and opposed-phase sequences
2. Coronal (and/or) axial T2: SS-SFE or HASTE
   - Instead, some sites still use alternate fast sequences:
   - STIR, with its uniform fat suppression, and radial fast spine echo imaging (PROPELLER, BLADE), which helps create motion-free image during free breathing
3. Additional options:
   - Fast T1(VIBE or LAVA) whole-body coronal—for bone lesions fat-saturation sequences
   - T1 postgadolinium contrast: whole body for myeloma or regional for other disease
   - Small FOV in areas of concern, such as female pelvis (depending on disease)
   - Axial or coronal DWI with two *b*-values
   - Dedicated T2-weighted sequences for chest and/or liver regions
   - May use respiratory gating
   - Regional MR scans: With/without contrast as indicated; scans/ADC map with high B values may minimize need or replace contrast images for some purposes, such as marrow evaluation in myeloma

ADC, Apparent diffusion coefficient; *FOV*, field of view; *DWI*, diffusion-weighted imaging; *GRE*, gradient echo; *HASTE*, half-Fourier acquisition single-shot turbo spin echo; *LAVA*, liver acquisition with volume acceleration; *MR*, magnetic resonance; *PET*, positron emission tomography; *PET/CT*, positron emission tomography with computed tomography; *PET/MR*, positron emission tomography with magnetic resonance; *SS-SFE*, single-shot fast spin echo; *STIR*, short-tau inversion recovery sequence; *VIBE*, volumetric interpolated breath-hold examination.

MRAC-corrected PET/MR data may vary significantly from those obtained using PET/CT. Therefore, direct comparison is not advised.

The Dixon sequence data can be reconstructed, fused to MR, and displayed as fat-weighted, water-weighted, in-phase, and opposed-phase sequences. Although these may be sufficient for some purposes, spatial resolution is lower than from standard MR sequences. Most sites will routinely obtain additional free-breathing whole-body axial and/or coronal T2-weighted (T2W) images done with a fast technique such as the more

rapid single-shot spin echo (single-shot fast spin echo [SS-FSE], single-shot turbo spin echo [SSh-TSE], or half-Fourier acquisition single-shot turbo spin echo [HASTE] depending on vendor). These images will demonstrate higher-quality anatomical resolution and tissue contrast, as well as better visualization of pathology, than can be seen with the MRAC data alone and can be completed perhaps 75% faster than standard sequences. Any additional sequences must be carefully considered in terms of the overall examination length, especially if a dedicated regional MR is also required.

IMAGE INTERPRETATION

Normal F-18 FDG Distribution

The brain is an obligate glucose user, so uptake is normally very high. The kidneys, ureters, and bladder also show intense activity from excreted radiotracer in urine. Moderate activity should be seen in the liver, mildly greater than the mediastinal background, and the spleen should be less intense than the liver. Bone marrow accumulation is normally low. Variable activity is seen in the bowel, muscle, heart, salivary glands, tonsils, testes, and uterus.

Pharyngeal and Parapharyngeal

Mild activity is normally present in the salivary glands. Marked uptake is often seen in oropharyngeal lymphoid tissue, including the palatine and lingual tonsils. Asymmetry can occur normally or as the result of therapy and inflammation but may make the evaluation for tumor more difficult. Diffuse marked uptake is often seen in the vocal cords and oropharynx and is increased from speaking. In vocal cord paralysis, unilateral uptake may occur in the normal vocal cord, along with decreased activity in the contralateral abnormal vocal cord (Fig. 12.6).

Myocardial Metabolism

Minimizing cardiac activity is desirable when evaluating cancer. The myocardium uses glucose as an optional fuel source. In a fasting state, fatty acid metabolism dominates over glycolysis, leading to decreased FDG uptake. However, fasting yields inconsistent results, and significant cardiac uptake is seen in up to 50% of fasting patients, often very heterogeneous in the left ventricle. Glucose loading, such as done for a cardiac viability study, increases glycolysis and, therefore, FDG uptake. Benign, fairly intense activity is occasionally seen in the intraatrial septal fat.

Urinary Excretion

Activity in excreted urine can create interpretation difficulties. Although the ureters usually appear as long, tubular structures, they can be seen as very focal areas of activity that may be confused with tumor or lymph node metastasis. Correlation with CT and MIP images can help confirm ureter activity or rule out a soft tissue lesion. In addition, activity in the filling bladder can obscure lesions in the pelvis, and urine contamination on the skin may be difficult to differentiate from an actual superficial lesion.

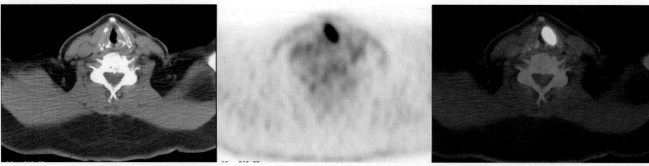

Fig. 12.6 F-18 fluorodeoxyglucose (FDG) positron emission tomography with computed tomography (PET/CT) images (computed tomography [CT], *left;* positron emission tomography [PET], *center;* fused, *right)* at the level of the larynx in a patient previously treated for lung cancer reveal marked asymmetrical increased activity in the left vocal cord but no mass—from right vocal cord paralysis and compensatory hypertrophy on the left.

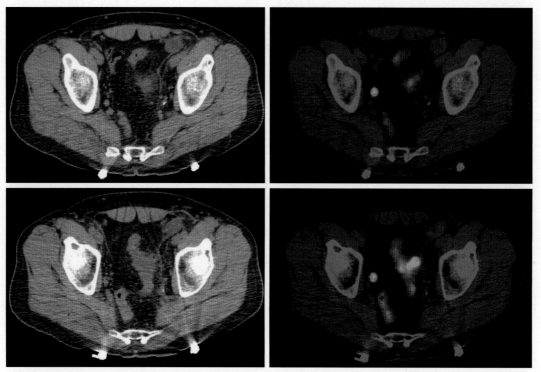

Fig. 12.7 Computed tomography (CT) and fused images from positron emission tomography with computed tomography (PET/CT) performed for lung cancer show stranding in the fat around the sigmoid colon on CT and focal radiotracer uptake in the area of a diverticulum, consistent with diverticulitis.

Gastrointestinal Tract

The esophagus normally shows no significant uptake. Nonspecific focal or more diffuse activity could be due to inflammation from reflux. In general, this is less than that seen with cancer or acute radiation. Significant activity in the stomach, especially when collapsed, can limit the usefulness of F-18 FDG in the evaluation of gastric adenocarcinoma or lymphoma. Highly variable activity in both the small and large bowel is especially problematic because it may obscure tumor in the bowel and mesentery. Focal transient activity is frequently seen in the small bowel, possibly the result of lymphoid tissue uptake. Marked uptake in the bowel can occur from metformin. Inflammation, such as from colitis, inflammatory bowel disease, appendicitis, and diverticulitis, can cause radiotracer accumulation (Fig. 12.7). However, these diseases should cause corresponding changes on CT: fat stranding, inflammatory fluid collections, changes in the bowel wall, and air within forming abscesses.

Reproductive Organs

Cyclical changes can be seen normally in the uterus and ovaries in premenopausal women (Fig. 12.8). Uniform, diffuse, mild to moderate endometrial uptake normally occurs, with maximal uptake occurring during menstruation (menstrual cycle days 0–4) and near ovulation (approximately day 14). Activity is lower during proliferative (days 7–13) and secretory (days 15–28) phases. Normal activity can occur in the ovaries related to ovulation and occasionally in association with follicle growth and the development of the corpus luteum cyst. Increased F-18 FDG uptake can be seen in benign uterine leiomyomas and endometrioma. In men, the testes vary widely but often show high-F-18 FDG levels normally.

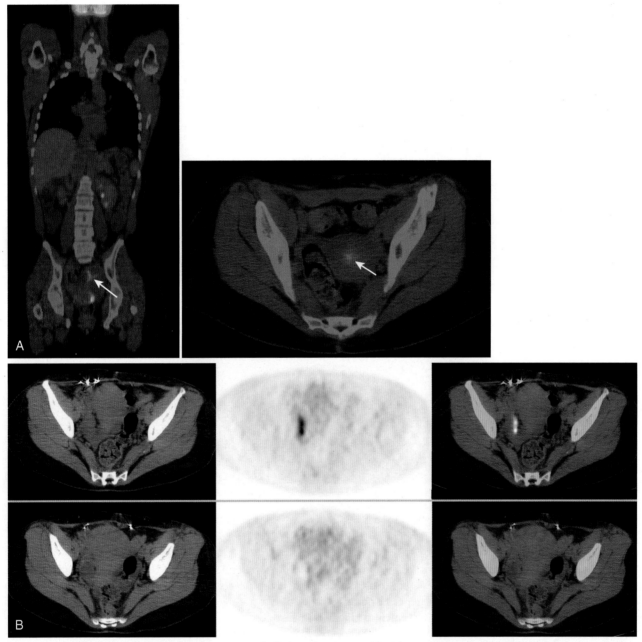

Fig. 12.8 Two different young women (with breast cancer and lymphoma in the chest) showing benign activity related to cyclical changes from the menstrual cycle in the uterus (A) and in the right ovary along the periphery of a small adnexal cyst related to ovulation (B). Follow-up studies performed to restage cancer were then performed at a different point in the cycle.

Benign F-18 FDG Distribution Variants
Thyroid Disease

Thyroid activity is normally low or absent; however, multiple uptake patterns can occur (Fig. 12.9). Diffusely increased uptake may be seen in thyroiditis, radiation thyroiditis, and Graves' disease. The significance of low-level diffuse activity in patients without identifiable thyroid disease is uncertain; it may be normal or the result of subclinical thyroiditis. Focal uptake can be seen in benign adenomatous nodules. However, focal activity can be the result of malignancy in 30% to 50% of cases, and evaluation with ultrasound is warranted to determine whether a biopsy is needed.

Brown Adipose Tissue Activation

Brown fat (or BAT) plays a role in nonshivering heat generation and can be stimulated by the adrenergic system as well as the cold (Fig. 12.10). It is particularly important in the young but is also occasionally seen in adults. When BAT stimulation is present, F-18 FDG uptake is seen in the fat of the supraclavicular region and neck and occasionally in the upper mediastinum and suprarenal regions. Uptake frequently occurs bilaterally in the region of costovertebral junctions. Sedatives (e.g., lorazepam or diazepam) and beta-adrenergic blockers (e.g., 20 mg oral propranolol) are sometimes used to decrease this uptake, although the effectiveness is variable. Rather, it is generally

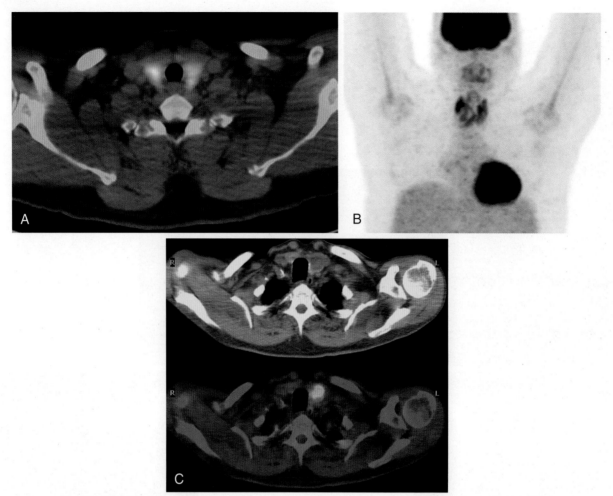

Fig. 12.9 Patterns of thyroid activity. The normal thyroid should show no significant fluorodeoxyglucose (FDG) uptake. (A) Diffuse activity can be seen in benign thyroiditis such as Graves' disease, and multifocal activity (B) can be due to multinodular goiter. (C) Focal activity, however, is associated with a malignant thyroid nodule in 30% to 50% of cases and requires follow-up by ultrasound and then possibly with fine-needle aspiration.

preferred to keep the patient warm for a period before injection until the examination is complete because this tends to be more effective. In some cases, a scan may have to be repeated because it may be difficult to rule out lymph node involvement such as from lymphoma (Fig. 12.11).

Inflammation, Infection, and Trauma

One of the greatest challenges that arises with F-18 FDG is uptake that occurs in infectious and inflammatory processes, which can be difficult to differentiate from malignancy. In infections, the cause has been attributed to glycolytic activity in leukocytes and the impact of molecules associated with inflammation (e.g., cytokines) on the glut-1 transporters. Infections such as pneumonia will have intense radiotracer accumulation. Inflammatory uptake in a lymph node or mass cannot be reliably differentiated from malignancy. Such findings are commonly problematic in sarcoidosis and granulomatous disease (e.g., histoplasmosis and tuberculosis) in the chest (Fig. 12.12 and Fig. 12.13). Other inflammatory processes in the lungs, such as occupational lung diseases and active interstitial fibrosis and pneumonitis, may also cause markedly abnormal uptake.

Low-level radiotracer can be seen in atherosclerotic plaque and higher levels in arteritis. Mild F-18 FDG may routinely localize to vascular bypass graft walls. However, if more focal intense activity is seen, the CT should be examined for signs of infection or abscess, such as gas, fluid collections, or stranding. Abdominal wall surgical mesh and biliary stents may remain hot indefinitely.

Healing fractures normally accumulate F-18 FDG, but evidence of fracture should be clear on CT (Fig. 12.14). Because PET is more sensitive than CT for bone metastasis, the lack of a fracture on CT could mean the activity is caused by metastatic disease, even if no lytic or blastic CT change is seen. Arthritis can cause increased activity, with activity on both sides of the joint, and increased activity can also be seen around the joint capsule or surrounding soft tissues, with CT fusion helping confirm lack of bone involvement.

Effects of Therapy

Therapy often causes an inflammatory response resulting in increased activity (Figs. 12.15 and 12.16). No definitive rules indicate how long to wait after therapy to perform a PET scan. At times, repeat or even serial imaging is needed to confirm that

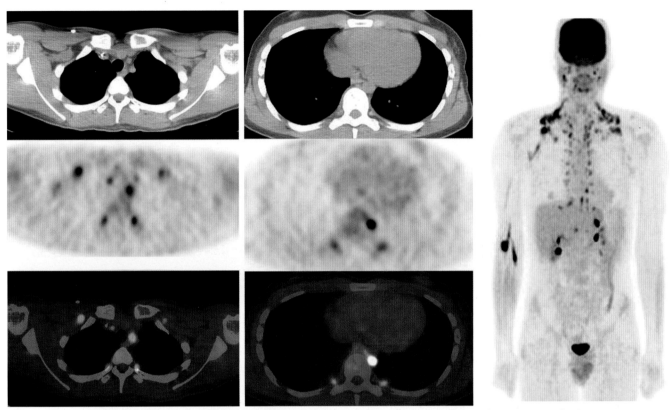

Fig. 12.10 Brown adipose tissue (BAT) or "brown fat," which helps generate heat (more common in the young), can cause benign activity in the fat of the neck and supraclavicular region, sometimes involving the thoracic inlet and fat around the diaphragm, along with bilateral costovertebral junction uptake, likely related to stimulation of the ganglia at the nerve root. Activity in the right antecubital region is residual from the injection.

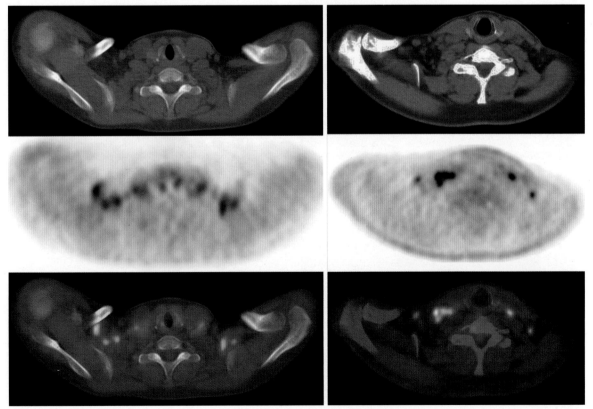

Fig. 12.11 In some cases, it may be difficult to exclude tumor involvement in lymph nodes when brown adipose tissue (BAT) activity *(left)* is present because the pattern may be nodular, as seen in lymphoma *(right),* or when the activity occurs in areas where lymph nodes seen on computed tomography (CT).

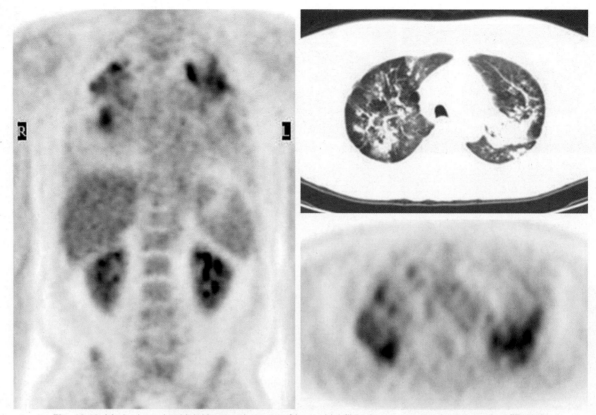

Fig. 12.12 Marked uptake *(right)* is seen in areas of interstitial fibrosis on computed tomography (CT) *(left)* as a result of occupational lung disease. This level of activity could also be seen from pneumonia or sarcoid.

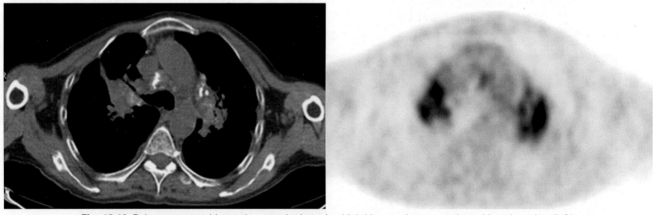

Fig. 12.13 Pulmonary sarcoid can show marked uptake *(right)* in prominent or enlarged lymph nodes *(left)*. Although this can be difficult to differentiate from lymphoma, evidence of granulomatous disease may be seen, such as partially calcified lymph nodes.

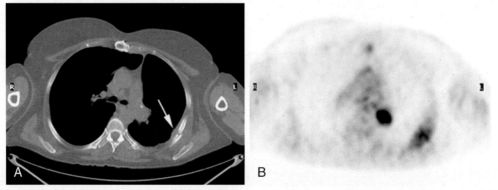

Fig. 12.14 F-18 fluorodeoxyglucose (FDG) uptake in fracture. (A) Computed tomography (CT) shows a left rib fracture *(arrow)* after biopsy of lung cancer. (B) Positron emission tomography (PET) shows uptake in the fracture and the left suprahilar mass, which is not well seen on the single noncontrast CT slice.

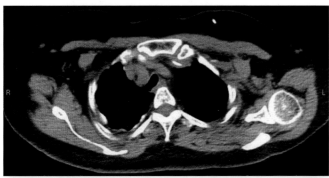

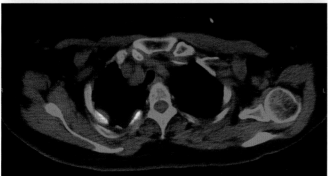

Fig. 12.15 Positive positron emission tomography (PET) scan from talc pleurodesis shows calcified pleura plaques on computed tomography (CT; *upper*) associated with marked uptake on PET *(lower)* that can last indefinitely. Posttherapy changes can be extensive or focal and can be difficult to distinguish from infection or mesothelioma.

a change is iatrogenic. Waiting 2 to 4 weeks or so after procedures will help minimize the impact of surgery (Fig. 12.17). Delaying the PET for 2 to 3 months is often recommended after external-beam radiation due to expected acute inflammation and increased uptake. Although this may allow soft tissues to return to background, activity intensifies and often remains high over time in the lungs. However, the pattern of radiation change will mirror the evolution of scarring, with air bronchograms occurring on the CT, and uptake is normally fairly homogeneous if no residual tumor is present (Fig. 12.18). Bones within the radiation port usually show decreased activity after a short interval.

F-18 FDG accumulates in the bone marrow as a result of marrow stimulation from anemia, marrow-stimulating drugs (filgrastim [Neupogen] or epoetin alfa [Procrit]), or certain cancer therapies. This activity may be intense enough to obscure underlying lesions, and although usually more homogeneous than changes from tumor (Fig. 12.19), it can be patchy and asymmetrical, particularly in the long bones. Because the duration of these marrow-stimulating agents is frequently long lasting, it may not be practical to delay a study until their effects subside.

Chemotherapy often causes a lesion to appear to worsen on PET. The impact can be minimized by delaying a study for at least 2 weeks after treatment, but in some cases, a several-week delay or waiting until just before beginning the next

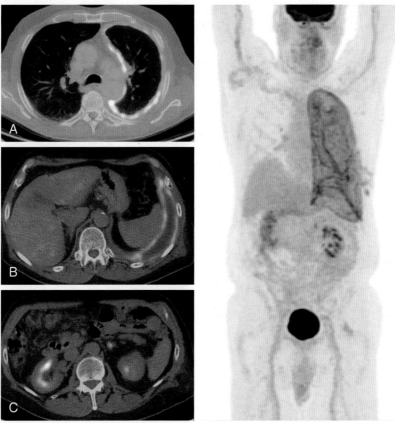

Fig. 12.16 Intense pleural activity is seen in mesothelioma (A, B) with early contralateral right hilar (A) and left adrenal metastases (C).

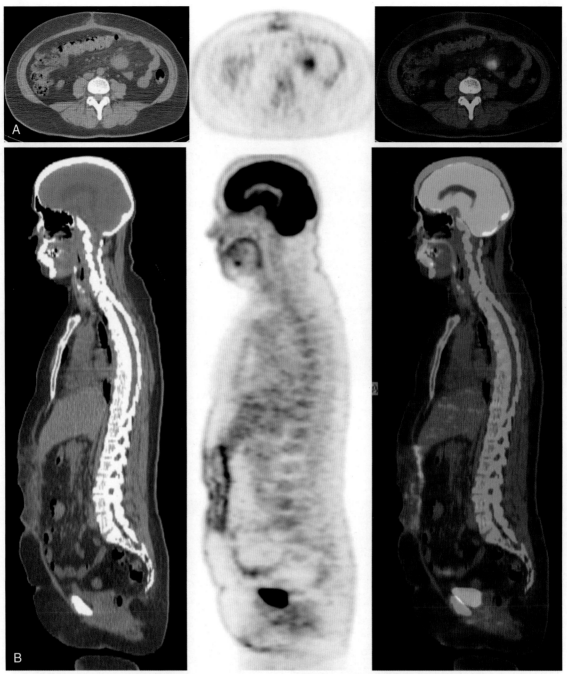

Fig. 12.17 Postoperative change. (A) Two weeks after laparotomy, the computed tomography (CT) scan shows secondary changes in the midline anterior abdominal wall. Stranding of the left-lower-quadrant peritoneal fat around a fluorodeoxyglucose (FDG)-avid tumor implant could be increased by the recent procedure. (B) Activity can be indefinitely increased when associated with mesh, as here in the midline abdominal wall.

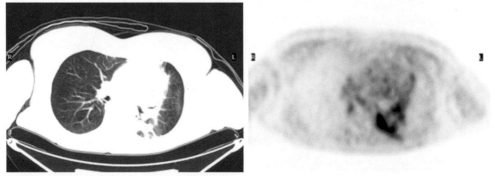

Fig. 12.18 Fluorodeoxyglucose (FDG) posttherapy uptake. Computed tomography (CT) and positron emission tomography (PET) images show radiation changes in the posterior medial left lung 3 months after external-beam radiation therapy. The uptake may decrease slightly on follow-up scans, but marked uptake typically persists in the lungs.

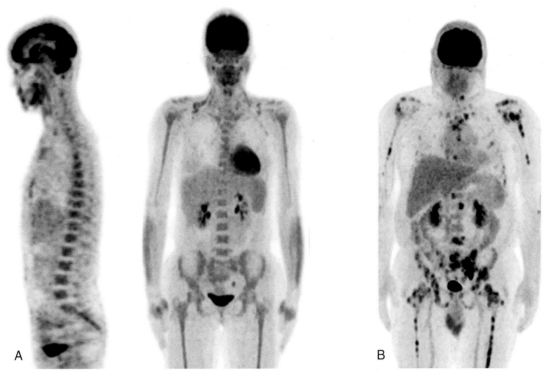

Fig. 12.19 Patterns of bone marrow fluorodeoxyglucose (FDG) uptake. (A) Diffuse uptake in the marrow is frequently seen in patients with cancer after therapy with colony-stimulating factors. (B) Osseous metastases usually present with heterogeneous focal lesions.

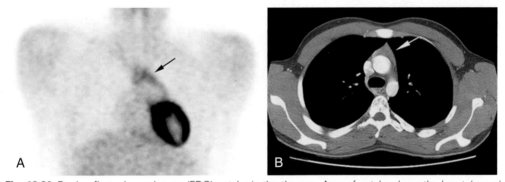

Fig. 12.20 Benign fluorodeoxyglucose (FDG) uptake in the thymus. Area of uptake above the heart *(arrow)* in the typical configuration of the thymus (A) corresponds to a normal thymus (B) on computed tomography (CT). After chemotherapy, this uptake may be even more intense, the so-called thymic rebound.

chemotherapy cycle is optimal. There is, however, some evidence suggesting that imaging early after chemotherapy can better predict long-term response in certain tumors, most notably in lymphoma. In some cases, therapy causes a change in the thymus, known as thymic rebound, where the normal low-level shield-shaped uptake in the anterior mediastinum in younger patients intensifies and the organ increases in size on CT (Fig. 12.20). It is important not to confuse this with residual active or worsening lymphoma.

Artifacts

When metal or dense-iodinated contrast is present, the attenuation-correction images may mistakenly show increased radiotracer activity around the area (Fig. 12.21). Correlation with CT helps identify the source of such artifacts, and examining the corresponding nonattenuation-correction images will show a

significant drop in activity that leads to the correct interpretation. Uptake in tumor or infection, on the other hand, will tend not to decrease on the nonattenuation-correction images (Fig. 12.22).

Hybrid PET/CT systems can generate certain artifacts. One common problem is misregistration of PET and CT images. Often, patients move their head or limbs between the two portions of the examination. Also, because the PET must be acquired in quiet respiration, the CT is usually performed by having the patient stop breathing for a few seconds or while in quiet respiration. Although this minimizes the significant organ shift that would be seen if the CT was done using maximal inspiratory effort, motion and low lung volumes can obscure lesions or make them project in an incorrect location. A well-known example of this can occur in lesions around the diaphragm, such as hepatic metastases that project over lung or rib

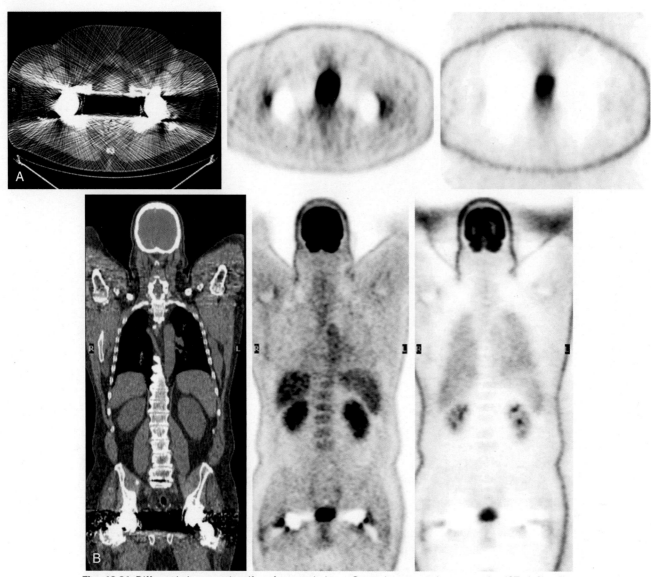

Fig. 12.21 Differentiating metal artifact from pathology. Coronal computed tomography (CT; *left*) scans demonstrate streak artifact in the pelvis from bilateral hip prostheses. On positron emission tomography (PET) attenuation-corrected images *(center)*, the effect of the metal manifests as linear increased activity along the edge of the metal. The nonattenuation-corrected images *(right)* confirm this is artifact because the activity is significantly decreased.

on the PET due to patient breathing (Fig. 12.23). Motion can additionally decrease lesion intensity as the counts are spread over adjacent voxels. Many systems possess respiratory gating capabilities where image acquisition is triggered only during one portion of the breathing cycle, resulting in decreased motion and improved lesion conspicuity. Because this technology requires extra time and radiation (from added CT slices), it is usually reserved for limited areas containing known smaller lesions (Fig. 12.24).

Patterns of Malignancy

Aggressive tumors usually have greater uptake because of higher levels of metabolic activity. This pattern must be differentiated from the intense activity often seen in infection or after radiation therapy. Low-level activity may be seen in low-grade tumors and tumors with a lower relative number of cells, such as

well-differentiated carcinoid and mucinous adenocarcinoma. Malignant pleural effusions most often have low-level F-18 FDG activity, and some are even negative, which may be due to the dispersion of tumor cells in the fluid so that uptake is not detected.

Areas of central necrosis, often seen in large malignant and inflammatory masses, will have diminished F-18 FDG accumulation. By localizing areas of necrosis and differentiating areas of increased activity, PET scans can help direct biopsy for increased sensitivity and more accurate sampling. It may not be possible to differentiate a cavitary infectious process from a necrotic tumor on PET because both will have a cold center and a peripheral rim of increased activity (Fig. 12.25).

Levels of background activity play a role in the detection of malignant lesions. For example, the high background activity of the brain contributes to limited sensitivity for metastatic disease, with

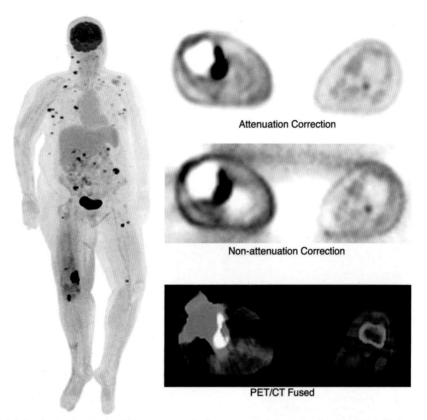

Attenuation Correction

Non-attenuation Correction

PET/CT Fused

Fig. 12.22 Infection or tumor should be suspected adjacent to metal prosthesis when it is fairly intense, such as this case of recurrent metastatic melanoma to the knee in a patient with widespread metastatic disease. The lack of change between nonattenuation-correction and attenuation-correction images also favors the presence of true pathology in the region.

perhaps only a third of lesions being visualized. Also, if background uptake is heterogeneous, as may happen in the bowel, liver, or bone marrow, it can make lesion detection more difficult.

Quantification: The Standard Uptake Value

Lesion activity can be described in comparison to contralateral background, blood pool, or liver activity. Areas can be graded as mild, moderate, or marked depending on the level compared with normal structures. However, it is often desirable to use a numerical value, and this is usually done with the standard uptake value, or SUV.

A region of interest (ROI) is drawn around an area or volume of tissue. The number of photons detected will reflect the actual radiopharmaceutical concentration in the body once differences in photon attenuation are compensated for by applying the attenuation-correction map from the CT data. This calculation also requires the precise knowledge of the injected activity, determined by subtracting the postinjection residual in the syringe from the known activity initially present and decay-correcting for time. Therefore, the dose calibrator quality control must be maintained, and dose infiltration must be avoided during injection. The formula used to determine SUV is:

$$SUV = (\text{Tissue activity (mCi/mL)}) / ((\text{Injected dose mCi})) / (\text{patient weight (grams)})$$

Activity in a lesion often is reported in terms of the SUV_{max}, or the value of the most intense pixel in the ROI. This allows the

exclusion of low counts from areas of necrosis or adjacent normal structures. An SUV_{mean} is an average of all counts in the ROI, which may be more representative because a spurious single hot area will not cause incorrect data to be recorded. Many experts advocate using an SUV_{peak}, which is calculated as an average of the counts from a circular volume (often 1 cm) surrounding the hottest pixel. The SUV_{peak} may more accurately represent maximal tumor metabolism with a higher degree of statistical significance than the SUV_{max}. In addition, a correction can be applied for body mass or body surface area (SUV_{lean} or SUV_{bsa}). This helps eliminate the problem created by the fact that the very low distribution of F-18 FDG in fat leads to higher activity values in tumor and normal tissues in heavier patients than in thin patients.

In general, an SUV greater than 2.5 has been considered suspicious for malignancy, although most tumors have an even higher level, and considerable overlap occurs with inflammatory processes. Numerous factors affect SUV levels (Table 12.3). When evaluating the response to therapy on serial scans or when comparing data from multiple sites participating in a trial, SUV accuracy is critical. All parameters that could alter the SUV must be controlled. However, variability still occurs, and most consider that the SUV must change at least 20% to be significant. Reports describe greater technical differences when considering a multicenter trial. Because of difficulties in maintaining protocol compliance and other issues, a 34% change was required before it could be considered significant.

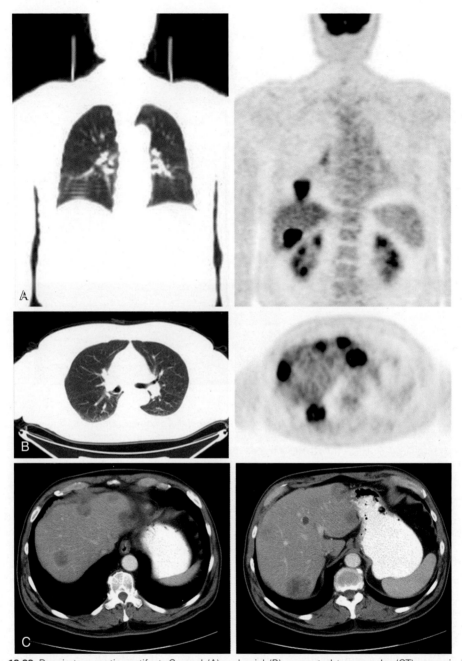

Fig. 12.23 Respiratory motion artifact. Coronal (A) and axial (B) computed tomography (CT) scans in lung windows and corresponding positron emission tomography (PET) scans show intense fluorodeoxyglucose (FDG) activity in liver metastases and the right lung base. However, no lung mass is seen on CT. (C) Two axial-enhanced CT images show liver metastases. Differences in respiration have caused misregistration, and a posterior liver lesion projects over the lung on PET.

CLINICAL F-18 FDG PET USE IN ONCOLOGY

Evaluation of lung cancer in solitary pulmonary nodules was the first clinical indication for F-18 FDG PET scanning in the United States approved by the CMS. Since that time, its use has rapidly evolved. It is important to understand the strengths and weakness of this examination for each type of tumor. F-18 FDG PET is very sensitive for many cancers (Table 12.4), whereas the examination is frequently less sensitive for others (Table 12.5). Several of the indications for PET are described in the following subsections. Brain tumor assessment with F-18 FDG is discussed in Chapter 13.

Cancers Not Localized to an Organ or Region
Lymphoma

Lymphomas can be divided into Hodgkin's lymphoma (HL) in approximately 10% of cases and non-Hodgkin's lymphoma (NHL) in the remainder. Characterization also depends on the type of lymphocyte the tumor arises from: NHL can originate from T cells or B cells, whereas HL involves the B lymphocytes, and numerous subtypes have been identified under these main groupings. Each individual cancer can follow an aggressive, moderate, or more indolent course, but even cases that initially behave in a low-grade manner can undergo malignant transformation, turning highly aggressive and frequently fatal. Patients may also relapse after remission, and in such cases, tumors are often refractory to therapies.

HL progression tends to involve contiguous nodal chains and lymphoproliferative structures. It most frequently presents with painless supraclavicular or cervical adenopathy (60%–80%), axillary adenopathy (30%), and/or mediastinal mass (50%–60%). Disease outside of the lymph nodes is rare (10% to 15%), but when it happens, involvement is most often in the lung, bone marrow, bone, or liver. Disease in NHL does not tend to spread in a similar orderly fashion, and patients frequently present initially with widespread disease.

Survival has improved over the years but is worse if disease is not localized. In HL, the overall 5-year survival rate of greater than 90% decreases to 77% for distant involvement, and for NHL, the overall survival rate of more than 86% falls to roughly 63% when disease is no longer localized. Accurate staging and assessment of treatment response can help prevent unnecessary or ineffective therapy, which, given the high cure rates and long survival times, may be especially important to decrease toxicity from therapy. However, the tumor, node, metastasis (TNM) system commonly used for solid tumors is not as useful for lymphoma.

Methods used for staging and assessment of therapy response have evolved over the years. The Ann Arbor staging system has

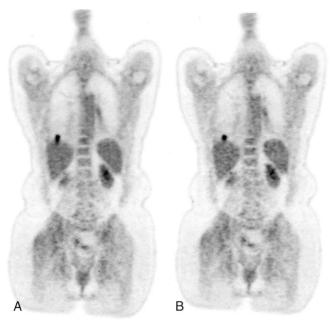

Fig. 12.24 Coronal slices of a lung nodule performed with normal quiet respiration (A) and then with respiratory gating (B) showed decreased blurring of the nodule. In addition, standardized uptake value (SUV) measurements of the nodule saw a mild but potentially significant 4% increase in the SUV_{max} that could improve lesion conspicuity.

TABLE 12.3 Factors Altering the Standard Uptake Value (SUV)

Factor	Change in SUV
↑ Serum glucose	↓
↑ Body mass	↑
↓ Dose from extravasation	↓
↑ Uptake period	↑
↓ Region-of-interest size	↑
↓ Pixel size	↑

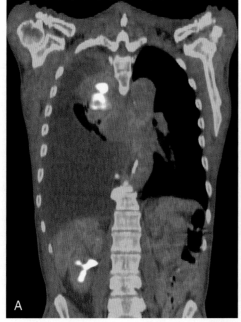
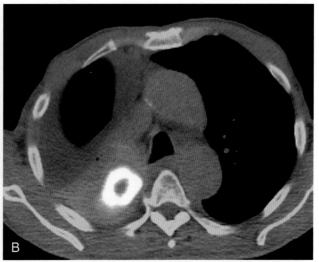

Fig. 12.25 Central tumor necrosis on positron emission tomography (PET). A left-upper-lung carcinoma seen as a solid mass on computed tomography (CT) actually contains significant central necrosis that is revealed as absent uptake on fused PET axial (A) and coronal (B) images. Visualization of regional differences in tumor metabolic activity with PET can help direct biopsy.

TABLE 12.4 F-18 Fluorodeoxyglucose (FDG) PET Common Applications in Oncology

TUMORS WITH GREATER UPTAKE/SENSITIVITY

Primary Tumor Region

Head and neck cancer	Squamous (most common) Adenocarcinoma	
Solitary lung nodule (SPN)	>7–8 mm	
Lung cancer	Non–small cell Small cell	Lower for ground-glass/ subsolid adenocarcinoma (formerly bronchoalveolar cancer)
	Small cell	
Mesothelioma		
Breast cancer	Moderate uptake—lower in lobular and in situ lesions	
Esophageal		
Gastric cancers	May be difficult to see due to background	
Colon cancer		
Rectal cancer		
Pancreatic adenocarcinoma		
Cervical cancer		
Endometrial cancer		
Uterine cancer		
Testicular cancer	Seminomatous +/– more than nonseminomatous	

Tumors With Primary Not Regionally Localized

Lymphoma	Non-Hodgkin's	Usually hot: Low-grade tumors may not be FDG+
	Hodgkin's	Almost always hot
Melanoma		
Multiple myeloma		
Sarcoma	(locations vary)	

Tumors With Moderate Sensitivity

Hepatocellular cancer	Use enhanced CT/MR using noncontrast, arterial phase, venous phase, and delayed washout timing
Ovarian cancer	
Glioblastoma multiforme	

CT, Computed tomography; *MR,* magnetic resonance; *PET,* positron emission tomography.

TABLE 12.5 Malignant Tumors With Lower Sensitivity on F-18 Fluorodeoxyglucose (FDG) PET

Cancer Type From Head to Toe	Comments
Low-grade glioma	Improved in GBM and lymphoma but accuracy < outside the brain Best assessed with enhanced MR
Brain metastases	Detects ≈1/3
Well-differentiated thyroid cancer	Imaging with radioiodine preferred
Pulmonary neuroendocrine tumor (carcinoid)	F-18 FDG is useful when Ga-68 DOTATATE uptake is poor (i.e., poorly differentiated tumor).
NSCLC bronchoalveolar	Lowest in ground-glass opacities FDG still commonly used
Lobular breast cancer	Detects ≈40% FDG still commonly used
Cholangiocarcinoma	
Bowel and pancreatic neuroendocrine tumors (NETs)	F-18 FDG is useful in when Ga-68 DOTATATE uptake is poor (i.e., poorly differentiated tumor).
Cystic borderline or low-grade pancreatic neoplasm	
Renal-cell carcinoma	
NSGCT testicular cancer	
Cystic, borderline, or low-grade ovarian tumor	
Prostate adenocarcinoma	FDG is useful when hormonal control/castration no longer inhibits growth (de-differentiates).
ENMZL (MALT lymphoma)	
Liposarcoma	

ENMZL, Extranodal marginal-zone lymphoma; *GBM,* glioblastoma; *MALT,* mucosa-associated lymphoid tissue lymphoma; *MR,* magnetic resonance; *NSCLC,* non–small-cell lung cancer; *NSGCT,* nonseminomatous germ-cell tumor; *PET,* positron emission tomography.

activity as opposed to the location of lesions. This is essential because the presence of fibrosis and scar can mean lesions seen on CT do not fully resolve, even after tumor has been successfully eradicated (Fig. 12.26). However, metabolic activity on PET tends to be proportional to tumor grade and can better identify and differentiate sites of active disease from scarring. Changes in F-18 FDG metabolic activity on PET/CT can be used to significantly improve the accuracy concerning changing disease status over anatomical measurement alone on CT or MR. In order to better standardize descriptions of lesion intensity, the Deauville Criteria established a 5-point scale, comparing maximal to background structures:

1 = no activity above background
2 ≤ mediastinal blood pool
3 > mediastinum
4 > liver (moderately)
5 >> liver (markedly)

been widely used for years, relying on lesion location and size changes in lymph nodes, lymphoproliferative tissue, and other organs (Box 12.4). Over the years, classification and grading systems have evolved to better reflect actual changes in tumor

The Lugano Criteria, which combine staging parameters based on the Ann Arbor system with the 5-point visual PET grading system, were published in 2014 and are now in widespread use (Table 12.6).

F-18 FDG PET imaging of lymphoma has been one of the most successful applications of F-18 FDG. It is clearly superior to the previous nuclear medicine examination for lymphoma assessment, Ga-67 (Fig. 12.27), and compares very favorably with CT scanning, which has been the preeminent lymphoma imaging examination for years. Overall, the reported sensitivity and specificity of PET/CT for detecting active tumor are approximately 86% and 96%, respectively, compared with a CT sensitivity of 81% and a specificity of 41% in HL. Viable NHL lymphoma is also almost always FDG avid, particularly in diffuse large B cell (DLBCL). A baseline examination is recommended, however, to confirm each tumor is FDG avid because some low-grade tumors do not accumulate significant amounts of radiopharmaceutical. In addition to facilitating interpretation of subsequent examinations, the pretreatment PET reportedly modifies the disease stage in 15% to 20% and may affect management in 5% to 15%. The sensitivity of FDG PET/CT for several types of lymphoma is outlined in Table 12.7. Tumors with lower sensitivity are often extranodal, and some of these include primary cutaneous T-cell lymphoma (40%), extranodal marginal-zone lymphoma (54%–66%), and gastrointestinal (GI) tract lymphoma (67%; Fig. 12.28). It has been known for a long time that posttherapy PET/CT can predict long-term outcomes in HL, with patients with positive examinations demonstrating markedly decreased survival compared with those whose areas of abnormal uptake clear (69% compared with 95%, respectively). Results with other tumors have varied somewhat. However, recent Lugano Criteria recommendations support the use of F-18 FDG PET/CT in all lymphomas that show positive uptake.

Potential challenges with F-18 FDG can at times include detection of bone marrow lesions. Because background bone marrow activity greatly varies, lesions may be difficult to detect. However, although the reported sensitivity has varied compared with bone marrow biopsy, the sensitivity has been reported as high as 90% to 92% with PET/CT (Fig. 12.29).

BOX 12.4   Ann Arbor Staging System With Cotswold Modifications

Stage I
Single lymph node region or lymphoid organ (i.e., spleen, Waldeyer's ring, thymus)
Stage IE involves a single extralymphatic site.

Stage II
Two or more lymph node regions on same side of diaphragm or localized contiguous involvement of one extranodal organ and its regional lymph nodes
Stage IIE involves other lymph node regions on the same side of the diaphragm.

Stage III
Lymph node involvement on both sides of the diaphragm
Stage IIIS also involves the spleen.
Stage IIIE involves one extranodal organ on one side of the diaphragm.
Stage IIISE involves one extranodal on both sides of the diaphragm.

Stage IV
Multifocal/dissemination of one or more extranodal organs (including marrow) or structures, with or without associated lymph nodes, *or*
Involvement of an isolated extralymphatic organ with nonregional/distant lymph node involvement
Additional designations:
  A—No symptoms
  B—Fever, drenching night sweats, unexpected >10% weight loss in 6 months
  X—Bulky disease
Decreased number of target lesions from 10 to 5

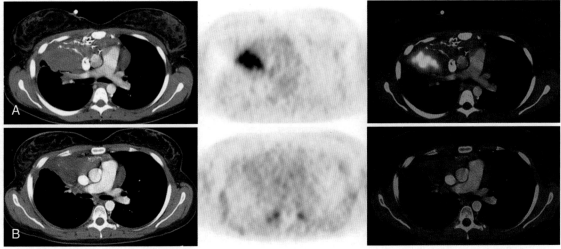

Fig. 12.26 Evaluation of a residual mass. (A) During chemotherapy for lymphoma, a large partially enhancing anterior mediastinal mass on computed tomography (CT) showed persistently abnormal fluorodeoxyglucose (FDG) accumulation in one region of the mass. (B) When the follow-up CT showed residual mass, a repeat positron emission tomography (PET) was done. No FDG uptake was seen, consistent with fibrosis and scar.

TABLE 12.6 Lugano Criteria for Lymphoma Response Assessment

Deauville Score	Definition of Score	Posttherapy PET Lugano Score (hottest lesion)	Posttherapy CT	Lymphoma Status
1 2 3	No abnormal ↑ activity ≤ Mediastinal blood pool > Mediastinal blood pool	Score 1, 2, or 3 (+/– residual mass) No new FDG+ lesion No FDG+ bone marrow disease	Lymph node ↓ ≤ 1.5 cm Radiographic lesions completely disappear	Complete response (CR)
4	Mildly > liver	Score 4 or 5 with↓ uptake compared with baseline and with residual mass(es) Bone marrow lesion activity ↓ from baseline but not cleared No new lesions	Lesion SPD or PPD ↓ ≥50% No progression of nonmeasured lesions	Partial response (PR)
5	>> Liver (2–3 times greater) New lesions	Score 4 or 5 w/o significant change in uptake No change in bone marrow uptake from baseline No new lesions	Lesions ↓ <50% No evidence of progression	Stable disease (SD) or no response
		Score 4 or 5 with ↑ uptake from baseline New lesions consistent with lymphoma New or recurrent FDG+ bone marrow	Lesion SPD or PPD ↑ ≥50% from nadir Lesions ≤2.0 cm ↑ by 0.5 cm and those >2 cm ↑ by 1.0 cm New or larger nonmeasured lesions Splenomegaly↑ 50% if no prior splenomegaly, length ↑2 cm	Progressive disease (PD)
X	Activity unlikely related to lymphoma			

Single CT lesion: PPD = product of perpendicular diameter (short axis × long axis) in cm; multiple CT lesions: SPD = sum of the product of each lesion's perpendicular diameter (SPD = lesion A [short axis × long axis] + lesion B [short axis × long axis] +..., etc.).
CT, Computed tomography; *FDG,* fluorodeoxyglucose; *PET,* positron emission tomography.

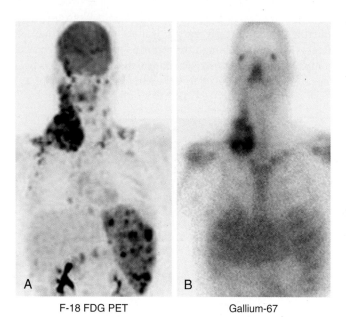

F-18 FDG PET   Gallium-67

Fig. 12.27 Improved sensitivity of fluorodeoxyglucose (FDG) positron emission tomography (PET) over gallium-67 (Ga-67). PET shows a large right neck mass and involvement in the left neck, spleen, and abdomen from lymphoma (A), whereas a 10-mCi Ga-67 scan at 96 hours has inferior image quality and fails to detect lesion outside of the right neck (B). Ga-67 was used extensively in the past to evaluate lymphoma but is less sensitive than F-18 FDG PET, as seen in this patient.

Another important issue to consider is the significance of residual masses after therapy, which can be seen in up to 85% of HL patients and 40% with NHL. In general, PET/CT is much more specific than CT (86% vs. 31%). However, such masses can show residual uptake, particularly when occurring in the anterior mediastinum, where nonspecific, mild residual activity is sometimes seen but represents active tumor in <50% of cases. In addition, postchemotherapy thymic rebound can cause a false positive with mild to moderately increased F-18 FDG activity and enlargement on CT. A follow-up examination may be needed if an anterior mediastinal soft tissue lesion does not have the characteristic shield-shaped configuration.

Melanoma

For patients with melanoma, survival strongly depends on the stage at the time of diagnosis, and the prognosis is extremely poor with nodal or distant metastases. Apart from the presence or absence of metastatic disease, the depth to which the primary lesion extends is the most important prognostic factor, and grading is based on thickness according to the Breslow classification. Metastases are frequently found in high-risk patients (i.e., >4-mm Breslow depth), but metastatic disease frequently occurs even in lower-risk patients. In high-risk cases, PET/CT often identifies lesions in unpredictable and unusual locations, often distant from

TABLE 12.7 F-18 Fluorodeoxyglucose (FDG) Activity in Lymphoma PET/CT

High FDG Uptake	Positive Lymphomas With More Variable FDG Uptake	Lower FDG Uptake
Hodgkin's lymphoma	Follicular lymphoma (ranges low to moderate)	CLL/SLL
Diffuse large B-cell lymphoma	Nodal marginal-zone lymphoma (none to high activity)	ENMZL (previously called MALT marginal-zone lymphoma)
Burkitt lymphoma	Mantle-cell lymphoma (low to high activity)	Splenic marginal-zone lymphoma
Lymphoblastic lymphoma		Primary cutaneous T-cell or B-cell lymphoma
Anaplastic large T-cell lymphoma		Mycosis fungoides
Peripheral T-cell lymphoma (variable sensitivity with positive lesions in 40%–98%)		Posttransplant lymphoproliferative disorder (PTLD)
NK/T-cell lymphoma		

CLL, Chronic lymphocytic leukemia; *ENMZL,* extranodal marginal-zone lymphoma; *MALT,* mucosa-associated lymphoid tissue lymphoma; *NK,* natural killer; *PET/CT,* positron emission tomography with computed tomography; *SLL,* small lymphocytic lymphoma.

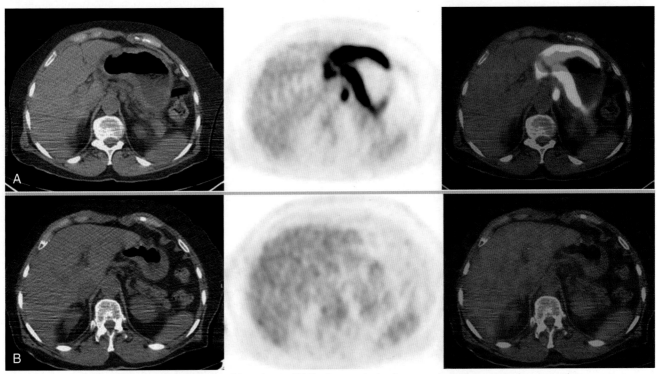

Fig. 12.28 Monitoring therapy of lymphoma. (A) Positron emission tomography with computed tomography (PET/CT) images show intense uptake in a gastric lymphoma and an adjacent lymph node. Gastric involvement may not be detected, but when present, positron emission tomography (PET) may be useful for follow-up. (B) After one cycle of chemotherapy, no tumor could be identified. This suggests a better prognosis than for a late responder or nonresponder.

the primary (e.g., other cutaneous and subcutaneous sites, spleen, distant nodes, liver, and gallbladder), and it often uncovers lesions not detected by CT (Fig. 12.30). Thus, many sites perform head-to-toe imaging on patients with melanoma. The sensitivity of FDG PET is reported to be greater than 90%, with a specificity of 87%. Lesions that are not detected are likely microscopic or in the brain, where enhanced MR is most effective. PET alters therapy in approximately 25% of patients and is useful in staging disease in patients at high risk for metastases or who relapse.

In terms of lymph node staging, however, PET does not replace sentinel lymph node scintigraphy with Tc-99m sulfur colloid or Tc-99m Tilmanocept in intermediate-risk (>1.4-mm Breslow depth) or high-risk patients diagnosed with melanoma. Evaluating the resected sentinel lymph node with histochemical staining is the most sensitive method to reveal microscopic disease. Although PET often identifies metastases in stage I or II patients, positive examinations are not seen in lower-risk patients without more extensive involvement in the area of the sentinel nodes.

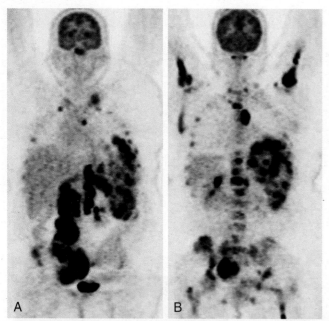

Fig. 12.29 Restaging lymphoma. (A) The initial positron emission tomography (PET) image in a patient with non-Hodgkin's lymphoma shows extensive abdominal adenopathy and involvement of the spleen, chest, and supraclavicular nodes. (B) After two cycles of chemotherapy, much of the adenopathy has resolved in the abdomen, but worsening disease is seen in the spleen, bone marrow, and mediastinum, requiring a change in therapy protocol.

Head and Neck Cancer

Squamous-cell tumors make up approximately 90% of all head and neck cancers (HNCs), with adenocarcinoma making up most of the remainder. Smoking and alcohol have long been recognized as the most important risk factors for squamous-cell cancer. In these tumors, the extent of lymph node involvement was historically the critical discriminating factor determining patient prognosis. Since 2007, however, the World Health Organization has officially recognized human papilloma virus (HPV) as a cause for HNC that can be identified by staining tissue for the immunohistochemical marker p16. It has become clear recently that HPV-positive HNC is a separate class of disease, showing unusually good response to therapy and positive outcomes even for stage III and stage IV disease using the prior standard classification system (TNM). Therefore, a different staging system was required with subgroups that better reflected differences in survival/prognosis (i.e., hazard discrimination) than the traditional system for squamous-cell cancer (i.e., HPV negative).

In 2018, the eighth edition of the American Joint Committee on Cancer (AJCC) *Cancer Staging Manual* went into effect for squamous-cell HNC using the TNM system. Restaging of HNC is broken down into three main groups: (1) nasopharynx (+/– Epstein–Barr virus [EBV]), (2) HPV-negative oro-/hypopharynx, and (3) HPV-positive oro-/hypopharynx. In addition to creating an entirely new staging system for HPV-positive oro-

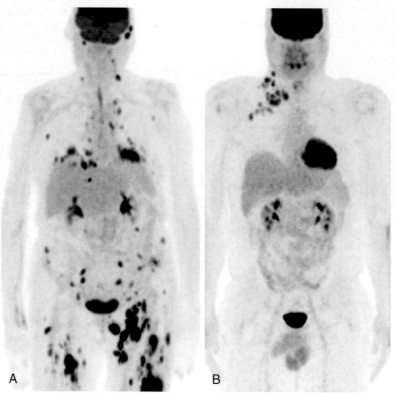

Fig. 12.30 Fluorodeoxyglucose (FDG) positron emission tomography (PET) in melanoma. (A) Diffuse tumor involvement including uptake near the primary tumor in the left thigh, multiple lymph nodes, organs, and soft tissue metastases from melanoma. This result led to changing the planned radiation therapy to systemic chemotherapy. PET can also identify subtle disease not found on computed tomography (CT). (B) Regional metastases are seen in numerous right cervical lymph nodes in a patient with a recently resected melanoma of the right ear.

TABLE 12.8 Staging/Restaging HPV-Negative Head and Neck Cancers[a]

Category	Oropharyngeal	Oral Cavity (includes DOI)
Tumor Size		
Tx	Cannot be assessed due to lack of information	Cannot be assessed due to lack of information
T0	(Deleted category)	
Tis	Carcinoma in situ	Carcinoma in situ
T1	≤2 cm	≤2 cm, DOI ≤5 mm
T2	>2 cm but ≤4 cm	≤2 cm, DOI >5 mm but ≤10 mm or >2 cm but ≤4 cm, ≤10 mm
T3	>4 cm or extension lingual surface epiglottis	>4 cm or any tumor DOI >10 mm
T4a	Tumor invades larynx, extrinsic tongue muscles, medial pterygoid, hard palate, or mandible	Invades lip or adjacent structures through bone; involves inferior alveolar nerve, floor of mouth, or skin of face
T4b	Any size invading lateral pterygoid muscle, skull base, pterygoid plates; or surrounds carotid artery or invades	Invades masticator space, pterygoid plates, or skull base and/or encases internal carotid artery

N Classification	Clinical LN Category	Pathological LN Category
NX	Cannot be assessed	Cannot be assessed
N0	No LN involvement	No LN involvement
N1	1 ipsilateral LN ≤3 cm, ENE–	1 ipsilateral LN ≤3 cm, ENE–
N2a	1 ipsilateral LN >3 cm but not >6 cm, ENE–	1 ipsilateral LN ≤3 cm, ENE+, *or* 1 LN >3 cm but not >6 cm, ENE–
N2b	Multiple ipsilateral LN, none >6 cm, ENE–	Multiple ipsilateral LN, none >6 cm, ENE–
N2c	Contralateral or bilateral LNs, none >6 cm, ENE–	Contralateral or bilateral LNs, none >6 cm, ENE–
N3a	1 ipsilateral LN >6 cm, ENE–	1 ipsilateral LN >6 cm, ENE–
N3b	Any LN(s) with clinically overt ENE+	1 ipsilateral LN >6 cm, ENE–, *or* Single ipsilateral LN >3 cm, ENE+, *or* Multiple ipsilateral, contralateral, or bilateral LNs if any are ENE+
M0	No distant spread	
M1	Distant spread	

DOI, Depth of invasion; *ENE,* extranodal extension; *HPV,* human papilloma virus; *LN,* lymph node.
[a]According to American Joint Committee on Cancer (AJCC) *Cancer Staging Manual*, eighth edition.

pharyngeal cancers, modifications were made for HPV-negative tumors, including determination of T by not only tumor size but also the depth of invasion (DOI), expanding nodal disease (N) classification to include extranodal extension, and modifying the "unknown primary" classification. The TNM classifications for HPV-negative and HPV-positive disease are outlined in Tables 12.8 and 12.9, respectively. The new staging systems for HNC are outlined in Table 12.10 for HPV-negative tumors and in Table 12.11 for HPV-positive tumors.

PET/CT is highly sensitive for these tumors and their metastases (Fig. 12.31) and is able to alter management in 15% to 25% of cases overall. Despite this sensitivity, most patients are initially diagnosed by contrast-enhanced CT or MR and physical examination. Up to 10% of patients, however, present with adenopathy from a "cancer of unknown primary" that escapes detection by standard means. Primary tumor identification allows the clinician to modify treatment and limit radiation fields. F-18 FDG is able to localize these lesions in an additional 25% to 56% of cases (sensitivity more limited in small tumors).

Although roughly 60% of cases present with locally advanced disease, distant metastases are unusual at the time of diagnosis (approximately 5%; Fig. 12.32). Although false positives from infection or inflammatory processes must be avoided, F-18 FDG has high sensitivity for lymph node involvement (90% compared with 82% for CT and 80% for MR). In high-risk

TABLE 12.9 AJCC TNM Classification for HPV-Positive Squamous-Cell Oropharyngeal Cancer

Category	Tumor Size
T0	No primary identified
T1	≤2 cm
T2	>2 cm but ≤4 cm
T3	>4 cm or growing into epiglottis
T4	Growing into larynx, extrinsic tongue muscle, mandible, hard palate, or medial pterygoid plate
	(Separation into T4a/b eliminated; no prognostic difference)

LYMPH NODE STATUS

Clinical Classification		Pathological Classification	
NX	Cannot assess regional LN	NX	Cannot be assessed
N0	No LN involvement	pN0	No regional LN
N1	≥1 LN, none >6 cm	pN1	≤4 LN involved
N2	Contralateral or bilateral LN; none >6 cm	pN2	>4 LN with metastasis
N3	≥1 LN >6 cm		

AJCC, American Joint Committee on Cancer; *HPV,* human papilloma virus; *LN,* lymph node; *TNM,* tumor, node, metastasis.

TABLE 12.10 Staging of HPV-Negative Squamous-Cell Oropharyngeal Head and Neck Cancer

Tumor Category	Node Category			
	N0	N1	N2a, b, c	N3a, b
T1	I	III	IVA	IVB
T2	II	III	IVA	IVB
T3	III	III	IVA	IVB
T4a	IVA	IVA	IVA	IVB
T4b	IVB	IVB	IVB	IVB

Also: IVC = M1 disease
HPV, Human papilloma virus.

TABLE 12.11 Clinical Staging in HPV-Positive Oropharyngeal Head and Neck Cancer

Tumor Category	Node Category			
T	N0	N1	N2	N3
T0	NA	I	II	III
T1	I	I	II	III
T2	I	I	II	III
T3	II	II	II	III
T4	III	III	III	III

HPV, human papilloma virus.

patients (T3–T4 and N2–N3 disease), PET is often used to better detect the distant metastases and can detect a second primary tumor in a significant number of patients.

PET is most commonly used for restaging and has consistently been found superior to conventional imaging modalities. Although a loss of symmetry and elevated background uptake posttherapy can make the evaluation for recurrence difficult, fusion images allow better identification of potential sources of error, such as increased uptake in normal structures, muscles, and brown fat. PET/CT has a known high negative predictive value (>90%–95%) and is superior to CT or MR in the detection of recurrent disease. The ability of FDG to predict survival is promising, but additional work is needed.

Consistent terms must be used to describe the location of HNC. In addition to an understanding of the key spaces of the region, this includes an accurate description of the station of involved nodes (Table 12.12; Figs. 12.33 and 12.34).

Thyroid Cancer

Thyroid cancer must be considered separately from other HNC. F-18 FDG may accumulate with equal intensity in benign thyroid adenomas and thyroiditis as well as malignant lesions. Although an incidentally detected F-18 FDG–avid nodule should be pursued to exclude malignancy, PET has no role in the diagnosis of thyroid cancer. Most thyroid cancers are derived from the follicular cells of the gland, giving rise to papillary,

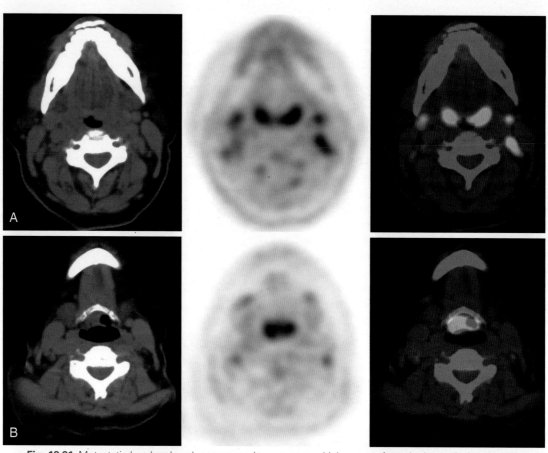

Fig. 12.31 Metastatic head and neck cancer can be seen as multiple areas of uptake in cervical nodes (A). Although the primary tumor may be hard to detect in areas of increased background from inflammation, biopsy, and normal lymphoid tissue, soft tissue fullness and asymmetrical uptake raises suspicions, as in this tumor involving the right epiglottis and tongue base (B).

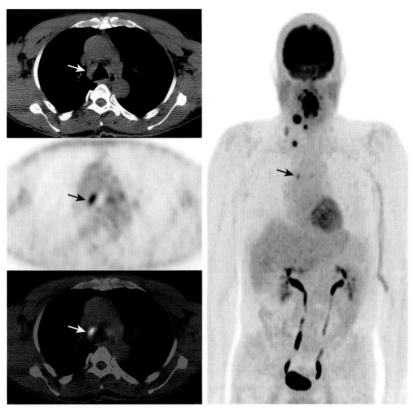

Fig. 12.32 Head and neck carcinoma staging. Positron emission tomography (PET) images reveal several abnormal lymph nodes in the right cervical and supraclavicular region and an unexpected mediastinal metastasis to a normal-size lower paratracheal node *(arrows)*.

TABLE 12.12   Lymph Node Imaging Stations in the Neck

Rouviere System	AJCC System	Imaging-Based System		
Submental	**I**	**IA:** Medial to medial edge anterior belly digastrics	Below mylohyoid muscle, above hyoid bone	
Submandibular	**I**	**IB:** Lateral to IA and anterior to back of submandibular gland		
Internal jugular	**II:** Skull base to hyoid, anterior to back edge sternocleidomastoid	**II:** Skull base to bottom of hyoid, anterior to back edge sternocleidomastoid	**IIA:** Anterior, lateral, or inseparable from internal jugular vein	
			IIB: Posterior to internal jugular vein with fat plane between	
Retropharyngeal	**III:** Hyoid to cricothyroid membrane, anterior to back edge sternocleidomastoid	**III:** Bottom of hyoid to bottom of cricoid arch, anterior to back edge sternocleidomastoid	Lateral to carotid, level VI nodes medial to carotids	
Midjugular	**IV:** Cricothyroid membrane to clavicle, anterior to back edge of sternocleidomastoid	**IV:** Bottom of cricoid arch to top of manubrium, anterior to back edge sternocleidomastoid	Lateral to carotids, level VI nodes medial to carotids	
Spinal accessory	**V:** Posterior to sternocleidomastoid, anterior to trapezius, above clavicle	**V:** Posterior to sternocleidomastoid, anterior to trapezius	**VA:** Skull base to bottom of cricoid arch	
			VB: Bottom cricoid arch to level clavicle	
Anterior compartment	**VI:** Below hyoid, above suprasternal notch, between carotid sheaths	**VI:** Below bottom of hyoid, above top of manubrium, medial to carotid arteries	Visceral nodes	
Upper mediastinal	**VII:** Below suprasternal notch Anterior compartment	**VII:** Below top manubrium and above innominate	Overlaps highest mediastinal nodes of chest classification between carotids	
Supraclavicular		Clavicles in field of view, above and medial to ribs		

All systems use facial, parotid, retropharyngeal, and occipital groups.
AJCC, American Joint Committee on Cancer.

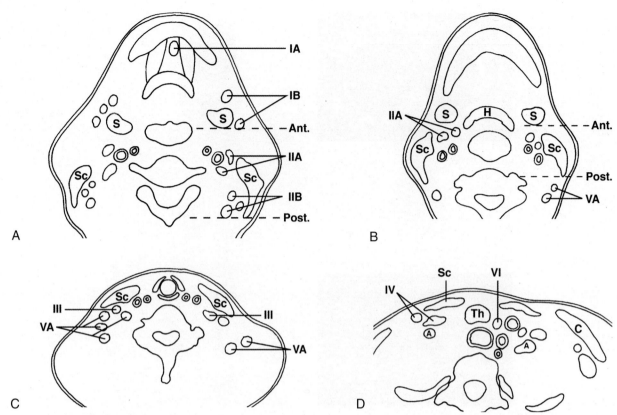

Fig. 12.33 Transaxial diagram of cervical lymph node stations at (A) the level of the floor of the mouth and submandibular gland *(S)*, (B) the hyoid bone *(H)*, (C) the thyroid cartilage and cricoid cartilage, and (D) just above the clavicles *(C)* with a portion of the thyroid gland *(Th)* in view. Note the appearance of the sternocleidomastoid muscle *(SC)*, which is a key landmark. *A*, Arteries; *Ant,* anterior.

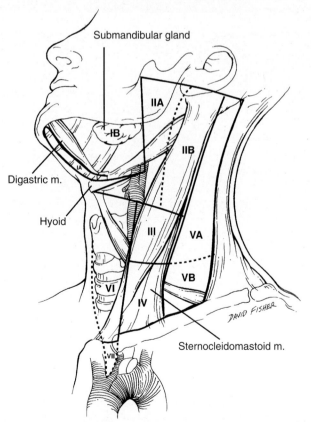

Fig. 12.34 Cervical lymph node levels according to the imaging-based classification system described in Table 12.12. *m,* Muscle.

follicular, or mixed-cellularity variants. These differentiated tumors accumulate iodine-131 (I-131) and are best evaluated and treated with radioactive iodine. The sensitivity of F-18 FDG in these patients is low.

The clinical utility of F-18 FDG PET scanning is generally limited to thyroid malignancies that do not accumulate I-131—that is, poorly differentiated, aggressive tumors. This may occur in metastatic and recurrent tumors that transform from previously well-differentiated, iodine-avid disease. In cases in which the I-131 scan is negative but serum thyroglobulin levels remain elevated, the sensitivity of PET is greater than 90%. PET has also shown sensitivity in the more aggressive Hürthle cell variant (up to 92%–95%, compared with 64% for iodine-131).

Medullary thyroid cancers are slow-growing neuroendocrine tumors (NETs) that arise from the calcitonin-producing parafollicular C cells and comprise 5% to 8% of thyroid cancers. Therapy is more challenging because they do not accumulate radioiodine. The sensitivity of F-18 FDG PET averages roughly 59%, but sensitivities are reportedly higher in recurrent disease when calcitonin levels are significantly increased (e.g., 75% when calcitonin >1000 ng/mL and 40% when <150). In fact, there is a complementary role for the PET somatostatin receptor analog, Ga-68 DOTATATE. Somatostatin-receptor–positive tumors tend to be lower grade, and imaging with receptor analogs is not only more sensitive but also identifies targets amenable to targeted radioactive somatostatin-receptor therapy. The more aggressive lesions not visualized with Ga-68 DOTATATE, on the other hand, tend to accumulate FDG.

Thoracic Cancers

Lung Carcinoma

Lung carcinoma is the most common malignancy and has the highest cancer-related death rate. Non–small-cell lung carcinoma (NSCLC) accounts for roughly 85% of cases, and small-cell lung carcinoma (SCLC) accounts for the remaining 20%. Approximately 75% of SCLC cases are initially diagnosed with disseminated disease. Therefore, surgery is rarely indicated, and chemotherapy and radiation therapy are used. NSCLC, on the other hand, is often resectable. Early diagnosis and proper staging are critical to therapeutic planning in NSCLC.

Presenting clinical and radiographic findings are variable in lung cancer. Patients may be asymptomatic or experience hemoptysis, cough, weight loss, and symptoms of metastatic disease. Radiographic findings are also nonspecific. A mass with an irregular, spiculated border is malignant in up to 85% of cases, but lesions with smooth margins may be cancerous over a third of the time. Larger and thick-walled cavitary lesions, especially in an upper-lobe location, must be considered suspicious. Workup for patients with these abnormal radiographs might include sputum cytology, bronchoscopy, transthoracic needle biopsy, and mediastinoscopy. Each of these procedures has limitations. For example, although bronchoscopy has a sensitivity of 85% for central tumors, it is much lower for small and peripheral lesions. The image-guided percutaneous transthoracic needle biopsy has an approximate sensitivity of 93% and a specificity 98%, although many lesions are too small or in an inaccessible location. Transthoracic needle biopsy also carries a 10% to 60% risk for pneumothorax (with a 2%–20% risk that it will require a chest tube). Patients may require thoracotomy and surgical biopsy for definitive diagnosis.

Diagnosis of Solitary Pulmonary Nodule

A pulmonary nodule is defined as a well-circumscribed lesion measuring less than 3 cm. With the increased use of CT, the detection of these nodules has risen tremendously; about half will prove to be malignant. The presence of central calcifications in a nodule indicates it is a benign granuloma. However, most pulmonary nodules are indeterminate based on radiographic appearance. Revised recommendations for the evaluation of incidentally discovered indeterminate nodules, based on number, size, and character, were released by the Fleischner Society in 2017. Patients are placed into risk groups (Box 12.5) that help guide follow-up, as noted in Table 12.13. The timing of follow-up imaging depends on a series of factors. The changes associated with malignancy that can be seen over the course of serial examinations include increasing size, spiculation, or irregularity as well as a ground-glass lesion that develops a solid component. Such changes should lead to a tissue diagnosis.

Characterization of a solitary pulmonary nodule (SPN) was one of the earliest clinical applications for F-18 FDG PET (Fig. 12.35). The specificity is hampered by the prevalence of granulomatous disease (e.g., sarcoid, histoplasmosis), which tends to be very FDG avid. In addition, the sensitivity is more limited in small nodules (i.e., less than 7 mm) and is very low for primary pulmonary carcinoid NETs. The sensitivity is mildly decreased in subsolid lung adenocarcinomas (formerly known as bronchoalveolar

cancer), which are often lower-grade, ill-defined ground-glass lesions rather than solid tumors. Often, these lesions show increasing size or density on serial CT (Fig. 12.36). Although the reported sensitivity in these tumors was 88% overall, the sensitivity increased to 96% when small and semisolid tumors were excluded (compared with a sensitivity of CT at 81%).

In fact, the sensitivity and high negative predictive value mean a negative examination virtually excludes malignancy, especially in a low-risk patient (<1%). Such patients with reasonably sized nodules (at least 8–10 mm) would not require further CT follow-up, unlike high-risk patients, who could still have up to a 10% risk of cancer. FDG can also help identify abnormal regional lymph nodes that might be good biopsy targets or visualize distant metastases that might change the type of diagnostic tissue sampling performed and would certainly affect further surgery and therapy decisions (Fig. 12.37). Although the current Fleischner recommendations include more limited use of PET/CT, many studies in the literature used in decision making were performed on older equipment: PET only or PET/CT without the more sensitive TOF capabilities. Also, it must be kept in mind that these guidelines apply to the incidentally discovered SPNs, and more aggressive follow-up is likely warranted in those with prior primary cancer.

Lung Cancer

Lung cancer is the leading cause of cancer deaths in both men and women, accounting for approximately 1.6 million deaths

TABLE 12.13 Fleischner Society Recommendations for Incidental Lung Nodule Imaging Follow-Up (FU)

A. SOLID NODULES

Nodule Type	<6 mm	6–8 mm	>8 mm	Comments
Single				
Low risk	No routine FU	CT 6–12 mo; then consider CT @ 18–24 mo	Consider CT 3 mo, PET/CT, or tissue sampling	Nodules <6 mm require no routine follow-up.
High risk	Optional CT @ 12 mo	CT 6–12 mo, then CT @ 18–24 mo	Consider CT 3 mo, PET/CT, or tissue sampling	A 12-mo CT may be warranted in some patients with suspicious morphology or upper-lobe location.
Multiple				
Low risk	No routine FU	CT 3–6 mo; then consider CT @ 18–24 mo	CT 3–6 mo; then consider CT @ 18–24 mo	Use the most suspicious nodule to guide management.
High risk	Optional CT @ 12 mo	CT 3–6 mo; then consider CT @ 18–24 mo	CT 3–6 mo; then consider CT @ 18–24 mo	Use the most suspicious nodule to guide management.

B. SUBSOLID NODULES

Nodule Type	<6 mm	≥6 mm	Notes
Single			
Ground glass	No routine FU	CT 6–12 mo to confirm persistence, then CT every 2 yr until 5 yr	In certain suspicious nodules <6 mm, consider FU @ 2 and 4 yr. If solid component or growth develops, consider resection.
Part solid	No routine FU	CT 3-6 mo to confirm persistence. If unchanged and solid component remains <6 mm, annual CT for 5 yrs	Part-solid nodules cannot be defined until ≥6 mm, and nodules <6 mm do not usually require FU. Persistent part-solid nodules with solid components should be considered highly suspicious.
Multiple	CT 3–6 mo; if stable, consider CT at 2 and 4 yr	CT 3-6 mo, subsequent management based on most suspicious nodule(s)	Multiple ground-glass nodules of <6 mm are usually benign, but consider FU in high-risk patients.

CT, Computed tomography; mo = months; PET/CT, positron emission tomography with computed tomography.

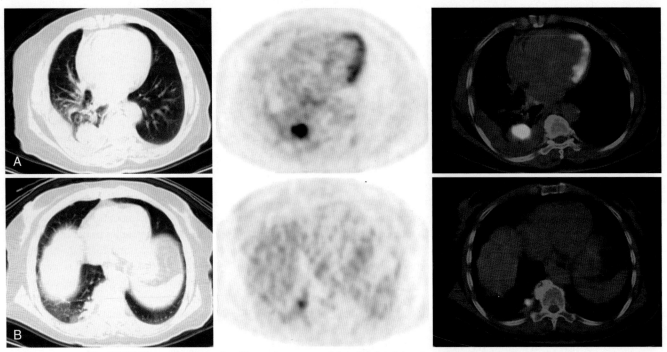

Fig. 12.35 Characterization of solitary pulmonary nodules. (A) A left lung nodule on computed tomography (CT) had no fluorodeoxyglucose (FDG) uptake on positron emission tomography (PET), consistent with a benign process. This lesion remained stable on CT follow-up, confirming this impression. (B) A small, well-circumscribed right-lower-lobe nodule with increased FDG accumulation on PET was later found to be an adenocarcinoma.

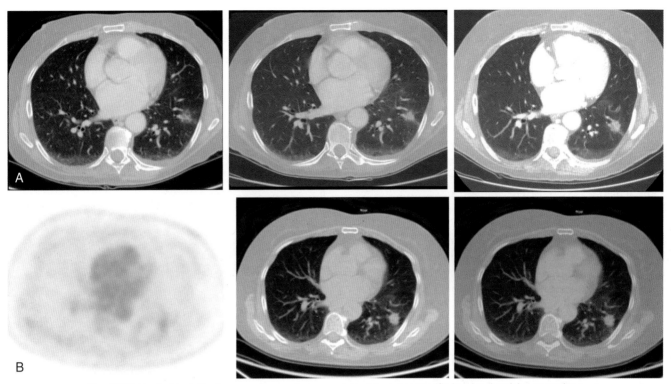

Fig. 12.36 An incidentally discovered ground-glass nodule shows nonspecific low-level activity on positron emission tomography with computed tomography (PET/CT; *upper*). However, given highly suspicious gradually increasing density on serial computed tomography (CT) images performed at 6- to 12-month intervals *(lower)*, biopsy was performed, revealing cancer.

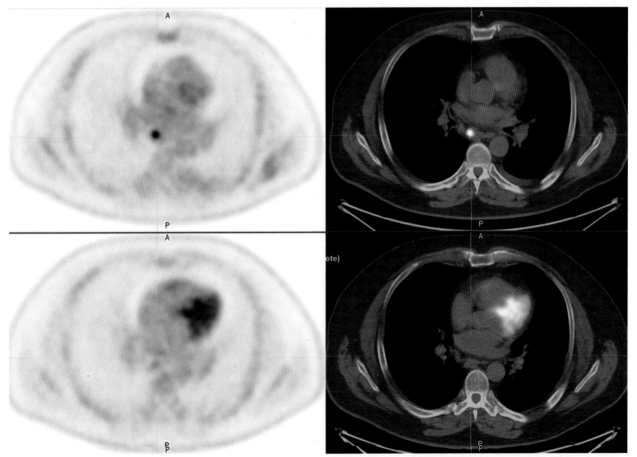

Fig. 12.37 Detection of metastatic disease with positron emission tomography (PET). *(Upper row)* Focal markedly increased fluorodeoxyglucose (FDG) uptake consistent with tumor involvement was seen in a normal-size lymph node. This was normal 6 months earlier *(lower row)*.

annually. Tumors originating from the airways or lung paren-chyma, also referred to as bronchogenic carcinomas, comprise roughly 95% of primary lung cancers and are broken down into two main groups: non–small-cell lung cancer (NSCLC) and small-cell lung cancer (SCLC). NSCLC is by far more common (80%–85%), and the most common types of lung cancers are both types of NSCLC: adenocarcinoma (40%–50%) and squamous-cell carcinoma (20%–30%).

The way lung cancers are organized and staged has recently evolved. Pathological lung cancer groupings put in place in 2015 recognize the importance of molecular and immunohisto-chemical markers as opposed to emphasizing only features seen with a microscope. In addition, there has been a redefinition of the adenocarcinoma category; elimination of the bronchoalve-olar tumor group, with those tumors reclassified as subtypes of adenocarcinoma; and the move of all NETs into a single class (Table 12.14).

An updated lung cancer staging system also went into effect in 2018, based on the TNM classification (Tables 12.15 and 12.16) and on updated chest lymph node descriptors (Table 12.17; Figs. 12.38 and 12.39). SCLC usually presents as systemic disease but is usually very sensitive to chemother-apy or, in locally advanced disease, to chemoradiation. Resection is only an option for a very limited number of patients who present early with a lung nodule but no nodal involvement. Most NSCLC (60%–75%) cases present with locally advanced (stage III) or advanced disease (stage IV). Although stage I and II tumors are generally considered resectable, up to 50% to 55% of these patients will suffer recurrence, often in less than a year. Better methods for determining risk and disease presence are needed. Imaging does play an increasingly important role in the management of lung cancer and could potentially improve staging accu-racy. Although chest CT is the primary examination most often utilized, it is known to be limited (sensitivity 55% and specificity 81%). Mediastinal lymph nodes with a short-axis length of >1 cm are considered abnormal. However, nor-mal-size nodes can harbor early metastatic disease, and enlarged nodes can be the result of a postinfectious or related inflammatory process. F-18 FDG PET/CT is more sensitive, but values in the literature vary. Although it is able to detect tumor in any one lymph node about 75% of the time, F-18 FDG averages 91% for the detection of overall mediastinal involvement. This still lacks sufficient accuracy to adequately stage the tumor, and the issue is compounded by the known specificity issues of PET/CT in the mediastinum. However, PET/CT can help direct biopsy away from locations typically sampled to focus on areas with the highest likelihood of yielding disease, even when nodes are normal in size.

In addition, F-18 FDG and chest CT have complementary roles in patient evaluation. CT better assesses tumor size, inva-sion of the pleura and mediastinum, and the distance of the tumor from the carina. Also, abnormalities such as atelectasis and aspiration pneumonia that can cause increased F-18 FDG uptake and are easily confused with malignancy are often iden-tifiable on CT. PET/CT leads to a reported change in manage-ment in 19% to 50% of cases, including a decrease in futile

TABLE 12.14 Changes in the World Health Organization (WHO) 2015 Classifications for Epithelial Lung Cancers

2004	2015
Adenocarcinoma	**Adenocarcinoma (40%–50%)**
Subtypes: Mixed, acinar, papillary, solid	Lepidic
Bronchoalveolar carcinoma	Acinar
Subtypes: Mucinous and nonmucinous	Papillary
Fetal	Micropapillary
Mucinous (colloid)	Solid
Signet ring	Invasive mucinous
Clear cell	Colloid
	Fetal
	Enteric
	Minimally invasive
	Preinvasive (atypical adenomatous hyperplasia
	Adenocarcinoma in situ (mucinous/nonmucinous)
Squamous-cell carcinoma	**Squamous-cell carcinoma (25%–30%)**
Papillary	Keratinizing
Clear cell	Nonkeratinizing
Small cell	Basaloid
Basaloid	
Small-cell carcinoma	**Neuroendocrine carcinoma**
	Small cell
Large-cell carcinoma	Large-cell neuroendocrine carcinoma
Large-cell neuroendocrine (NE) carcinoma	Carcinoid (typical and atypical)
Large-cell carcinoma with NE morphology	
	Large-cell carcinoma (10%)
Adenosquamous carcinoma	**Adenosquamous carcinoma**
Sarcomatoid carcinoma	**Sarcomatoid carcinoma (0.1%–0.4%)**
	Pleomorphic, spindle cell, giant cell, carcinosarcoma, pulmonary blastoma

Travis WD, Brambilla EW, Burke AP, et al. WHO classification of tumors of the lung, pleura, thymus, and heart. *J Thorac Oncol.* 2015;10(9):1243–1260.

thoracotomies. This is often the result of the superiority of PET over conventional modalities for the detection of unsuspected distant metastases, which occur 10% to 14% of the time. This includes bone metastases not visible on CT, which occur in 6% to 20% of cases in the literature. Bone involvement is also detected with a somewhat higher sensitivity and a considerably greater specificity than with bone scan. Other common sites of

TABLE 12.15 Revised Tumor, Node, Metastasis (TNM)[a] Characterization for Lung Carcinoma

Designation	Parameters
Tumor Description (T)	
TX	Cannot be assessed or proven by cells from sputum or bronchoscopy
T0	No evidence of primary
Tis	Carcinoma in situ
T1	≤3 cm surrounded by lung or visceral pleura, no invasion proximal to lobar bronchus
T1a	>3 cm but ≤5 cm; or involvement main bronchus, or visceral pleura invasion, or associated with partial or complete lung atelectasis or pneumonitis
T1b	>3 cm but ≤2 cm
T1c	>2 cm but ≤3 cm
T2	>3 cm but ≤5 cm; or involvement main bronchus, or visceral pleura invasion, or associated with partial or complete lung atelectasis or pneumonitis
T2a	>3 cm but ≤4 cm
T2b	>4 cm but ≤5 cm
T3	>5 cm but ≤7 cm; or directly invades parietal pleura, chest wall, parietal pericardium, or a separate nodule of same lobe
T4	>7 cm that invades any of the following: mediastinum, diaphragm, heart, great vessels, trachea, recurrent laryngeal nerve, esophagus, vertebra, carina, or separate nodule(s) in different lobe of the same lung
Lymph Node Description (N)	
NX	Cannot be assessed
N0	No regional LN metastasis
N1	Ipsilateral peribronchial and/or ipsilateral hilar and intrapulmonary LN (including by direct extension)
N2	Ipsilateral mediastinal and/or subcarinal LN
N3	Contralateral: mediastinal, hilar, or supraclavicular nodes Ipsilateral or contralateral scalene or supraclavicular
Distant Metastases (M)	
M0	No distant metastasis
M1	Distant metastasis
M1a	Separate tumor nodule(s) contralateral lung, malignant pleural effusion, pericardial thickening/nodules/masses
M1b	Single distant (extrathoracic) metastasis in single organ
M1c	Multiple distant metastases in single or multiple organs

LN, Lymph node.

[a]According to American Joint Committee on Cancer (AJCC) *Cancer Staging Manual*, eighth edition.
Modified from Goldstraw P, Chansky K, Crowley J, et al. The IASLC Lung Cancer Staging Project: Proposals for revision of the TNM stage groupings in the forthcoming (eighth) edition of the TNM Classification for lung cancer. *J Thorac Oncol.* 2016;11(1):39–51; and Detterbeck FC. The eighth edition TNM stage classification for lung cancer: what does it mean on the main street? *J Thorac Cardiovasc Surg.* 2018;155:356–359.

involvement include retroperitoneal and pelvic lymph nodes as well as soft tissue lesions (Fig. 12.40). Assessment of the adrenal glands is particularly important because they are a frequent site of lung cancer metastasis. CT reveals adrenal lesions in approximately 20% of cases, but the majority are later proved to be benign adenomas. PET can detect metastases in normal-size adrenals and can also help differentiate benign from malignant adrenal gland lesions based on the level of uptake (Fig. 12.41). Care must be taken when activity is only mild and not greater than liver background because nodular hyperplasia and benign adenomas can lead to mildly increased uptake. There is no absolute SUV measurement to use when deciding if metastases are present.

Restaging Non–Small-Cell Lung Cancer and Assessing Response to Therapy. PET/CT can also increase accuracy during restaging and when evaluating the response to therapy, with changes in radiotracer uptake noted earlier than in lesion size (Fig. 12.42). Tumor masses and lymph nodes may remain enlarged after disease has resolved and the PET scan has normalized. Perhaps more importantly, PET/CT can more often visualize patients who have progressive disease during therapy. Thereby, unnecessary time, expense, and exposure to toxicity can be avoided from an ineffective drug while potentially allowing nonresponders to be switched to an alternative regimen.

When surgery and therapy distort anatomy, PET can detect residual and recurrent tumor not found on CT. Caution must be used because increased F-18 FDG accumulation may occur after therapy, most significantly after radiation. Immediately after radiation, patchy areas of uptake can be seen, corresponding to ground-glass-appearing infiltrates. With time, these coalesce and contract, with a final appearance on CT of a sharply marginated infiltrate containing air-bronchograms. The PET findings also change over time, but intense activity often does

TABLE 12.16 Revised Lung Cancer Staging[a]

T/M	Subcategory	N0	N1	N2	N3
	T1a	IA1	IIB	IIIA	IIIB
	T1b	IA2	IIB	IIIA	IIIB
T1	T1c	IA3	IIB	IIIA	IIIB
	T2a	IB	IIB	IIIA	IIIB
T2	T2b	IIA	IIB	IIIA	IIIB
T3	T3	IIB	IIIA	IIIB	IIIC
T4	T4	IIIA	IIIA	IIIB	IIIC
M1	M1a	IVA	IVA	IVA	IVA
	M1b	IVA	IVA	IVA	IVA
	M1c				

T/M, Tumor/metastasis.

[a]According to American Joint Committee on Cancer (AJCC) *Cancer Staging Manual*, eighth edition.

From Detterbeck FC. The eighth edition TNM stage classification for lung cancer: what does it mean on the main street? *J Thorac Cardiovasc Surg*. 2018;155:356–359.

not resolve. It is generally advised to delay F-18 FDG PET until at least 3 months after therapy, although imaging can be done sooner if needed. Even given these limitations, PET can provide valuable information by identifying residual disease or relapse. For example, distant recurrence after complete resection of tumor occurs more than 20% of the time. PET restaging frequently leads to changes in management.

Small-Cell Lung Cancer. SCLC staging usually involves categorizing the disease as limited or extensive. If disease is confined to one hemithorax, it can be treated more successfully by adding radiation to the chemotherapy. Small-cell lung carcinoma shows intense F-18 FDG accumulation. In general, data on the use of F-18 FDG PET in SCLC are more limited than for NSCLC. PET may help detect additional metastasis and lead to upstaging of disease in some patients originally thought to be surgical candidates with localized disease.

Breast Carcinoma

Breast cancer is classified as being a noninvasive or invasive tumor, usually of ductal or lobular type. Of invasive carcinomas,

TABLE 12.17 Mediastinal Lymph Node Definitions From the IASLC Lymph Node Map

Station	Borders/Description
Supraclavicular Zone	
1 Lower cervical	Lower cervical, supraclavicular, sternal notch *Upper border:* lower margin of cricoid *Lower border:* clavicles laterally and upper manubrium at midline
Upper Zone	
2 Upper paratracheal	Borders: *On right:* Superiorly right lung apex and pleural space to inferior border at top of manubrium and medially to the left lateral tracheal wall *On the left:* Superiorly left lung apex and pleural space and upper manubrium medially; inferiorly to top of aortic arch
3A Prevascular	*Upper border:* apex of chest *Lower border:* level of carina *Anterior border:* posterior sternum *Posterior border:* On right—anterior SVC On left—left carotid artery
3P Retrotracheal	Posterior to trachea *Upper border:* apex of chest *Lower border:* carina
4R Right lower paratracheal	*Upper border:* intersection caudal margin innominate vein with trachea *Lower border:* lower border azygous vein *Medial border:* left lateral margin trachea
4L Left lower paratracheal	*Upper border:* upper margin aortic arch *Lower border:* upper rim main pulmonary artery
Aortopulmonary Zone	
5 Subaortic	Aortopulmonary (AP) window Lateral to ligamentum arteriosum *Upper border:* lower margin aortic arch *Lower border:* upper rim left main pulmonary artery
6 Paraaortic	Anterior and lateral to ascending aorta and aortic arch *Upper border:* line tangential to upper border aortic arch *Lower border:* lower margin aortic arch

TABLE 12.17	Mediastinal Lymph Node Definitions From the IASLC Lymph Node Map—cont'd
Station	**Borders/Description**
Subcarinal Zone	
7 Subcarinal	Upper border: carina of trachea Lower border: On left—upper border of the left lower lobe bronchus On right—lower border bronchus intermedius
Lower Zone (Lower Mediastinal)	
8 Paraesophageal	Lateral to esophagus below subcarinal nodes Upper border: On left—upper border of lower lobe bronchus On right—lower border bronchus intermedius
9 Pulmonary ligament	Lie within pulmonary ligament Upper border: inferior pulmonary vein Lower border: diaphragm
Hilar and Interlobar Zone	
10 Hilar	Immediately adjacent to mainstem bronchus and hilar vessels Upper border: On right—lower rim azygous On left—upper rim pulmonary artery Lower border: interlobar regions bilaterally
11 Interlobar	Between origin of lobar bronchi: 11Rs (right upper bronchus) and 11Ri (right middle and lower lobes)
Peripheral Zone (Pulmonary Nodes)	
12 Lobar	Adjacent lobar bronchi
13 Segmental	Adjacent to segmental bronchi
14 Subsegmental	Adjacent subsegmental bronchi

IASLC, International Association for the Study of Lung Cancer; *SVC,* superior vena cava.

ductal carcinoma accounts for ??, lobular for 10%, and medullary for 5%. Noninvasive carcinoma, or carcinoma in situ, may be detected by mammography when microcalcifications are present (i.e., ductal carcinoma in situ [DCIS]) but may be difficult to detect when it presents as architectural distortion as found in lobular carcinoma in situ (LCIS). Prognosis is related to many staging factors, as well as the genomic breakdown of the tumor. Hormone receptor expression (estrogen, progesterone, and HER-2 receptor expression) and overexpression of tumor markers have been found to be highly predictive of outcome. In fact, the updated eighth edition of the AJCC staging system now includes not only routine anatomical prognostic groups but also a pathological prognostic system that includes such markers and clinical prognostic staging groups. The majority of patients (61%) present with localized disease confined to the primary, whereas 32% have spread to the regional nodes, and about 5% have metastatic disease.

Diagnosis. Mammography is the primary mode of breast cancer diagnosis and screening, with a sensitivity of approximately 81% to 90 %, depending on factors such as tumor type and size, breast density, and availability of prior examinations. The specificity of this modality creates some challenges. More than 50% of women undergoing annual mammography for a decade will have a false-positive result,

frequently leading to biopsy as well as added cost and stress. Newer techniques such as tomosynthesis can improve tumor-detection rates, but with increased radiation exposure. MR and ultrasound are excellent problem-solving tools that do not involve ionizing radiation. MR has a high sensitivity (up to 90%–95%) for the detection of breast cancer, although its specificity is lower. It is particularly useful in high-risk patients and those with dense breasts but can also better visualize multifocal disease, recurrence, and cancer in patients with implants. Ultrasound has added considerably to the evaluation of the breast in cases of palpable masses and discrete masses found on the mammogram.

The role of nuclear medicine is limited for breast cancer diagnosis. Although dedicated breast cameras have reportedly improved sensitivity with Tc-99m sestamibi molecular breast imaging (MBI)/breast-specific gamma imaging (BSGI) or F-18 FDG positron emission mammography (PEM), whole-body PET/CT is not recommended for breast cancer diagnosis apart from the breast carcinoma incidentally detected during the evaluation of other malignancies. One meta-analysis of the literature suggests that the sensitivity of PET is 88%, and the specificity 79%, for detecting primary tumors (Figs. 12.43 and 12.44) However, the ability of F-18 FDG PET to detect primary breast cancer is related to tumor size. The reported sensitivity of PET is

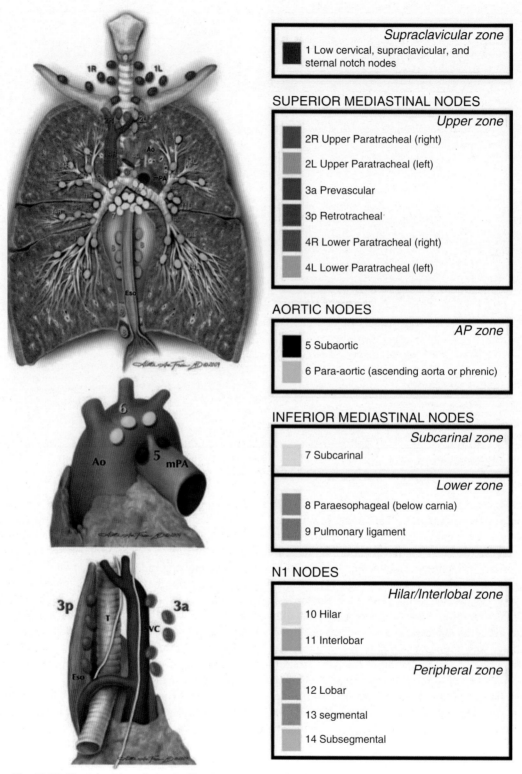

Fig. 12.38 Chest lymph node levels. The International Association for the Study of Lung Cancer (IASLC) lymph node map, including grouping of lymph node stations into "zones" for purposes of prognostic analyses. (From Rusch VW, Asamura H, Watanabe H, et al. The IASLC lung cancer staging project: a proposal for a new international lymph node map in the forthcoming seventh edition of the TNM classification for lung cancer. *J Thorac Oncol.* 2009;4:568–577.)

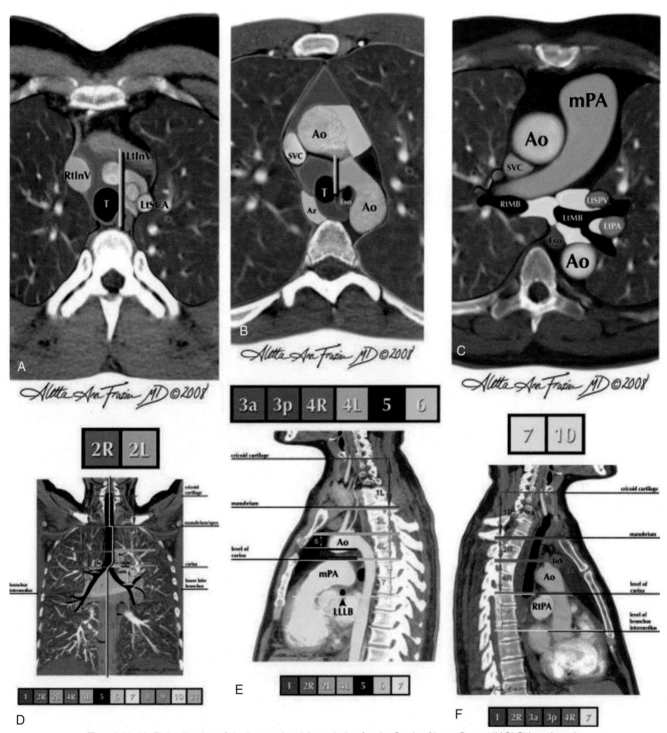

Fig. 12.39 (A–F) Application of the International Association for the Study of Lung Cancer (IASLC) lymph node map to computed tomography (CT). (From Rusch VW, Asamura H, Watanabe H, et al. The IASLC lung cancer staging project: a proposal for a new international lymph node map in the forthcoming seventh edition of the TNM classification for lung cancer. *J Thorac Oncol.* 2009;4:568–577.)

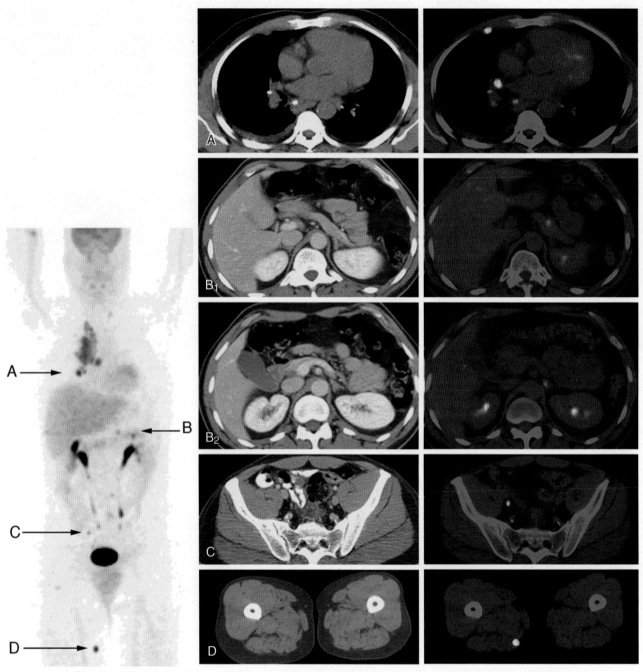

Fig. 12.40 Fluorodeoxyglucose (FDG) positron emission tomography with computed tomography (PET/CT) can be used to detect subtle and unexpected lesions, such as these in a patient with recurrent lung cancer. (A) Small right anterior pleural implant (note low-level activity in malignant right effusion). (B₁) Peripancreatic metastasis. (B₂) Left adrenal gland (unremarkable on computed tomography [CT]). (C) Normal-size pelvic node lateral to the ureter and (D) right thigh. Soft tissue metastases are often overlooked on contrast-enhanced CT. *Note:* Some images shown are from the enhanced CT performed 2 weeks earlier.

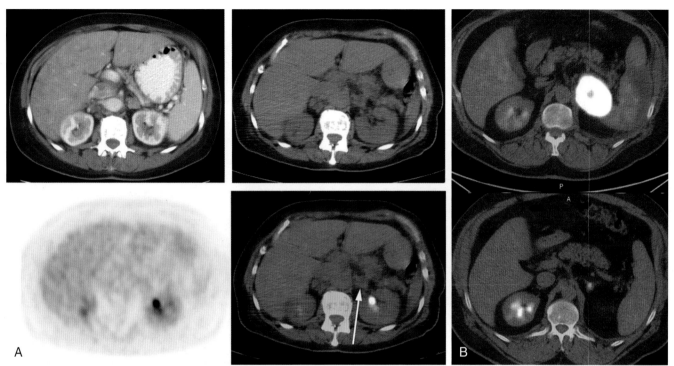

Fig. 12.41 Adrenal metastases are common in lung cancer, and nodules are frequently found on computed tomography (CT). (A) However, many of these lesions are benign fat-poor adenomas, as seen in the left adrenal lesion on enhanced CT, which then showed no F-18 fluorodeoxyglucose (FDG) activity. (B) Positron emission tomography with computed tomography (PET/CT) can also identify metastases earlier than CT, such as the small metastases on positron emission tomography (PET) in a normal-appearing adrenal gland *(lower row)*. The diagnosis was confirmed 3 months later with a centrally necrotic mass developing in the gland *(upper row)*.

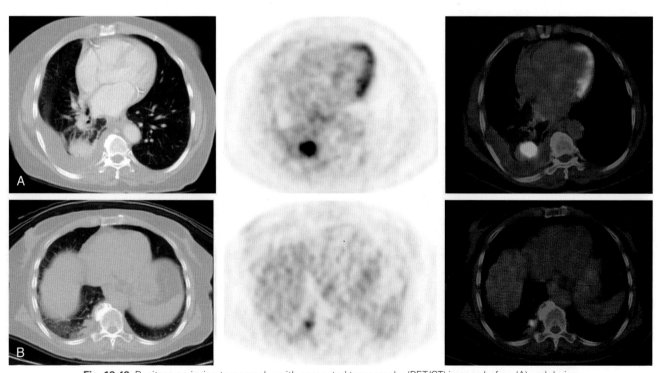

Fig. 12.42 Positron emission tomography with computed tomography (PET/CT) images before (A) and during (B) chemoradiation therapy for a non–small-cell lung cancer with mediastinal involvement *(not shown)* reveal the value of positron emission tomography (PET) for monitoring therapy, with some residual active disease seen on PET even though a residual mass was not well seen on computed tomography (CT).

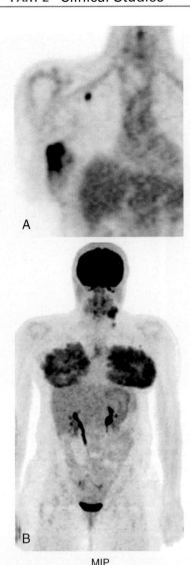

MIP

Fig. 12.43 Breast cancer staging. (A) F-18 fluorodeoxyglucose (FDG) positron emission tomography (PET) often identifies malignant adenopathy in advanced and recurrent breast cancer. In this case, the large right breast tumor shows markedly increased uptake, as does an axillary lymph node. (B) This postpartum patient presented with lymphoma in the left cervical region. Intense breast uptake was seen, resulting from hormonal stimulation rather than tumor.

92% for tumors measuring 2 to 5 cm but is only 68% for tumors smaller than 2 cm. The false-negative rate of F-18 FDG PET is insufficient for a screening test, especially because the detection of early tumors is critical. The histological type of the tumor also affects the sensitivity of F-18 FDG PET. For example, the detection of LCIS and DCIS is limited in comparison with invasive ductal carcinoma (the reported sensitivity for lobular cancers is approximately 40%).

Staging and Restaging. Lymph node involvement has important prognostic and therapeutic implications in breast carcinoma. Axillary lymph node dissection fully evaluates the draining lymph nodes. However, this is a highly invasive procedure with potentially serious side effects (e.g., lymphedema). F-18 FDG PET imaging is able to visualize lymph node metastases by detecting changes in metabolism, often before any anatomical change occurs on CT. However, not all lymph nodes are visualized because microscopic metastases will not be seen. In patients with nonpalpable lymph nodes, sentinel lymph node localization with Tc-99m sulfur colloid or Tc-99m Tilmanocept, with or without blue dye, is still the best method to select which lymph nodes to selectively biopsy. Additionally, if scans are interpreted in a highly sensitive mode, the specificity is lowered because inflammatory conditions frequently affect the axillary lymph nodes and cause increased FDG accumulation.

Although the sensitivity of FDG is limited for the detection of metastatic involvement in any individual lymph node and not generally recommended for initial breast cancer diagnosis or screening, it has proven useful for staging in patients with locally advanced/advanced disease (stage IIIA or stage IV). FDG can identify more positive internal mammary, mediastinal, and supraclavicular nodes than other methods (Fig. 12.45). In bone, PET is best able to identify more aggressive or lytic lesions, complementing the technetium bone scan, which visualizes sclerotic disease. Clinical guidelines may not recommend the use of PET for lower stages of disease, but studies have shown that it is able to add information in up to 29% of these cases. In stage IIB disease, several reports demonstrated a significant change in management in up to 37% (detecting occult N3 spread, detecting distant metastases, or even downstaging some patients).

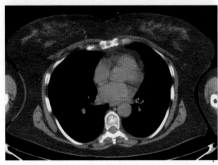
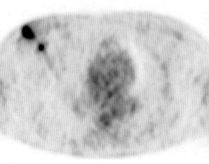
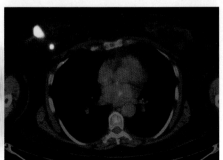

Fig. 12.44 Fluorodeoxyglucose (FDG) positron emission tomography with computed tomography (PET/CT) can detect primary lesions as well as satellite lesions within the breast, as in this patient with an unsuspected second hypermetabolic focus of tumor posterior to the known cancer. The sensitivity is related to lesion size.

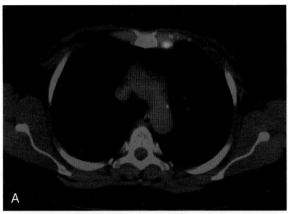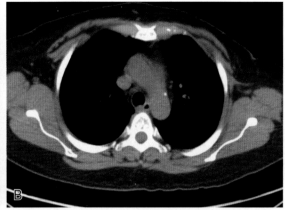

Fig. 12.45 Recurrent breast carcinoma in an internal mammary lymph node. F-18 fluorodeoxyglucose (FDG) positron emission tomography with computed tomography (PET/CT; A) is more sensitive than computed tomography (CT; B) when changes are often subtle. Positron emission tomography (PET) can identify metastases to regional lymph nodes and distant disease. Internal mammary node involvement is frequent in cancers of the inner or medial breast.

More accurate assessment of tumor response to therapy is possible with PET. It is superior to conventional imaging techniques for the detection of residual active or recurrent tumor after surgery or radiation, altering management as much as 51% of the time. During the course of therapy, performing the PET midcourse appears to result in the greatest accuracy in differentiating nonresponders from responders and predicting final outcome or response.

The assessment of bone lesions can be complicated by not only high background activity but also the posttreatment flare phenomenon. This paradoxical increase in radiotracer accumulation despite clinically responding disease and sclerosis of healing lesions on CT can also be seen with technetium bone scans. This pattern occurs not only with traditional chemotherapy but also with hormonal therapy.

Gastrointestinal Cancers
Esophageal Carcinoma

Esophageal carcinoma is most commonly due to squamous-cell cancer in the upper two-thirds of the esophagus, whereas adenocarcinoma typically occurs in the lower third. It frequently presents as dysphagia or is detected by endoscopic biopsy in patients with Barrett esophagus, a known precursor of many cases of esophageal cancer. Because whole-body scanners have limited sensitivity and specificity for detecting tumor in patients with Barrett esophagus, PET has not proved useful in screening these patients. However, F-18 FDG PET has been used in cases of equivocal biopsy or to assess patients with biopsy-confirmed tumor.

Diagnosis. Overall, the sensitivity of PET is greater than 90% in esophageal cancer. The diagnosis of primary esophageal tumors by PET may be limited by a small tumor volume. In adenocarcinoma, 10% to 15% of patients may have false-negative PET results because of the low uptake in mucinous- and signet-cell varieties. PET is not able to determine the extent of the primary tumor and may not offer any substantial advantage over the standard diagnostic modalities such as endoscopic ultrasonography.

Staging and Response to Treatment. Esophageal cancer most commonly spreads to the regional lymph nodes. The location of these nodes depends to a certain extent on the level of the primary tumor. For example, cervical metastases are more common in proximal tumors, and abdominal lymph node involvement may be more frequent in distal masses. However, disease spread may occur in unexpected locations.

The accuracy of detecting lymph node involvement with F-18 FDG PET, particularly with PET/CT, has been consistently shown to be higher than that of CT and MRI alone. Nodes may be inseparable from the primary mass, and small lesions may be below the resolution of the PET detection systems (Fig. 12.46). However, skip metastases can occur in 20% beyond local lymph nodes, and PET is commonly used for tumor staging due to its high sensitivity for the detection of regional and distant metastases compared with CT.

The ability to detect residual and recurrent disease is also significant. PET has proven value in assessing patients during therapy and after therapy for recurrence or interval development of distant metastatic disease. A scan following neoadjuvant chemotherapy may better predict patient survival than standard imaging methods (Fig. 12.47). However, caution must be taken when evaluating patients immediately after therapy because an artifactual increase in activity may be seen. After radiation therapy, this is frequently intense (Fig. 12.48).

Normal physiologic activity or uptake related to inflammation in the esophagus may confound interpretation. Similarly, moderate F-18 FDG uptake in a normal stomach limits the usefulness of PET in evaluating tumors of the stomach and gastroesophageal junction. Some gastric adenocarcinomas may show only low-level activity on PET/CT. However, when a gastric tumor is F-18 FDG avid, PET scanning may be used in monitoring therapy.

Colorectal Carcinoma

Colon cancer develops in colon polyps, with dysplastic elements found in approximately one-third of adenomatous polyps. A progression to invasive cancer occurs slowly. Tumor staging is

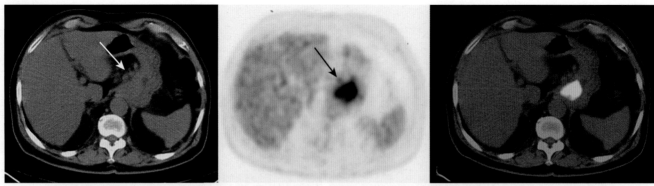

Fig. 12.46 Identification of regional lymph nodes in esophageal cancer. *(Left)* Small but suspicious nodes along the lesser curvature of the stomach *(arrow)* are seen on computed tomography (CT). *(Middle)* Marked F-18 fluorodeoxyglucose (FDG) uptake is present in the primary tumor at the gastroesophageal junction. However, as best seen on fused images *(right),* only low-level FDG activity was present despite the presence of metastases on endoscopic biopsy. The difficulty in identifying regional nodes may relate to activity in adjacent tumor or microscopic amounts of tumor present.

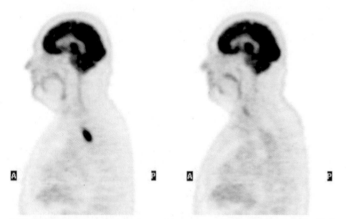

Fig. 12.47 Monitoring esophageal tumor response to therapy. Sagittal F-18 fluorodeoxyglucose (FDG) positron emission tomography (PET) scans *(left)* before and *(right)* after chemotherapy show rapid resolution of the abnormal activity within an esophageal tumor. This type of response has been linked to a better prognosis.

outlined in Table 12.18. The diagnosis of colorectal carcinoma depends on direct visualization by colonoscopy as well as imaging with CT and barium enema. When determining suitability for resection, CT often identifies regional adenopathy and distant metastases. Subsequently, 30% to 40% of patients suffer a recurrence, most often detected by CT and serum carcinoembryonic antigen (CEA).

Although more frequently recommended as a consideration in anal cancers, the National Comprehensive Cancer Network (NCCN) clinical guidelines include limited situations where PET/CT use is recommended for colorectal carcinomas (e.g., assessment of potentially resectable M1 disease, differentiation of presacral fibrosis from recurrent disease, and anal cancers with more advanced disease). However, multiple studies have consistently shown PET/CT to be superior to conventional imaging for the detection of liver and other distant metastases. FDG affects treatment decisions during initial planning and restaging (up to 39% in one study; Fig. 12.49). Additional and unexpected sites of involvement are frequently found, especially advanced rectal and anal cancers. Changes in activity correlate with prognosis, but this has not translated to definite survival benefits.

Cancer in lymph nodes may not be uncovered when immediately adjacent to the primary tumor or when containing either a small volume of disease or high mucin content. Care must be taken because recurrence can occur at the anastomosis, and the activity can be mistaken for normal bowel uptake. In addition, any activity in the colon should not be attributed to colitis, inflammatory bowel disease, or diverticulitis without inflammatory stranding, abscess, or suspicious fluid collection on CT.

Hepatobiliary and Pancreatic Tumors

The use of F-18 FDG PET in other tumors of the GI tract is more limited, and CT remains critical in the analysis of these tumors. However, PET may be helpful in tumors of pancreatic, biliary, and hepatic origin. PET is often used in patients with CT scans that are difficult to evaluate or in patients with elevated serum tumor markers, including alpha-fetoprotein in hepatocellular carcinoma and Ca 19-9 in pancreatic cancer.

PET is highly sensitive for the detection of adenocarcinoma of the pancreas (Fig. 12.50). However, CT is essential in defining tumor extent and vascular involvement, as well as in determining resectability. The detection of hepatic and lymph node metastasis is usually done with CT or MRI. However, PET may identify lymph nodes difficult to visualize on CT, such as in the upper portal regions, and can identify undiagnosed distant metastases in 14% of cases. These factors can lead to alterations in surgical management in a significant number of cases. PET is often limited by poor sensitivity in small tumors and in acute pancreatitis. The uptake in acute pancreatitis can be as intense as in malignancy and can mask underlying tumor. Acute pancreatitis often accompanies therapy or obstruction by tumor, and PET in these cases is often nondiagnostic.

Some pancreatic masses seen on CT are benign, and PET can often differentiate benign and malignant processes (with accuracies of 85%–93%). This can support a negative fine-needle biopsy finding. PET may also detect occult cancers not seen on CT in symptomatic patients.

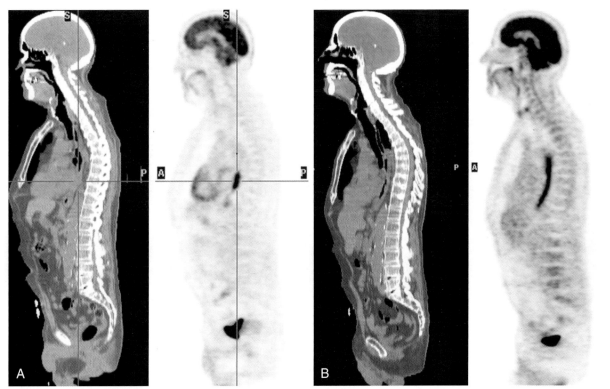

Fig. 12.48 Effects of radiation therapy on positron emission tomography (PET) interpretation. (A) Initial sagittal computed tomography (CT) and F-18 fluorodeoxyglucose (FDG) PET images reveal abnormal uptake in the esophagus from tumor. (B) Two months after radiation therapy, diffusely increased activity is seen in an extensive region of thickened esophagus. Although this was presumed secondary to therapy, underlying tumor could go undetected, and further follow-up was suggested.

TABLE 12.18	TNM Staging of Colorectal Cancer	
AJCC Stage	**Stage Grouping**	**Stage Description**
0	Tis N0 M0	Carcinoma in situ or intramuscular carcinoma
I	T1 or T2 N0 M0	Growth through muscularis mucosa into submucosa (T1) and maybe into muscularis propria (T2) but not spread to nearby nodes or distant sites
IIA	T3 N0 M0	Growth into outermost layers but not through them and not to nearby organs, nearby nodes, or distant sites
IIB	T4a N0 M0	Grown through bowel wall but not into nearby organs or tissues and no spread to nodes or distant sites
IIC	T4b N0 M0	Grown through bowel wall and grown into nearby organs but not to nodes or distant sites
IIIA	T1 or T2 N1/N1c M0 **or** T1 N2a M0	Grown through mucosa into submucosa or muscularis propria; spread to 1–3 nearby nodes (or into fat near nodes- N1c) but no distant sites Grown through mucosa into submucosa and spread to 4–6 nodes but not to distant sites

Continued

TABLE 12.18   TNM Staging of Colorectal Cancer—cont'd

AJCC Stage	Stage Grouping	Stage Description
IIIB	T3 or T4a N1/N1c M0	Grown into outermost bowel wall layers (T3) or through visceral peritoneum (T4a) but not into nearby organs; spread to 1–3 nodes or fat near nodes but not to distant sites
	or	
	T2 or T3 N2a M0	Grown into muscularis propria (T2) or into outermost bowel layers (T3); spread to 4–6 nearby nodes (N2a) but not to distant sites
	or	
	T1 or T2 N2b Mo	Grown through mucosa into submucosa (T1) and maybe into muscularis propria (T2) and spread to 7 or more nodes (N2b) but not to distant sites
IIIC	T4a N2a M0	Grown through bowel wall including visceral peritoneum but not to nearby organs; involves 4–6 nodes but not distant sites
	or	
	T3 or T4a N2b M0	Grown into outermost bowel layers (T3) or through visceral peritoneum (T4a) but not spread to nearby organs; involves 7 or more nodes but not distant sites
	or	
	T4b N1 or N2 M0	Grown through bowel wall and attached to or grown into nearby organs (T4b); has spread to at least 1 node or into fat near nodes but not to distant sites
IVA	Any T Any N M1a	Any T and any N with tumor in 1 distant organ but not to distant parts of peritoneum
IVB	Any T Any N M1b	Any T and any N with spread to more than 1 distant organ or distant nodes but not to distant parts of peritoneum
IVC	Any T Any N M1c	Any T and any N and spread to distant parts of peritoneum and may or may not have spread to distant organs or distant nodes

AJCC, American Joint Committee on Cancer; *TNM,* tumor, node, metastasis.

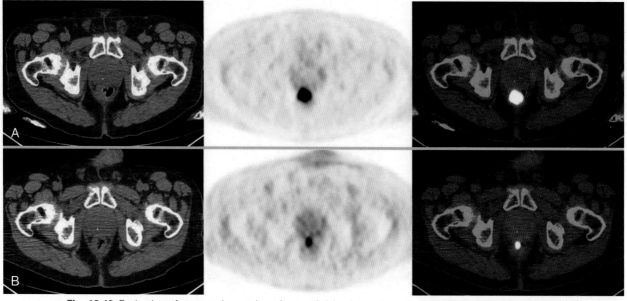

Fig. 12.49 Evaluation of metastatic rectal carcinoma. Axial-enhanced computed tomography (CT) and positron emission tomography (PET) images before (A) and after (B) chemotherapy show a decrease in activity in a malignant rectal mass. (C) Coronal images before *(left)* and after therapy *(right)* in this patient show a decrease in hepatic lesions, only one of which was ever detected by CT.

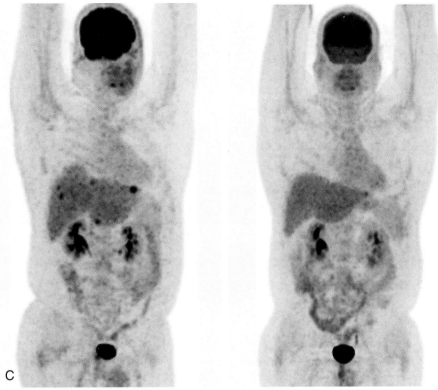

Fig. 12.49, cont'd

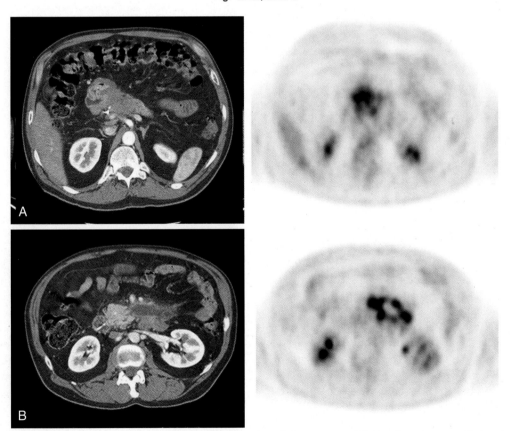

Fig. 12.50 Positron emission tomography (PET) imaging of the pancreas. (A) A malignant pancreatic head mass seen on contrast-enhanced computed tomography (CT) had a high level of F-18 fluorodeoxyglucose (FDG) uptake, consistent with malignancy. However, the inflammation that accompanies pancreatitis also can cause intense uptake. (B) CT following biopsy of a pancreatic mass showed inflammatory changes around the pancreatic tail positive on PET. Note the central "cold" area corresponding to a pancreatic duct dilated as a result of proximal obstruction from the mass.

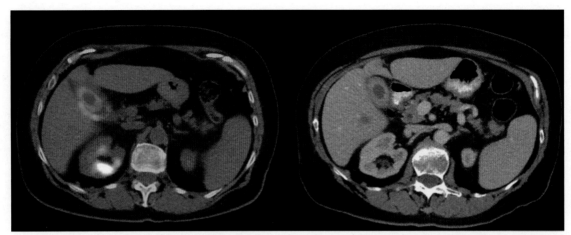

Fig. 12.51 Gallbladder cancer can present as a focal mass or as more diffuse wall thickening, as seen here on fused positron emission tomography with computed tomography (PET/CT; *left*). Enhanced computed tomography (CT) from 2 weeks prior in this patient *(right)* showed gallbladder wall thickening without fluid or inflammatory changes that might be expected if acute cholecystitis were the cause of the positron emission tomography (PET) abnormality. An indeterminate low-attenuation liver lesion on the enhanced CT was stable over time and non-FDG avid, consistent with benign a cyst.

Primary tumors of the liver are much less common than metastases and are most often evaluated by CT. The two most common primary liver tumors are hepatocellular carcinoma and cholangiocarcinoma. F-18 FDG PET is highly accurate for detecting metastases to the liver but has relatively low sensitivity for the detection of primary hepatocellular carcinomas (50%–70%). Despite this, in patients with a tumor known to accumulate FDG, PET/CT may be useful in evaluating treatment and potential recurrence in patients who undergo ablation, such as with transarterial chemoembolization (TACE) or intraarterial Yttrium-90 labeled microspheres (Y-90 TheraSphere).

Cholangiocarcinoma is a rare cancer of the bile ducts that may not be detected on CT. It may occur in extrahepatic or intrahepatic locations. Tumors arising peripherally have a better prognosis because they may be resected, whereas those near the hilum are infrequently resectable. Tumors can be infiltrating, exophytic, or a polypoid intraluminal mass. The sensitivity of PET is lower for the infiltrating type in particular. Gallbladder cancer is a rare tumor that is generally diagnosed late in the course of disease and usually shows significant F-18 FDG uptake (Fig. 12.51). PET usually shows intense uptake and may identify nodal metastases difficult to detect with CT, including distant nodes and those high along the common biliary duct.

One tumor in which PET has proved quite useful is the gastrointestinal stromal tumor (GIST; Fig. 12.52). These tumors usually show high levels of F-18 FDG accumulation. In cases in which tumors respond to imatinib (Gleevec) therapy, markedly decreased F-18 FDG accumulation is seen with PET in a matter of days. PET more accurately assesses early response than CT and predicts improved patient survival.

Genitourinary Tumors
Ovarian Cancer
Ovarian carcinoma diagnosis is challenging because physical examination may not reveal disease, and symptoms do not present until late in the course of disease. Hematogenous spread is rare, but direct invasion and seeding of the omentum and organ surfaces is common. Lymphatic spread can lead to malignant pleural effusions. Tumor staging is outlined in Table 12.19. Although patients with localized disease have a survival chance of more than 90%, most patients present with stage III or IV disease. The prognosis of ovarian carcinoma is poor, with overall survival of only 46% at 5 years.

Preoperative evaluation of patients often includes imaging with sonography, CT, and MRI. Staging with CT has 70% to 90% accuracy. However, small peritoneal lesions found with surgical exploration are frequently overlooked or undetectable by CT. PET/CT often highlights many of these abnormalities.

F-18 FDG PET has been used for staging and restaging but is most widely used to detect recurrent disease. Often, this involves patients with elevated serum markers (Ca-125, Ca 19-9, alpha-fetoprotein, and human chorionic gonadotropin) and negative or inconclusive CT findings. The reported sensitivity of PET varies from 50% to 90%, and the specificity varies from 60% to 80%. The accuracy of PET depends on tumor size and cell type. As with CT, small peritoneal nodules seen during laparoscopy and small primary tumors confined to the ovary may be missed. Well-differentiated and mucinous tumors may not be seen, causing false-negative results, and many of the tumor types listed in Box 12.6 fall under this umbrella. Also, PET scanning may not be useful for initial tumor diagnosis because several benign conditions may accumulate F-18 FDG Box 12.7. Despite these limitations, PET is especially helpful in cases in which CT is negative but suspicion for recurrence is high (Fig. 12.53). Overall, PET alters management in approximately 15% of cases.

Cervical Carcinoma
Cervical carcinoma is the most common gynecological cancer. It may be treated effectively by surgery when localized, but radiation and chemoradiation may be required for locally advanced disease. Cervical carcinoma usually spreads by local extension or

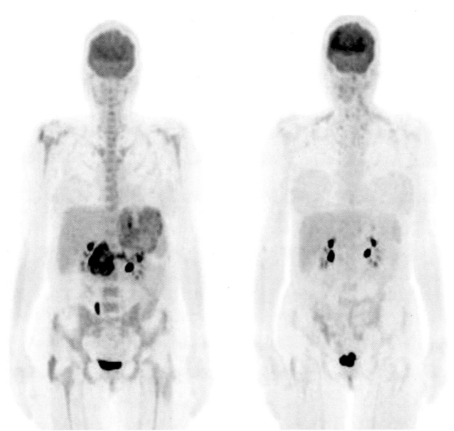

Fig. 12.52 Fluorodeoxyglucose (FDG) positron emission tomography (PET) in gastrointestinal stromal tumor (GIST). PET has proved useful in monitoring the remarkable effects of imatinib (Gleevec) therapy on GIST tumors. A baseline study *(left)* is needed to confirm the tumor is FDG avid. Unlike with computed tomography (CT), rapid improvement is often seen within days of therapy. In this case *(right)*, uptake has resolved even though the mass has decreased on CT only after 4 weeks of therapy.

lymphatic spread to pelvic, paraaortic, and retroperitoneal lymph nodes. However, distant metastases occur, such as to the supraclavicular lymph nodes. The detection of nodal involvement is important in planning therapy but may be difficult by CT. PET was first approved for use in cervical cancer to improve staging accuracy for patients with disease apparently confined to the pelvis on CT or MRI by identifying potential disease that might otherwise be outside of the treatment field for radiation therapy.

F-18 FDG PET has shown a sensitivity of greater than 90% for the detection of cervical cancer, with marked uptake in primary tumors and lymph node metastasis. PET may help identify recurrent tumors and is especially helpful in differentiating posttreatment scan on CT from tumor (Fig. 12.54). Evaluation may be complicated by inflamed superficial tissues, urinary contamination, and normal uptake in the urinary tract and bowel. Although increased uptake can occur in tissues affected by radiation therapy, the tumor response is usually evident.

Testicular Carcinoma

Most testicular cancers fall into either the seminoma or nonseminoma germ-cell tumor groups. Tumor usually presents as a painless mass and spread first through the lymphatics to the retroperitoneal lymph nodes and then hematogenously to the lungs. Although the overall prognosis for these tumors is

excellent, accurate staging and surveillance can optimize treatment and planning. For example, disease initially classified as stage I is commonly then found to have nodal involvement at surgery. Other patients placed incorrectly in high-risk groups may undergo unnecessary therapy. For example, it has been common practice to treat all patients with seminoma with radiation.

The primary tumor is usually adequately assessed by ultrasound or, in complex cases, by MR. CT is the primary imaging modality used for staging because it can visualize adenopathy and lung metastases with reasonable accuracy.

In general, FDG has shown a sensitivity of greater than 90% and a specificity of around 75% in lymph node assessment for testicular cancer. In comparison with CT, PET has shown superior sensitivity (80% vs. 70%), specificity (100% vs. 74%), positive predictive value (100% vs. 37%), and negative predictive value (96% vs. 92%) in the multicenter SEMPET trial. The high negative predictive value of PET is useful for the evaluation of residual masses, which are frequently seen on CT after therapy. Some studies have shown the sensitivity of PET to be greater for seminomas in comparison with nonseminomas (at perhaps 59%). However, other studies do not support this data and show no difference or improved detection in nonseminomas. The detection of small tumors and well-differentiated teratomas is especially limited with PET. Relapse of testicular carcinoma is a frequent occurrence, and PET is useful for surveillance.

TABLE 12.19 Staging of Ovarian Carcinoma

AJCC Stage	Stage Grouping	FIGO Stage	Stage Description
I	T1 N0 M0	I	Contained in ovaries or fallopian tubes
IA	T1a N0 M0	IA	Cancer in one ovary or fallopian tube; no cancer on their outer surfaces; no cells in ascites
IB	T1b N0 M0	IB	Tumor in both ovaries or tubes but not on surfaces; no cells in ascites or peritoneal washings
IC	T1c N0 M0	IC	Involves 1 or both ovaries/tubes and any of the following: • Tissue capsule disrupted • Tumor on surface ovaries/tubes • Cancer cells in ascites or peritoneal washings
II	T2 N0 M0	II	One or both ovaries/tubes with spread to other pelvic organs (uterus, bladder, sigmoid colon, rectum) or there is primary peritoneal cancer
IIA	T2a N0 M0	IIA	Cancer spread to or invaded uterus, fallopian tube, or ovaries
IIB	T2b N0 Mo	IIB	Cancer on surface or grown into nearby organs
IIIA1	T1 or T2 N1 M0	IIIA1	Cancer on one or both ovaries/tubes *or* there is primary peritoneal cancer (T1) and spread to other pelvic organs—uterus, bladder, sigmoid colon, rectum (T2)
IIIA2	T3a N0 or N1 M0	IIIA2	Cancer on one or both ovaries/tubes *or* there is primary peritoneal cancer *and* microscopical tumor deposit in abdomen spread to organs outside pelvis; may involve retroperitoneal nodes or not
IIIB	T3b N0 or N1 M0	IIIB	Cancer on one or both ovaries/tubes *or* there is primary peritoneal cancer *and* visible tumor deposit in abdomen spread to organs outside pelvis (none >2 cm); may involve retroperitoneal nodes or not
IVA	Any T Any N M1a	IVA	Cancer cells in pleural effusion
IVB	Any T Any N M1b	IVB	Cancer spread to spleen, liver, nodes beyond retroperitoneum, and/or organs outside peritoneal cavity (e.g., lung, bones)

AJCC, American Joint Committee on Cancer; *FIGO,* International Federation of Gynecology and Obstetrics.

BOX 12.6 World Health Organization (WHO) Histopathological Classification of Ovarian Tumors

Epithelial-Stromal Tumors
Serous tumors
   Benign cystadenoma, borderline serous tumor, malignant mucinous adeno-carcinoma
Mucinous tumors
   Benign cystadenoma, borderline mucinous tumor, malignant mucinous adenocarcinoma
Endometrioid
   Benign cystadenoma, borderline endometrioid tumor, malignant endometrioid adenocarcinoma
Clear-cell tumors
   Benign, borderline tumors, malignant clear-cell adenocarcinoma
Transitional-cell tumors
   Brenner tumor, Brenner tumor of borderline malignancy, malignant Brenner tumor, transitional-cell carcinoma (non-Brenner type)
Epithelial-stromal
   Adenosarcoma
   Carcinosarcoma (formerly Müllerian tumors)

Sex Cord–Stromal Tumors
Granulosa tumors
   Fibromas, fibrothecomas, thecomas
Sertoli-cell tumors
   Leydig-cell tumors
   Others

Germ-Cell Tumors
Teratoma
   Immature, mature, solid, cystic (dermoid cystic)
Monodermal (struma ovarii, carcinoid)
Dysgerminoma
Yolk sac tumor (endodermal sinus tumor)
Mixed germ-cell tumor

Malignant Tumors Not Otherwise Specified
Colonic, appendiceal
Gastric
Breast

Prostate Carcinoma

F-18 FDG PET has very limited sensitivity for prostate carcinoma. Uptake in primary tumor is often low and similar to that in benign prostatic hypertrophy, whereas focal uptake is most often due to inflation or infection. In terms of staging, F-18 FDG PET detected fewer than two-thirds of osseous metastases found on bone scintigraphy and approximately half of nodal metastases found on CT. CT is superior to F-18 FDG for the detection of pulmonary metastases. Many patients are now being evaluated with F-18 FACBC (approved by the Food and Drug Administration [FDA]) or Ga-68 prostate-specific membrane antigen (PMSA; not yet FDA approved) PET/CT (discussed in Chapter 13). However, F-18 FDG PET is often abnormal in advanced prostate carcinoma that has escaped hormonal control. In such cases, abnormal lesions may be identified in many areas, including bone and lymph nodes.

Renal and Bladder Carcinoma

Renal cell cancers are divided into histopathological groups: clear cell (60%–80%), papillary (10%), chromophobe oncocytic (5%), and a variety of other cell types. These lesions are increasingly being detected by CT, and CT remains the most common imaging modality used for the diagnosis and staging. F-18 FDG PET is not generally useful in the diagnosis of primary tumors. Although there is high sensitivity for papillary sarcomatoid tumors, overall sensitivities are only approximately 60% to 69%. In addition, benign renal oncocytomas, which cannot be differentiated from renal-cell tumors by CT, may show marked FDG uptake. Tc-99m sestamibi is taken up with high sensitivity and specificity in oncocytomas (discussed in Chapter 13).

Although some have suggested that the urinary excretion of F-18 FDG might obscure adjacent tumors, these masses often show no radiotracer uptake. The cause for this finding, such as variations in glucose transporter expression, is being investigated. However, PET may play a role in diagnosing distant metastases and detecting recurrent disease. Although a negative result is not meaningful in a patient suspected of recurrent or metastatic disease, PET may identify positive lesions.

In bladder tumors, more than 90% of cases are transitional-cell tumors of uroepithelial origin, with the remaining

---

BOX 12.7 F-18 Fluorodeoxyglucose (FDG) Processes Mimicking Ovarian Cancer

Gastrointestinal activity
Infection/inflammation
Benign tumors
Germ cell: Benign teratomas
Epithelial tumors: Mucinous cystadenoma, serous cystadenoma
Dermoid cysts, hemorrhagic follicle cyst, corpus luteum cyst
Endometrioma
Fibroma
Benign thecoma
Schwannoma

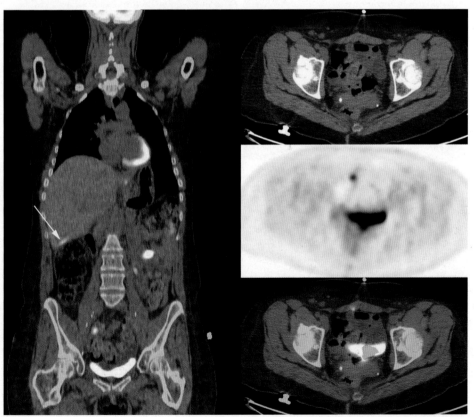

Fig. 12.53 Recurrent ovarian carcinoma. A patient with a rising CA-125 had numerous metastases on the coronal positron emission tomography (PET; *left*), including metastases studding the surface of the liver *(arrow)* and an anterior peritoneal lesion studding the right colon on axial images *(right)*.

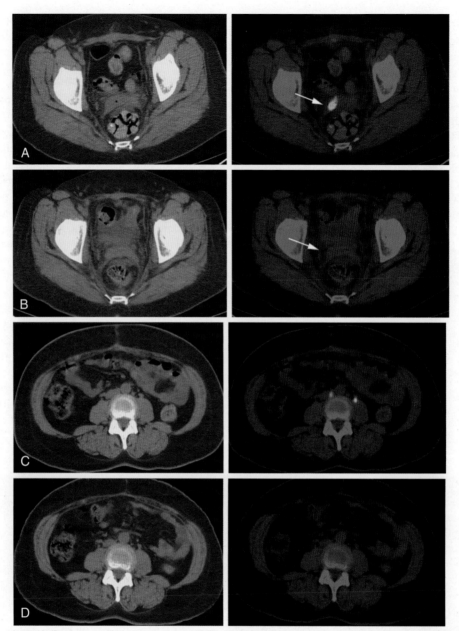

Fig. 12.54 (A) Positron emission tomography (PET) images of vaginal cuff show tumor (arrow) responding to radiation therapy (B) in a patient with cervical cancer. In the same patient, the detection of F-18 fluorodeoxyglucose (FDG) uptake in a normal-size right paraaortic lymph node (C) led to the disease being upstaged, requiring chemotherapy in addition to radiotherapy of the pelvis. (D) Follow-up showed resolution of the active tumor.

consisting of squamous-cell cancer (5%) and adenocarcinomas (2%). Although transitional-cell tumors are usually FDG avid, excreted activity in urine may limit detection, and PET has shown no benefit over other tests for diagnosis. It does, however, detect more metastatic lesions and recurrent tumors than conventional imaging, potentially changing management in as many as 68% of patients undergoing staging and 17% for restaging. Sensitivities reported in the literature vary but range from 65% to 84% for PET, with an accuracy of about 92% compared with roughly 80% with CT. Cell type may affect sensitivity.

Musculoskeletal Tumors

Malignant primary bone tumors are usually F-18 FDG avid, as are many benign conditions. Benign tumors such as giant-cell

tumor, fibrous dysplasia, and eosinophilic granulomas, for example, have been shown to accumulate F-18 FDG. PET may be useful for the evaluation of patients who cannot undergo MRI and for monitoring the effects of therapy. If a nonresponder is identified early by showing little change in SUV values on PET, the course of therapy can be altered. F-18 FDG may influence therapy by identifying other sites of disease, such as in patients with plasmacytoma.

For the evaluation of soft tissue sarcomas, the accuracy of F-18 FDG PET appears to be related to tumor grade. The increased uptake in high-grade tumors such as malignant fibrous histiocytoma allows detection with a high degree of sensitivity. Low-grade tumors, on the other hand, show minimal or nonexistent uptake, leading to poor sensitivity. Although MRI

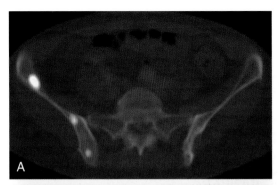
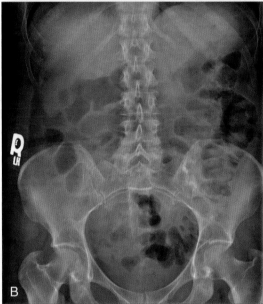

Fig. 12.55 F-18 fluorodeoxyglucose (FDG) positron emission tomography with computed tomography (PET/CT; A) is more sensitive than radiographs for skeletal survey or computed tomography (CT; B) for the detection of active disease.

remains the main imaging modality of the primary tumor, the ability of MRI to detect recurrence is limited in the postoperative patient. PET may help detect recurrent tumors, although the effects of surgery and radiation therapy lower sensitivity.

Multiple Myeloma

Several diseases are included in the spectrum of plasma-cell neoplasms, ranging from benign to highly aggressive tumors. These diseases originate from a single B cell and secrete monoclonal proteins. Multiple myeloma accounts for 101,000 deaths per year worldwide, with an incidence of 4 to 5 per 100,000. Patients may present with increased protein in the urine, monoclonal protein in blood or urine, hypercalcemia, anemia, bone pain, and/or renal failure. The patient workup consists of the evaluation of immunoglobulin levels, 24-hour urine protein evaluation, serum and urine electrophoresis, a whole-body skeletal survey, and bone marrow aspiration. Radiographic findings may begin with osteoporosis, but numerous lytic lesions are eventually seen. Because lesions are lytic rather than osteoblastic, bone scans are relatively insensitive, detecting 15% of lesions. The standard evaluation includes a whole-body skeletal survey. F-18 FDG PET/CT is clearly superior to skeletal surveys (Fig. 12.55), detecting bone

involvement in 25% of newly diagnosed patients with negative skeletal surveys and extramedullary involvement in up to 25%. As seen with other cancers that metastasize to bone, it is also more sensitive than CT. Although F-18 sodium fluoride (F-18 NaF) PET/CT bone imaging is most sensitive, F-18 FDG has good sensitivity for lytic lesions and can detect extraosseous disease. FDG PET/CT is routinely performed when plasmacytoma is of concern. The ease of whole-body PET imaging frequently results in added information to that seen on MRI, and hybrid PET/MR is an excellent option where available. PET/CT scans are often negative in patients in remission or in patients with monoclonal gammopathy not related to malignant myeloma. However, in chronically ill patients, the elevated marrow background may make it difficult to detect subtle change or differentiate stimulated marrow from low-level active disease.

SUGGESTED READING

PROTOCOL

Adams MC, Turkington TG, Wilson JM, Wong TZ. A systematic review of factors affecting accuracy of SUV measurements. *AJR.* 2010;195:310–320.

Surassi S, Bhambhvani P, Baldwin JA, Almodovar SE, O'Malley JP. 18F-FDG PET and PETCT patient preparation: a review of the literature. *J Nucl Med Technol.* 2014;42:1–9. https://doi.org/10.2967/jnmt.113.132621.

Tsai LL, Grant AK, Mortele KJ, Kung JW, Smith MP. A practical guide to MR imaging safety: what radiologists need to know. *Radiographics.* 2015;35:1722–1737. https://doi.org/10.1148/rg.2015150108.

PET/MR

Galgano S, Viets Z, Fowler K, et al. Practical considerations for clinical PET/MR imaging. *Magn Reson Imaging Clin N Am.* 2017;25:281–296.

IMPACT

Coleman RE, Hillner BE, Shields AF, et al. PET and PET/CT reports: observations from the National Oncologic PET Registry. *J Nucl Med.* 2010;51(1):158–163.

Hillner BE, Siegel BA, Liu D, et al. Impact of positron emission tomography/computed tomography and positron emission tomography (PET) alone on expected management of patients with cancer: initial results from the National Oncologic PET Registry. *J Clin Oncol.* 2008;26.

LYMPHOMA

Barrington SF, Qian W, Somer EJ, et al. Concordance between four European centres of PET reporting criteria for use in multicentre trials in Hodgkin lymphoma. *Eur J Nucl Med Mol Imaging.* 2010;37(10):1824–1833.

Cheson BD, Fisher RI, Barrington SF, et al. Recommendations for initial evaluation, staging, and response assessment of Hodgkin and non-Hodgkin lymphoma: the Lugano classification. *J Clin Oncol.* 2014;32:3059–3068.

Cheson BD, Pfistner B, Juweid ME, et al. Revised response criteria for malignant lymphoma. *J Clin Oncol.* 2007;(5):579–586.

Eisenhauer EA, Therasse P, Bogaerts J, et al. New response evaluation criteria in solid tumors: Revised RECIST guideline (1.0). *Eur J Cancer.* 2009;45:228–247.

Kulkarni NM, Pinho DF, Narayanan S, et al. Imaging for oncologic response assessment in lymphoma. *AJR.* 2017;208:18–31.

Moghbel MC, Mittra E, Gallamini A, et al. Response assessment criteria and their applications in lymphoma: part 2. *J Nucl Med.* 2017;58:13–22.

MELANOMA

Wong AN, McArthur GA, Hofman MS, Hicks RJ. The advantages and challenges of using FDG PET/CT for response assessment in melanoma in the era of targeted agents and immunotherapy. *Eur J Nucl Med Mol Imaging.* 2017. https://doi.org/10.1007/s00259-017-3691-7.

HEAD AND NECK

Denaro N, Russi EG, Merlano MC. Pros and cons of the new edition of TNM classification of head and neck squamous cell carcinoma. *Oncology.* 2018;95:202–210. https://doi.org/10.1159/000490415.

Gamss C, Gupta A, Chazen L, Philips C. Imaging evaluation of the suprahyoid neck. *Radiol Clin N Am.* 2015;53:133–144. https://doi.org/10.1016/j.rcl.2014.09.009.

Goel R, Moore W, Sumer B, Khan S, Sher D, Subramanian RM. Clinical practice in PET/CT for the management of head and neck cancer. *AJR.* 2017;209:289–303. https://doi.org/10.2214/AJR.17.18301.

Lydiatt W, O'Sullivan B, Patel S. Major changes in head and neck staging for 2018. *Ca Cancer J Clin.* 2017;67:122–137. Ascopubs.org/. https://doi.org/10.full/10.1200/EDBK_199697.

Plaxton NA, Brandon DC, Corey AS, et al. Characteristics and limitations of FDG PET/CT for imaging of squamous cell cancer of the head and neck: a comprehensive review of anatomy, metastatic pathways, and findings. *AJR.* 2015;205:W519–W531.

Salto N, Nadgir RN, Nakashira M, et al. Posttreatment CT and MR imaging in head and neck cancer: what the radiologist needs to know. *Radiographics.* 2012;32:1261–1282. https://doi.org/10.1148/rg.325115160.

Som PM, Curtin HD, Mancuso AA. Imaging-based nodal classification for evaluation of neck metastatic adenopathy. *AJR.* 2000;174:837–844.

THYROID

Marcus C, Whitworth PW, Surasi DS, Pai SI, Subramanian RM. PET/CT in the management of thyroid cancers. *AJR.* 2014;2023:1316–1329.

CHEST

Lung Nodule Evaluation

Bankier AA, MacMahon H, Goo JM, et al. Recommendations for measuring pulmonary nodules at CT: a statement from the Fleischner Society. *Radiology.* 2017;285(2):584–600. https://doi.org/10.1148/radiol.2017162894.

Bueno J, Landeras L, Chung JH. Updated Fleischner society guidelines for managing incidental pulmonary nodules: common questions and challenging scenarios. *Radiographics.* 2018;38:1337–1350. https://doi.org/10.1148/rg.2018180017.

Detterbeck FC. The eighth edition TNM stage classification for lung cancer: what does it mean on the main street? *J Thorac Cardiovasc Surg.* 2018;155:356–359. https://doi.org/10.1016/j.jtcvs.2017.08.138.

Evangelista L, Panunzio A, Polverosi R, Pomerri F, Rubello D. Indeterminate lung nodules in cancer patients: pretest probability of malignancy and the role of 18-F-FDG PET/CT. *AJR.* 2014;202:507–513.

MacMahon H, Naidich DP, Goo JM, et al. Guidelines for management of incidental pulmonary nodules detected on CT images: from the Fleischner Society 2017. *Radiology.* 2017;284:228–243. https://doi.org/10.1148/radiol.2017161659.

Revel MP, Mannes I, Benzakoun J, et al. Subsolid lung nodule classification: a CT criterion for improving interobserver agreement. *Radiology.* 2018;286:316–325. https://doi.org/10.1148/radiol.2017170044.

LUNG CANCER

Carter BW, Lichtenberger JP, Benveniste MK, et al. Revisions to the TNM staging of lung cancer: rationale, significance, and clinical application. *Radiographics.* 2018;38:374–391. https://doi.org/10.1148/rg.2018170081.

El-Sherief AH, Lau CT, Wu CC, Drake RL, Abbott GF, Rice TW. International Association for the Study of Lung Cancer (IASLC) lymph node map: radiological review with CT illustration. *Radiographics.* 2014;34:1680–1691. doi:10.1148/rg.346130097.

Rusch VW, Asamura H, Watanabe H, et al. The IASLC lung cancer staging project: a proposal for a new international lymph node map in the forthcoming seventh edition of the TNM classification for lung cancer. *J Thorac Oncol.* 2009;4:568–577.

Sheikhbahaei S, Mena E, Yanamadala A, et al. The value of FDG PET/CT in treatment response assessment, follow-up, and surveillance of lung cancer. *AJR.* 2017;208:420–433. https://doi.org/10.2214/AJR.16.16532.

BREAST CANCER

Koolen BB, Valdes RA, Vogel WV, et al. Pre-chemotherapy 18F-FDG PET/CT upstages nodal stage II-III breast cancer patients treated with neoadjuvant chemotherapy. *Breast Cancer Res Treat.* 2013;141(2):249–254. https://doi.org/10.1007/s10549-013-2678-8.

Rosen EL, Eubank WB, Mankoff DA. FDG PET, PET/CT, and breast cancer imaging. *Radiographics.* 2007;27:S215–S229. https://doi.org/10.1148/rg.27si075517.

GASTROINTESTINAL AND GENITOURINARY

Gade M, Kubik M, Fisker RV, Thorlacius-Ussing O, Petersen LJ. Diagnostic value of 18F-FDG PET/CT as first choice in the detection of recurrent colorectal cancer due to rising CEA. *Cancer Imaging.* 2015;15:11–18. https://doi.org/10.1186/s40644-015-0048-y.

Gayed I, Vu T, Iyer R, et al. The role of 18F-FDG PET in staging and early prediction of response to therapy of recurrent gastrointestinal stromal tumors. *J Nucl Med.* 2004;45:17–21.

Patel MD, Ascher SM, Paspulati RM, et al. Managing incidental findings on abdominal and pelvic CT and MRI, part 1: white paper of the ACR incidental findings committee II on adnexal findings. *J Am Coll Radiol.* 2013;10(9):675–681. https://doi.org/10.1016/j.acr.2013.05.023.

MUSCULOSKELETAL TUMORS

Cavo M, Terpos E, Nanni C, et al. Role of 18F-FDG PET/CT in the diagnosis and management of multiple myeloma and other plasma cell disorders: a consensus statement by the international myeloma working group. *Lancet Oncol.* 2017;18(4):e206–e217. https://doi.org/10.1016/S1470-2045(17)30189-4.

13

Oncology—Beyond Fluorodeoxyglucose

This chapter reviews tumor scintigraphy using radiopharmaceuticals other than F-18 fluorodeoxyglucose (FDG), as well as therapeutic radiopharmaceuticals for specific malignancies (Box 13.1). *Theranostics* is a topic of increasing importance as it relates to nuclear oncology. The term refers to a pharmaceutical that is labeled with one radionuclide for diagnostic imaging and another radionuclide for therapy, for example, Ga-68 dotatate and Lu-177 dotatate for neuroendocrine tumors and Ga-68 PSMA or F-18 prostate-specific membrane antigen (PSMA) and Lu-111 PSMA for prostate cancer. Although this approach is not really new, with radioiodine being the first theranostic agent used for diagnosis and treatment, the field is rapidly growing thanks to the many new agents entering the clinical arena.

PSMA, Prostate-specific membrane antigen.

NEUROENDOCRINE TUMOR IMAGING AND PEPTIDE RECEPTOR RADIOTHERAPY

Gastroenteropancreatic and Lung Neuroendocrine Tumors

Neuroendocrine tumors (NETs) are a diverse group of epithelial neoplasms that may occur in almost any organ but most commonly arise in the gastroenteropancreatic region (70%) and lung (20%). Well-differentiated neuroendocrine tumors in these regions were previously called carcinoids (Fig. 13.1). Although they often produce specific clinical syndromes due to their unique secretory products ("carcinoid syndrome"), the majority of the tumors are nonfunctioning. Many NET tumors are well differentiated, and these patients have prolonged survival; however, some grow more aggressively and become metastatic. The initial clinical diagnosis can be difficult because of their nonspecific clinical manifestations, depending on the specific amines/peptides secreted, and their small size (Table 13.1). Gastroenteropancreatic NETs are classified on the basis of the Ki-67 proliferation index or the mitotic count (Table 13.2).

Resection of NETs can potentially cure the patient of the malignancy and amine/peptide production; however, this is often not possible due to the extent of disease. Management guidelines emphasize that resection should be the first-line treatment for patients with advanced tumors if 90% of the disease burden is resectable. However, only 5% to 20% of patients meet this criterion. Liver-directed therapies (embolization, radiofrequency ablation, chemoembolization, and radioembolization) are used in appropriate cases. Chemotherapy has not been very effective, but somatostatin (Sandostatin), mTOR inhibitors (everolimus), and tyrosine kinase inhibitors (sunitinib) can extend survival. With metastatic disease, 5-year survival rates are less than 50%.

Computed tomography (CT), ultrasonography, and magnetic resonance imaging (MRI) are used for initial evaluation, but detection rates are not high due to the small size of the tumors and variable location. Because well-differentiated NETs express high levels of somatostatin receptors (SSTRs), SSTR-targeted radionuclide imaging (e.g., In-111 pentetreotide or Ga-68 dotatate) can detect and functionally characterize these tumors. The primary tumor and regional or distant metastases can also often be detected. Expression of SSTRs is associated with a good prognosis, whereas lack of expression of SSTRs and overexpression of GLUT (FDG uptake) is predictive of poor prognosis and survival.

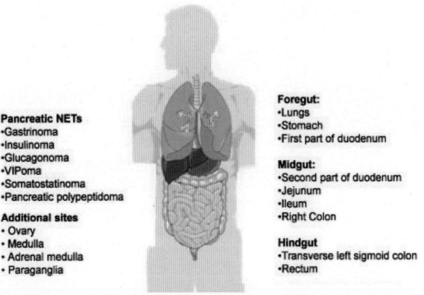

Pancreatic NETs
- Gastrinoma
- Insulinoma
- Glucagonoma
- VIPoma
- Somatostatinoma
- Pancreatic polypeptidoma

Additional sites
- Ovary
- Medulla
- Adrenal medulla
- Paraganglia

Foregut:
- Lungs
- Stomach
- First part of duodenum

Midgut:
- Second part of duodenum
- Jejunum
- Ileum
- Right Colon

Hindgut
- Transverse left sigmoid colon
- Rectum

Fig. 13.1 Primary sites of neuroendocrine tumors. (Redrawn from Oronsky B, Ma PC, Morgensztern D, et al: Nothing But NET: A Review of Neuroendocrine Tumors and Carcinomas. *Neoplasia* 19, Issue 12, 2017, pp. 991-1002. Source: An Elsevier journal.)

TABLE 13.1 Secretory Products of Neuroendocrine Tumors

Site	Tumor	Peptide/Amine	Clinical Features
Foregut	Carcinoids: Bronchi, thymus, stomach, first part of duodenum, pancreas	Histamine, ACTH, CRH, GH, gastric, 5 HIAA, 5 HTP	Pulmonary obstruction, flush, hormone syndrome
Midgut	Carcinoids: Second part of duodenum, jejunum, ileum, right colon	5-HT, tachykinins, prostaglandins, bradykinins, 5-HIAA	Bowel obstruction, flush, wheeze, diarrhea
Hindgut (distal third of transverse colon and splenic flexure, descending colon, sigmoid colon, and rectum)	Insulinoma	Insulin, proinsulin	Whipple' triad
	Gastrinoma	Gastrin	Zollinger, Ellison
	VIPoma	VIP	Watery diarrhea, hypokalemia
	Glucagonoma	Glucagon	DM, cachexia
	Somatostatinoma	SS	Gallstones, DM, steatorrhea
	GRFoma	GRF	Acromegaly
	ACTHoma	ACTH	Cushing' syndrome

ACTH, Adrenocorticotropin; *CRH,* corticotropin-releasing hormone; *DM,* diabetes mellitus; *GH,:* growth hormone; *GRH,* growth hormone–releasing hormone; *5-HIAA,* 5 hydroxyindoleacetic acid; *HTP,* hydroxytryptamine; *SS,* somatostatin; *VIP,:* vasointestinal peptide.

TABLE 13.2 Histopathology of Neuroendocrine Tumors

Histological Classification	Well Differentiated (Low Grade)	Moderately Differentiated (Intermediate Grade)	Poorly Differentiated (High Grade)
Prognosis	Prolonged survival	Intermediate	Poor
Mitotic rate	<2	2–20	>20
Ki-67 index	<3%	3–20%	>20%
Necrosis	Absent	Not well defined	Present

The normal human hormone *somatostatin* is a 14-amino-acid peptide produced in the hypothalamus, pituitary gland, brainstem, gastrointestinal tract, and pancreas. Somatostatin receptors are found on many normal cells as well as tumors of neuroendocrine origin. In the central nervous system, somatostatin acts as a neurotransmitter. Outside of the brain, it inhibits the release of growth hormone, insulin, glucagon, gastrin, serotonin, and calcitonin. It also inhibits angiogenesis, is involved in the immune function of leukocytes, and has an antiproliferative effect on tumors.

Five different subtypes of human SSTRs have been identified, expressed to varying degrees on different tumors. Therapeutic drugs have been developed that readily bind to these receptors. Octreotide (Sandostatin) and lanreotide (Somatuline) are somatostatin analogs used clinically to inhibit growth in acromegaly and to control symptoms of carcinoid syndrome. Radiopharmaceuticals have also been developed that bind to SSTRs.

Diagnostic SSTR Radiopharmaceuticals
Indium-111 Pentetreotide (OctreoScan)

OctreoScan was approved by the U.S. Food and Drug Administration (FDA) in 1994 for imaging of NETs. This radiolabeled SSTR

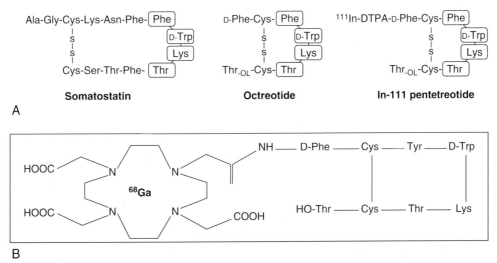

Fig. 13.2 Comparison of somatostatin analogs.

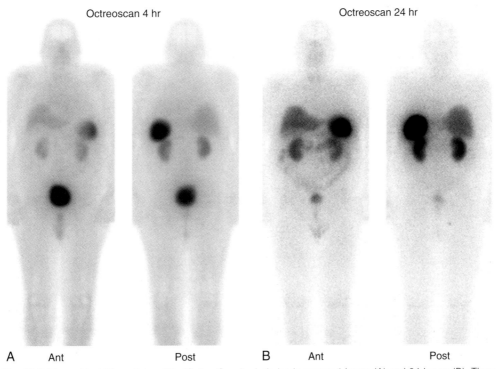

Fig. 13.3 Normal In-111 pentetreotide (OctreoScan) whole-body scans: 4 hours (A) and 24 hours (B). There is no intestinal activity at 4 hours, but it is present at 24 hours. Normal prominent renal and spleen uptake are both more intense than the liver uptake. *Ant,* Anterior; *Post,* posterior.

binding agent has high affinity for subtypes 2 and 5 (Fig. 13.2). It has high-energy emissions (171, 245 keV), relatively slow pharmacokinetics, and thus unfavorable dosimetry (see Appendix 1), which limits the administered dose to 6 mCi (222 MBq) and adversely affects image quality.

Normal Distribution. Splenic and renal uptake is quite high. Lesser uptake is seen in the liver. Low-level hepatobiliary excretion increases intestinal clearance over time (Fig. 13.3). The kidneys rapidly excrete the radiopharmaceutical, with 85% of the dose cleared from the body by 24 hours after injection. Uptake may be seen in the pancreas in the region of the uncinate process; this must not be confused with tumor. Radiotracer

uptake is also be seen with benign inflammatory conditions (e.g., thyroiditis, granulomatous disease, inflammatory bowel disease, postradiation therapy, and at sites of recent surgery) due to the SSTRs present on human immune cells (e.g., mononuclear leukocytes, peripheral blood lymphocytes, and macrophages).

Methodology. An imaging protocol is described in Box 13.2. Early planar imaging at 4 hours after injection permits visualization of tumor uptake before bowel excretion; however, 24-hour imaging has a higher tumor-to-background ratio and is more sensitive for tumor detection (Fig. 13.4). Delayed imaging at 48 hours can further confirm tumor uptake versus bowel

BOX 13.2   Indium-111 Pentetreotide (OctreoScan): Protocol Summary

Patient Preparation
None

Radiopharmaceutical
Children: 0.14 mCi/kg (5 MBq/kg)
Adults: 6 mCi (222 MBq) In-111 octreotide, intravenously

Instrumentation
Gamma camera: Large field of view
Collimator: Medium energy
Windows: 20% centered at 173 keV and 247 keV

Acquisition
Imaging: Planar whole body and SPECT or SPECT/CT of abdomen and or other
    indicated site at 24 hours
    If only planar imaging: 4 and 24 hours; 48-hour images may occasionally
        be useful

Whole-Body Images
Dual-head camera 6 cm/min (approximately 40 minutes head to below hips)
1024 × 512 word matrix

SPECT
128 × 128 matrix, 3-degree angular sampling, 360-degree rotation, 35 sec/stop
Fusion to CT or SPECT/CT preferable

CT, Computed tomography; *SPECT,* single-photon emission computed tomography; *SPECT/CT,* single-photon emission computed tomography with computed tomography.

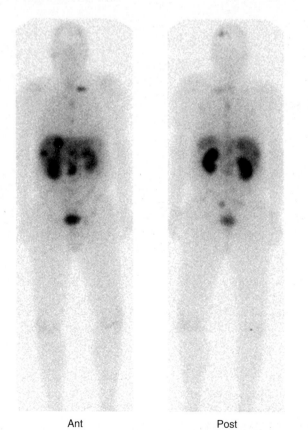

Ant   Post

Fig. 13.4 In-111 pentetreotide whole-body study in a patient with metastatic carcinoid, at 24 hours after injection. Metastases are seen in left supraclavicular region and liver, nodal disease in the abdomen and pelvis, and skull metastasis. *Ant,* Anterior; *Post,* posterior.

activity. With single-photon emission computed tomography with computed tomography (SPECT/CT), imaging only at 24 hours is routine, and it improves tumor identification and localization (Fig. 13.5).

Accuracy. The sensitivity of In-111 pentetreotide for tumor detection is reported to be high for carcinoid tumors (85%–95%; Box 13.3). However, a lower sensitivity of approximately 75% occurs with pancreatic NETs (e.g., gastrinomas, glucagonomas, vasoactive intestinal polypeptide-secreting tumors [VIPomas], and nonfunctioning islet cell tumors). Because of high normal liver uptake, liver metastases are not always detected. Detection may be reduced in patients on octreotide therapy; thus, the study should be performed immediately before the patient's monthly therapeutic injection.

Gallium-68 (Ga-68) Dotatate (DOTA-0-Tyr3-Octreotate)

Several Ga-68-labeled somatostatin receptor positron emission tomography (PET) imaging agents have been investigated, including Ga-68 dotatoc, dotanoc, and dotatate (see Fig. 13.2). These short amino acid–chelator conjugates demonstrate superior affinity for somatostatin receptors compared with In-111 pentetreotide. The three dota agents are similar in imaging accuracy. Ga-68 dotatate (NetSpot) was approved by the FDA in 2016 for imaging of neuroendocrine tumors. The radionuclide, Ga-68, is produced in a Germanium 68/Ga-68 generator, similar to a Molybdenum-99/Tc-99m generator. The parent Ge-68 has a half-life of 271 days; thus, the generator can be used for at least a year. The Ga-68 daughter has a half-life of 68 minutes. In a high-volume clinic, a generator can make sense. Alternatively, some commercial radiopharmacies maintain a generator and distribute individual radiopharmaceutical doses on a regional basis. The recommended dose is 0.054 mCi/kg (2 MBq/kg) up to 5.4 mCi (200 MBq).

Normal Distribution. Ga-68 dotatate binds with high affinity to SSTR-2 receptors. Uptake is seen in the pituitary, thyroid, and salivary glands; spleen; adrenals; kidney; prostate; and liver (Fig. 13.6). Normal uptake may also be seen in the uncinate process, similar to that seen with In-111 pentetreotide. There is no brain uptake, but focal activity in the nonenlarged pituitary is normal. Cardiac uptake is absent, and lung uptake is low. Twelve percent of the administered dose is excreted in the urine by 4 hours postinjection.

Methodology. A Ga-68 dotatate PET/CT study requires considerably less patient time than SPECT/CT In-111 pentetreotide. PET/CT imaging begins approximately 1 hour after injection of the radiopharmaceutical. The total time from injection to the completion of imaging is about 2 hours, similar to routine F-18 FDG oncologic imaging. The radiation dose to the patient is less with Ga-68 dotatate compared with In-111 pentetreotide (see the Appendix).

Accuracy. In a large retrospective study of 728 patients with NETs, Ga-68 dotatate had a sensitivity of 94% and a specificity of 92%. The highest accuracy was for primary midgut tumors. In a comparison study of 131 patients with NETs and unknown primaries, Ga-68 dotatate PET/CT had a higher detection rate (95%) compared with In-111 pentetreotide SPECT/CT (31%)

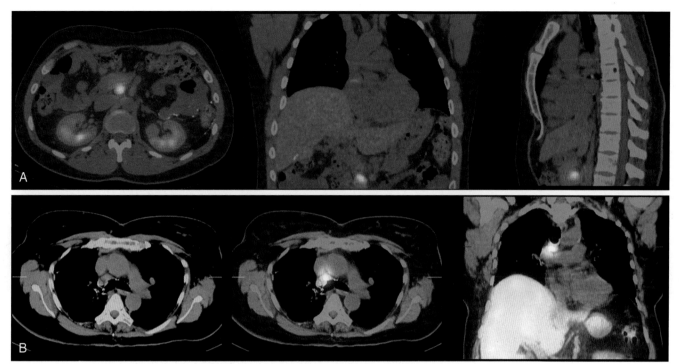

Fig. 13.5 In-111 pentetreotide SPECT/CT. (A) Fused images localize a small focus of activity to a peripancreatic retroperitoneal lymph node, which was difficult to see on planar images (not shown), and (B) shows marked uptake in a precarinal nodal metastasis, which would likely be falsely called normal by computed tomography (CT) size criteria.

BOX 13.3 Sensitivity of Indium-111 Pentetreotide (OctreoScan) for Various Applications

High
Carcinoid (86–95%)
Islet cell tumors (75–100%)
  Gastrinoma, glucagonoma, VIPoma
Adrenal medullary tumors (>85%)
  Pheochromocytoma, neuroblastoma, paragangliomas
Small-cell lung cancer (80–100%)

Moderate
Medullary thyroid (50–75%)
Insulinoma (25–70%)
Medulloblastoma (61–93%)
Meningioma (50% and 100% reported)

Low
Pituitary adenoma
Astrocytoma grade IV (higher in grades I and II)
Breast cancer
Melanoma
Renal cell carcinoma

VIPoma, Vasoactive intestinal polypeptide-secreting tumor.

---

or CT or MRI (46%) (Fig. 13.7). Additional clinical information is found in 70% to 80% of Ga-68 dotatate cases compared with pentetreotide (OctreoScan), and a change in clinical management is reported to occur in greater than 40% of patients (Figs. 13.8 and 13.9). Patients with poorly differentiated tumors may not have uptake and may benefit from F-18 FDG PET, although these patients have a poorer prognosis. The use of intravenous contrast with SSTR PET/CT increases the detection rate for liver metastases and small bowel primaries. SSTR PET/MRI is also reported to provide improved detection of liver metastases.

Other Neuroendocrine Tumors

Because neuroendocrine cells are spread throughout the body, NETs can develop in many different places, including in endocrine glands. Other NETs include medullary carcinoma that starts in the C cells of the thyroid, parathyroid carcinoma or parathyroid adenoma, thymic neuroendocrine cancer, pheochromocytoma that starts in the chromaffin cells of the adrenal glands, paraganglioma, neuroblastoma, pituitary gland tumors, neuroendocrine tumors of the ovaries and testicles, Merkel cell carcinoma, a type of nonmelanoma skin cancer, and small-cell lung cancer.

Therapeutic Radionuclides Bound to SSTRs

High doses of In-111 pentetreotide have been investigated for peptide receptor radionuclide therapy (PRRT) of NETs, taking advantage of the radionuclide's Auger and conversion electron emissions. Although showing effectiveness, more promising results were found using a pure beta emitter, Yttrium-90 (Y-90), bound to other SSTRs, dotatoc and dotatate. In spite of increased survival, bone marrow and renal toxicity were a significant problem.

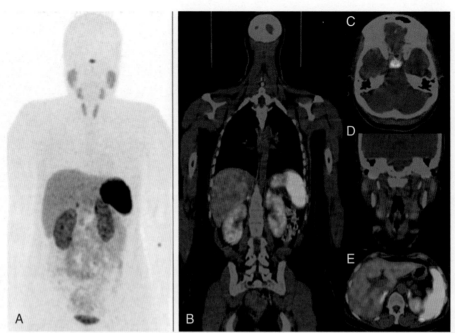

Fig. 13.6 Ga-68 dotatate normal distribution. *(Left)* Maximum-intensity projection (MIP) image. *(Right)* Fused SPECT/CT coronal *(left)* and selected transverse images *(right)*. Note normal uptake in pituitary and adrenals. (With permission, Kuyumcu S, Özkan ZG, Sanli Y, et al. Physiological and tumoral uptake of (68) Ga-DOTATATE: standardized uptake values and challenges in interpretation. *Ann Nucl Med.* 2013;27[6]: 538–545.)

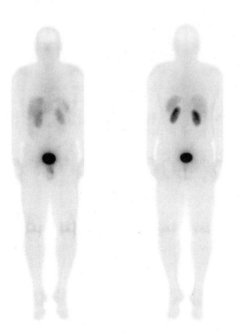

Fig. 13.7 Comparison of maximum-intensity projection (MIP) whole-body image of Ga-68 dotatate *(left)* and In-111 pentetreotide (Oct-reoScan) anterior and posterior whole-body scans in the same patient *(right)*, illustrating the clear superiority of Ga-68 dotatate compared with the In-111 OctreoScan. Although a liver metastasis is seen on OctreoScan, many more are seen on the Ga-68 dotatate study, as well as multiple other intraabdominal nodal disease locations. (Courtesy of Corina Millo, MD.)

Lutecium-177 (Lu-177) Dotatate (Lutathera) Therapy for Neuroendocrine Tumors

As an alternative to Y-90, Lu-177 labeled to dotatate, a beta and gamma emitter, was investigated. Retrospective studies had shown similar effectiveness without the side effects of Y-90. In 2017 a phase 3 multicenter randomized prospective controlled trial of Lu-177 dotatate (Fig. 13.10) was published that studied therapeutic effectiveness in patients with advanced midgut (jejunum, ileum, proximal colon) NETs who had disease progression while on standard first-line octreotide therapy. The investigation reported that compared with octreotide therapy, Lu-177 dotatate resulted in longer progression-free survival (65% vs.11% at 20 months), a significantly higher response rate (18% vs. 3%), and a lower risk of progression, 79% lower than high-dose octreotide therapy. Clinically significant myelosuppression occurred in <10% of patients. Risk of death was 60% lower. Renal toxicity was not a problem with amino acid infusion. Lutathera was approved for clinical use by the FDA in early 2018.

Methodology. Lu-177 dotatate, 200 mCi (7.4 MBq), is infused intravenously over 30 minutes. Patients receive at least four infusions at 8-week intervals. The amino acid solution is infused simultaneously for renal protection. However, significant nausea accompanies the amino acid solution and requires simultaneous antinausea therapy. Reports suggest that the combination of lysine and arginine has far fewer side effects than the amino acid solution.

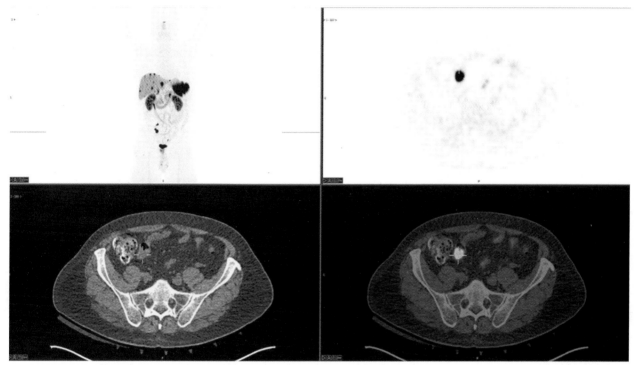

Fig. 13.8 Ga-68 dotatate positron emission tomography with computed tomography (PET/CT) scan in a 65-year-old male patient with abdominal pain. Ultrasonography showed liver lesions, and biopsy diagnosed well-differentiated neuroendocrine tumor (NET). The primary tumor was not detected. The Ga-dotatate PET/CT scan shows the primary lesion in the terminal ileum and additional metastases in the abdomen and liver. (Courtesy of Corina Millo, MD.)

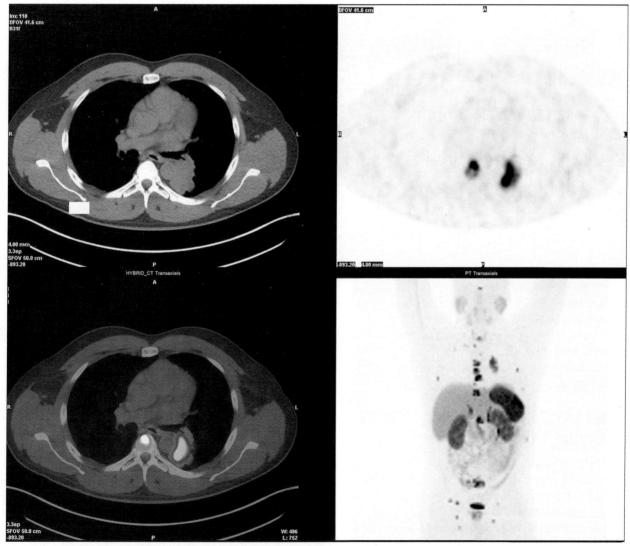

Fig. 13.9 Bronchopulmonary carcinoid with Ga-67 dotatate positron emission tomography with computed tomography (PET/CT). Image shows radiotracer avid mass in the superior segment of the left lower lobe and extensive osseous metastases throughout the axial skeleton, worst in the thoracic spine.

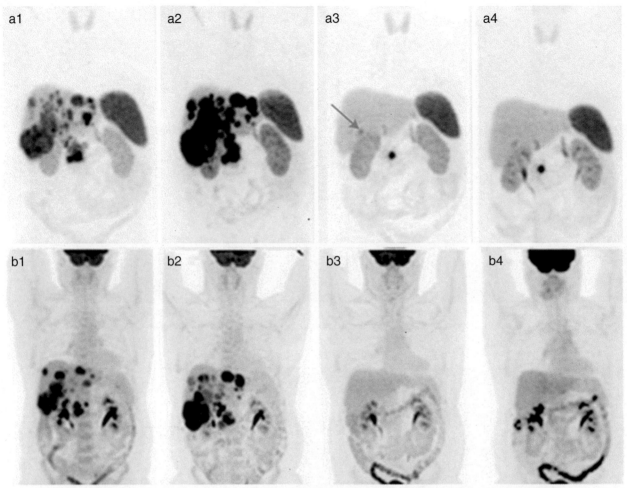

Fig. 13.10 Peptide receptor radionuclide therapy (PRRT). Primary pancreatic neuroendocrine tumor (NET) with extensive metastases. Serial Ga-68 dotatate maximum-intensity projection (MIP) images *(above)* and F-18 fluorodeoxyglucose (FDG) positron emission tomography (PET; *below*). Baseline study *(a1, b1)*, after three cycles of chemotherapy *(a2, b2)*, after one cycle of Y-90 dotatate and three cycles of Lu-177 dotatate (Lutathera; *a3, b3*). At this time point, complete response is seen on F-18 FDG and near-complete response on Ga-68 dotatate *(arrow shows small area of residual disease)* and on similar images 6 months posttherapy *(a4, b4)*. (With permission, Kong G, Callahan J, Hofman MS, et al. High clinical and morphological response using 90Y-DOTA-octreotate sequenced with 177Lu-DOTA-octreotate induction peptide receptor chemoradio-nuclide therapy [PRCRT] for bulky neuroendocrine tumors. *Eur J Nucl Med Mol Imaging.* 2017;44[3]:476–489.)

F-18 Fluorodeoxyglucose PET/CT

The sensitivity of F-18 FDG PET/CT for tumor detection is low in well-differentiated NETs. However, FDG PET has an important role in the imaging of aggressive, poorly differentiated tumors. If Ga-68 dotatate is negative, FDG imaging should be performed. Some advocate using both because tumors can be quite heterogeneous.

I-123 AND I-131 MIBG ADRENERGIC TUMOR IMAGING AND THERAPY

Radiolabeled metaiodo-benzyl-guanidine (mIBG) adrenal medullary scintigraphy has been used clinically since the 1980s for diagnosis and staging of neural crest tumors (e.g., pheochromocytomas, paragangliomas, and neuroblastomas). I-131-labeled mIBG was the original diagnostic agent; however, I-123-labeled mIBG is now widely available and preferable because of its superior image quality with an optimal 159-keV

gamma-ray energy and lower patient radiation given a lack of β⁻ emissions and shorter half-life of 13 hours as opposed to I-131 with a 364-keV gamma-ray energy, β⁻ emissions, and 8-day half-life (see Appendix 1). I-131 mIBG is reserved for therapy.

I-123 mIBG (AdreView)

I-123 mIBG (AdreView) was approved by the FDA in 2003 for the detection of primary or metastatic pheochromocytoma and neuroblastoma, as an adjunct to other diagnostic tests. As an analog of the drugs bretylium and guanethidine, mIBG shares structural features and biological behavior with the adrenergic neurotransmitter hormone norepinephrine. Both norepinephrine and mIBG are taken up in cells rich in sympathetic neurons by an active process mediated by the norepinephrine uptake-1 transporter. Once in the cytoplasm, it is actively transported into the presynaptic nerve terminal and catecholamine storage granules by the vesicular monoamine transporter (Fig. 13.11).

Uptake and Distribution

I-123 mIBG avidly localizes in organs with high adrenergic innervation, including the heart, salivary glands, kidneys, and liver. (Fig. 13.12). Variable activity is seen in the lungs, gallbladder, salivary glands, and nasal mucosa. Mild to moderate adrenal uptake often occurs with planar I-123 mIBG imaging and is nearly always seen with SPECT. No uptake occurs in the normal skeleton. It is cleared through the colon and kidneys.

Methodology

Numerous drugs interfere with mIBG uptake. The most common include tricyclic antidepressants, reserpine, cocaine, and the alpha- and beta-blocker labetalol (Table 13.3). A detailed

imaging protocol is summarized (Box 13.4). Pretreatment with saturated potassium iodide (SSKI) or Lugol's solution is recommended in the package insert and in procedural guidelines to block thyroid uptake (Table 13.4). Although the 159-keV photopeak can be imaged with a low-energy collimator, a fraction of the photons (<3%) are high energy (440–625 keV [2.4%] and 625–784 keV [0.15%]), reducing the image quality. Although a low-energy collimator is often used, a medium-energy collimator is preferable. Images are routinely acquired 24 hours after injection. Whole-body imaging is standard in order to detect an

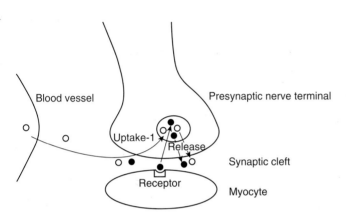

Fig. 13.11 Uptake mechanism of mIBG. It is actively taken up in the presynaptic nerve terminal and retained in catecholamine storage granules, similar to norepinephrine. In the nerve terminal, norepinephrine is converted from tyrosine to DOPA to dopamine and then to norepinephrine (noradrenaline) and then secreted in response to acetylcholine. (With permission, Scott LA, Kench PL. Schematic representation of the 123I-MIBG uptake mechanism. *J Nucl Med Technol.* 2004;32:66–71.)

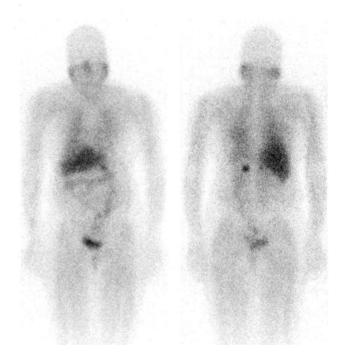

Fig. 13.12 Pheochromocytoma. Planar I-123 mIBG whole-body scan. Patient with poorly controlled hypertension and very elevated serum and urinary catecholamines. Distribution is normal except for focal markedly increased uptake in the region of the left adrenal, best seen in posterior view *(right),* consistent with pheochromocytoma.

TABLE 13.3	Medications Recommended to Be Held Before I-123 mIBG Study		
Drug	**Related Drugs**	**Mechanism**	**Discontinue for:**
Antihypertensive/cardiac agents	Bretylium, guanethidine, reserpine	Deplete granules	7 days
	Calcium channel blockers (amlodipine, nifedipine, nicardipine)	Deplete granules	14 days
	Labetalol	Deplete granules and inhibit uptake Beta-blocker	21 days
Antipsychotics	Butyrophenones (droperidol, haloperidol)	Inhibit uptake	21 days
	Loxapine	Inhibit uptake	
	Phenothiazines (chlorpromazine, fluphenazine, promethazine)	Inhibit uptake	
Cocaine/opioids		Inhibit uptake	7 days
Sympathomimetics	Amphetamine, dopamine, ephedrine, isoproterenol, fenoterol, phenylephrine, phenylpropanolamine, pseudoephedrine, salbutamol, terbutaline, xylometazoline	Deplete granules	7 days
Tramadol		Inhibits uptake	14 days
Tricyclic antidepressants	Amitriptyline (and derivatives), amoxapine, doxepin	Inhibit uptake	21 days

mIBG, Metaiodobenzylguanidine.

BOX 13.4   Iodine-123 mIBG: Summary Protocol

Patient Preparation
Discontinue interfering medications (Table 13.3).
Potassium iodide or Lugol's solution to prevent thyroid uptake (Table 13.4)

Radiopharmaceutical
Intravenous injection over 30 seconds
I-123 MIBG
　　Children: 0.14 mCi/kg (5.2 MBq/kg); minimum 1.0 mCi (20 MBq) and maximum 10 mCi (400 MBq)
　　Adults: 10 mCi (400 MBq)

Instrumentation
Gamma camera: Large field of view for planar images
Planar imaging and SPECT/CT as indicated
Collimator: Medium energy, parallel hole; low energy can be used.

Acquisition
I-123: Image at 24 hours.
Whole-body planar images (8 cm/sec)
SPECT: 3-degree steps, 35 sec/step, 180 projections, 128 × 128 matrix

mIBG, Metaiodo-benzyl-guanidine; *SPECT*, single-photon emission computed tomography; *SPECT/CT*, single-photon emission computed tomography with computed tomography.

TABLE 13.4   Daily Doses of Thyroid Blockade Compounds

Drug	Adults	Child (15–50 kg)	Child (5–15 kg)	Child (<5 kg)
Capsules[a]				
Potassium iodate	170	80	40	20
Potassium iodide	130	65	32	16
Potassium perchlorate	400	300	200	100
Solution				
Lugol solution 1%	1 drop/kg to max 40 (20 drops twice daily)			

[a]Dose in milligrams per day.
Data from Giammarile F, Chiti A, Lassmann M, et al. EANM procedure guidelines for I-131 MIBG therapy. *Eur J Nucl Mol Imaging.* 2008;35:1039–1047.

extraadrenal pheochromocytoma, malignant metastases, or primary and metastatic neuroblastoma. SPECT/CT is very useful for anatomical localization.

Clinical Applications of I-123 mIBG

Pheochromocytoma. This catecholamine-secreting tumor is derived from chromaffin cells. It can precipitate life-threatening hypertension or cardiac arrhythmias secondary to its excessive catecholamine secretion. When these tumors arise outside of the adrenal gland, they are called *paragangliomas* and can be found anywhere from the bladder up to the base of the skull. Ten percent of pheochromocytomas are bilateral, 10% are extraadrenal, and 10% are malignant. They may be associated with multiple endocrine neoplasia (MEN) types IIA and IIB,

von Hippel–Lindau disease, neurofibromatosis, tuberous sclerosis, and Carney syndrome. Adrenomedullary hyperplasia occurs in patients with MEN type IIA.

Pheochromocytomas often present with elevated blood or urinary catecholamines and metanephrines, usually three times or greater than normal. If an adrenal mass is demonstrated with morphological imaging in patients with evidence for the disease, the diagnosis is often inferred, and further workup before surgery is not always necessary. However, I-123 mIBG can confirm the adrenergic etiology of a detected adrenal mass on anatomical imaging, detect extraadrenal paragangliomas, and diagnose medullary hyperplasia and metastatic pheochromocytoma.

The characteristic I-123 mIBG scintigraphic appearance of a pheochromocytoma, extraadrenal paraganglioma, or metastatic disease is intense focal uptake with a high tumor-to-background ratio (Fig. 13.12). The sensitivity and specificity for detection are 90% and 95%, respectively. Planar imaging is often diagnostic, although SPECT/CT can be helpful (Figs. 13.13 and 13.14). F-18 FDG has only a limited role but can be useful with high-grade adrenal cancers or malignant pheochromocytoma.

Neuroblastoma. This embryonal malignancy of the sympathetic nervous system most commonly occurs in children younger than 4 years of age. Over 70% of tumors originate in the retroperitoneal region, either from the adrenal or the abdominal sympathetic chain, whereas approximately 20% occur in the chest, derived from the thoracic sympathetic chain. Patients with localized tumors can have a good prognosis and outcome; those with metastatic disease fare poorly. At the time of diagnosis, more than 50% of patients present with metastatic disease, 25% have localized disease, and 15% have regional extension. Metastatic disease involves the lymph nodes, liver, bone marrow, and bone. I-123 mIBG is valuable for staging, detecting metastatic disease, restaging, and determining patient response to therapy. The sensitivity for detection of neuroblastoma is reported to be >90%, and the specificity is about 95%. Whole-body scanning is routine (Figs. 13.15 and 13.16). SPECT and SPECT/CT aid in detection and localization (Fig. 13.17). NETs and medullary carcinoma of the thyroid also take up mIBG, however, with lower sensitivity than for neuroblastoma or pheochromocytoma.

Bone scans have long been used to detect osseous metastases in neuroblastoma. A common location for metastases is in the bilateral metaphyses of long bones. This could be overlooked because of their symmetrical appearance and high normal growth-plate uptake in children. However, I-123 mIBG has superior sensitivity for the detection of metastases compared with bone scans because the tumors initially involve the bone marrow.

Therapy With High-Dose I-131 mIBG. Conventional therapies for metastatic pheochromocytoma and neuroblastoma include surgery, chemotherapy, and tyrosine kinase inhibitors. The 5-year survival rate has been <50%. The high uptake of mIBG in neuroectodermal tumors has led to therapy with high-dose I-131 mIBG in patients who have failed conventional therapies and have progressive or symptomatic disease, utilizing its 606-keV I-131 beta emissions. The 5-year survival rate has been reported to be increased; however, complete response rates are not high. This therapy, although performed for many years at

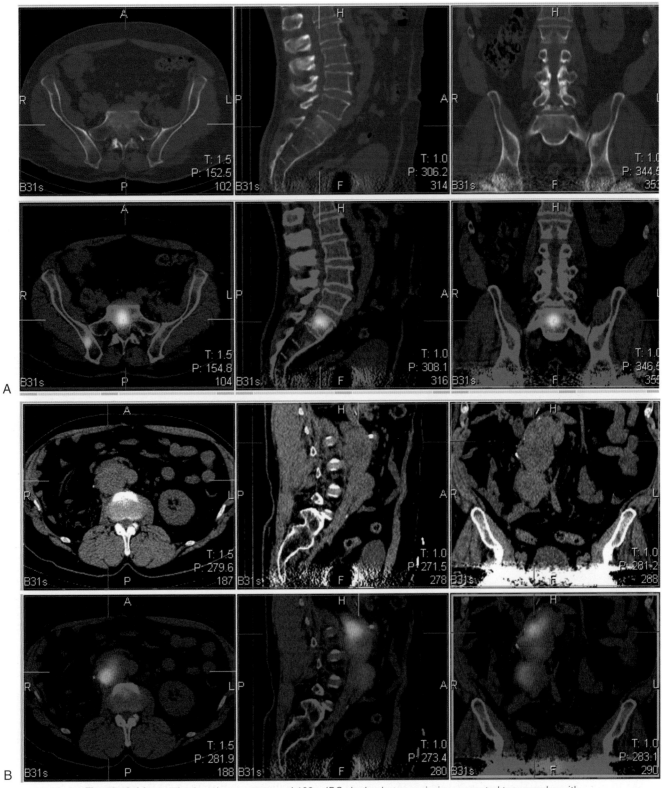

Fig. 13.13 Metastatic pheochromocytoma—I-123 mIBG single-photon emission computed tomography with computed tomography (SPECT/CT). (A) A 70-year-old man with extensive metastases. CT *(above)* and fused images *(below)*, transverse *(left)*, sagittal *(middle)*, and coronal *(right)* selected images. Metastases noted in the ischium, sacrum, and lumbar spine. (B) Conglomeration of retroperitoneal nodes with metastases.

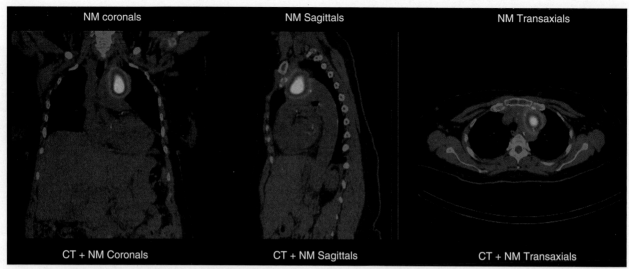

Fig. 13.14 Mediastinal paraganglioma—I-123 mIBG single-photon emission computed tomography with computed tomography (SPECT/CT). A 68-year-old woman found to have anterior mediastinal mass and elevated metanephrines. On fused images, intense uptake is seen in large superior anterior mediastinal mass along the lateral border of the aortic arch. On CT, the tumor is seen to extend superiorly and encase the left subclavian and common carotid arteries. No metastases were seen.

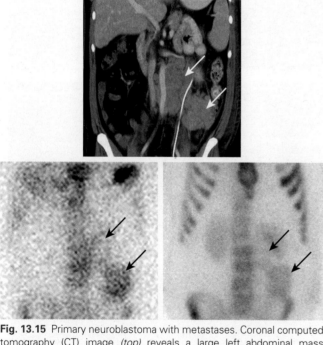

Fig. 13.15 Primary neuroblastoma with metastases. Coronal computed tomography (CT) image *(top)* reveals a large left abdominal mass *(arrows)* that had arisen from the retroperitoneum. I-131 mIBG images *(bottom left)* show increased uptake in the mass as well as throughout the skeleton, with diffuse metastases. Tc-99m methyl diphosphonate (MDP) bone scan *(bottom right)* shows abnormal soft tissue uptake in the mass. Skeletal metastases are also seen.

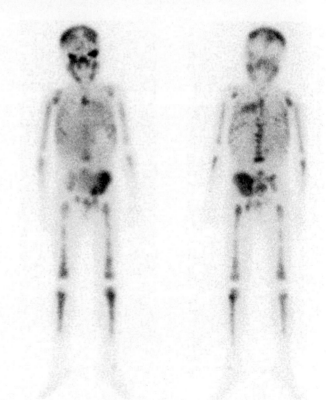

Fig. 13.16 Metastatic neuroblastoma on I-123 mIBG whole-body scan. A 7-year-old boy with stage IV tumor after two bone marrow transplants. Extensive metastases are seen throughout the skeleton.

selected centers in the United States and Europe, has been considered investigational. However, in 2018 the FDA approved iobenguane I-131 (Azedra) for adult and pediatric patients aged ≥12 years with a positive I-123 MIBG scan and unresectable, locally advanced, or metastatic pheochromocytoma or paraganglioma. Toxicity cincludes nausea, myelosuppression, and fatigue but less than that seen with more traditional chemotherapy.

For therapy with I-131 mIBG, patients must be pretreated with potassium iodide or other thyroid-blocking medications beginning 24 to 48 hours before injection to minimize uptake of free radioiodine by the thyroid (Table 13.4). It should be continued for 10 to 15 days posttreatment. In spite of doing this, hypothyroidism occurs in 11% to 20% of patients. Before initiating therapy, excess catecholamines should be managed with alpha

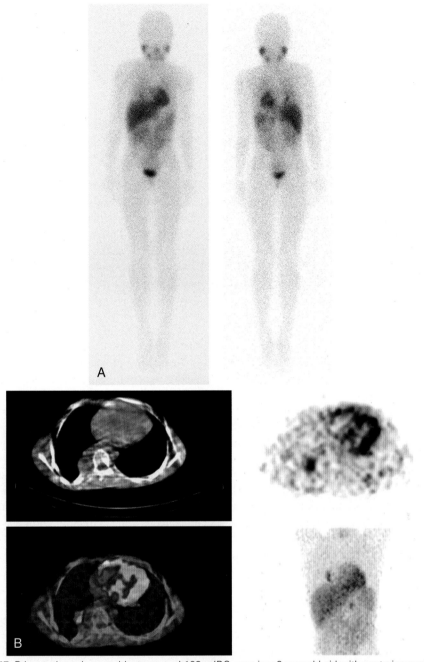

Fig. 13.17 Primary thoracic neuroblastoma on I-123 mIBG scan in a 9-year-old girl with posterior mediastinal mass. (A) Planar anterior and posterior whole-body images. The posterior planar image shows focal uptake in the chest just above the liver. (B) Single-photon emission computed tomography with computed tomography (SPECT/CT) clearly localizes the paraspinal mass.

blockade and atenolol. Drugs that interfere with mIBG uptake must be discontinued, including labetalol, reserpine, tricyclic antidepressants, sympathomimetics, and cocaine (Table 13.3). The most significant toxicity is hematologic.

PROSTATE CANCER DIAGNOSTIC IMAGING AND THERAPY

Prostate cancer is the most frequent malignant tumor in men and the second leading cause of death. Routine blood testing showing an elevated serum prostate-specific antigen (PSA) often brings the patient to medical attention. Examination and biopsy can confirm the diagnosis. For staging, restaging, diagnosis of recurrence, and therapeutic monitoring, noninvasive tests such as MRI, contrast-enhanced CT, and Tc-99m bone scans have been standard. However, all of these have significant limitations for pretherapy risk stratification, for staging patients at risk for pelvic lymph node metastases or systemic disease, and for the detection of biochemical recurrence at low PSA levels in patients previously treated with curative intent. The specificity of magnetic resonance (MR) within the prostate can be compromised by postbiopsy change and inflammation, and both CT and MR are limited for the detection of lymph node metastases by the need to wait until disease causes lymph node enlargement for diagnosis.

Prostate cancer staging is based on the combination of physical examination, histopathological Gleason score, and the serum PSA level. Therapy with radical prostatectomy is not undertaken when there is nodal involvement or distant spread. The lymph nodes are the most common site of metastatic disease, usually occurring in a stepwise fashion from the periprostatic or obturator nodes to internal or external iliac nodes, and then to the common iliac and periaortic nodes. However, this sequence is not invariable. Frequent sites of distant metastases are the skeleton, liver, and lungs.

If the PSA fails to decline after prostatectomy or begins to rise (biochemical failure), then residual or recurrent tumor is suspected. If disease is localized to the prostate fossa or pelvis, radiation therapy offers the potential for effective treatment. However, if recurrence involves periaortic lymph nodes or other distant sites outside the therapy field, radiation therapy exposes the patient to significant morbidity without the potential for cure. Staging has limitations. Bone scans are most likely to detect metastases if the serum PSA is >20 ng/mL and in patients with a high Gleason score. However, post–hormonal therapy PSAs are a less useful guide because they are often low even in the setting of residual tumor. CT and MRI have limited value because of their low sensitivity for detecting nodal involvement. F-18 FDG PET has poor sensitivity for detecting prostate cancer. It plays a limited role in staging or detecting recurrence, only showing significant sensitivity when recurrent disease has transformed, escaping hormonal control, and has become more aggressive.

For recurrent prostate cancer therapy planning, it must be determined whether disease is confined to the prostate/prostate bed or is extraprostatic. Identification of metastatic pelvic disease requires modification of the radiation field to cover the pelvic lymph nodes; extrapelvic disease changes the approach from potential curative salvage therapy to system hormonal therapy.

Molecular imaging has the potential to better characterize primary prostate cancer, perform staging before radiotherapy or surgery, localize the site of recurrence in patients with a rising PSA level after primary therapy, monitor tumor response to therapy, and select patients for targeted radionuclide therapy. Approaches have included C-11 acetate (fatty acid analog), C-11 and F-18 choline (cell membrane analogs), and F-18 fluorocholine (amino acid analog).

F-18 Fluciclovine (FACBC, Axumin)

F-18 fluciclovine (FACBC, Axumin) was approved by the FDA in 2016 for the diagnosis of suspected recurrent prostate cancer in patients with elevated PSA after initial therapy. F-18 fluciclovine is an amino acid analog of leucine (Fig. 13.18). Amino acid transport is upregulated in carcinomas because of increased amino acid use for energy requirements and protein synthesis.

Primary tumor characterization is not an approved indication because there is poor specificity for uptake in primary prostate cancer and benign prostate tissue as well as low sensitivity

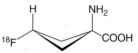

Fig. 13.18 F-18 fluciclovine (Axumin)—molecular structure. Chemical name, *Anti*1-amino-3-F-18-fluorocyclobutane-1-carboxylic acid. *(Left to right)* F-18 radiolabel, cyclic side chain, amino terminus, and carboxy terminus.

for nodal disease. For identifying disease in the treated prostate bed, fluciclovine demonstrates high sensitivity but low specificity and moderate positive predictive value (PPV).

The radiopharmaceutical is most useful in patients with biochemical failure and suspected recurrent locoregional and distant metastatic disease. F-18 fluciclovine PET/CT has demonstrated superiority to CT for the detection of local and distant disease in the clinical setting of biochemical failure. F-18 fluciclovine has uptake in osteolytic and osteoblastic lesions, and sometimes this may be seen before morphological changes detected on CT. Limited studies suggest equivalent or better results than bone scintigraphy. The radiopharmaceutical has shown superior diagnostic performance compared with CT, In-111 ProstaScint, and C-11 choline.

Regarding preparation, 4-hour fasting is recommended before injection. Unlike FDG PET/CT, no prolonged uptake phase is necessary. Imaging begins approximately 4 minutes after injection of 10 mCi (370 MBq) F-18 fluciclovine. Normal biodistribution includes marked pancreatic uptake, with somewhat lesser uptake in the liver. The pituitary, salivary glands, lymphoid tissue of Waldeyer's ring, thyroid gland, breast, esophagus, stomach and bowel, adrenal glands, and renal parenchyma may all have mild to moderate uptake. Excretion is via the urinary tract (Figs. 13.19 and 13.20). Bone marrow may show heterogeneous uptake. Inflammation may show varying degrees of uptake. Preliminary data suggest F-18 fluciclovine may have a role in other malignancies (e.g., breast cancer, gliomas, and lung cancer). Guidelines for F-18 fluciclovine image interpretation are summarized in Box 13.5.

Investigations have shown that preprostatectomy sensitivity depends on the PSA level, being limited for low PSA values. However, postprostatectomy, sensitivity improves. The higher the PSA, the higher the likelihood of detection.

Prostate-specific membrane antigen (PSMA) is overexpressed in primary and metastatic adenocarcinomas of the prostate. The level of PSMA expression rises with increasing tumor dedifferentiation and in hormone-refractory cancers.

In-111 Capromab Pendetide (ProstaScint)

In-111 capromab pendetide (ProstaScint) is a monoclonal antibody to PSMA approved by the FDA for clinical use in 1996 as a diagnostic imaging agent in patients with localized prostate cancer at risk for tumor spread and in postprostatectomy patients who might relapse. ProstaScint targets an intracellular epitope of PSMA. In retrospect, this limited its ability to localize to intact cancer cells. Its sensitivity for the detection of metastatic prostate cancer has been found suboptimal, even with SPECT and SPECT/CT, with difficulty differentiating uptake in lymph nodes from high levels of background blood-pool activity in adjacent vessels

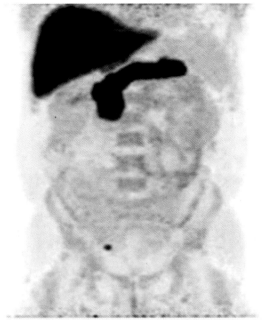

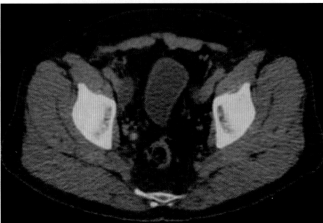

Fig. 13.19 F-18 fluciclovine (FACBC)—patient with history of radical prostatectomy, now rising PSA, suspected recurrence. Internal iliac/pelvic sidewall lymph node seen on maximum-intensity projection (MIP) image *(above)* and transverse positron emission tomography (PET) slice *(below)*. (Courtesy of Bital Savir-Baruch.)

and lower resolution in the prostate bed. Newer generations of PSMA-targeted radiotracers that interact with the extracellular domain of the enzyme have subsequently been developed.

Ga-68, F-18, and Tc-99m PSMA-Targeted Imaging Radiopharmaceuticals

PSMA is an enzyme *(glutamate carboxypeptidases, GCP, Type II)* that is highly expressed in primary and metastatic prostate cancer. The target of these small-molecule radiopharmaceuticals is the enzyme active site within the extracellular domain. This approach has been found to be much superior to that of ProstaScint because it allows these radiotracers to target intact prostate cancer cells. After antigen binding to PSMA in the cell membrane, it is internalized by endocytosis, leading to concentration and retention in the cells, which can create very high-contrast-resolution images and allow the detection of even small-volume disease.

Generator-produced Ga-68 labeled to PSMA-targeted agents (PSMA-11, PMSA-617, or PSMA I&T) has been extensively studied and successfully used clinically in Europe. Also, F-18-labeled PSMA radiopharmaceuticals (DCFPyL and PSMA-1007) are under investigation in Europe and the United States. Ga-68 has disadvantages, such as the need for a Ge-68/Ga-68 generator and sufficient patient volume to utilize it cost-effectively. The image quality of Ga-68 and F-18 PSMA is superior to that of F-18 fluciclovine and C-11 choline. The F-18 radiolabel for PSMA will likely be preferable to Ga-68 because of F-18's superior imaging characteristics and PET/CT's wide availability.

The normal distribution of Ga-68, F-18, and Tc-99m PSMA-targeted agents includes the prominent uptake in the salivary glands, kidney cortex, and duodenum, with lesser uptake in the spleen, lacrimal glands, and liver (Fig. 13.21).

These radiolabeled PSMA-targeted radiopharmaceuticals have reported high accuracy for the detection of local, regional, and distant metastases. They can detect sites of recurrent disease that were occult or equivocal by conventional imaging modalities, especially in the pelvic/periprostatic tissues, in subcentimeter lymph nodes, and bone metastases (Figs. 13.22–13.24). A higher detection rate and sensitivity have been reported compared with conventional imaging in hormone-naïve and castration metastatic prostate cancer and in the setting of biochemical recurrence, even in patients with low PSA. A prospective investigation of 431 patients found that Ga-68-targeted PSMA PET/CT led to a change in planned management in 51% of patients. Unsuspected disease was found in the prostate bed in 27%, locoregional positive nodes in 39%, and distant metastatic disease in 16% of patients (see Figs. 13.22 and 13.24).

However, false positives may occur, and uptake may be seen in ganglia, granulomatous disease, hemangiomas, healing bone fractures, Paget's disease, and tumors of neurogenic origin. False negatives may occur in nodal metastases <5 mm in diameter. PSMA is also expressed in the neovasculature of nonprostate tumors, including clear-cell renal carcinoma, thyroid cancer, breast cancer, and colon cancer.

Lutetium-177 (Lu-177) PSMA-Targeted Therapy of Prostate Cancer (Lutathera)

An important application of radiotargeted PSMA diagnostic imaging is the selection of patients for radionuclide therapy. Experience with Lu-177 PSMA-targeted radiotherapy in patients with castration-resistant prostate cancer has been very positive to date, even in advanced cases. Retrospective studies have demonstrated significant benefits for overall survival and progression-free survival, improvement in clinical symptoms, and excellent pain palliation compared with other pharmacological therapies. The most common side effect has been hematologic, a bystander effect with bone metastases. Prospective studies are needed.

SENTINEL NODE MAPPING WITH LYMPHOSCINTIGRAPHY

Cancers such as melanoma and breast carcinoma metastasize first to regional lymph nodes. Mapping the lymphatic drainage

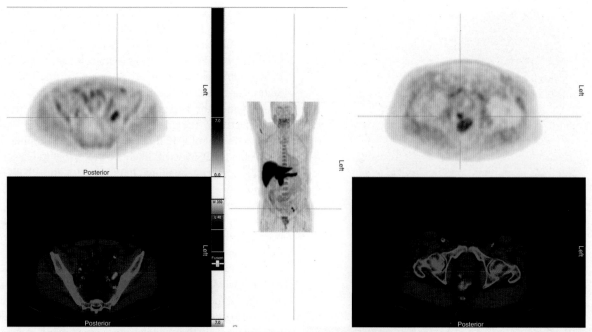

Fig. 13.20 F-18 fluciclovine (FACBC)—a patient with prostate cancer who received brachytherapy, now with rising prostate-specific antigen (PSA). Uptake seen in (A) a left obturator node and (B) seminal vesicle. (Courtesy of Bital Savir-Baruch.)

BOX 13.5 Interpretative Guidelines for F-18 Fluciclovine (FACBC, Axumin)

Nonprostatectomy Prostate Bed

Moderate focal asymmetrical uptake ≥ bone marrow is suspicious for cancer recurrence. Small foci (<1 cm) are suspicious if uptake is > blood pool. Diffuse heterogeneous or homogenous uptake > blood pool and bone marrow is suspicious for cancer.

Prostate Bed Postprostatectomy

Focal uptake ≥ bone marrow in areas suspicious for cancer—interpret as positive.
Small foci (<1 cm) are suspicious if uptake is > blood pool.

Lymph nodes

Typical sites for recurrence, uptake ≥ bone marrow is suspicious for cancer.
Small foci should be > bone marrow to call positive.
Atypical nodal sites (inguinal, distal external iliac, hilar, axillary) should usually be considered physiological.

Focal Bone Uptake

Is suspicious for cancer if seen on MIP images or PET-only images.
A CT bone abnormality without uptake does not exclude metastasis.

CT, Computed tomography; *MIP*, maximum-intensity projection; *PET*, positron emission tomography.

---

of a tumor has improved staging in patients with early cancer (those with no clinically evident nodal involvement) by identifying the sentinel lymph node (SLN). The SLN is the first node that drains the region of the tumor and is the one most likely to reveal occult metastases. Once identified with scintigraphy, it can be detected at surgery with a portable gamma probe and excised for pathological evidence of nodal spread. If there is no sentinel nodal spread of tumor, resection of the remaining lymph node basin is unnecessary. This process has proved more accurate for staging than routinely dissecting all nodes in the clinically perceived drainage basin and has markedly decreased morbidity from lymphadenectomy, most commonly lymphedema. This procedure is widely used for melanoma and breast cancer but is also now being be used for a variety of other tumors, including head and neck, cervix, vaginal, colon, and thyroid cancer. Some surgeons also inject blue dye at the time of surgery for a similar purpose, however, usually in conjunction with scintigraphy.

Radiopharmaceuticals

A number of radiopharmaceuticals have been investigated and used for this purpose. In the United States, filtered Tc-99m sulfur colloid (SC) has been most commonly used. The range of particle size varies. Small particles migrate quickly and have shorter lymph node residence times; larger particles may not migrate. Because particle sizes for Tc-99m SC (Tc-99m SC) tend to be large (0.1–1.0 μm), the administered dose is commonly first filtered through a 0.22-micron Millipore filter. In Europe, Tc-99m-labeled nanocolloid of human serum albumin is most commonly used, and in Australia, Tc-99m antimony trisulfide.

Tc-99m tilmanocept (Lymphoseek) was approved by the FDA in 2013 for sentinel node lymphoscintigraphy for melanoma, breast, and oral cavity cancers. This small molecule carries multiple units of mannose with high affinity for receptor proteins (CD206) found on the surface of macrophages and dendritic cells. By tightly binding to these mannose receptors, it accumulates in lymphatic tissue and localizes in draining nodes. It clears rapidly from the injection site, has high SLN extraction, and has low distal node accumulation. Detection rates are said to be similar. Lymphatic channels are more commonly seen with Tc-99m SC.

However, studies directly comparing Tc-99m tilmanocept with Tc-99m SC are few and small. Lymphoseek has been claimed to result in less pain to the patient on injection, although pain is usually caused by the intracutaneous bleb and is very transient with Tc-99m SC. Because Tc-99m tilmanocept is cleared via the bladder, it is not ideal for vulvovaginal locations.

Clinical Indications
Malignant Melanoma

Factors influencing prognosis include the primary lesion's thickness (millimeter depth of tumor invasion), lesion ulceration, and mitotic rate and are useful for staging early tumors and predicting occult lymph node involvement. Lymph node involvement is the most important independent predictor of survival. Patients without clinically detected adenopathy but with intermediate-thickness tumors (Breslow >1.0 mm and <4.0 mm) benefit most from SLN biopsy. With tumors <1.0 mm (stage I), the procedure is sometimes performed if there are other high-risk factors, such as a high mitotic biopsy rate (≥1 mitosis/mm^2) or lesion ulceration.

Methodology. An intradermal injection is performed either the morning of surgery or in the afternoon before the next-morning surgery. An intradermal injection that raises a wheal generally results in good dose migration through the lymphatic vessels. Filtered Tc-99m SC radiopharmaceutical is typically injected in four divided doses within 1 cm and around the lesion/biopsy scar, and images are acquired for approximately 30 minutes. Occasionally, delayed images are needed, for example, to differentiate a lymphatic channel from nodal uptake. Lymph nodes may be visualized in remote, unexpected locations, so vigilance is warranted. Various imaging methodologies have been described. One is summarized in Box 13.6.

For Tc-99m tilmanocept (Lymphoseek), 0.5 mCi is injected intradermally the morning of surgery or 2 mCi the afternoon before next-morning surgery. Multiple-view images can be obtained as early as 15 minutes after injection.

Image Interpretation. The first retained "hot spot" seen is the sentinel node. Subsequent ones are secondary nodes. It is possible to have two sentinel nodes if they have separate lymphatic drainage paths (Fig. 13.25). Care must be taken to differentiate temporary retention in a lymphatic channel from a node. Further delayed imaging can often clarify the issue. *In-transit nodes,* most commonly in the extremities in the antecubital or popliteal fossa, should be carefully looked for when injecting distally because they would be considered the sentinel node (Fig. 13.26). SPECT/CT can be helpful in some cases, particularly in the head and neck (Fig. 13.27).

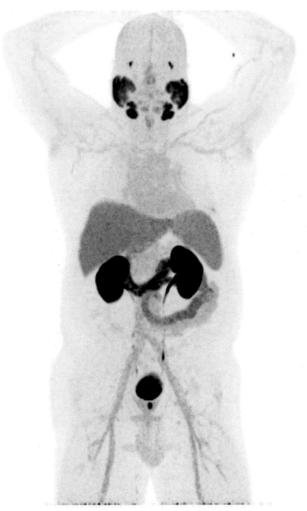

Fig. 13.21 Normal distribution—F-18 DCFPyL prostate-specific membrane antigen (PSMA)-targeted radiopharmaceutical, maximum-intensity projection (MIP) image. Greatest uptake in the parotids and salivary glands, kidney, and duodenum and lesser activity in the lacrimal glands, liver, and spleen, and urinary clearance.

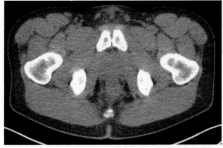
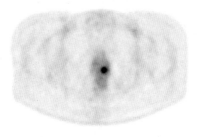
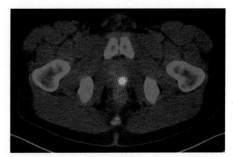

Fig. 13.22 F-18 DCFPyL prostate-specific membrane antigen (PSMA)-targeted positron emission tomography with computed tomography (PET/CT) in a patient with newly diagnosed Gleason 8 prostate cancer with focal uptake detected in left prostate apex. (Courtesy, Steven P. Rowe, MD, PhD and Michael A. Gorin, MD.)

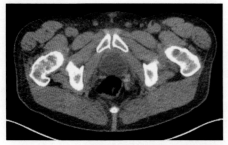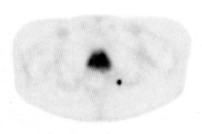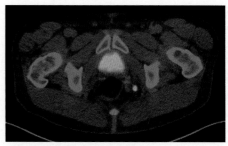

Fig. 13.23 Prostate bed uptake on F-18 DCFPyL prostate-specific membrane antigen (PSMA)-targeted radiopharmaceutical positron emission tomography with computed tomography (PET/CT) images. Rising prostate-specific antigen (PSA) postsurgery for prostate cancer. A recurrence of prostate cancer is detected in the posterolateral left aspect of the prostate bed. Conventional imaging was negative. (Courtesy, Steven P. Rowe, MD, PhD and Michael A. Gorin, MD.)

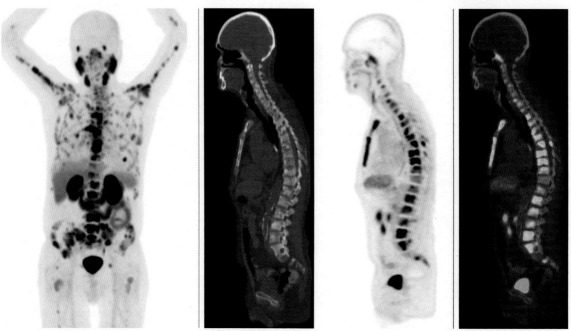

Fig. 13.24 Metastatic prostate cancer to bone on F-18 DCFPyL prostate-specific membrane antigen (PSMA)-targeted radiopharmaceutical positron emission tomography with computed tomography (PET/CT). Patient was on therapy. This is a follow-up scan. Widely metastatic to bone, seen on maximum-intensity projection (MIP) and sagittal (left to right) CT, PyL, and fused images. (Courtesy, Steven P. Rowe, MD, PhD and Michael A. Gorin, MD.)

SLN biopsy accuracy is much higher than clinical and standard imaging assessment. False-negative rates (a sentinel node not detected) for SNL lymphoscintigraphy are quite low, <5%. Importantly, surgical complication rates are much lower with the SLN biopsy approach than for complete nodal basin dissection, in two trials, 10.1% versus 37.2% and 4.6% versus 23.2%. A metanalysis of nonrandomized studies reported better survival for those who had SLN biopsy. However, the Multicenter Selective Lymphadenectomy Trial showed no definite survival advantage. Quality of life is improved for those with negative sentinel nodes for metastases because they do not require a complete axillary node dissection and its common complications.

Breast Cancer

Axillary lymph node status is a major prognostic factor in early-stage breast cancer. Even in small, T1 tumors (≤2 cm), axillary nodes are involved at initial staging 10% to 30% of the time, and this increases to 45% for T2 lesions (2.1–3.0 cm). Some centers limit SLN biopsy to those with unifocal tumors smaller than 2 to 3 cm; others offer the procedure to patients with large T2 or T3 lesions (>5 cm) and multifocal or multicentric lesions. In breast cancer, the use of the sentinel node biopsy has largely replaced initial axillary lymph node dissection. Usually, the SLN is identified in the axillary region, detected at surgery with a miniaturized gamma probe, and removed. Lymphoscintigraphy detects the SLN in >90% of cases. False-negative rates of are <10%. Surgeons do not perform confirmatory axillary dissection if the SLN is free of tumor. The risk for lymphedema is lower after SLN biopsy than from axillary dissection (5% vs. 13%). At some centers, imaging is not performed.

Methodology. Various injection methods have been used, including intradermal, subdermal, subcutaneous, peritumoral, periareolar, and subareolar injections. Although peritumoral injection with ultrasound guidance is recommended for deep tumors, subdermal or intradermal injections are sufficient in most cases, resulting in rapid dose migration. Periareolar injections can be used if the tumor is in the upper outer quadrant, to avoid confusion or crosstalk between the injection

---

BOX 13.6   Sentinel Node Lymphoscintigraphy

Patient Preparation
None

Procedure Tray
4 syringes with 1 mCi Tc-99m SC or Tc-99m tilmanocept (Lymphoseek) 0.5 mCi divided into four 0.1-mL-volume tuberculin syringes
Alcohol wipes, gauze, needle discard basin, blue chuck, Lidocaine cream, Tegaderm

Procedure
Blue absorbent chuck with center cut out to expose primary site
Gloves should be worn and injection sites cleaned.
Inject radiopharmaceutical intradermally at four sites within 1 cm of the periphery of lesion or surgical resection.
The needle should be withdrawn with negative pressure to prevent contamination.

Image Acquisition Protocol
Tc-99m sulfur colloid:
　Acquire images for 30 minutes (six sets of five 1-minute frames) in 128 × 128 matrix
　Obtain transmission scan with Co-57 sheet source during 1-minute frame for each 5- minute acquisition.
　Additional 5-minute acquisitions as needed
　If no drainage is seen, heat and massage may be helpful.
　For back or abdominal lesions, image both axillary and inguinal nodal regions.
　In-transit nodes should be looked for in extremities and marked. Thus, good images of the lower and upper leg or arm are necessary.
Tc-99m Tilmanocept:
　Similar protocol except that only static images 15 minutes after injection are required.
　SPECT/CT can be helpful for localization, particularly for the head and neck and pelvis.

SPECT/CT, Single-photon emission computed tomography with computed tomography.

---

site and any nodes. Massage of the injection site promotes dose movement. The presence of internal mammary nodes may be demonstrated with greater frequency with periareolar injections. Disagreement exists on surgical management of these nodes, with many not including the findings in their assessment at staging. Because internal mammary nodes are frequently involved in breast cancer, it would seem that attention to this region is warranted, particularly in medially located primary tumors, when restaging, such as with PET/CT.

Imaging begins immediately after injection. Protocols vary, but with Tc-99m SC, sequential images are performed at 5-minute intervals until the node is detected, usually within 30 to 60 minutes. Lymphoseek imaging begins at 10 to 15 minutes and requires only multiple-view static images. SPECT or SPECT/CT may be helpful. Transmission images using a cobalt-57 sheet source placed between the patient and the camera for 10 to 15 seconds can provide anatomical landmarks. Visualized nodes are marked on the skin. An intraoperative gamma probe is used at surgery for detection. The sentinel node usually has uptake >2 times background. Although intraoperative vital blue dye injection and radiolabeled colloids have been used independently, sensitivity is highest if they are used together.

Lymphedema—Extremity Lymphoscintigraphy

The lymphatic system removes interstitial fluid from all parts of the body and returns lymph to the blood circulation. Lymphedema results from impaired lymphatic transport, which can be caused by injury, infection, or a congenital abnormality of the lymphatics. Arm lymphedema is a frequent complication of breast cancer therapy with axillary node dissection, with an estimated frequency of 5% to 30%. Lower extremity lymphedema results from treatment of pelvic cancer, with a reported frequency of ranging from 10% to 49%. The most common cause worldwide is due to filariasis. However, in developed countries, postsurgical and postphlebitic lymphedema is most common. Congenital causes are much less common. Delay in diagnosis and treatment allows for secondary fibrosis and lipid deposition, which is much more difficult to treat. Untreated lymphatic stasis results in inflammation, fibrosis, and a decrease in the number of functioning lymphatic channels and lipid deposition. In the extremities, the lymphatic system consists of a superficial system that collects

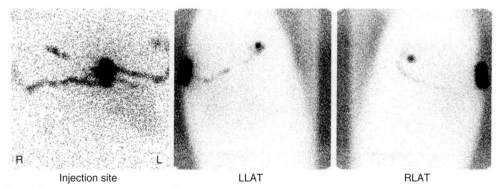

R　　　　　　　　　　　L
Injection site　　　　　　　　　　LLAT　　　　　　　　　　RLAT

Fig. 13.25 Sentinel node lymphoscintigraphy in a patient with melanoma in the midback demonstrates its value for detecting unpredictable patterns of drainage. Activity moves from the region of the lesion in the midback to sentinel lymph nodes in the right and left axilla. *L,* Left; *LLAT,* left lateral; *R,* right; *RLAT,* right lateral.

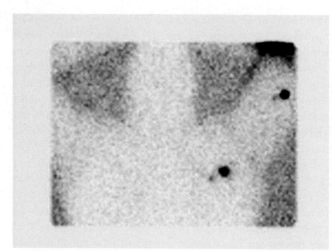

Fig. 13.26 In-transit epitrochlear sentinel node. Recently diagnosed melanoma of the left forearm. Scatter from the injection site can be seen in the upper left. An in-transit node is seen just below that in the epitrochlear region. Uptake is also seen in the axilla. The epitrochlear node is the sentinel node.

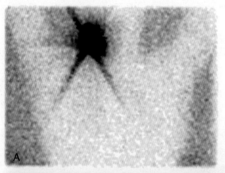

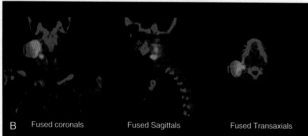

Fused coronals   Fused Sagittals   Fused Transaxials

Fig. 13.27 Sentinel node, advantage of single-photon emission computed tomography with computed tomography (SPECT/CT). Melanoma neck lesion. (A) Planar image after Tc-99m SC intradermal injection shows intense uptake at site of injection in right neck. No definite sentinel node was detected. (B) Fused SPECT/CT image shows a sentinel lymph node immediately medial to the injection site.

lymph from the skin and subcutaneous tissue and a deeper system that drains muscle, bone, and deep vessels. The two drainage systems merge in the pelvis and in the axilla. There are nonsurgical and surgical approaches to the treatment of lymphedema, which include manual lymphatic massage, pneumatic compression, hyperthermia, pharmacological interventions, liposuction, and microsurgery.

Lymphoscintigraphy has largely replaced the invasive and technically difficult technique of lymphangiography. Scintigraphy to determine whether the patient's edema is lymphatic in

origin has a long history. The protocol has never been standardized, but various radiopharmaceuticals and methodologies all seem to work well. Filtered Tc-99m SC is most commonly used in the United States; however, various other radiocolloids have been used worldwide, including Tc-99m antimony SC, Tc-99m albumin colloid, and Tc-99m human serum albumin (HAS). The radiotracer is injected in the webs of the toes or fingers intracutaneously or subcutaneously. Scans are obtained at 30 minutes to 2 hours and at 4 to 6 hours after tracer administration, imaging from the toes to the level of the liver.

The diagnostic criteria for lymphatic dysfunction include delay, asymmetrical or absent visualization of deep lymphatic channels and regional lymph nodes, and the presence of a "dermal backflow" pattern (Fig. 13.28). Other findings that may be seen include collateral lymphatic channels, interrupted vascular structures, lymphatic leaks, and lymph nodes deep to the lymphatic system.

MOLECULAR BREAST IMAGING— SCINTIMAMMOGRAPHY

Radiography mammography has long been the primary breast cancer screening method, with a sensitivity of approximately 85% but that decreases to 68% in women with dense breasts. Specificity is a major problem. Many patients undergo biopsy for lesions detected by mammography that are ultimately diagnosed as benign. The positive predictive value of mammography for breast cancer ranges from 20% in women under age 50 to 60% to 80% in women age 50 to 69. Ultrasonography similarly has a low positive predictive value. Contrast-enhanced MRI is sensitive for breast cancer detection and advocated for screening high-risk groups with *BRCA1* and *BRCA2* genetic mutations. However, it has a quite variable reported sensitivity and specificity. Patients cannot undergo the examination if they have renal failure, claustrophobia, implanted devices, or large body habitus.

F-18 Fluorodeoxyglucose PET Mammography

Whole-body F-18 FDG PET/CT is useful for the staging and restaging of locally advanced breast carcinoma. However, the sensitivity of the standard FDG PET study is more limited in breast cancer than in many other tumors, especially in low-grade breast tumors. The reported sensitivity is 85%, and the specificity is 76%. The sensitivity is less than 50% for small (≤1 cm) low-grade invasive cancers and ductal carcinoma in situ (DCIS).

Dedicated F-18 Fluorodeoxyglucose PET Breast Mammography

Dedicated F-18 FDG PET breast mammography (PEM) has a high intrinsic resolution of 1 to 2 mm and is superior to whole-body scanners for the detection of primary tumors. However, PEM still has the disadvantages of whole-body FDG PET imaging, including the same preparation (fasting, controlled serum glucose levels), a 50- to 60-minute delay after injection, and the need for significant dosing-room shielding. The sensitivity is

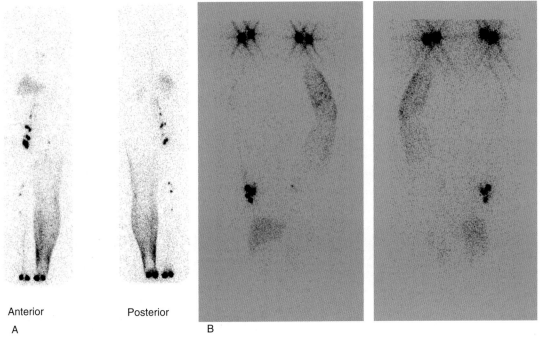

Fig. 13.28 Lymphedema. (A) Lymphoscintigraphy of the lower extremities. A 60-year-old male with history of malignant melanoma and nodal excisions of the left knee over 20 years ago presented with left lower extremity edema. Scan at 4 hours after injection of Tc-99m SC in webs of feet. Normal nodal drainage is seen on the right. The enlarged left lower extremity has an obstructive dermal pattern of distribution, and no nodal drainage is seen. (B) Patient with past history of breast cancer. Anterior and posterior images, upper extremities. The left arm has a dermal pattern, and no transit to nodes is seen on that side.

87%, and the specificity is 85%, but the specificity is 73% for subcentimeter cancers and DCIS. Direct comparison studies of dedicated FDG PET with whole-body FDG PET have found higher sensitivity for dedicated breast PET (92–95%) versus whole-body PET (56–58%) and PET/CT (87%). False positives occur with fibrocystic changes and fibroadenomas. Dedicated FDG PET/CT can be valuable to follow the effects of therapy, identify tumor recurrence, and visualize multifocal or synchronous lesions in the ipsilateral and contralateral breast.

Tc-99m Sestamibi Scintimammography

Tc-99m sestamibi (methoxy-isobutyl-isonitrile, Cardiolite) is most commonly used for cardiac perfusion imaging and parathyroid scintigraphy. For breast imaging, the same radiopharmaceutical is marketed as Miraluma. This Tc-99m sestamibi–labeled lipophilic cation passively diffuses into the cell. The positively charged lipophilic molecule is attracted to the negatively charged mitochondria, where it is retained. Cell clearance is slow, allowing time for imaging. Uptake occurs in various other benign and malignant tumors.

Standard breast gamma camera imaging with Tc-99m sestamibi can detect breast cancers, even in dense breasts (Fig. 13.29). Patients are positioned prone, with the breast hanging off the table or through a special holder cutout. The sensitivity and specificity are about 83%, but they are lower for lesions less than 2 cm. *Dedicated breast gamma camera imaging* is now commercially available, which provides high-resolution images with a reported sensitivity of >92% and a specificity of 71% to 80% (Fig. 13.30). These solid-state detector cameras are available with single- and dual-head configurations and optional

biopsy device attachments. Detection is not affected by breast density, but sensitivity is decreased for cancers <1 cm, DCIS, and nonpalpable lesions. Additional foci of mammographically occult (<1 cm) breast cancers are detected in 9% of women with newly diagnosed breast cancer. Standard mammographic positioning (craniocaudal and mediolateral oblique) is used, with the breast in direct contact with the gamma camera.

The breast is highly radiation sensitive. The risk for radiation-induced cancers from imaging studies such as mammography has been of concern. Originally, 20 mCi Tc-99m sestamibi was used for Scintimammography; however, the dose has been reduced to as low as 8 mCi without loss of sensitivity (see Fig. 13.30), and even lower doses are being investigated. The presently recommended dose is 10 mCi, which results in a breast radiation dose approximately 10 times the effective dose of digital mammography (see Appendix 1).

A protocol summary for scintimammography is described (Box 13.7). Normal breast parenchyma shows low-level activity. Small focal areas of uptake are suggestive of malignancy (Fig. 13.30); patchy uptake is likely benign. However, the intensity of the uptake may not parallel the aggressiveness of the lesion. Uptake in the axilla may represent nodal metastasis if there is no dose infiltration, but the sensitivity for nodal disease is not high.

RADIONUCLIDE MONOCLONAL ANTIBODY THERAPY—B-CELL LYMPHOMA

Non-Hodgkin lymphoma is the most common hematological cancer. Whereas high-grade non-Hodgkin lymphoma is often

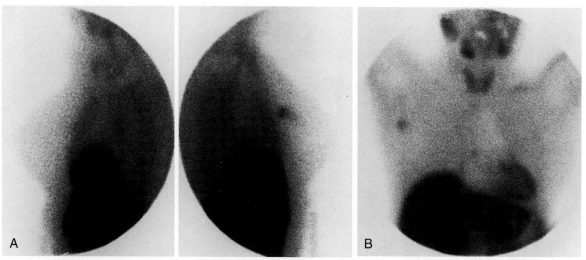

Fig. 13.29 Gamma camera scintimammography. A palpable right breast mass shows obvious accumulation of Tc-99m sestamibi in the upper outer breast on lateral (A) and anterior (B) images on a routine gamma camera scan.

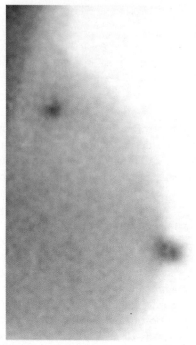

Fig. 13.30 Dedicated scintimammography. Tc-99m sestamibi scan of 7-mm invasive ductal carcinoma using only 8 mCi (296 MBq). (With permission, Even-Sapir E, Golan O, Menes T, et al. Breast imaging utilizing dedicated gamma camera and 99mTc-MIBI: experience at the Tel Aviv Medical Center and review of the literature breast imaging. *Semin Nucl Med.* 2016;46[4]:286–293.)

BOX 13.7   Tc-99m Scintimammography With Tc-99m Sestamibi: Summary Protocol

Patient Preparation
Nil per os (NPO) 4 to 6 hours, except water

Radiopharmaceutical
Tc-99m sestamibi intravenously—8 mCi (296 MBq)
Consider lower doses (4 mCi [74–148 MBq]) for dual-head cadmium zinc telluride detector small-field-of-view dedicated breast cameras.

Instrumentation and Acquisition
Small-field-of-view dedicated single-head or dual-head breast camera:
    Begin imaging 5 to 10 minutes after injection.
    Immobilize breast with light compression.
    Image 7 to 10 min/view (craniocaudal [CC] and mediolateral oblique [MLO]).
    Image injection site.
    Additional views optional: True (90-degrees) lateral, axillary tail, cleavage view, exaggerated CC, implant displacement
Standard gamma camera (not preferred):
    Begin imaging 5 to 10 minutes after injection.
    Place patient prone on table with breasts hanging dependent, preferably in holder through cutouts.
    Image 10 min/view for prone lateral and supine anteroposterior chest, including axilla.
    Image injection site.
    Obtain marker view of any palpable nodule.

---

curable, low-grade disease is generally incurable. Patients ultimately relapse after initial positive responses, tumors become refractory, and transformations to high-grade tumors are common. The mean survival is 8 to 10 years with conventional radiation and chemotherapy. Numerous treatment options are available, including chemotherapy, radiation therapy, vaccines, interleukin-2, stem cell transplants, surgical intervention, immunotherapy, and radioimmunotherapy. The standard first-line therapy of non-Hodgkins lymphoma is usually CHOP-R (cyclophosphamide, doxorubicin, vincristine, and prednisone) in combination with rituximab, a monoclonal antibody.

Antibodies are immune proteins produced by lymphocytes and plasma B cells in response to exposure to foreign antigens. IgG antibodies have two identical heavy (H) and two light (L) chains linked by a disulfide bridge (Fig. 13.31). Each chain is made up of a *variable* region (Fab'), responsible for binding to a cell-surface antigen and the *constant* region (Fc), involved with cell destruction by complement fixation and antibody-dependent cell cytotoxicity.

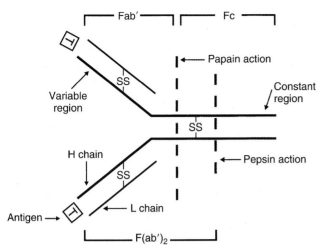

Fig. 13.31 IgG antibody. The molecule can be digested enzymatically by papain, resulting in three parts, two Fab′ fragments and one Fc fragment, or by pepsin to produce one F(ab′)₂ and one Fc subfragment. Fab′ may be produced by splitting the disulfide bond of F(ab′)₂SS.

TABLE 13.5 Lymphoma Therapy Radiopharmaceuticals—Y-90 Rituximab and I-131 Tositumomab		
Therapeutic Radiopharmaceutical	**Y-90 Rituximab (Zevalin)**	**I-131 Tositumomab (Bexxar)[a]**
Radionuclide half-life	64 hr	8 days
Beta particle	2.293 MeV 5-mm path	0.606 MeV 8-mm path
Gamma emission	No	Yes, 364 keV
Pretreatment dosimetry	No	Yes
Pretreatment unlabeled antibody	Rituximab chimeric	Tositumomab murine
HAMA	1–2%	60%
Outpatient therapy	+	+/−

HAMA, Human antimouse antibody.
[a]Bexxar is no longer commercially available.

A specific monoclonal antibody can be produced by fusing myeloma cancer cells with lymphocytes from the spleen of a mouse immunized with a particular antigen. These "hybridoma" cells have the specific antibody-production capacity of the lymphocytes and the immortality of cancer cells. However, the human immune system recognizes these murine monoclonal antibodies as foreign and may mount an immunological response with a human antimouse antibody (HAMA). This may be mild, with fever and hives, or severe, with shortness of breath, hypotension, or even fatal anaphylaxis. Antibody fragments formed from smaller active regions contribute less to the HAMA response; however, the potential for serious reactions remains. Chimera monoclonal antibodies that replace the murine Fc portion of the antibody with a human component and fully human monoclonal antibodies can potentially lessen this problem. The therapeutic radiolabeled monoclonal antibody currently available clinically, Y-90 ibritumomab tiuxetan (Zevalin), is derived from whole murine antibodies.

CD20 is an antigen expressed on the surface of mature and malignant B cells and is widely expressed in many B-cell malignancies, including lymphoma, chronic lymphocytic leukemia, and some forms of Hodgkin disease. Because of its high expression, several antibodies targeting CD20 expressing lymphoma have been developed. Rituximab was the first monoclonal antibody drug approved by the FDA for the treatment of CD20-expressing lymphoma.

Similar antibodies labeled with beta-emitters such as Y-90 and I-131 can directly kill the tumor cell (Table 13.5). Because beta radiation travels only a short distance, only nearby cells are irradiated. This limits damage to normal cells, but it still produces a *crossfire* effect, killing adjacent tumor cells not bound by the antibody. Thus, radiolabeled monoclonal antibody therapies can result in a better tumor response than nonradiolabeled monoclonal antibody therapies.

Yttrium-90 Ibritumomab Tiuxetan (Zevalin)

Y-90 Zevalin was the first radiolabeled antibody therapeutic agent approved by the FDA, in 2002. The murine immunoglobulin IgG1 kappa monoclonal CD20 antibody uses the chelator molecule tiuxetan to form a stable link to Y-90, a pure beta emitter. Y-90 has a high-energy (2.29 MeV) beta-particle that travels only 5 mm, depositing an effective dose of radiation close to the binding site. Zevalin was initially approved for the treatment of relapsed, refractory, or transformed CD20 + non-Hodgkin lymphoma but is now also approved as a first-line therapy. It is contraindicated in patients with a known hypersensitivity reaction to murine proteins (HAMA), >25% tumor involvement of marrow, or impaired marrow reserves. Patients must not have had myelotoxic therapies with autologous bone marrow transplant or stem-cell rescue. External-beam radiation should not have involved >25% of the marrow. The neutrophil count must be >1500 cells/mm³, and the platelet count must be >100,000.

Zevalin has an average physical half-life in the blood of 27 hours and a biological half-life of 48 hours, resulting in a dose to the tumor of 15 to17 Gray. There is some urinary excretion (7%), although most of the agent remains in the body. No special shielding is needed with this pure beta-emitter, and treatment can be performed as an outpatient. Few radiation safety precautions are required.

Methodology

Unlabeled rituximab (Rituxan) is administered before therapy to block CD20 antigens on cells circulating in the blood and spleen, thus limiting potential off-target toxicity. Patients should be closely monitored during the infusion because serious potentially fatal reactions can occur. Hydration and frequent voiding are important. Even though radiation exposure to others is low, patients should limit prolonged close contact, sleep apart, and restrict time in public places for the first 4 to 7 days. Exchange of bodily fluids in the first week should be discouraged, and careful bathroom hygiene should be encouraged.

Toxicity

Within 7 to 9 weeks, blood counts reach a nadir, with a 30% to 70% reduction in platelets and neutrophils, which may last 7 to 35 days. Approximately 7% of neutropenic patients are prone to fever and infections. Thrombocytopenia can result in hemorrhage. Only 1% to 2% of patients treated with Zevalin experience an HAMA response. Myelodysplasia or acute myelogenous leukemia occurs in 1.4% of patients. Seventy-five percent of patients experience some response, with 15% to 37% showing complete remission. This is significantly better than the results of nonlabeled Rituxan monoclonal antibody therapy alone. The duration of response ranges from 0.5 to 24.9 months.

I-131-labeled tositumomab (Bexxar) is a murine IgG2a therapeutic monoclonal antibody developed to target CD20, the same target as for Zevalin. It was also approved by the FDA in 2002. It has shown excellent efficacy and safety profiles in clinical trials; however, a more recent large clinical trial showed no significant improvement in response rate or survival between patients receiving Bexxar and CHOP and those receiving rituximab and CHOP. This resulted in declining sales that led to the discontinuation of the product by the manufacturer in 2014.

TC-99M SESTAMIBI RENAL IMAGING— ONCOCYTOMA VERSUS RENAL CELL CARCINOMA

The widespread use of CT has led to the increased detection of renal masses. Preoperative differentiation of aggressive forms of renal cell carcinoma from benign etiologies is a diagnostic dilemma. Without a definite diagnosis, most patients with solid renal lesions undergo partial or radical nephrectomy. Up to 20% of renal masses treated with nephrectomy are benign, with oncocytomas accounting for half of these. Tc-99m sestamibi uptake is a marker of mitochondrial metabolism and is useful for imaging of renal lesions with rich mitochondrial content, such as oncocytomas and hybrid oncocytic/chromophobe tumors, but not renal cell carcinoma. Published investigations have found good accuracy for making this differentiation. Tc-99m sestamibi SPECT/CT has the potential to spare patients unnecessary invasive procedures and surgery (Fig. 13.32). In a recent study 50 patients with a solid clinical T1 renal mass with subsequent surgical confirmation, Tc-99m sestamibi correctly identified 5/6 (83%) of oncocytomas and 2/2 (100%) of oncocytic/chromophobe adenomas. F-18 FDG has also shown marked uptake in oncocytomas, although this has not been extensively studied. Renal cell cancers, on the other hand, most frequently show low or background activity, with a sensitivity of 50% to 70%.

GALLIUM-67 TUMOR IMAGING

Gallium-67 (Ga-67) citrate was originally used as a bone-imaging agent, then subsequently used for infection and tumor imaging. Before FDG PET, Ga-67 was often used to help stage and restage various tumors, most commonly lymphoma. The imaging characteristics of Ga-67 are not optimal, due to its high-energy photons, high background activity, and 48-hour

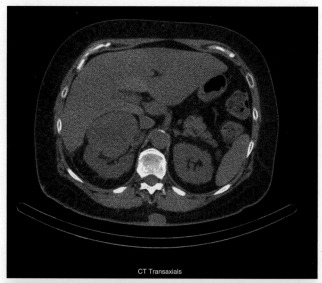

CT Transaxials

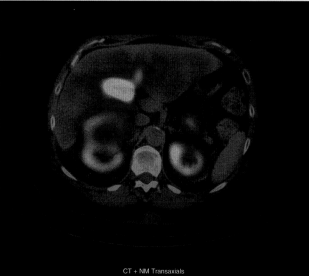

CT + NM Transaxials

Fig. 13.32 Tc-99m sestamibi single-photon emission computed tomography with computed tomography (SPECT/CT) for renal mass. The mass seen on CT *(above)* has definite sestamibi uptake. This rules out a renal cell carcinoma and is consistent with an oncocytoma or oncocytic/chromophobe adenoma.

imaging. Today it is rarely used for tumor imaging unless FDG PET imaging is not available. It still has a limited role for inflammatory and infection imaging for specific indications, as discussed in the chapter on infection.

SUGGESTED READING

SOMATOSTATIN RECEPTOR IMAGING AND THERAPY

Barrio M, Czernin J, Fanti S, et al. The impact of somatostatin receptor-directed PET/CT on the management of patients with neuroendocrine tumor: a systematic review and meta-analysis. *J Nucl Med*. 2017;58:756–761.

Bodei L, Ambrosini V, Hermann K, Modlin I. Current concepts in 68Ga-DOTATATE imaging of neuroendocrine neoplasms: interpretation, biodistribution, dosimetry, and molecular strategies. *J Nucl Med*. 2017;58:1718–1726.

Deppen SA, Blume J, Bobbey AJ, et al. Ga-68 DOTATATE compared with In-11-DTPA-Octreotide and conventional imaging for pulmonary and gastroenteropancreatic neuroendocrine tumors: a systematic review and meta-analysis. *J Nucl Med.* 2016;57:872–878.

Horch D, Ezziddin S, Haug A, et al. Effectiveness and side effects of peptide receptor radionuclide therapy for neuroendocrine neoplasms in German: a multi-institutional registry study with prospective followup. *Eur J Cancer.* 2016;58:41–51.

Kulkarni Harshad R, Singh A, Baum RP. Advances in the diagnosis of neuroendocrine neoplasms. *Semin Nucl Med.* 2017;46:395–404.

Oronsky B, Ma PC, Morgenstern D, Carter CA. Nothing but NET: a review of neuroendocrine tumors and carcinomas. *Neoplasia.* 2017;19:991–1002.

Sadowski SM, Neychev V, Millo C, et al. Prospective study of Ga-68-DOTATATE positron emission tomography/computed tomography for detecting gastro-entero-pancreatic neuroendocrine tumors and unknown primary sites. *J Clin Onc.* 2016;34:588–596.

Strosberg J, El-Haddad E, Wolin A, et al. Phase 3 Trial of Lu-177-Dotatate for midgut neuroendocrine tumors. *NEJM.* 2017;376:125–135.

ADRENAL IMAGING AND THERAPY

Carrasquillo JA, Pandit-Taskar N, Chen CC. I-131 metaiodobenzylguanidine therapy of pheochromocytoma and paraganglioma. *Semin Nucl Med.* 2016;46:203–214.

Castellani MR, Aktolun C, Buzzoni R, et al. Iodine-131 metaiodobenzylguanidine (I-131 MIBG) diagnosis and therapy of pheochromocytoma and paraganglioma: current problems, critical issues, and presentation of a sample case. *Q J Nucl Med Mol Imaging.* 2013;57:146–152.

Pepe G, Bombardieri E, Lorenzoni A, Chiti A. Single photon emission computed tomography tracers in the diagnosis of neuroendocrine tumors. *PET Clin.* 2014;9:11–26.

Wilson JS, Gains JE, Moroz V, et al. A systematic review of 131 I-meta iodobenzylguandine molecular radiotherapy of neuroblastoma. *Eur J Cancer.* 2014;50:801–815.

PROSTATE CANCER IMAGING

Fendler WP, Matthias Eiber, Beheshti M, et al. 68Ga-PMSA PET/CT: Joint EANM and SNMMI procedure guideline for prostate cancer imaging: version 1.0. *Eur J Nucl Med Mol Imaging.* 2017;44:1014–1024.

Fendler WP, Schmidt D, Wenter V, et al. 68Ga-PSMA PET/CT detects the location and extent of primary prostate cancer. *J Nucl Med.* 2016;57:1720–1725.

Parent EE, Schuster DM. Update on 18F-fluciclovine PET for prostate cancer. *J Nucl Med.* 2018;59(5):733–739.

Perera M, Papa N, Christidis D, et al. Sensitivity, specificity, and predictors of positive 68Ga-prostate-specific membrane antigen positron emission tomography in advanced prostate cancer: a systematic review and meta-analysis. *Eur Urol.* 2016;70:926–937.

Rabbar K, Ahmadzadehfar H, Kratochwil C, et al. German multicenter study investigating 177Lu-PMSA-617 radioligand therapy in advanced prostate cancer patients. *J Nucl Med.* 2017;58:85–90.

Roach PJ, Francis R, Emmett L, et al. The impact of 68Ga-PSMA PET/CT on management intent in prostate cancer: results of an Australian prospective multicenter study. *J Nucl Med.* 2018;59:82–88.

Rowe SP, Drzezga A, Neumaier B, et al. Prostate-specific membrane antigen-targeted radiohalogenated PET and therapeutic agents for prostate cancer. *J Nucl Med.* 2016;57:90S–96S.

Rowe SP, Macura KJ, Mena E, et al. PSMA-based [(18)F]DCFPyL is superior to conventional imaging for lesion detection in patients with metastatic prostate cancer. *Mol Imaging Biol.* 2016;18:411–419.

BREAST IMAGING

Berg WA. Nuclear breast imaging: clinical results and future directions. *J Nucl Med.* 2016;57:46S–52S.

Berg WA, Madsen KS, Schilling K, et al. Comparative effectiveness of positron emission mammography and MRI in the contralateral breast of women with newly diagnosed breast cancer. *AJR Am J Roentgenol.* 2012;198:219–232.

Brem RF, Ruda RC, Yang JL, et al. Breast-specific imaging for the detection of mammographically occult breast cancer in women at increased risk. *J Nucl Med.* 2016;57:678–682.

Conners AL, Hruska CB, Tortorelli CL, et al. Lexicon for standardized interpretation of gamma camera molecular breast imaging: observer agreement and diagnostic accuracy. *Eur J Nucl Med Mol Imaging.* 2012;39:971–982.

Even-Sapir E, Golan O, Menes T, et al. Breast imaging utilizing dedicated gamma camera and 99mTc-MIBI: experience at the Tel Aviv medical center and review of the literature breast imaging. *Semin Nucl Med.* 2016;46:286–293.

Fowler AM. A molecular approach to breast imaging. *J Nucl Med.* 2014;55:177–180.

Surti S. Radionuclide methods and instrumentation for breast cancer detection and diagnosis. *Semin Nucl Med.* 2013;43:271–280.

SENTINEL NODE LYMPHOSCINTIGRAPHY

Gershenwald JE, Ross MI. Sentinel-lymph-node biopsy for cutaneous melanoma. *N Engl J Med.* 2011;364:1738–1745.

Moncayo VM, Alazraki AL, Alazraki NP, Aarsvold JN. Sentinel lymph node biopsy procedures. *Semin Nucl Med.* 2017;47:595–617.

Pasquali S, Mocellin S, Campana LG, et al. Early (sentinel lymph node biopsy-guided) versus delayed lymphadenectomy in melanoma patients with lymph node metastases: personal experience and literature meta-analysis. *Cancer.* 2010;116:1201–1209.

Wong SL, Balch CM, Hurley P, et al. Sentinel lymph node biopsy for melanoma: American Society of Clinical Oncology and Society of Surgical Oncology joint clinical practice guideline. *Ann Surg Oncol.* 2012;19:3313–3324.

ANTIBODY THERAPY

Eskian M, Khorasanizadeh M, Kraeber-Bodere F, Rezaei N. Radioimmunotherapy in non-Hodgkin lymphoma: prediction and assessment of response. *Crit Rev Oncol Hematol.* 2016;107:182–189.

Rizzieri D. Zevalin (ibritumomab tiuxetan): After more than a decade of treatment experience, what have we learned? *Crit Rev Oncol/Hematol.* 2016;105:5–17.

TC-99M SESTAMIBI—RENAL ONCOCYTOMA/CHROMOPHOBE ADENOMA VERSUS RENAL CELL CARCINOMA

Gorin MA, Rowe SP, Baras AS, et al. Prospective evaluation of 99mTc-sestamibi SPECT/CT for the diagnosis of renal oncocytomas and hybrid oncocytic/chromophobe adenomas. *Eur Assoc. Urology.* 2015;69:413–416.

14

Central Nervous System

Molecular imaging examinations using positron emission tomography (PET) and single-photon emission computed tomography (SPECT) are frequently used in the brain because they can complement the anatomical information from magnetic resonance (MR) imaging and computed tomography (CT). By examining cellular function, disease is often detected at an earlier stage, or the extent of disease may be more accurately demonstrated with nuclear medicine techniques. Hybrid cameras combining PET and SPECT with CT or MR (PET/CT, SPECT/CT, and PET/MR) allow optimal image acquisition so that structural and physiological data can be accurately correlated. Some indications for nuclear medicine imaging in the central nervous system (CNS) include the following: characterization of dementia, diagnosis of parkinsonian syndromes, presurgical seizure focus localization, confirmation of tumor recurrence, brain death identification, stroke risk evaluation in vascular disorders (e.g., following carotid occlusion or in Moya Moya), and assessment of cerebrospinal fluid (CSF) flow or ventricular shunt function. The most common indications are listed in Box 14.1.

The blood–brain barrier (BBB) makes imaging the CNS more complicated. When diseases such as glioblastoma disrupt the BBB, traditional agents, such as thalium-201 (Tl-201) and technetium-99m (Tc-99m) sestamibi, can be used. The intact BBB, however, prevents most radiopharmaceuticals from entering the brain (Fig. 14.1). There are two lipophilic SPECT agents currently available clinically, Tc-99m hexamethylpropyleneamine oxime (Tc-99m HMPAO) and Tc-99m ethyl cysteinate diethylester (Tc-99m ECD), that are able to traverse the barrier and are taken up in viable neurons. The most commonly used PET agent, F-18 fluorodeoxyglucose (F-18 FDG), is a glucose analog and is actively taken up by the brain using the same pathways as the glucose that the brain requires for fuel. Other radiotracers have been created that are able to exploit other uptake mechanisms, such as those for key amino acids. For example, imaging nigrostriatal function in Parkinson's disease can be performed with F-18 F-DOPA PET or with the SPECT dopamine transporter (DAT) analog iodine-123 ioflupane (I-123 DaTscan).

PET imaging has made significant contributions to our understanding of dementia. The impact of PET radiopharmaceuticals approved for the detection of abnormal beta-amyloid protein deposits (F-18 florbetapir, F-18 flutemetamol, F-18 florbetaben) is being investigated in multicenter trials looking at Alzheimer's and mild cognitive impairment (MCI). Other proteins that accumulate in the brain in other dementia subtypes, such as the protein Tau, are also being explored with targeting radiotracers. Additional imaging biomarkers are being sought for neuroinflammation and other processes that contribute to neurodegenerative diseases.

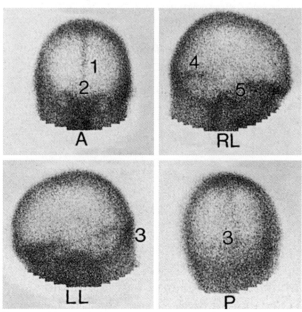

• **Fig. 14.1** Normal delayed technetium-99m (Tc-99m) diethylenetriaminepentaacetic acid (DTPA) planar images. Anterior *(A)*, right lateral *(RL)*, left lateral *(LL)*, and posterior *(P)* projections. The superior sagittal sinus *(1)* is seen on anterior and posterior views. The floor of the frontal sinus *(2)*, confluence of sinuses *(3)*, transverse sinuses *(4)*, and sphenoid sinus *(5)* are faintly seen.

BOX 14.1 Indications for Molecular Imaging of the Brain With Nuclear Medicine Techniques

Epileptic seizure focus identification
Dementia diagnosis
Parkinson's disease/parkinsonian syndrome differentiation from essential tremor
Recurrent glioma
Differentiate tumor from opportunistic infection in ring-enhancing lesions
Vascular reserve assessment in patients at high stroke risk
Acute stroke: select candidates for thrombolytic therapy
Brain death diagnosis
Ventricular shunt function
Normal-pressure hydrocephalus
Cerebrospinal fluid leak
Investigational
   Psychiatric diseases
   Head trauma
   Neuroinflammation
   Tau and other proteinopathies in various types of dementia

TABLE 14.1 Clinically Approved Radiopharmaceuticals for Functional Brain Imaging Able to Cross Intact Blood–Brain Barrier

Agent	Localizing Mechanism	Use
F-18 fluorodeoxyglucose (F-18 FDG)	Glucose metabolism: Cellular activity and viability	• Neurodegenerative disease diagnosis • Assess viability and ischemia • Tumor (recurrent) diagnosis • Interictal seizure focus identification
Technetium-99m (Tc-99m) hexamethyl propyleneamine (Tc-99m HMPAO, Ceretec) Tc-99m ethyl cysteinate dimer (Tc-99m ECD, Neurolite)	Perfusion and metabolism mirror cellular activity and viability	• Neurodegenerative disease diagnosis • Assess viability and ischemia • Ictal/interictal seizure focus identification
I-123 Ioflupane (DaTscan)	Presynaptic dopamine transporter (DAT) binding	Diagnose parkinsonian syndromes/Parkinson's disease
F-18 florbetapir (F-18 AV-45) F-18 florbetaben (F-18 AV-1) F-18 flutemetamol (F-18-3′-F-PIB)	Beta-amyloid (Aβ) deposition	Excluding or identifying potential Alzheimer's disease
Thallium-201 (Tl-201) Tc-99m sestamibi (MIBI)	Nonspecific uptake relates perfusion and activity • Tl-201 Na+/K+ pump • MIBI mitochondrial activity	Differentiating recurrent brain tumor from MRI-enhancing posttreatment scar

MRI, Magnetic resonance imaging.

This chapter reviews commonly performed scintigraphic brain-imaging procedures. Radiopharmaceuticals able to cross the intact BBB for clinical use in PET and SPECT are listed in Table 14.1. Several experimental PET agents are listed in Table 14.2.

Knowledge of brain anatomy is critical in understanding patterns of disease and image interpretation. The brain consists of two hemispheres, further segmented into lobes, above the tentorium and the cerebellum below in the posterior fossa. The lobes of the brain are illustrated in Fig. 14.2. Within these lobes, key functional centers, or regions, have been identified that are important when trying to assimilate clinical changes with anatomical and functional images (Fig. 14.3). Studies such as dynamic radionuclide brain flow and brain death examination allow visualization of the vascular supply of the brain to a limited degree, so understanding the arterial and venous anatomy is important (Figs. 14.4 and 14.5). Even more important for image interpretation is familiarity with the cerebral regions these vessels supply (Fig. 14.6).

RADIOPHARMACEUTICALS

The brain is an obligate glucose user, and it is possible to determine the level of activity in different areas of the brain when imaging with the glucose analog F-18 FDG. The level of regional cerebral glucose metabolism (rCGM) usually closely correlates with regional cerebral blood flow (rCBF), and both parameters reflect activity in the neuron.

F-18 FDG is able to cross the BBB using glucose transporter systems. After entering the neuron, rapid phosphorylation by hexokinase-1 occurs. F-18 FDG cannot proceed further along the glucose metabolism pathway, and once phosphorylated, it cannot cross back through the cell membrane. Approximately 4% of the administered dose is localized to the brain. By 35 minutes after injection, 95% of peak uptake is achieved. Urinary excretion is rapid, with 10% to 40% of the dose cleared in 2 hours. F-18 FDG can be shipped from regional cyclotron

TABLE 14.2 Brain Positron Emission Tomography (PET) Radiopharmaceuticals for Experimental Use

Agent	Imaging Target
C-11 PIB	Beta-amyloid (Aβ) deposition
F-18 FDDNP	Aβ, tau, other proteins (e.g., Huntingtin)
F-18 flortaucipir (F-18 AV-1451)	Tau deposition
F-18 MISO Cu-64 ATSM	Tumor hypoxia
F-18 fluorothymidine (F-18 FLT)	DNA synthesis/tumor diagnosis
F-18 fluoroethyl L-tyrosine thymidine (18F-FET) C-11 methionine	Amino acid metabolism/peptide synthesis/tumor diagnosis
F-18 fluoro-L-dopa	Peptide synthesis (tumor) and Neurotransmitter (clinical use at limited sites)
C-11 dihydrotetrabenazine (C-11 DTBZ) F-18 fluoropropyldihydrotetrabenazine (F-18 DTBZ)	Vesicular monoamine transporter 2
C-11 raclopride F-18 fallypride	D2/D3 dopamine receptor activity
C-11 carfentanil	Mu opiate receptor activity
F-18 FDPN	Opiate receptor (nonspecific) activity
C-11 flunitrazepam	Benzodiazepine receptor activity
C-11 scopolamine	Muscarinic cholinergic receptor activity
C-11 ephedrine	Adrenergic terminals
O-15 H2O	Blood flow
O-15 O2	Oxygen metabolism and flow
O-15 or C-11 carboxyhemoglobin	Blood volume

F-18 FDDPN, 2-(-(6-((2-[18F]fluoroethyl)(methyl)-amino)-2-napthyl)ethylideine) malonitrile; *FDPN*, fluoroethyl-6-O-diphrenorphine; *F-18 MISO*, fluoromisonidazole; *PIB*, Pittsburgh B compound.

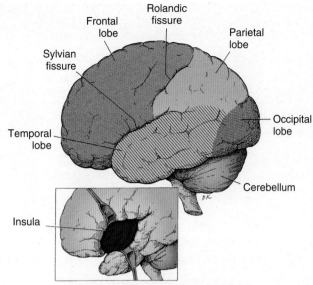

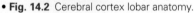

• **Fig. 14.2** Cerebral cortex lobar anatomy.

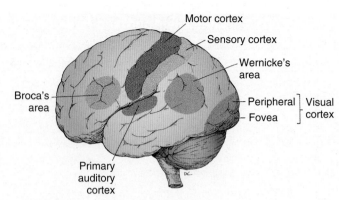

• **Fig. 14.3** Motor, sensory, visual, speech, and auditory functional and associative centers of the brain.

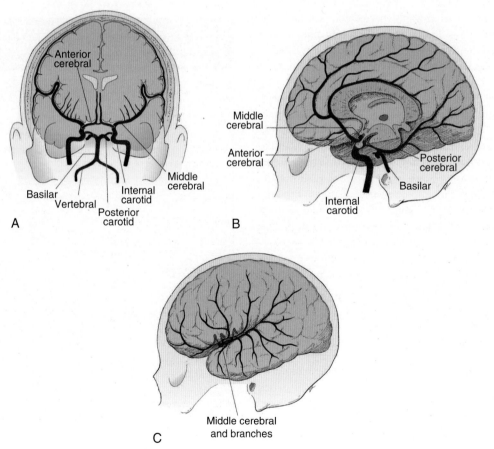

• **Fig. 14.4** Cerebral arterial anatomy on (A) coronal and (B) midline sagittal sections. Vertebral arteries join to form the basilar artery posteriorly. The basilar artery and the two anterior internal carotid arteries then form the circle of Willis in the base of the brain. From there, two anterior cerebral arteries anteromedially, the middle cerebral arteries laterally, and two posterior cerebral arteries posteromedially are seen. The anterior cerebral artery supplies the anterior cerebrum along its *medial* margin above the corpus callosum and extends posteriorly to the parietal fissure and to anterior portions of the basal ganglia centrally. The posterior cerebral arteries also lie medially and supply the occipital lobe and cerebellum. The middle cerebral arteries run laterally in the sylvian fissure, then backward and upward on the surface of the insula, where they divide into branches to the lateral cerebral hemispheres. (C) Left lateral view shows its superficial course over the cortex.

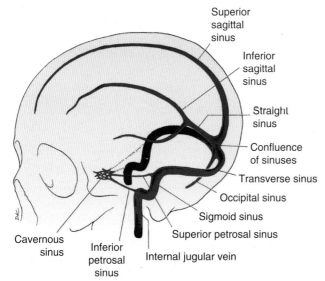

• **Fig. 14.5** Cerebral venous anatomy. The superior sagittal sinus runs along the falx within the superior margin of the interhemispheric fissure. The inferior sagittal sinus is smaller, courses over the corpus callosum, and joins with the great vein of Galen to form the straight sinus, which drains into the superior sagittal sinus at the confluence of sinuses (torcular herophili) at the occipital protuberance. Transverse sinuses drain the sagittal and occipital sinuses into the internal jugular vein.

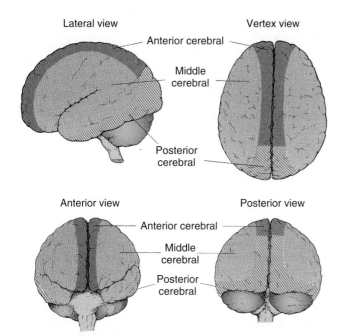

• **Fig. 14.6** Regional cerebral cortical perfusion of the anterior, middle, and posterior cerebral arteries.

production facilities due to its 110-minute half-life. As with all PET emitters, its decay results in two high-energy 511-keV gamma photons traveling at 180 degrees, which are best detected by a dedicated PET/CT or PET/MR camera.

The two SPECT agents currently used to assess regional cerebral blood flow are Tc-99m HMPAO and Tc-99m ECD. Favorable characteristics of these two neutral, lipophilic agents include high first-pass extraction across the BBB, distribution corresponding to rCBF, and desirable 140-keV gamma photons. However, both slightly underestimate true rCBF, especially at

high-flow states. The Tc-99m perfusion agents are relatively fixed once inside in the neuron. Therefore images can be delayed and still show what the perfusion pattern looked like at the time of injection. For example, if the agent is injected during an epileptic seizure, images can be performed after the seizures are brought under control (within a few hours).

Tc-99m HMPAO (Tc-99m exametazime [Ceretec]) was first introduced in the mid-1980s. It was originally available as a kit requiring use within 30 minutes of radiolabeling; however, stabilizers have since been added, allowing a 4-hour shelf life after addition of the radiolabel. Doses from the radiopharmacy should be labeled with fresh generator eluate (<2 hours old) just before delivery. Tc-99m HMPAO has an approximately 80% first-pass extraction; 3.5% to 7% of the injected dose localizes in the brain within 1 minute of injection. Once across the BBB, it enters the neuron and becomes a polar hydrophilic molecule trapped inside the cell. However, some of the radiopharmaceutical may be present in different isomeric forms that are not trapped. Although up to 15% of the dose washes out in the first 2 minutes, little loss occurs over the next 24 hours. SPECT images can be acquired from 20 minutes to 2 hours after injection. Excretion is largely renal (40%) and gastrointestinal (15%).

Tc-99m ECD (Tc-99m bicisate, Neurolite) is a neutral lipophilic agent that passively diffuses across the BBB like Tc-99m HMPAO. Once prepared, the Tc-99m ECD dose is stable for 6 to 8 hours. It has a first-pass extraction of 60% to 70%, with peak brain activity reaching 5% to 6% of the injected dose. The blood clearance is more rapid than Tc-99m HMPAO, resulting in better brain-to-background ratios. At 1 hour, less than 5% of the dose remains in the blood, compared with more than 12% of a Tc-99m HMPAO dose.

Once inside the cell, Tc-99m ECD undergoes enzymatic deesterification, forming polar metabolites unable to cross the cell membrane. However, slow (roughly 6% per hour) washout of some labeled metabolites occurs, with almost 25% of the brain activity cleared by 4 hours. Although images may be superior to those with Tc-99m HMPAO at 15 to 30 minutes after injection, they may be suboptimal if imaging is delayed.

PET Image Acquisition

Patient preparation for F-18 FDG brain imaging is similar to that for oncology applications. Patients should fast for 4 to 6 hours before injection, have serum glucose less than 200 mg/dL, have had insulin withheld for 2 hours (short-acting insulin) to 8 to 12 hours (long-acting insulin), and avoid strenuous exercise for a few days before the test. Exercise and insulin cause radiotracer to be shunted into muscle, decreasing activity in the brain.

F-18 FDG should be injected in a quiet, dimly lit room with the patient remaining still and undisturbed during the uptake period (at least 30-35 minutes). CT images are limited, particularly in the posterior fossa, because low-dose protocols are used and the fixed camera gantry angle contributes to noise and streak artifact, respectively. The posterior fossa also poses a problem when PET/MR is used if calculated attenuation correction is not performed properly. Without the CT for attenuation correction, mathematical or atlas-based attenuation-correction methods are used that could result in substantial artifacts on the

BOX 14.2 Example Protocol for F-18 FDG Brain PET/CT Imaging

Patient Preparation

- Patient should fast 4 to 6 hours, avoid carbohydrates, and maintain normal blood glucose.
- Encourage oral hydration.
- If patient takes insulin, delay injection until effects have worn off (e.g., 2 hours after short-acting insulin, 8-12 hours for long acting).
- Check blood glucose. If less than 180 to 200 mg/dL, continue.
- Elevated glucose: Consider rescheduling, administer insulin, recheck, and delay 2 hours.
- If patient experiences seizures, an interictal scan is recommended. EEG may be used to avoid erroneous interpretation in postictal or occult ictal periods.
- If conscious sedation is required, administer short-acting benzodiazepine >20 minutes after injection, as close to scan acquisition as possible.

Radiopharmaceutical

- F-18 FDG 8 mCi (296 MBq) intravenous (IV) (range 5-12 mCi [185-444 MBq])
- Inject in a quiet, dimly lit room, with the patient's eyes open.
- Wait 35 to 60 minutes (adhere to this same delay on any subsequent scan).

Image Acquisition

- Low-dose CT scan for attenuation correction/anatomical localization (contrast optional)
- Acquisition: 7 to 12 minutes per bed position for one bed position
  - Serial dynamic scans can be acquired if significant motion artifact is anticipated (e.g., five 2-minute frames).

Processing

- Orient brain along the anterior commissure–posterior commissure plane.
- Iterative (or analytic) reconstruction, automated software
- Pixel size < 2 mm

CT, Computed tomography; *EEG,* electroencephalogram; *FDG,* fluorodeoxyglucose; *PET,* positron emission tomography.

BOX 14.3 Single-Photon Emission Computed Tomography (SPECT) Cerebral Perfusion Imaging Protocol

Patient Preparation

None; start intravenous (IV) line in advance.

Radiopharmaceutical

Tc-99m HMPAO (Ceretec) or Tc-99m ECD (Neurolite)
Adults: 20 to 30 mCi (740-1100 MBq) IV
Pediatric dose: 0.2 to 0.3 mCi/kg (7.4-11.1 MBq); minimum dose 3 to 5 mCi (111-185 MBq) IV
Make sure dose falls within recommended 6-hour shelf-life parameter.
Inject in a quiet, dimly lit room, with the patient's eyes open.

Positioning

Maintain the minimum distance possible between camera heads and patient. A head-holder extension beyond the table end allows closer positioning of the camera heads.

Camera Setup

Orbit: Circular
Collimator: High resolution, parallel hole
Acquisition: Angle 3 degrees/step, 40 stops/head, 40 seconds/stop (total time, 27 minutes)
Computer: Matrix size: 128 × 128, zoom: 1.5 to 2 (for pixel size ≤ 3.5 mm)
Processing: Filtered back-projection or iterative reconstruction
Filter: Hamming, 1.2 high-frequency cutoff, or other low-pass (e.g., Butterworth) filter
Attenuation correction: Can be used

PET. Although time-of-flight technology is commonly used on the latest generation of scanners, this technique is less helpful than in the body, where scatter and attenuation are generally greater. A sample protocol is listed in Box 14.2.

For perfusion brain SPECT exams, no particular preparation is needed. As with PET, patients are injected in a quiet, dimly lit room. For the best-quality image, a delay of 30 to 60 minutes for Tc-99m ECD and 30 to 90 minutes for Tc-99m HMPAO should be used to improve the signal-to-noise ratio. A gamma camera with multiple heads creates images superior to single-headed systems. Patient positioning is just as important as the equipment used. The heads of the camera must come as close to the patient as possible, or resolution is reduced. A head-holder attachment extending from the end of the table allows the camera heads to come in closer than the width of a table or the patient's shoulders. In heavy patients and those whose shoulders obstruct the view, the posterior fossa may not be seen. The SPECT images can be processed with either iterative reconstruction or filtered back-projection. A filter is applied to smooth the image. In general, filters can be sampled and modified for each patient in the postprocessing stage to achieve an optimal image. A protocol for Tc-99m SPECT imaging is given in Box 14.3.

Tc-99m HMPAO SPECT images generally reflect cortical rCBF because it is determined by the oxygen demands of the brain. In addition, the blood-flow distribution is usually similar to the metabolism seen with F-18 FDG. Areas with more synaptic activity require greater blood flow. Activational studies can therefore target areas of the brain showing increased flow when stimulated by a certain task. Although findings on both SPECT and PET scans will closely correlate with neuronal activity, many studies have shown that the superior PET images are significantly more sensitive. Given this superiority, PET has largely replaced SPECT for several applications.

There is a 2:1 to 4:1 differential in uptake in gray matter compared with white matter. Lesions in the white matter are often undetectable or cannot be differentiated from adjacent CSF spaces, so magnetic resonance imaging (MRI) or CT correlation is necessary for identifying white-matter changes and enlarged ventricles. Although anatomy seen on CT and MRI is much more detailed, many structures are clearly visualized with scintigraphy (Fig. 14.7, *A, D*). Typically, activity is fairly evenly distributed between the lobes of the brain. However, this is dependent on the conditions at the time of injection. For example, bright lights will increase occipital lobe activity, falsely causing the frontal lobes to appear decreased.

The distribution of Tc-99m HMPAO differs only slightly from that of Tc-99m ECD. Tc-99m HMPAO accumulates more in the frontal lobes, thalamus, and cerebellum, whereas Tc-99m ECD shows a higher affinity for the parietal and occipital lobes. Although the differences are not usually noticeable, it would be

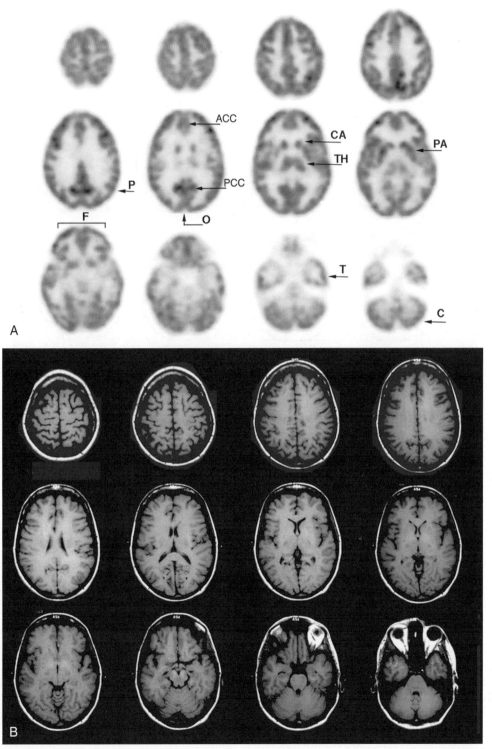

• **Fig. 14.7** Normal distribution of F-18 fluorodeoxyglucose (FDG). High-resolution (A) transverse positron emission tomography (PET) images with corresponding levels on T1-weighted magnetic resonance imaging (MRI) (B). Coronal PET

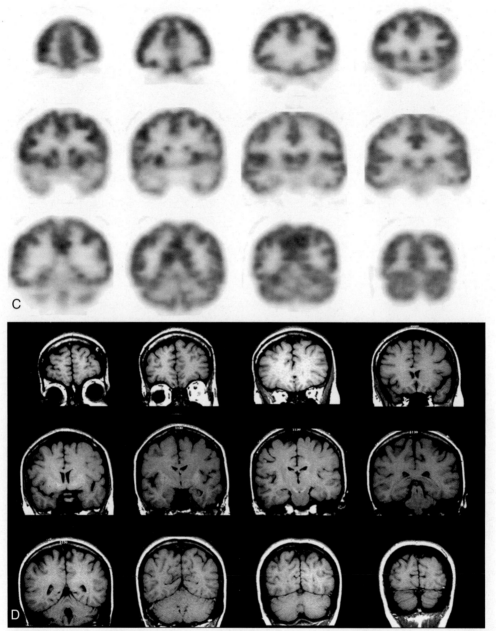

Fig. 14.7, cont'd (C) and comparable T1-weighted MRI (D). *ACC,* anterior cingulate cortex; *C,* Cerebellum; *Ca,* caudate; *F,* frontal lobe; *O,* occipital lobe; *P,* parietal lobe; *PA,* putamen; *PCC,* posterior cingulate cortex; *T,* temporal lobe; *Th,* thalamus.

best to use the same agent for serial examinations, and most clinicians use the agent with which they are most familiar.

The normal distribution of SPECT and PET agents also changes with age. In infants, a relative decrease is seen in frontal lobe perfusion. This frontal activity increases over time, reaching an adult level by about 2 years of age. In adults, global activity decreases with age, and this decrease is more prominent in the frontal regions. Given these changes, using comparison age-matched normal databases and computer programs that quantitate rCBF may help improve interpretation accuracy.

Although dementia can be the result of many conditions (Box 14.4), it is usually caused by a neurodegenerative disease (Box 14.5). Neurodegenerative disorders, also referred to as *proteinopathies,* are a varied group of disorders caused by the

BOX 14.4 **Common Causes of Dementia**

Degenerative dementias/neurodegenerative proteinopathies
Vascular dementia: stroke or multiinfarct dementia
Vitamin B$_{12}$ deficiency
Medication (drug abuse, overdose, or from side effects)
Alcohol abuse
Depression
Thyroid disorder
Infection (e.g., HIV/AIDS, Lyme disease)
Subdural hematoma
Normal-pressure hydrocephalus
Brain tumor
Multiple sclerosis
Renal failure, heart disease, chronic obstructive pulmonary disease, dehydration

BOX 14.5 Neurodegenerative Diseases

- Alzheimer's disease (AD)
  - Classic, late-onset "amnestic" AD
  - AD variants: Posterior cortical atrophy, corticobasal syndrome/corticobasal degeneration, frontal variant AD, logopenic variant primary progressive aphasia
- Frontotemporal dementia (FTD)/frontotemporal lobar degeneration (FTLD)
  - Behavioral variant FTLD (e.g., Pick's disease)
  - Primary progressive aphasia (PPA): Semantic variant PPA, nonfluent variant PPA
- Parkinsonian syndrome
  - Parkinson's disease (PD)
  - Atypical parkinsonian syndromes: Progressive supranuclear palsy, multisystem atrophy, corticobasal syndrome
- Dementia with Lewy bodies (DLB)
- Others:
  - Chronic traumatic encephalopathy (CTE)
  - Cerebral amyloid angiopathy (CAA)
  - Down's syndrome (trisomy 21)
  - Huntington's chorea
  - Creutzfeldt–Jakob disease (prion diseases not always included)

buildup of neurotoxic, misfolded proteins over time. These disorders can be grouped not only on the basis of the symptoms (Box 14.6) that they cause but also by the key proteins underlying each disorder as well (Fig. 14.8, *A*, *B*).

Abnormal Proteins in Alzheimer's Disease

Alzheimer's disease (AD) is associated with two abnormal proteins that make up the extracellular "senile" plaques and intracellular *neural fibrillary tangles (NFTs)* found histopathologically. NFTs are composed of a protein called tau, whereas the plaques are largely made up of abnormally folded amyloid protein, beta-amyloid (also referred to as amyloid-β or Aβ). The abnormal configuration of Aβ causes fragments to autoaggregate, forming pleated sheets and insoluble fibrils.

The *amyloid cascade hypothesis* proposes that Aβ deposition is the central event that incites the neuroinflammation, NFT formation, vascular damage, and synaptic loss that ultimately lead to neuronal death in AD. This theory is supported by studies showing that the Aβ fibrils are neurotoxic. Additionally, the genetic defects found in familial forms of AD cause an increase in abnormal Aβ by altering amounts of the *amyloid precursor*

BOX 14.6 Primary or Key Early Features of Common Neurodegenerative Disorders

Dementia

Episodic memory loss, becoming lost in familiar places, difficulty performing multistep tasks
- Alzheimer's disease (AD):
  - Classic Alzheimer's (amnestic AD): Memory loss—presents early in disease
    - Typical late-onset form (≥65), sporadic (familial forms uncommon)
    - Early-onset form (<60-65), may be familial, rapid progression compared with late-onset form
  - AD variants: Amyloid-positive disorders, commonly early onset, with memory usually intact initially, instead presenting with other key features (see following points)
    - Posterior cortical atrophy (visual variant), logopenic variant primary progressive aphasia (verbal variant), corticobasal syndrome (motor variant), behavioral or frontal variant AD
- Dementia with Lewy bodies (DLB)
  - Fluctuating decreased cognition, visual hallucinations, rapid eye movement sleep disorder
  - Parkinsonism: Bradykinesia, rigidity, and/or rest tremor
  - Supporting signs: Autonomic dysfunction, severe reactions to antipsychotics, falls/postural instability
- Parkinson's disease dementia (PDD): Frequent development in Parkinson's disease (PD)
  - PD, PDD, and DLB may represent a spectrum of disease and can overlap with AD.

Personality and Behavior

Personality change, disinhibition, loss of judgment, apathy
- Behavioral variant frontotemporal lobar degeneration (bvFTLD)
- Frontal variant AD: Clinical presentation like FTLD, with underlying histopathology similar to AD (e.g., tau neurofibrillary tangles, amyloid)

Speech and Language
- FTLD primary progressive aphasia (PPA)
  - Semantic variant primary progressive aphasia (svPPA)
    - Inability to understand/remember meaning of words, understand sentences

- Nonfluent variant progressive aphasia (NFPA) or progressive nonfluent aphasia (PNFA)
  - Ungrammatical and/or hesitant (nonfluent) speech, difficulty pronouncing/getting words out, speech may slur or voice may change
- Alzheimer's variant (verbal variant AD):
  - Logopenic variant PPA (lvPPA) or logopenic variant progressive aphasia (LVPA)
    - Deficits in naming objects and repetition, with sparing of semantic, motor, syntactic abilities
    - Speech slows as patient searches for words, but word meanings are preserved, and speech is not physically effortful.

Motor Abnormalities: Parkinsonism and Motor Neuron Pathology
- Parkinsonism: Resting tremor, rigidity, bradykinesia, falls, postural instability/balance issues
- PD
  - Parkinsonism, olfactory loss, or cardiac sympathetic denervation
  - Responds to dopaminergic medication
  - Dementia frequent (PDD)
  - Differentiating PD from atypical parkinsonian syndromes (APSs) may be clinically difficult.
- DLB
  - Dementia, visual hallucinations, parkinsonism
- Multisystem atrophy (MSA)
  - Atypical parkinsonian syndrome: Ataxia, long tract signs
  - MSA-P: Parkinsonism symptoms dominate
  - MSA-C: Cerebellar ataxia, autonomic nervous system dysfunction
- Progressive supranuclear palsy (PSP)
  - Most common of the APSs
  - Oculomotor abnormalities and deficits in vertical gaze
  - Rigidity, falls, gait disorder, bulbar symptoms
- Corticobasal degeneration (see following points)
- Motor neuron/motor cortex
- *Corticobasal syndrome (CBS):* Term used for a constellation of symptoms, multiple potential etiologies

Continued

BOX 14.6 Primary or Key Early Features of Common Neurodegenerative Disorders—cont'd

- Corticobasal degeneration (CBD): CBS with tauopathy at autopsy (causes 50% of CBS)
- *Asymmetric,* usually begins with one limb
- Motor cortex/premotor affected: Progressive rigidity and apraxia, alien limb phenomena
- Striatal (basal ganglia)/extrapyramidal dysfunction: Parkinsonism
- May also show: Myoclonus, dysphagia, visuospatial disorientation, acalculia, dementia
- Symptoms may overlap other neurodegenerative diseases with motor deficits (PSP, PD, and MSA)
- Others:
  - Amyotrophic lateral sclerosis (ALS): upper and lower motor neurons
  - Huntington's chorea

Visual Abnormalities
- Visual field deficits
  - Posterior cortical atrophy (PCA): Visual variant AD
    - Presenting abnormalities from asymmetric, lateral occipital involvement; memory initially relatively preserved
    - Asymmetric atrophy in the occipital lobe may be seen on magnetic resonance imaging
- Visual hallucinations
  - DLB
  - AD: Later finding in up to 20%
  - Sometimes seen in posterior cortical atrophy (PCA)

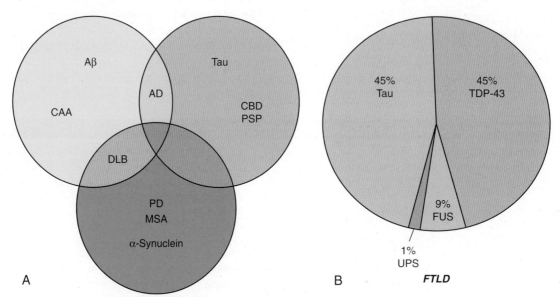

• **Fig. 14.8** (A) Degenerative brain disease (proteinopathies) can be categorized by the presence of abnormal proteins produced. *Beta-amyloid (Aβ)* was first characterized in Alzheimer's disease (AD) plaques. Perivascular amyloid is present in cerebral amyloid angiopathy (CAA) and dementia with Lewy bodies (DLB). The *tauopathies* result from abnormal tau protein deposition and include the tau subtype of frontotemporal lobar dementia (FTLD-t), corticobasal degeneration (CBD), and progressive supranuclear palsy (PSP). *Alpha-synuclein* is the primary component of Lewy bodies found in DLB and Parkinson's disease (PD) and is present in the abnormal neurites of multisystem atrophy (MSA). (B) The proteins in FTLD, in addition to tau, commonly include either TDP-43 or fused in sarcoma (FUS) proteins in tau-negative cases. These two entities might be labeled "U" for unknown or "UPS" for ubiquitin protease system markers in older literature because they have been characterized more recently.

protein (APP) or by changing the way APP is cleaved during posttranslational processing. The abnormal Aβ (i.e., Aβ42) fragments have a different configuration that leads to the auto-aggregation and formation of insoluble fibrils and pleated sheets found in Alzheimer's.

In the search for a cure for AD, attention has focused on the extracellular fibrillar plaques in accordance with the amyloid cascade hypothesis. However, clinical trials with new therapies that correct amyloid buildup have so far failed to correct cognitive decline or alter the course of disease. Several other facts are difficult to explain if the amyloid cascade hypothesis is entirely correct. First, significant Aβ deposition is seen in 15% to 30% of cognitively normal elderly patients. Also, amyloid volume and distribution fail to reflect the stage or severity of symptoms. For

example, anteromedial temporal lobe dysfunction develops very early in the course of AD, but plaques are not detected there until later (first occurring in the basal temporal lobe, anterior cingulate, and parietal operculum). Also, Aβ plaque appears decades before the disease is clinically manifest and plateaus many years before the symptoms peak.

Despite the conflicting information as to the importance of amyloid, detecting its presence with PET or measuring changes in CSF amyloid concentration can help with the diagnosis of dementia, particularly in differentiating AD from frontotemporal lobar degeneration (FTLD). Other contributing factors that could play a role in dementia include inflammation from overactive microglial cells, decreased phagocytosis of toxic debris, and toxicity related to the combination of abnormal proteins present. In AD, the relationship between abnormal Aβ and tau proteins is increasingly attracting interest.

The protein tau is normally involved in the regulation of intracellular transport by the cellular microtubules and is encoded for by the *MAPT* gene located on chromosome 17. NFTs are largely composed of an insoluble, abnormally phosphorylated (hyperphosphorylated) form of the microtubule-associated protein tau (MAPT or tau).

In AD, tau accumulates in a pattern that mirrors the progression of functional changes. Filaments are first found in the anteromesial temporal lobe and hippocampus, then spread to involve the lateral temporal and temporoparietal cortex. The posterior cingulate cortex (PCC) and superior posterior parietal lobe are next involved. Unlike amyloid, the amount of tau present appears to correlate with the severity of disease, and evidence increasingly points to tau as a critical factor in the development of the AD.

Different forms of tau accumulate have been found to be characteristic in several other neurodegenerative disorders. These disorders are cumulatively referred to as "tauopathies" and include the behavioral variant frontotemporal lobar dementia (bvFTLD), corticobasal degeneration (CBD), and progressive supranuclear palsy (PSP). In the past, FTLD was referred to as Pick's disease, but that term is now used to refer to the subset of frontotemporal dementia (FTD) cases where Pick bodies, intracellular inclusions containing tau, are seen in tissue specimens.

Lewy bodies are another type of intracellular inclusion, composed largely of abnormal α-synuclein protein. Lewy bodies were originally described in Parkinson's disease (PD), but they are also found in dementia with Lewy bodies (DLB) and Parkinson's disease dementia (PDD). It is likely that DLB and PDD are related on a spectrum of disease. Neuronal involvement in each disease progresses in a predictable pattern marked by the spread of the abnormal protein. For example, Lewy bodies in DLB are found in the brainstem and substantia nigra before moving rostrally to dopaminergic neurons in the striatum. This is followed by the cingulate region, insula, and finally widely through the cortex. Lewy bodies are not specific to diseases of striatal or motor neurons and are found in other conditions, including 50% of patients with AD. In fact, the overlap between AD and DLB is significant in other ways, with patients with DLB frequently showing AD cellular pathology (i.e., amyloid), and the F-18 FDG PET patterns of the two disorders are sometimes difficult to differentiate in clinical cases. Abnormal α-synuclein can be found in forms other than as Lewy bodies. For example, glial intracellular inclusions, primarily in oligodendrocytes, are the hallmark of the atypical parkinsonian syndrome, multisystem atrophy (MSA).

Roughly 50% of FTLD cases are tau negative. The abnormal proteins related to these cases have been characterized recently, with two proteins being involved in almost all cases: TAR-DNA binding protein of 43 kDa (TDP-43) and fused in sarcoma (FUS) protein. These two proteins also often occur in a subset of amyotrophic lateral sclerosis (ALS), and accumulations of FUS are found in some patients with essential tremor. The two

proteins can also be seen as secondary proteins in other degenerative diseases when more than one protein is present.

Abnormal protein accumulation characterizes several other diseases. In Huntington's chorea, an abnormal protein, Huntingtin, is found. Prion disease, such as in Creutzfeldt–Jakob disease, will also result in abnormally folded protein deposition. The dementia of Down's syndrome (trisomy 21) is associated with AD pathology because of the presence of the amyloid precursor protein gene on chromosome 21. In addition, traumatic brain injury that leads to chronic traumatic encephalopathy (CTE) is strongly associated with NFT deposition. Understanding the different abnormal proteins found in the dementias may help uncover new diagnostic tests and therapies.

AD typically occurs after age 60 to 65 and is characterized primarily by progressive cognitive decline with episodic memory loss, difficulty navigating familiar places, and organizational problems (i.e., amnestic AD). AD is the most common cause of dementia, accounting for 60% to 80% of cases diagnosed in the United States and affecting 10% of the population over 65 years of age and nearly 50% in those over 85 years of age. In those under 65, dementia is rare (comprising roughly 5% of diagnosed cases), but when it occurs, early-onset dementia is most commonly caused by AD. Roughly half the cases are caused by AD, and most of the remainder are a result of FTLD/FTD. Early-onset AD is more frequently associated with familial inherited patterns of disease and demonstrates a more aggressive clinical course than the classic late-onset form.

More than 80% of AD cases are sporadic, but in those cases of inherited forms of disease, three important autosomal-dominant genetic defects have been found (Table 14.3). In nonfamilial and late-onset disease, a strong correlation has been found with abnormalities in the genes for apolipoprotein (ApoE). Specifically, an increased incidence of AD is seen in those who carry the ApoE ε_4 allele, and the risk increases when more than one copy of the ApoE ε_4 is present. In both early- and late-onset disease, defects result in the buildup of abnormal forms of Aβ related to these genes. Other factors that have been linked to Alzheimer's are diabetes mellitus, elevated serum glucose/hyperinsulinemia, hypertension, and head injury.

Occasionally, AD will present clinically in an atypical fashion with symptoms other than memory loss dominating early in the course of disease. These disorders include aphasia in logopenic primary progressive aphasia (verbal variant AD), visual deficits in posterior cortical atrophy (visual variant), corticobasal degeneration (motor variant), and personality or behavioral changes (frontal lobe variant). Although clinical findings and corresponding F-18 FDG PET (or Tc-99m HMPAO/ECD SPECT) imaging findings vary widely in cases of atypical AD, the AD variants demonstrate the same underlying histopathological findings typical of amnestic AD (i.e., increased Aβ and NFT buildup and decreased CSF Aβ or tau).

Different phases of disease are now recognized in AD: preclinical, prodromal mild cognitive impairment, and dementia from Alzheimer's (Table 14.4). Preclinical amyloid deposition begins years before patients demonstrate symptoms. Such patients may be identified by genetic markers or abnormal imaging or CSF biomarker findings. In the early stages of

TABLE 14.3 Genetic Mutations in Familial Alzheimer Dementia

Chromosome	Gene	Notes
Early-Onset Dementia (<60-65 years of age)		
21	Amyloid precursor protein (APP) gene mutations	Improper APP cleavage: ↑Aβ42 fragment (↑Aβ42 to ↑Aβ420 ratio).
		Trisomy 21: Triplicate genes and ↑ APP expression related to early-onset AD in Down's syndrome
14	Presenilin 1 (PSEN1)	Both part of the γ-secretase
1	Presenilin 2 (PSEN2)	complex that cleaves APP
		Majority of early-onset familial AD mapped to chromosome 14
Late-/Senile-Onset Dementia (>65 years of age)		
19	Apolipoprotein E (ApoE):	ApoE₄ is the major risk for late-onset AD
	3 isoforms (ε₂, ε₂, ε₂)	Found in 65%-80% of sporadic and familial cases
		Multiple copies E₄ ↑↑ risk 2 copies by age 85, 12%; 4 copies, 91% by age 85
		E3 neutral risk E2 protective ↓ risk 50%
	Triggering receptor on myeloid cells 2 (TREM2)	Less common; expression limited to microglia; critical for response to injury/Aβ
	Others (very rare)	

Aβ, Beta-amyloid; *AD,* Alzheimer's disease

disease progression, memory and cognitive issues are usually not serious enough to affect daily living activities. These patients are said to have MCI. MCI is present in 15% to 20% of the population over 65 years of age and can be caused by multiple etiologies. Patients may not develop dementia in 35% to 40% of cases. However, patients with MCI are at high risk for the development of AD, with 15% of patients with MCI converting to AD in 2 years and more than a third in 5 years (up to perhaps half of the cases). When MCI is caused by the early stages of AD, F-18 FDG PET (or sometimes SPECT) will often reveal abnormal patterns similar to AD. Additionally, amyloid PET scans will usually be positive in these cases. Thus, these scans can help predict which MCI cases will progress to actual AD. Once neurologic deficits have worsened to a level that affects daily living activities, the clinical diagnosis of dementia is made.

In the 2011 revision of the National Institute on Aging and the Alzheimer's Association (NIA-AA) workgroup criteria for the diagnosis of AD, the importance of the underlying histopathology is recognized as opposed to only relying on clinical findings. Patients are classified as either possible or probable AD based on clinical factors, and the degree of certainty can be increased by obtaining evidence of abnormal biomarkers for Aβ deposition (positive amyloid PET scan or low concentrations of CSF Aβ₄₂), disproportionate atrophy of the entorhinal cortex on MR, or other signs of typical neuronal injury (elevated CSF tau [both total and phosphorylated tau], decreased F-18 FDG in the temporoparietal cortex). When patients meet the core clinical criteria for AD, biomarker evidence can increase the certainty of the diagnosis (Table 14.5). F-18 FDG PET/CT detection of AD (Fig. 14.9) has a reported sensitivity of up to 94% and a specificity of 83%. The accuracy of SPECT is also high, but it is less than PET, with a sensitivity of 65% to 85% and a specificity of 72% to

TABLE 14.4 Stages in Alzheimer's Dementia Diagnosis

Category		Stage	CLINICAL Cognitive Change	BIOMARKERS Aβ PET or CSF	Neuronal Injury (Tau, MR, FDG)
Normal	0	AD biomarkers normal	−	−	−
Preclinical AD	1	Amyloidosis	−	+	−
	2	Amyloidosis and neurodegeneration	−	+	+
	3	Plus early cognitive change	+ (subtle—doesn't meet MCI criteria)	+	+
	SNAP	Neurodegeneration without amyloid	−	−	+
MCI		Symptomatic predementia—daily living activities not affected	+ (mild)	+	+
Alzheimer's Dementia	Symptomatic dementia	Affects daily living activities	+	+	+

Aβ, Beta-amyloid; *AD,* Alzheimer's disease; *CSF,* cerebrospinal fluid; *MCI,* mild cognitive impairment; *MR,* atrophy hippocampus, entorhinal cortex, amygdala; *PET,* positron emission tomography; *SNAP,* suspected non-Alzheimer pathophysiology; *tau,* tau-total and tau-P (phosphorylated tau). Based on National Institute on Aging Criteria 2011 with subsequent modifications.

TABLE 14.5 National Institute on Aging and Alzheimer's Association (NIA-AA) Criteria for Alzheimer's Disease (AD) as the Cause for Dementia

Is Dementia related to AD?	Biomarker Evidence of AD Pathophysiological Process		Add "↑ level of clinical certainty" with any of the following:
	Aβ PET (+) or CSF Aβ↓	Tau ↑ or (+) MR atrophy or FDG PET	
Uncertain	No (+) biomarker or conflicting biomarkers		
Intermediate probability	(+) Aβ	**OR** (+): tau or MR or FDG	• Documented cognitive decline
High probability	(+) Aβ	**AND** (+): tau or MR or FDG	• Carrier AD genetic mutation
Prodromal AD	Clinically (−) but shows (+) Aβ **or** tau/Aβ		

Aβ, Beta-amyloid; *CSF*, cerebrospinal fluid; *FDG*, F-18 FDG PET/CT ↓ posterior cingulate/precuneus and anteromesial temporal; *MR*, magnetic resonance; *MR atrophy*, hippocampal/anteromesial temporal atrophy; *PET*, positron emission tomography.

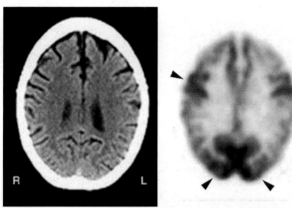

• **Fig. 14.9** F-18 fluorodeoxyglucose (FDG) positron emission tomography (PET)/computed tomography (CT) in Alzheimer's disease shows typical parietal hypometabolism and sparing *(arrowheads)* of the sensorimotor cortex and occipital lobes. Symmetrical frontal lobe involvement is consistent with fairly advanced disease.

TABLE 14.6 Accuracy of Biomarkers in Alzheimer's Disease Diagnosis[a]

Examination	Sensitivity (%)	Specificity (%)
MR	83 (79-87)	85 (80-89)
CT	80 (68-88)	87 (78-93)
SPECT	79 (72-85)	84 (78-88)
PET/CT	91 (86-94)	85 (79-91)
CSF-Aβ	76 (72-80)	77 (72-82)
CSF-tau (total/phosphorylated)	78 (73-83)	85 (76-89)

[a]95% Confidence interval.

Aβ, Beta-amyloid; *CSF*, cerebrospinal fluid; *CT*, computed tomography; *MR*, magnetic resonance; *PET*, positron emission tomography; *SPECT*, single-photon emission computed tomography.
Adapted from Shivamurthy V, Tahari A, Marcus C, Subramanian R. Brain PET and the diagnosis of dementia. *AJR*. 2015;204(1):W76-W85. DOI: 10.2214/AJR.13.12363.

87% (Table 14.6). Imaging tests have been shown to be more accurate in the diagnosis of dementia than clinical exam alone. In some cases, the etiology of dementia may not be clear clinically or based on biomarker findings. Postmortem tissue biopsy remains the gold standard for the diagnosis of AD.

The first steps in the complex process of PET image analysis are as follows:

1. Exclude significant vascular disease (usually evident on MR), or confirm that vascular disease is present; clinical determination is needed if a secondary process may be present in addition.
2. Determine if cortical uptake is sufficient to categorize disease; when cortical disease becomes severe, decreased uptake becomes more generalized with atrophy, and changes progress beyond the point where they can be categorized.
3. Attempt to categorize the scan into the posterior (parietal or occipital) or frontal (Fig. 14.10), or temporal (Fig. 14.11) categories.

Table 14.7 outlines typical F-18 FDG PET imaging findings of AD and other neurodegenerative disorders. In Fig. 14.12, a systematic approach to the interpretation of these scans is diagramed. As shown, it is generally best to first determine if the disease pattern can be placed into a primarily posterior category. Even if the anterior regions are involved, when deficits are greater posteriorly than those anteriorly, processes such as AD or DLB are more likely than FTLD.

Image Analysis in AD

Gliosis and neuronal loss begin in the anteromesial temporal lobe entorhinal cortex (Fig. 14.13). Although these earliest findings may be difficult to visualize, increasing the angle of the patient's head 30 to 40 degrees, with the nose up from the canthomeatal line during scanning, can make hippocampal and anteromesial temporal deficits more apparent.

AD is most often evident after involvement of the temporoparietal association cortices, posterior cingulate cortex (PCC), and precuneus regions (Fig. 14.14). As disease progresses, changes spread to the frontal lobes, sparing the sensory-motor cortex and occipital lobes (Fig. 14.15) until the disease is very advanced. Changes in classic amnestic AD may begin with moderate asymmetry in each area involved, but findings then usually become symmetric (Fig. 14.16). Persistent or significant asymmetries can be caused by the presence of mixed pathologies or when disease is the result of an atypical or variant form of AD. Changes on F-18 FDG PET may be apparent before atrophy is seen on MR.

Recognizing the location of PCC and precuneus is important (Fig. 14.17) because their involvement is not only the most easily visualized abnormality in early AD, but it is also the most specific finding when attempting to differentiate AD from FTLD. The position of these structures may be difficult to identify in the different planes on the MR. As noted previously,

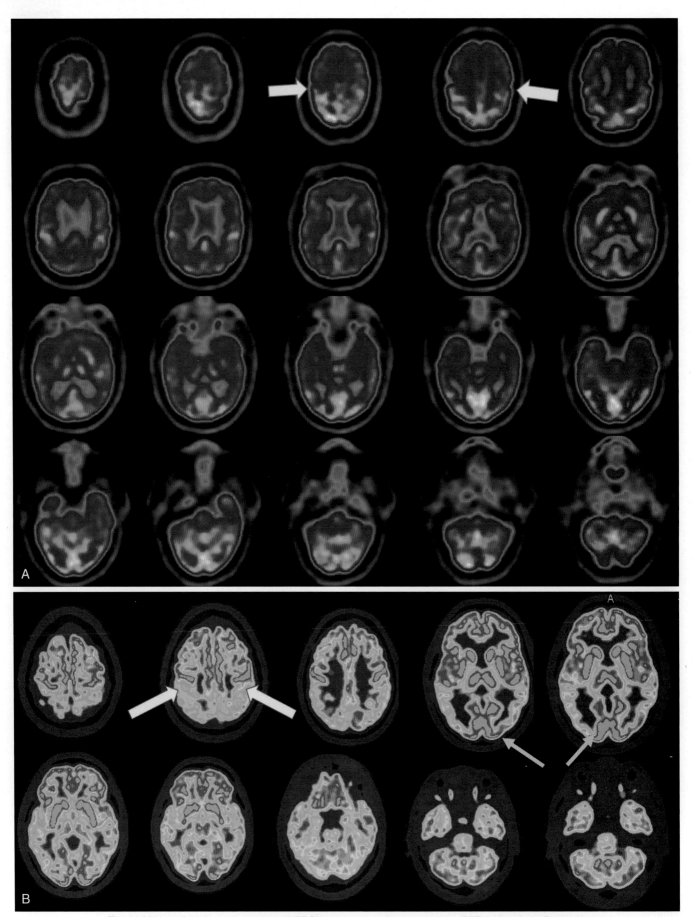

• **Fig. 14.10** Axial F-18 fluorodeoxyglucose (FDG) positron emission tomography (PET) in dementia. Even when advanced, degenerative disease usually fits in a major category: anterior, posterior, temporal. On axial F-18 FDG PET, a sharp front-to-back demarcation *(yellow arrows)* will differentiate (A) frontotemporal lobar degeneration from a posterior (posterior parietal or occipital) dementia. (B) The superior parietal lobe is most commonly affected in Alzheimer's disease (AD), which spares the occiput until very late *(orange arrows)*. Prominent bilateral occipital involvement is expected in dementia with Lewy bodies (DLB). In another severely abnormal case

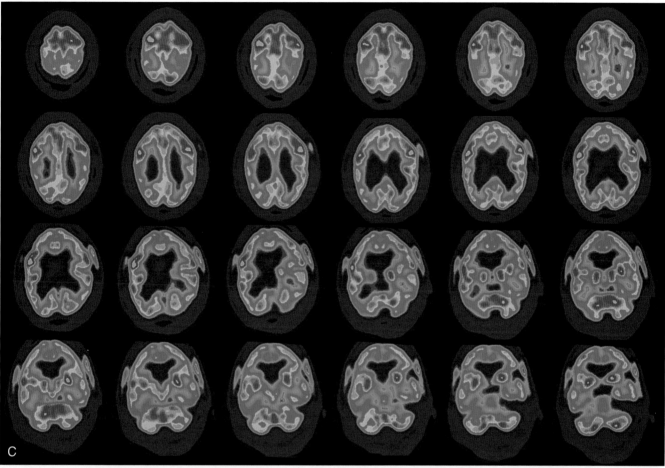

Fig. 14.10, cont'd (C), greater posterior involvement is seen than frontal, and because the frontal involvement would typically be more severe than the occipital/cerebellar abnormalities in AD, the likely etiology is DLB. Posterior cortical atrophy, an AD variant that also frequently involves the occipital region, is usually more asymmetrical and lateral than DLB.

posterior cingulate and temporoparietal cortex hypometabolism on PET has also been shown predictive of which MCI cases will convert to AD. Although the reported accuracy varies from 58% to 100%, there is a high negative predictive value, and accuracy is reportedly greater than MR.

Dementia With Lewy Bodies

DLB is the second-most-common cause of neurodegenerative dementia, causing 15% to 25% of cases. Patients classically demonstrate a fluctuating dementia, visual hallucinations, and rapid eye movement (REM) sleep behavior disorder. Consensus criteria include these symptoms under the "core features" category of disease. Additional "suggestive features" are postural instability, neuroleptic sensitivity, significant autonomic dysfunction, parkinsonism, and other psychiatric symptoms (delusions, depression, other types of hallucinations). Supportive features also include abnormal functional imaging exams with decreased activity in the basal ganglia uptake on the dopamine transporter (DAT) I-123 ioflupane SPECT (DaTscan), in the occipital lobes on F-18 FDG PET, and/or in myocardium with I-123 metaiodobenzylguanidine (I-123 MIBG) SPECT.

DLB scan findings are typically bilateral and may be extensive. In many ways, the pattern on F-18 FDG PET is usually similar to AD, with symmetric involvement of the posterior temporoparietal cortices bilaterally, increasingly abnormal-appearing frontal lobe as disease progresses, and sparing of the sensorimotor cortex. The primary difference between AD and DLB is that DLB usually shows early occipital lobe involvement (Fig. 14.18). In addition, the activity in the underlying PCC may be relatively preserved in DLB (i.e., the "cingulate island sign"). Other variations between DLB and AD include cerebellar involvement in some cases of DLB and frontal lobe involvement that is often earlier than is seen in AD. However, the occipital hypometabolism is the most specific abnormality.

In some cases, it is not possible to differentiate AD and DLB because clinical, F-18 FDG PET imaging, amyloid PET findings, and even histopathologic findings (e.g., Lewy bodies and amyloid) can overlap. However, differentiating the cause of dementia when DLB is present is important—not only to ensure correct treatment but to also prevent serious side effects from improper treatment (Table 14.8). In cases where the etiology is unclear, an abnormal I-123 ioflupane brain SPECT can usually differentiate DLB from AD and FTLD, showing decreased basal ganglia uptake with DLB. The accuracy of imaging is much greater than clinical assessment (sensitivity of 78%-88% and specificity of 90%-100% compared with a clinical sensitivity of 75% and specificity of

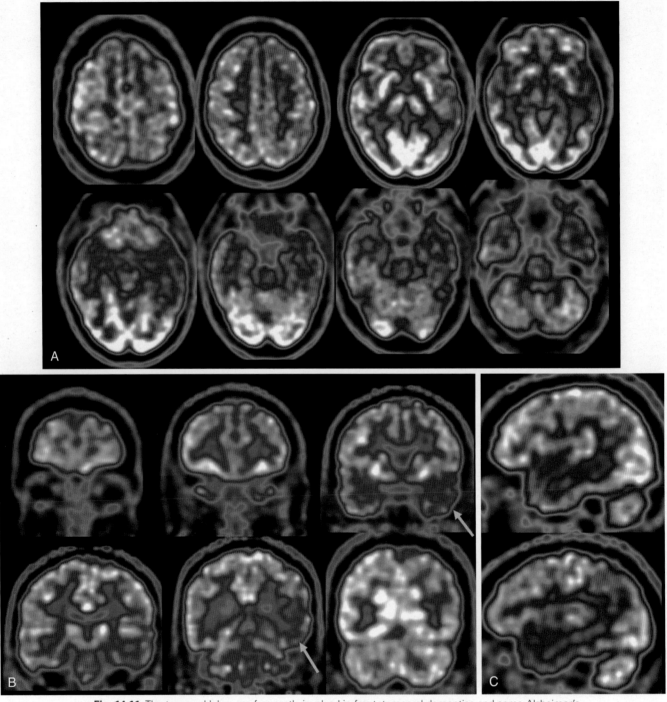

• **Fig. 14.11** The temporal lobes are frequently involved in frontotemporal dementias and some Alzheimer's disease variants. When asymmetrical temporal lobe involvement is the main or only finding, the semantic variant primary progressive aphasia, one type of frontotemporal lobar degeneration (FTLD), is a likely cause. As seen here, the left side is more commonly affected: (A) axial, (B) coronal, and (C) left lateral F-18 fluorodeoxyglucose (FDG) positron emission tomography (PET) images.

TABLE 14.7 F-18 FDG PET Findings in Dementia and Neurodegenerative Diseases

Area	AD	DLB	PCA	bvFTLD	PPA	CBD
PCC	↓	↓	↓	Initially no Δ	Varies—↓ if related AD and no Δ if FTLD	↓ asymmetrical
Posterior/Superior parietal (precuneus)	↓	↓	↓ (may be asymmetrical)	No Δ (may ↓ later)	Varies-↓ if related AD and No Δ if FTLD	Varies (asymmetrically ↓ or preserved)
Posterior temporal	↓	↓	↓	No Δ	↓ (varies and may be asymmetrical)	Varies (asymmetrically ↓ or preserved)
Occipital	No Δ	↓ especially medial	↓ lateral (often asymmetrical)	No Δ	No Δ	No Δ
Frontal	Midlate ↓	↓ (often)	No Δ (varies)	↓	May be↓ often asymmetrical	↓ asymmetrical
ACC	No Δ	varies	No Δ	↓	May	↓
Anterior temporal	No Δ	varies	No Δ	↓	↓ (often asymmetrical)	No Δ
Sensorimotor cortex	No Δ	No Δ	No Δ	No Δ	No Δ	↓ asymmetrical
Basal ganglia or Thalamus	No Δ	No Δ	No Δ	Varies	No Δ	↓ asymmetrical

ACC, Anterior cingulate cortex; *AD,* Alzheimer's disease; *bvFTLD,* behavioral variant frontotemporal lobar degeneration; *CBD,* corticobasal degeneration; *DLB,* dementia with Lewy bodies; *No Δ,* unchanged; *PCA,* posterior cortical atrophy; *PCC,* posterior cingulate cortex; *PPA,* primary progressive aphasia (as a result of AD or FTLD).

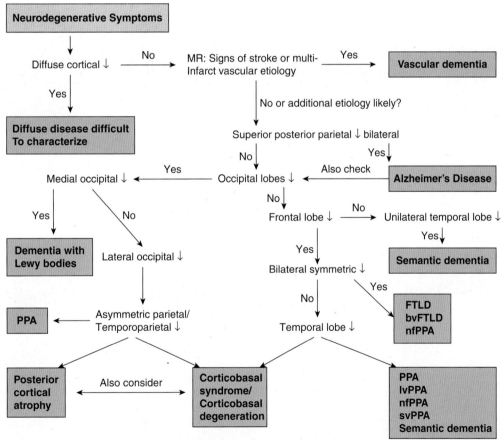

• **Fig. 14.12** A system for F-18 fluorodeoxyglucose (FDG) positron emission tomography (PET) interpretation in neurodegenerative disease. Image interpretation in neurodegenerative disease requires a systematic approach. If the posterior parietal or occipital regions are most heavily involved, the etiology is most likely not a frontotemporal dementia, even when the frontal lobes are involved. *bvFTLD,* Behavioral variant FTLD; *FTLD,* frontotemporal lobar degeneration; *lvPPA,* logopenic variant PPA; *nfPPA,* nonfluent PPA; *PPA,* primary progressive aphasia; *svPPA,* semantic variant PPA ("semantic dementia").

42%). In some cases, a cardiac I-123 MIBG may also be of benefit because uptake will also be decreased in DLB.

The occipital lobe can be involved in other disorders besides DLB. Although rare, *posterior cortical atrophy (PCA),* which is most often an AD variant, classically affects the occipital lobes. (Fig. 14.19, A, B). PCA often presents in younger patients (50-65 years), with asymmetric signs typically involving visual field or visual processing but with preservation of memory and cognitive processes (at least initially). PCA will usually present with at least mildly asymmetric hypometabolism that tends to involve the more lateral occipital lobe (see Fig. 14.19, C, D). DLB, on the other hand, will affect the midline region (and may affect the lateral occipital lobe as well). PCA may also affect the parietal and temporoparietal regions more asymmetrically than is typical of DLB or classic AD. Patients may present with findings of severe focal atrophy on MR in the parietooccipital region. Although the frontal lobe is abnormal in some cases, it is likely less severely affected than with DLB or FTLD. The severity is also usually less severe in the frontal portions of the temporal lobe and anterior cingulate cortex (ACC) compared with various types of FTLD.

Frontotemporal Dementia/Frontotemporal Lobar Degeneration

The frontotemporal dementias are a diverse group of diseases in which memory issues are generally less significant initially as compared with other symptoms, unlike AD. FTLD is the cause of almost half of dementia cases occurring in younger patients (<60-65 years). Frontal lobe involvement results in personality changes, including loss of judgment, apathy, and inappropriate behavior with loss of inhibitions. These are the predominant findings in behavioral variant FTLD (bvFTLD) (Fig. 14.20).

When speech difficulties are the predominant presenting symptom, the temporal lobes and speech areas of the brain are involved, although frontal and other areas may also be abnormal. Three types of degenerative aphasias, often referred to as primary progress aphasia (PPA), are generally now recognized. Two of these are associated with FTLD pathology: semantic variant

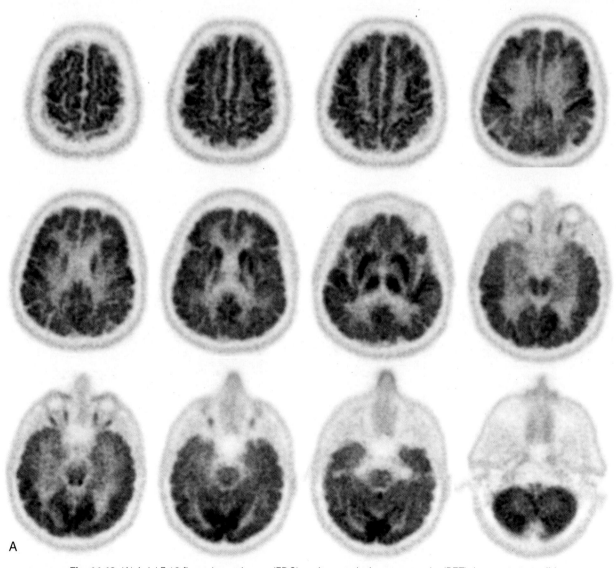

A

• **Fig. 14.13** (A) Axial F-18 fluorodeoxyglucose (FDG) positron emission tomography (PET) demonstrates mild decreased activity in the mesial temporal lobes in a patient with early Alzheimer's disease.

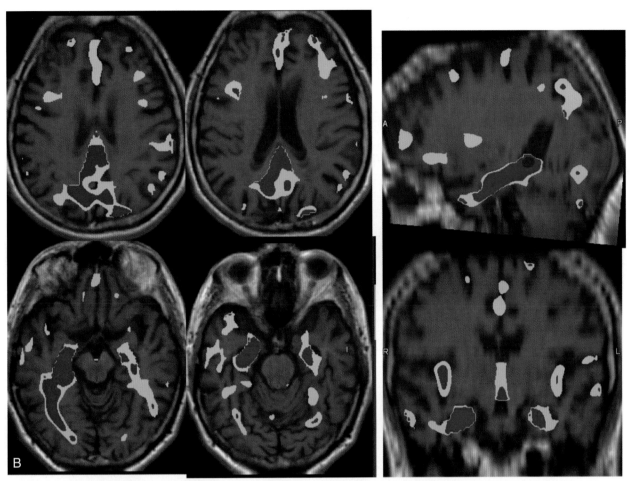

Fig. 14.13, cont'd (B) A topographical representation of the comparison of this case to a normal database confirms the temporal lobe is statistically significantly decreased and also highlights early involvement posteriorly and medially in the posterior cingulate gyrus (posterior cingulate cortex [PCC]).

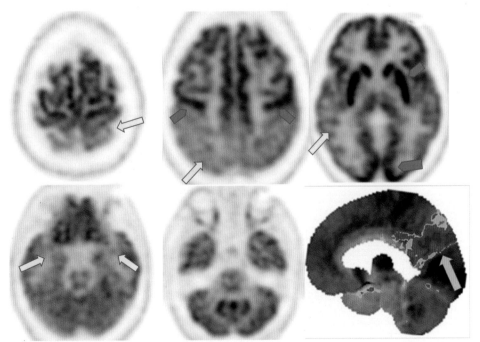

• **Fig. 14.14** Axial positron emission tomography (PET) images in Alzheimer's disease demonstrate decreased uptake *(yellow arrows)* in the parietal, temporoparietal, and anteromesial temporal cortex. Preserved activity *(blue arrows)* is noted in the sensorimotor cortex, occiput, and basal ganglia.

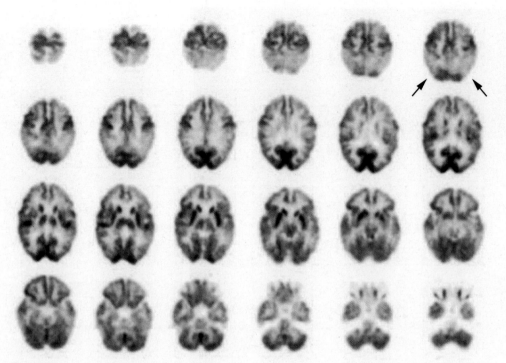

• **Fig. 14.15** Alzheimer's disease (AD). Transaxial positron emission tomography (PET) images reveal expected hypometabolism in the temporoparietal cortex, especially high in the posterior parietal region *(arrows)*, and sparing of the sensorimotor cortex. Frontal lobe involvement is consistent with fairly advanced disease.

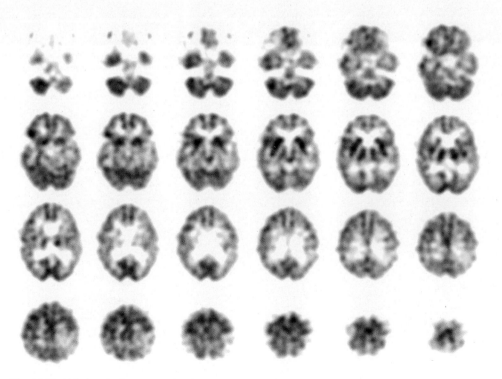

• **Fig. 14.16** Alzheimer's disease can begin asymmetrically in a region, but change becomes more symmetrical over time. In this case, decreased activity is seen bilaterally in the posterior parietal cortex, but the left is slightly worse than the right. If the asymmetry is marked, it may be secondary to an Alzheimer's variant or vascular disease superimposed on a degenerative process.

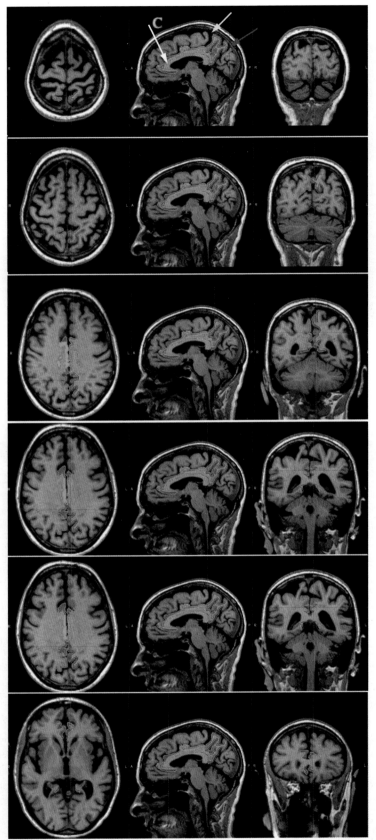

• **Fig. 14.17** The *precuneus* and *posterior cingulate cortex* (*PCC*) in the medial posterior parietal lobe may be difficult to recognize, especially when only a single image from an example is shown. T1-weighted magnetic resonance (MR) from top to bottom *(axial images, left)* and from back to front *(coronal right)* with a fixed sagittal reference *(middle)*, just to the left of the longitudinal fissure. The *precuneus (pink, left hemisphere; yellow, right hemisphere)* is almost all hidden from the brain surface in the longitudinal fissure; it is bordered anteriorly by the cingulate sulcus marginal ramus *(yellow arrow)* and parieto-occipital sulcus posteriorly *(red arrow)*; the cingulate sulcus separates it from the underlying cingulate gyrus *(blue)*. The posterior cingulate cortex is above the corpus callosum *(white arrow)*, with the sulcus of the corpus callosum between them. The PCC extends anteriorly to the level of the marginal ramus of the cingulate sulcus and posteriorly to the parieto-occipital sulcus. The PCC contains Brodman's areas 23, 29, and 31 (anteriorly) and the retrosplenial cortex (posteriorly).

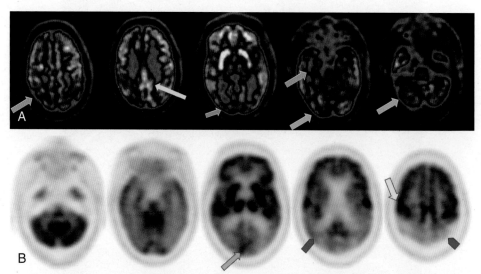

• **Fig. 14.18** Dementia with Lewy bodies (DLB). (A) Decreased activity is seen in the parietal and temporal cortices *(blue arrows)*. Classic Alzheimer's is unlikely given mild decreases in the occipital lobe (mildly asymmetrical; right > left) and cerebellum *(green arrows)*, and frontal regions and the posterior cingulate cortex *(yellow arrow)* are still preserved. The pattern suggests early DLB. Although an atypical Alzheimer's was a possible explanation, the developing clinical findings supported the diagnosis of DLB. (B) Marked deficits posteriorly involve the occiput but also the temporoparietal and superior frontal regions, with sparing of the sensorimotor and inferior frontal cortices. These changes could be from advanced DLB, but the severe parietooccipital atrophy on CT is suggestive of the Alzheimer variant posterior cortical atrophy.

TABLE 14.8	Potential Side Effects of Incorrect Therapies in Neurodegenerative Diseases	
Disease	**Treatment**	**Result**
Dementia with Lewy bodies	Neuroleptics—contraindicated	• Irreversible parkinsonism or autonomic dysfunction • Impaired consciousness
	Antipsychotics—use with caution	• Anticholinergic effects could exacerbate extrapyramidal symptoms and worsen cognitive status
Frontotemporal dementia	Acetylcholinesterase inhibitors (Donepezil)—avoid use	• Activating/alerting properties can ↑ psychiatric symptoms/worsen behavioral symptoms • No benefits
Multisystem atrophy	Deep-brain stimulators	Clinical worsening
Corticobasal degeneration	Thalamotomy	Clinical deterioration
General use Alzheimer's disease	Anticholinesterase inhibitor (approved for use)	Typical side effects: Nausea, vomiting, diarrhea, sleep disturbance, urinary incontinence, cramps, bradycardia

FTLD (svFTLD or semantic dementia) and nonfluent progressive aphasia (NFPA) or progressive nonfluent aphasia (PNFA). The third condition, logopenic progressive aphasia (or logopenic variant progressive aphasia [LVPA]), is usually an AD variant.

Three main patterns of hypometabolism are seen on F-18 FDG in FTLD: (1) bilateral frontal lobe, with anterior temporal lobes and anterior cingulate cortex (ACC); (2) frontal involvement with temporal lobe sparing; and (3) temporal lobe predominant, with bilateral but often asymmetric or unilateral findings. It should be noted that svFTLD is often more asymmetric than the other forms of PPA. Also, in bilateral frontal/anterior temporal lobe involvement, Pick body inclusions may be found at biopsy (i.e., FTLD was formerly known as Pick's disease). When changes in the frontal lobes are significant or affect motor/premotor cortical areas, the contralateral cerebellum may show neuronal loss as crossed-cerebellar diaschisis (Fig. 14.21).

When marked asymmetry is seen, without change from ischemic infarct, the two processes that should be considered first are semantic dementia and corticobasal degeneration (CBD). These patients have very different clinical presentations, with speech issues central to semantic dementia and unilateral motor abnormalities (and/or unilateral phantom limb) typical of CBD. On F-18 FDG PET, CBD will classically affect the primary sensorimotor strip, ipsilateral basal ganglia, or thalamus. CBD is often the result of atypical AD but can also be a result of FTLD processes. Additionally, semantic variant PPA and PCA may also be considered in situations where findings are fairly asymmetric.

Scan interpretation is complex when the pattern is not consistent with classic AD or FTLD. In many situations, the etiology of scan findings can only be narrowed down. For example, it might be possible to exclude classic AD or DLB while

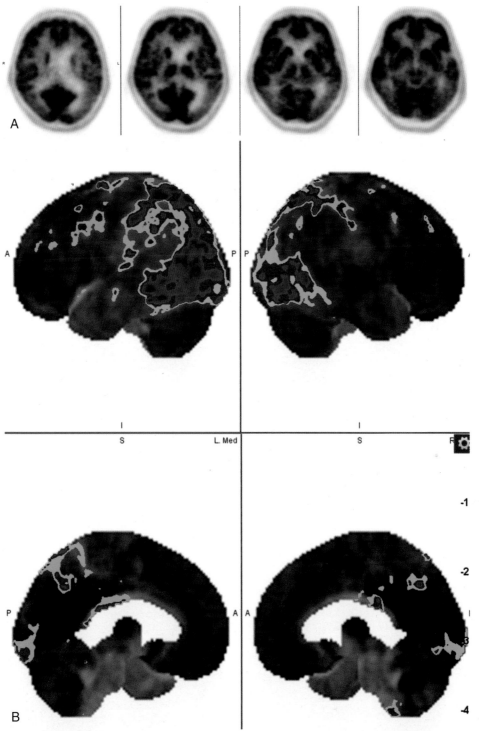

• **Fig. 14.19** (A) *Posterior cortical atrophy* (PCA) is also known as visual variant Alzheimer's disease (AD) because occipital involvement causes visual field changes. It is often very asymmetrical and involves the occipital lobe, usually more laterally. There is asymmetrical involvement of structures typically affected in classic AD, such as the temporal lobe. Compared with a normal database (B), statistically significant abnormalities appear as blue to purple on a brain map, which can help confirm the presence of subtle changes.

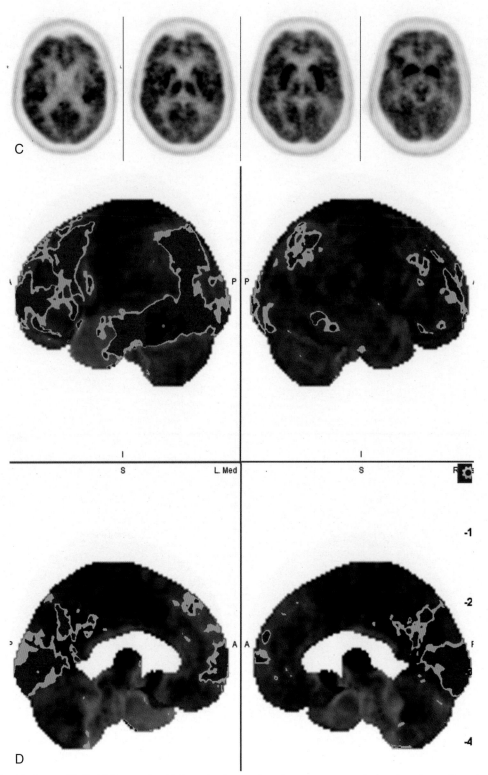

Fig. 14.19, cont'd (C, D) *Dementia with Lewy bodies* tends to be more symmetrical and tends to affect the central/midline occiput. (Images courtesy Dr. Kirk Frey, MD, PhD, University of Michigan.)

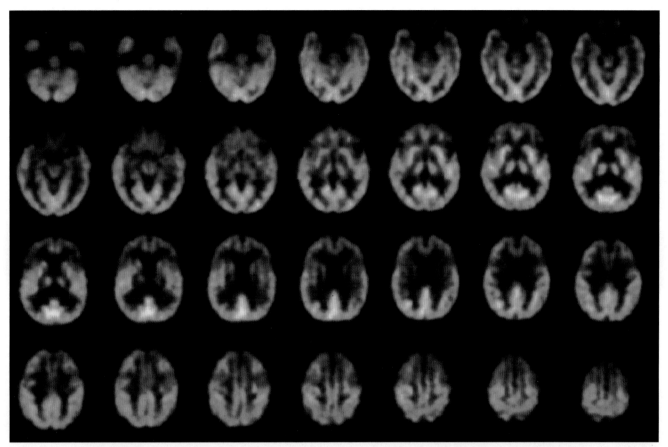

• **Fig. 14.20** Frontotemporal dementia/frontotemporal lobar degeneration (FTLD). Behavioral frontotemporal lobar degeneration is the most common FTLD type and includes most cases previously referred to as Pick's disease. F-18 fluorodeoxyglucose (FDG) positron emission tomography (PET) demonstrates bilateral decreased activity in the frontal lobes, including the anterior cingulate, and the anterior temporal lobes.

suggesting findings may be related to an AD variant or combination of an FTLD with an AD variant (Fig. 14.22). In some instances, other imaging tests may be helpful. For example, amyloid PET is negative in cases related to FTLD and positive with underlying AD. Other AD variants, in addition to logopenic PPA and posterior cortical atrophy, can occur. Both classic and variant forms of AD are typically amyloid positive, and both may show decreases in perfusion or metabolism in the posterior parietal/temporoparietal cortices. Variant forms of AD, however, more often demonstrate asymmetric decreases on F-18 FDG PET. The specific areas will usually reflect symptoms: occipital lobe for visual changes, frontal lobes for behavioral and executive symptoms, temporal for language, and basal ganglia or motor cortex for motor symptoms.

If metabolic changes occur in Parkinson's disease or an atypical parkinsonian syndrome, they are often subtle, and their diagnosis is not a currently approved indication for F-18 FDG PET. The use of dopamine transporter imaging (e.g., I-123 ioflupane) will be more sensitive and specific when differentiating such cases from AD or FTLD.

In some patients with known vascular abnormalities, there may be clinical concern for a superimposed degenerative dementia. In such cases, imaging is appropriate but must be closely compared with MR findings and clinical signs. Vascular disease may cause a greater impact in the frontal and

frontoparietal cortex because of the large area the middle cerebral artery affects (Fig. 14.23).

Several PET radiopharmaceuticals have been developed that bind to Aβ. The first and most studied of these is C-11 Pittsburgh B compound (PIB), developed from thioflavin T, a fluorescent dye used to evaluate amyloid. C-11 PIB binding is seen in more than 90% of patients with AD. In normal volunteers, background cortical uptake is identified, similar to that in the cerebellum, which is used as the usual normal reference. Clinical use, however, is limited by the short, 20-minute half-life of C-11.

An initial significant development in amyloid imaging was the formulation of the F-18 labeled radiopharmaceutical F-18 FDDNP (an F-18 6-dialkylamino-2-naphthyethylidene derivative). This lipophilic agent crosses the BBB and binds to Aβ. However, many studies have shown that F-18 FDDNP has less specific binding than C-11 PIB, with uptake also seen in NFTs and other proteins in addition to Aβ.

Three F-18–labeled amyloid binding agents have since been approved for use in the United States: F-18 florbetapir (Amyvid, AV-45), F-18 florbetaben (Neuraceq, AV-1), and F-18 flutemetamol (Vizamyl, F-18-3′-F-PIB). Protocol modifications compared with the standard F-18 FDG PET protocol are listed in Box 14.7. Each agent is able to cross the BBB and shows specific high-affinity binding for Aβ. Patterns of uptake will vary

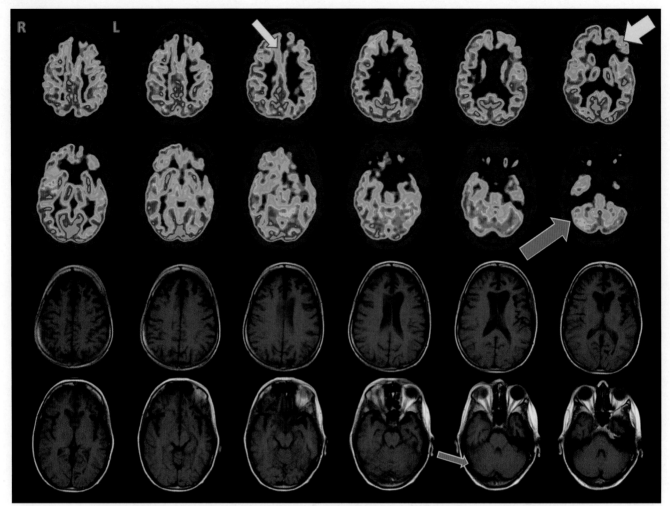

• **Fig. 14.21** Distal effects of neuronal loss on F-18 fluorodeoxyglucose (FDG) positron emission tomography (PET). *(Top)* Frontotemporal lobar degeneration (FTLD) with marked hypometabolism *(wide yellow arrow)* in the frontal and temporal lobes (left > right) with characteristic involvement of the anterior cingulate *(thin yellow arrow)*. Diaschisis is seen with decreased activity *(orange arrows)* in the left (opposite) cerebellum (i.e., crossed cerebellar diaschisis). *(Bottom)* Corresponding axial T1-weighted MR slices show only minimal atrophy in the affected frontal cortex and left cerebellum *(orange arrow)*, disproportionate to metabolic change, and no underlying major infarct as a cause.

somewhat between the agents, but each of these agents functions with similar accuracy in the clinical setting. As noted previously, the distribution of amyloid does not necessarily equate with F-18 FDG PET abnormalities, the presence of amyloid is seen long before symptoms begin, and activity peaks long before clinical signs and symptoms.

Interpretation guidelines specify that abnormal activity must be seen in more than one cortical area in order for a study to be read as positive. They also recommend the use of the following phrases: equates with "no to sparse amyloid plaque" in negative exams (Fig. 14.24) or "moderate to severe amyloid plaques" when positive (Box 14.8). Because early deposition of amyloid occurs in the deeper cortical levels, the amount of white-matter binding seen in these radiopharmaceuticals may cause diagnostic difficulties. Interpretation may be difficult in cases where severe atrophy is seen. Due to the complexities of interpretation, physicians are required to undergo additional training prior to interpretation of clinical exams.

A positive amyloid exam (Fig. 14.25) helps confirm the diagnosis of AD and differentiate AD from FTLD. The negative predictive value of these exams is high. Amyloid PET scans are reportedly 96% sensitive and 100% specific for the presence of amyloid plaque. However, a positive study is not diagnostic of AD because Aβ accumulation can occur in asymptomatic patients: increasing from 10% in those younger than 70 to up to 30% to 40% by age 80. Appropriate use criteria have been developed by the Society of Nuclear Medicine and Molecular Imaging and the Alzheimer's Association, with concerns in mind that referring physicians may not fully understand the limitations of the exam or how to interpret results (Box 14.9).

Amyloid PET imaging has been widely accepted in Europe as a suitable biomarker for assessing disease in research trials and in diagnostic criteria. Use in the United States continues to evolve, with long-standing difficulties obtaining payment from insurers. In April 2019, results from over 11,400 patients with dementia or MCI in the multicenter Imaging

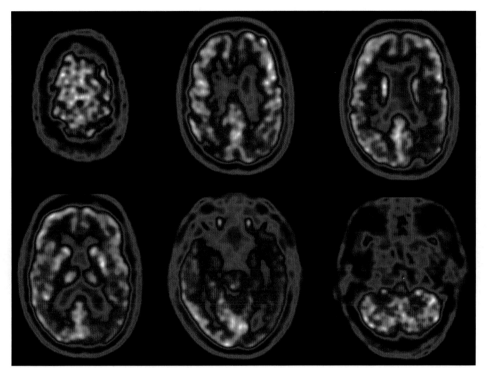

• **Fig. 14.22** A patient with symptoms including speech and memory difficulties for several months. Striking asymmetrical activity in the left temporal lobe favors primary progressive aphasia (PPA). Although this could be the result of the semantic variant frontotemporal dementia, involvement of the left occiput and bilateral posterior parietal regions is suggestive of an Alzheimer's variant (logopenic PPA). Beta-amyloid positron emission tomography (PET) imaging may be helpful because it is expected to be positive in AD variants and not in FTLD (although this is not definitive because roughly 15%-20% of asymptomatic patients are also positive).

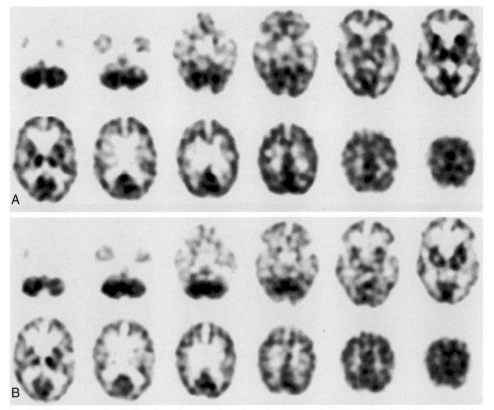

• **Fig. 14.23** Vascular dementia often shows a frontal predisposition similar to other frontotemporal dementias. (A) Vascular dementia may be more diffuse, as seen in this patient, and difficult to differentiate from other causes, including severe Alzheimer's disease. (B) Slow progression was seen in this patient clinically and on a repeat scan 5 years later.

BOX 14.7 PET/CT Imaging Protocol Modifications for Amyloid PET Scan

Preparation

No fasting, glucose control, or change in insulin scheduling

Radiopharmaceutical

5 to 12 mCi (185-444 MBq) intravenous (IV), flush 10 mL 0.9% sterile sodium chloride

Delay scan for 30 to 50 minutes.

F-18 florbetapir (Amyvid) 10 mCi (370 MBq) IV, delay 10 minutes; acquisition 10 minutes.

F-18 florbetaben (Neuraceq) 8 mCi (300 MBq) IV, delay 45 to 130 minutes; scan 10 to 20 minutes.

F-18 flutemetamol (Vizamyl) 5 mCi (185 MBq) IV injected over 40 seconds, 5 to 15 mL 0.9% NaCl flush. Delay 90 minutes; acquisition 10 to 20 minutes.

Note: Clearance is 37% renal, 52% hepatobiliary; plasma levels decrease 75% in first 20 minutes, 90% in 180 minutes.

Patient Positioning

After voiding bladder, patient is placed supine with head immobilized and in center field of view, neck relaxed, nose pointed upward.

PET Image Acquisition

Three-dimensional (3-D) data acquisition, 1 bed position for 10 minutes; pixel size 2 to 3 mm, slice thickness 2 to 4 mm; matrix 256 ×256, zoom 2.

Note: Patient should be encouraged to void bladder postscan to decrease exposure.

CT, Computed tomography; *PET,* positron emission tomography.

Dementia-Evidence for Amyloid Scanning (IDEAS) trial were published (Rabinovici GD, et al. *JAMA*, 2019). The results of the trial showed that amyloid PET exams resulted in a diagnosis change from non-AD to AD in 10.5% and from AD to non-AD in 25.1%. In addition, the composite endpoint changed in 63.5% of patients with dementia and in 60.2% of patients with MCI. It was noted that further work needed to be done to see if these exams would result in a change in clinical outcomes.

Parkinson's disease (PD) is the most common of the movement disorders, affecting approximately 1.5% of people over 65 years and 2.5% of those over the age of 80. As the dopaminergic neurons in the substantia nigra degenerate, patients classically experience a triad of symptoms: resting tremor, rigidity, and bradykinesia. However, diagnosis may be difficult, especially earlier in the course of disease when all signs are not always present. The three groups of parkinsonian syndromes are idiopathic PD, secondary PD (caused by etiologies such as Wilson's disease or other extrinsic agents such as carbon monoxide poisoning and neuroleptic drugs), and neurodegenerative syndromes (atypical Parkinson's or AP) such as multisystem atrophy (MSA) and progressive supranuclear palsy (PSP). In many cases, clinically differentiating idiopathic PD from AP may be especially difficult when patients do not respond to L-dopa therapy. In addition, it may be helpful to have a noninvasive test to help better differentiate PD and parkinsonian syndromes from essential tremor.

PET has been a research tool in movement disorders for decades, using the classic agent F-18 6-fluorodopa (F-18

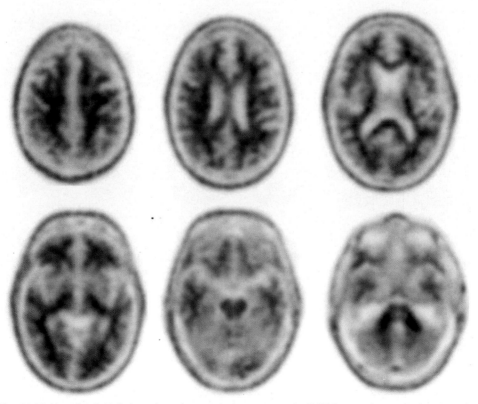

• **Fig. 14.24** Negative F-18 florbetapir positron emission tomography (PET) images in a control patient show the expected nonspecific white-matter binding but no significant cortical accumulation in gray matter.

dopa). F-18 dopa enters the dopamine metabolism pathway early as an analog of L-dopa. Imaging assesses uptake in the corpus striatum, made up by the posterior lentiform nucleus (putamen and globus pallidus) and anterior caudate nucleus. It is estimated that there is a 2% to 10% decrease in striatal activity per year in PD. However, the use of F-18 dopa is complex, with challenges including its tendency to underestimate loss.

BOX 14.8 Amyloid PET Imaging Findings

Interpretation

No cortical uptake
    Equates with no to sparse Aβ
    Interpreted as negative scan
Cortical gray-matter uptake in at least two brain regions
    Correlates with moderate to severe Aβ plaques
    Interpreted as positive scan
Amount of activity: AD > MCI > normal subjects
Normal patients: 22% to 30% show positive scans
    Aβ burden increases with aging.
AD patients: Higher amounts of amyloid and typically higher uptake rates than MCI
MCI patients: Greater uptake volume and higher rates than cognitively normal patients
    Positive scans are associated with poorer memory than MCI patients with lower amounts, but levels do not directly correlate with cognitive test results.

AD, Alzheimer's disease; *MCI,* mild cognitive impairment; *PET,* positron emission tomography.

Newer PET and SPECT agents have been developed to image different components of the dopamine neurotransmitter system (Fig. 14.26). These radiopharmaceuticals are grouped based on the location or mechanism of dopamine metabolism they image and measure dopamine neuron integrity and loss. Other agents target the vesicular monoamine transporter type 2 (VMAT2), presynaptic membrane dopamine transporter (DAT), and postsynaptic dopamine receptors (D2 and D1). Tropane agents derived from cocaine have been developed to image DAT activity. These include F-18/C-11 β-CIT and SPECT agents such as I-123 FP-CIT (I-123 ioflupane, I-123 DaTscan).

U.S. Food and Drug Administration (FDA) approval for I-123 ioflupane was initially complicated by the U.S. Drug Enforcement Agency (DEA) requirement that it be treated as a Schedule II controlled substance. I-123 ioflupane was initially approved in the United States for the differentiation of essential tremor from parkinsonian syndromes.

After injection, uptake in the brain is 7% at 10 minutes but decreases slightly to 3% after 5 hours. Activity accumulates in the striata, remaining fairly stable for 3 to 6 hours. The main route of excretion is through the urine, with 60% of the injected dose excreted by 48 hours. Fecal excretion accounts for roughly 14% of the dose. Dosimetry of I-123 ioflupane is listed in Appendix 1.

A protocol for I-123 ioflupane is presented in Box 14.10. Patient medications should be reviewed for any drug that might interfere with the examination (Box 14.11). Patient preparation consists of blocking thyroid uptake with potassium iodide (400 mg) or Lugol solution (equivalent 100 mg iodide) at least 1 hour

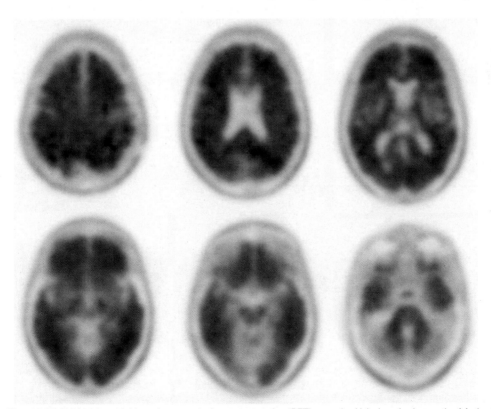

• **Fig. 14.25** Positive amyloid positron emission tomography (PET) scan in Alzheimer's dementia. Marked cortical gray-matter activity is seen diffusely in addition to nonspecific white-matter binding on axial F-18 florbetapir images.

before injection. The patient should be well hydrated and void frequently in the first 48 hours after the examination. After radiotracer injection, a 3- to 6-hour delay is needed before SPECT imaging.

As the dopaminergic striatal neurons degenerate, effects downstream in the globus pallidus occur.

I-123 ioflupane normally shows significant uptake in the basal ganglia with very low background in the surrounding brain (Fig. 14.27, A). Generally, it is not possible to separate the components of the lentiform nucleus into the putamen and globus pallidus by PET or SPECT. Over the course of the disease, decreased uptake occurs in the posterior striatum initially that then moves anteriorly—posterior putamen first, then anterior putamen, and then finally the caudate nucleus (see Fig. 14.27, B). The abnormality is often asymmetric, especially in patients with early disease. Although it is not possible to use the I-123 ioflupane findings to differentiate PD from atypical parkinsonian syndromes (progressive supranuclear palsy, multisystem atrophy, corticobasal degeneration), because the patterns of decreased uptake in the substantia nigra overlap significantly, atypical parkinsonian cases tend to involve the caudate earlier and may be more symmetric. In PD, abnormalities can be greater on the side contralateral to the side of the most severe symptoms (Fig. 14.28). Abnormal decreased radiotracer binding can often detect preclinical disease.

Interobserver variability is good for positive and negative examinations. Although only 78% of patients with PD had a positive scan, a negative scan (NPV) effectively excludes the diagnosis of PD, with 97% of patients with a non-PD, such as essential tremor, showing a normal examination. In addition, following I-123 ioflupane imaging, clinicians report changing diagnosis in up to 30% of patients and significantly altering

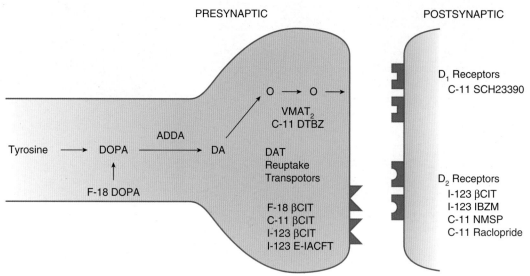

• **Fig. 14.26** Striatal dopamine production and metabolism. The sites of positron emission tomography (PET) and single-photon emission computed tomography (SPECT) agent uptake are shown. *AAAD,* Aromatic amino acid decarboxylase; *DAT,* dopamine reuptake transporter; *VMAT₂,* vesicular monoamine transporter type 2.

BOX 14.10 I-123 Ioflupane (I-123 DaTscan) SPECT Imaging Protocol

Patient Preparation
Stop interfering medications.
Thyroid blocking: Potassium iodide Lugol solution (equivalent to 100 mg iodide) or potassium perchlorate 400 mg, at least 1 hour before injection

Radiopharmaceutical
I-123 ioflupane 3 to 5 mCi (111-185 MBq) slow intravenous (IV) infusion
Delay to scan: 3 to 6 hours

Instrumentation
Multiple-head gamma camera; attenuation correction recommended (e.g., CT in SPECT/CT)
Collimators: Low energy, high resolution
Energy window: Peak 159 keV ± 10%
Matrix and zoom to a pixel size of 3.5 to 4.5 mm and 1 pixel thick

Positioning
Supine with head in center of the field of view in a head holder extending beyond bed to allow tight camera head orbit (11-15 cm)

Acquisition
Step-and-shoot: 3-degree steps, 30 to 40 seconds/step, 180 degrees/head (360-degree rotation); continuous acquisition also acceptable
Minimum 1.5 million counts for optimal image

Processing
Iterative or filtered back-projection reconstruction, Butterworth or other low-pass filter; motion-correction software can be used as needed; alignment of the anterior commissure–posterior commissure (AC/PC) line parallel to the transverse slice axis
Quantification software can be implemented or the striatal binding ratio can be calculated after placing a region of interest (ROI) around each basal ganglia and a background ROI in occipital cortex or other area of low DAT concentration.
Striatal binding ratio = (mean striatal counts − mean background counts)/(mean background counts)

CT, Computed tomography; *DAT,* dopamine transporter; *SPECT,* single-photon emission computed tomography.

BOX 14.11 Medications Potentially Interfering With Iodine-123 Ioflupane

Cocaine
Amphetamines
  d-amphetamine
  methamphetamine
  methylphenidate
CNS stimulants
  Phentermine
  Ephedrine
  Methylphenidate
Modafinil
Antidepressants
  Amoxapine
  Mazindol
  Bupropion
  Radafaxine
  Sertraline
Adrenergic agonists
  Phenylephrine
  Norepinephrine
  Phenylpropanolamine
Anticholinergic: Benztropine
Opioids
  Fentanyl
Anxiolytic
  Buspirone
Anesthetics
  Ketamine
  PCP
  Isoflurane
Anti-parkinsonian drugs: no significant interference
  Dopamine agonists (Levodopa), MAO B inhibitors, amantadine, N-methyl-D-aspartate receptor blockers
Effects uncertain:
  Serotonin reuptake inhibitors: paroxetine, citalopram

CNS, Central nervous system; *MAO,* monoamine oxidase.

clinical management in 50% to 60% of cases. I-123 ioflupane can also help differentiate DLB from AD, with decreased uptake in DLB.

Intractable or medically refractory partial complex seizures may require surgery for therapy. Precise seizure localization often requires a combination of scalp electroencephalogram (EEG), MRI, magnetoencephalography (MEG), and nuclear medicine imaging for evaluation. These noninvasive studies are important in directing the invasive intracranial EEG grid placement in the operating room and determining therapeutic options. Although MRI often reveals abnormalities at the site of seizure foci, such as mesial temporal hippocampal sclerosis, it is rare for structural imaging to fully visualize the actual extent of the abnormally activated neurons by structural imaging. In addition, although EEG remains critical in seizure localization, it is often inconclusive, localizing the ictal focus in only 50% of patients and incorrectly localizing the abnormal area 5% to 10% of the time.

PET and SPECT may play important roles in seizure evaluation. In the ictal state, activated foci show increased activity, representing increased rCBF and glucose metabolism. Interictal images, however, show normal or decreased activity. In the immediate postictal state, activity is changing and may show areas of increased and decreased activity. Therefore, it is essential to know the clinical status of the patient at the time of injection. This is best accomplished with continuous EEG monitoring prior to injection. In addition, because patients may have more than one type of seizure, the EEG and clinical presentation can help determine whether the seizure of interest was actually occurring during the ictal state.

Although ictal studies are most sensitive, they are technically highly demanding (Fig. 14.29). Patients are admitted and continuously monitored off medication. Once the seizure is identified, trained personnel must inject the radiotracer within seconds of seizure onset. Because the radiotracer is essentially trapped once taken up into the brain, imaging can be delayed for a few hours until the seizure is controlled. Ictal PET would not be practical given the shorter half-life of F-18 FDG.

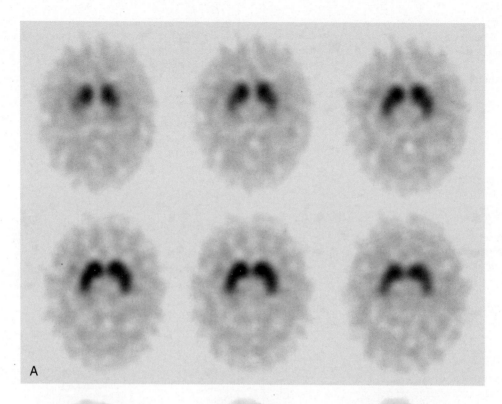

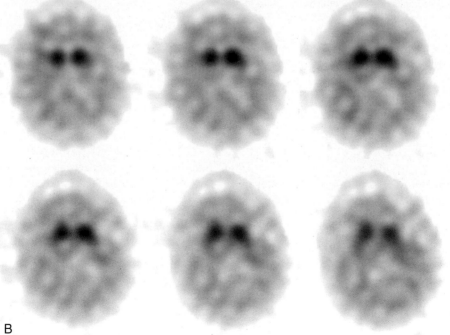

• **Fig. 14.27** (A) Normal distribution of the dopamine transporter agent I-123 ioflupane showing high striatal uptake relative to cortex. (B) Abnormal single-photon emission computed tomography (SPECT) in a patient with Parkinson's disease shows absent posterior uptake bilaterally and asymmetrical decreased activity beginning in the right caudate. Eventually, caudate activity will also vanish in severe disease.

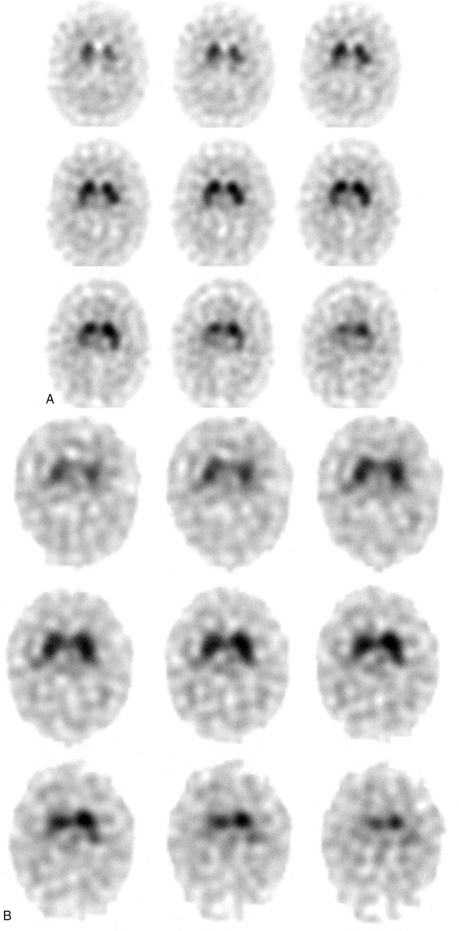

• **Fig. 14.28** I-123 ioflupane single-photon emission computed tomography (SPECT) images initially (A) show subtle abnormal decreased activity in the posterior right basal ganglia. (B) A repeat examination confirms the case was abnormal, with disease progression on the right, now with a mild decrease anteriorly in the caudate, and subtle decreased activity in the left putamen.

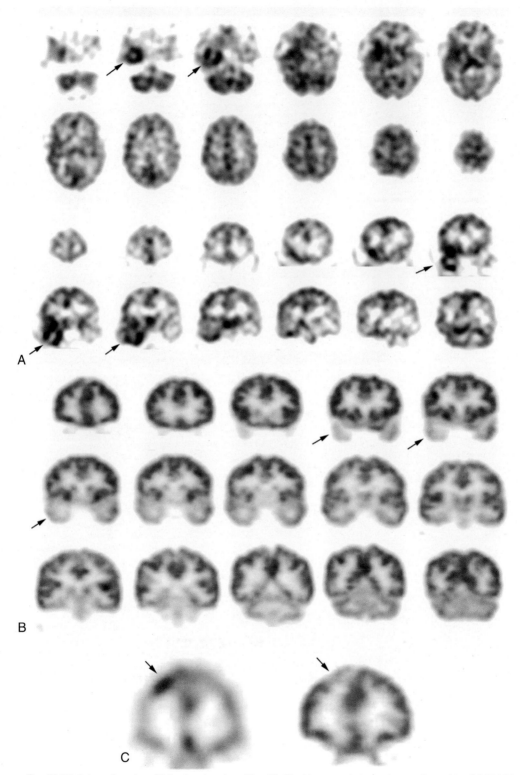

• **Fig. 14.29** Seizure imaging. (A) Ictal technetium-99m (Tc-99m) hexamethylpropyleneamine oxime (HMPAO) single-photon emission computed tomography (SPECT) axial *(top)* and coronal *(bottom)* images reveal increased perfusion *(arrows)* to the right temporal region from an active seizure. (B) The abnormal temporal region is a subtle area of hypometabolism *(arrows)* on the interictal fluorodeoxyglucose (FDG) positron emission tomography (PET). (C) Ictal SPECT in a second patient demonstrates hyperperfusion *(arrow)* in the right parasagittal region *(left)* corresponding to an area of hypometabolism *(arrow)* on interictal PET *(right)* from a seizure focus.

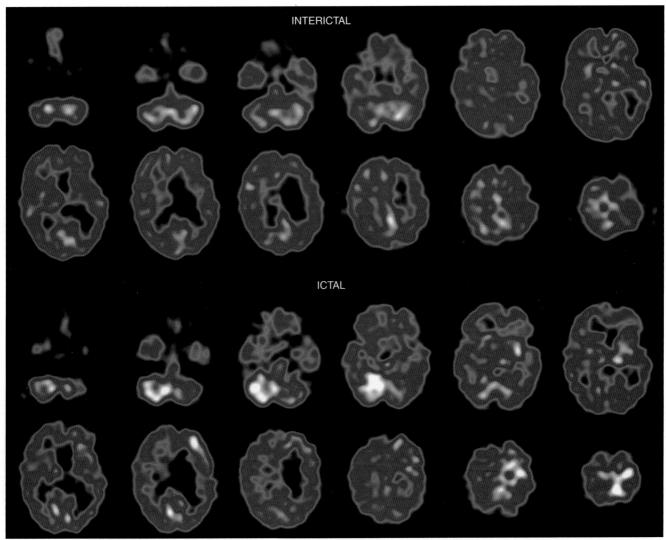

• **Fig. 14.30** Interictal technetium-99m (Tc-99m) hexamethylpropyleneamine oxime (HMPAO) single-photon emission computed tomography (SPECT) reveals extensive hypoperfusion in a congenitally malformed cortex. Ictal images show increased activity throughout much of the frontal and parietal lobes, without a resectable focus, and increased uptake in the right cerebellum from diaschisis.

Interictal studies are far less sensitive than ictal exams, although interictal PET is superior to interictal SPECT. Clinical knowledge of the most recent seizure is needed to be sure that a study is truly ictal or interictal. Ictal SPECT has a sensitivity of roughly 90% in temporal lobe seizures, and the abnormal areas are generally more extensive than any structural abnormality on MRI. However, the sensitivity for extratemporal seizures is lower, on the order of 50% to 75%. Interictal FDG PET identifies a hypometabolic ictal focus in roughly 80% of patients, although this is higher if a discrete MR abnormality is seen. Interictal SPECT may identify the focus in approximately 70% of cases involving the temporal lobes. In some cases, extensive or multifocal abnormalities are seen without an excisable lesion (Fig. 14.30).

Although MRI and CT are the preeminent modalities for diagnosing stroke, PET and SPECT can be useful in several situations. They might help evaluate stroke risk in certain patients, indicate those patients most likely to benefit from intervention, and even predict stroke recovery. Relationships such as distant neuronal activity loss (diaschisis), neuron recruitment, and recovery through neuronal plasticity can be studied. In acute stroke, Tc-99m HMPAO SPECT has been used to identify which patients will most likely benefit from thrombolytic therapy, although this can be done with newer MRI techniques.

Functional imaging can also assess the expected complications that might arise if arterial blood supply is compromised by disease or surgically altered. Finally, planar perfusion exams are frequently used to aid in the diagnosis of brain death.

After arterial blood flow enters the brain, the vessels join at the circle of Willis in the base of the brain, allowing blood from one side to provide flow to areas that are otherwise being underserved. In theory, this anatomy should protect patients who require internal carotid artery sacrifice (such as in the treatment of glomus tumor or intracranial aneurysm) or who suffer occlusion following endarterectomy or complication from bypass. However, a small but significant proportion of these patients will suffer a stroke despite an intact circle of Willis and adequate cross-filling on arteriogram. Additional testing to assess risk

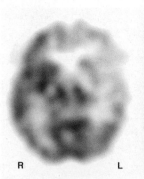
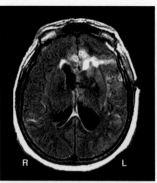

• **Fig. 14.31** *Left,* hexamethylpropyleneamine oxime (HMPAO) single-photon emission computed tomography (SPECT) performed after a carotid balloon occlusion injection shows severe left middle cerebral artery territory hypoperfusion, identifying a high risk for stroke. The patient underwent permanent left carotid occlusion using gradual occlusion with a Selverstone clamp rather than bypass. *Right,* This gradual occlusion was not sufficient to protect the patient, and the patient had a stroke in the same distribution as the SPECT on follow-up computed tomography (CT) performed after the procedure.

can include transcranial doppler and Wada neurological testing. During the Wada test, the patient's speech and memory function are examined after half the brain is anesthetized by intracarotid sodium amobarbital infusion and temporary occlusion by a balloon catheter. The risks of complications from permanent carotid occlusion can be further reduced through the addition of a Tc-99m HMPAO or Tc-99m ECD SPECT scan to the preoperative workup, with previous reports of a decrease of up to 20% in morbidity and mortality.

The radiopharmaceutical is injected intravenously in the angiography suite at the time of temporary internal carotid artery balloon occlusion. The balloon is then deflated after 1 minute. Imaging is done later, after the catheter has been removed and the patient has been stabilized. Patients at risk for stroke are easily identified by a significant drop in perfusion to the occluded side compared to baseline on SPECT images. Carotid bypass is generally warranted in these patients because the remaining vessels cannot meet the needs of the side that will be occluded (Fig. 14.31).

The acetazolamide SPECT study is a pharmacological vascular stress test for the brain that can help evaluate the risk for stroke in patients with prior stroke, transient ischemic attack (TIA), atherosclerotic stenosis, vascular malformations, or vascular compromise such as in moyamoya. The vascular reserve of these patients can be assessed by Tc-99m HMPAO or Tc-99m ECD SPECT imaging after intravenous administration of 1 gram of the carbonic anhydrase inhibitor and antihypertensive agent acetazolamide (Diamox). The drug causes vasodilation through an increase in carbon dioxide, which in turn leads to an increase in rCBF. Although global blood flow is increased, abnormal vessels cannot dilate, and blood is shunted away. This will accentuate any abnormality and better demonstrate territories at risk for infarction as areas of relatively decreased activity on SPECT images (Fig. 14.32). It is important to compare the resting state to the stress state.

Accuracy and speed in making the diagnosis of brain death become critical when organ donation is considered and life support systems must be used. Although the diagnosis of brain

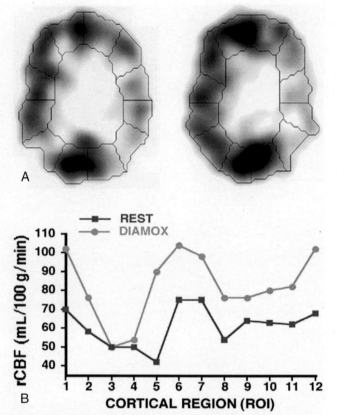

• **Fig. 14.32** Semiquantitative analysis of ischemia with acetazolamide (Diamox) single-photon emission computed tomography (SPECT). (A) Baseline technetium-99m (Tc-99m) hexamethylpropyleneamine oxime (HMPAO) SPECT before acetazolamide *(left)* shows mild left parietal hypoperfusion. After acetazolamide *(right),* the brain shows increased activity in response to vasodilation, with the exception of the left parietal defect, and the decreased activity from ischemia is even more apparent. (B) Regional cerebral blood flow curves generated from region of interest (ROI) boxes placed over summed SPECT images (positioned as on a clock, numbered from 1 o'clock to 12 o'clock). After acetazolamide administration, counts are increased relative to rest perfusion with the exception from 2 o'clock to 4 o'clock where the postdiamox curve dips, signifying an area at high risk for infarction because it is unable to respond to the vasodilation.

death is by definition a clinical one, clinical diagnosis may be difficult. The specific criteria necessary to make the diagnosis of brain death are as follows:
1. The patient must be in deep coma with a total absence of brainstem reflexes or spontaneous respiration.
2. Potentially reversible causes such as drug intoxication, metabolic derangement, or hypothermia must be excluded.
3. The cause of the brain dysfunction must be diagnosed (e.g., trauma, stroke).
4. The clinical findings of brain death must be present for a defined period of observation (6-24 hours).

Although confirmatory ancillary tests are used by clinicians to increase certainty, they cannot themselves establish the diagnosis of brain death. An isoelectric EEG alone does not establish brain death, and at least one repeat study is required. In the patient with intoxication from barbiturates or other depressive drugs or with hypothermia, the EEG may be flat, even though cerebral perfusion is still present and recovery is possible.

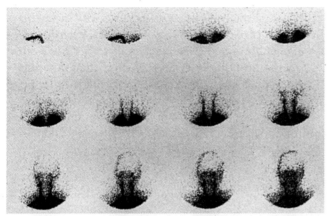

• Fig. 14.33 Brain death. This technetium-99m (Tc-99m) diethylenetri-aminepentaacetic acid (DTPA) brain blood-flow study shows radiotracer transiting the internal carotids; however, there is no intracerebral blood flow. Only external carotid blood flow to the scalp is seen.

In brain death, edema, softening, necrosis, and autolysis of brain tissue lead to increased intracranial pressure. As pressure rises, it eventually prevents intracranial perfusion. On cerebral arteriography, this is seen with flow that does not extend beyond the internal carotid arteries in the neck into the brain above. However, catheter angiography is invasive, resource intensive, and unnecessary. The radionuclide brain death study is a rapid and simple alternative that can be performed at the bedside. It is usually indicated when the EEG and clinical criteria are equivocal or if urgent decisions need to be made. Scintigraphy is not affected by drug intoxication or hypothermia, and an abnormal radionuclide angiogram showing no cerebral perfusion is more specific for brain death than an isoelectric EEG.

Technetium-labeled radiopharmaceuticals are used to assess dynamic flow. In the past, Tc-99m DTPA was often used because it clears rapidly from the blood, allowing a repeat study if necessary. However, optimal technique is mandatory, and interpretation may be extremely difficult. Blood flow through the external carotid system that drains via intracranial veins can be confused with internal artery flow to the cortex because of the lack of anatomic landmarks (Fig. 14.33).

Tc-99m HMPAO and Tc-99m ECD studies are easier to interpret and are now preferred because they rely only on delayed images, which are not as dependent on adequate bolus technique (Fig. 14.34). Delivery of these agents requires blood flow to be present, and because uptake only occurs in living brain cells, delayed images showing the fixed presence or absence of brain uptake require flow to the brain. If no CBF is present, no cerebral uptake will occur.

Tc-99m DTPA requires diagnostic-quality imaging of the arteriographic phase following injection, done as dynamic planar images after injection. Tc-99m HMPAO, on the other hand, is injected intravenously, and although flow images can be obtained, they are unnecessary. Delayed planar images can be obtained at the bedside, and SPECT is unnecessary. Images of the injection site can be performed to ensure the dose was adequate and not infiltrated. A radionuclide protocol used in brain death is outlined in Box 14.12.

With brain death, flow to both common carotid arteries is seen extending up only to the level of the base of the skull. No visualization of the brain is seen with Tc-99m HMPAO, making it the easiest test to interpret.

A secondary finding of the "hot-nose" sign is sometimes seen. This has been reported as being a result of the diversion of intracranial blood flow into external carotid circulation because of the increased pressure, resulting in relatively increased flow to the face and nose. However, lateral views have shown the activity lies far posteriorly, along the brainstem and posterior fossa region.

PET

Although enhanced MR is the best imaging exam for the diagnosis of primary brain tumors, F-18 FDG PET has long been used as a problem-solving tool in their assessment, with F-18 FDG uptake being related to metabolic activity and therefore to tumor grade. Although low-grade gliomas (World Health Organization [WHO] grades I and II) typically show uptake similar to that of white matter, and high-grade tumors (WHO grade III) may be difficult to separate from the high background activity of gray matter, grade IV tumors (glioblastoma multiforme) should show uptake increased above gray-matter background (Fig. 14.35).

F-18 FDG PET can be used to help direct biopsy to the most aggressive areas in a lesion. Additionally, because the evolution of radiation changes in a tumor often leads to increasing enhancement and even nodularity on MR after a few months, PET can help differentiate recurrent tumor from post-therapy change. Direct, side-by-side comparison with the MRI is critical for image interpretation, and actual fusion of PET images to the MRI is even better. In the case of high-dose radiation therapy, increased F-18 FDG activity can be seen and may persist. Although this activity is generally mild and not greater than normal cortical uptake, serial images to look for any areas of increasing activity may be necessary to exclude early recurrence. Recurrent gliomas are typically highly aggressive and therefore likely to show more intense radiotracer accumulation. Interestingly, important exceptions to the rule that uptake is directly related to tumor grade are seen in low-grade pilocytic astrocytomas and benign pituitary tumors, which both can show significantly increased F-18 FDG accumulation.

Protocols for F-18 FDG imaging in the brain usually involve a shorter delay after injection (30-45 minutes) compared with whole-body oncology cases (55-65 minutes). However, in primary brain tumor assessment, longer delays (e.g., 2-4 hours) have been reported to improve sensitivity. Lengthy delays such as this are often not practical in a busy clinic.

Although F-18 FDG PET is a valuable clinical tool in the workup of many types of malignancy outside of the CNS, nearly two-thirds of intracranial metastatic lesions are not seen on PET because of the high background activity (Fig. 14.36). Therefore, MRI remains the standard for metastatic lesion detection.

Other experimental PET radiopharmaceuticals have been used in research protocols to assess aspects of tumor cellular activity other than glucose metabolism. The evaluation of DNA

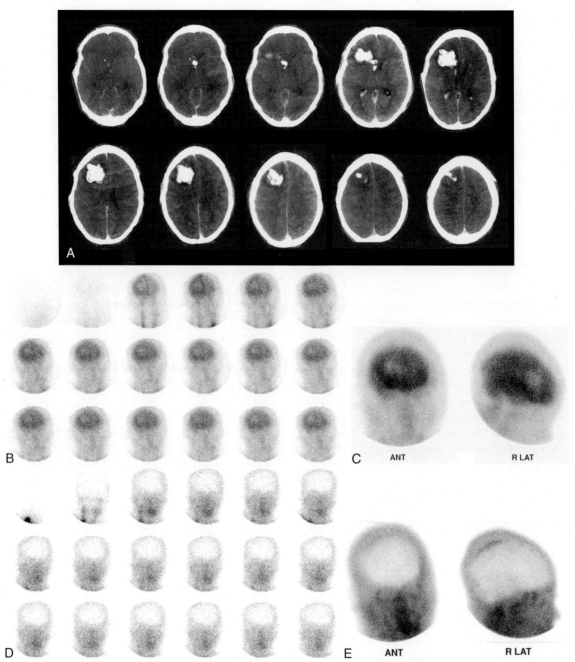

• **Fig. 14.34** Brain death evaluation. (A) Computed tomography (CT) images of a head trauma victim show a right frontal parenchymal hemorrhage extending into the ventricles. (B) In the evaluation for brain death, initial technetium-99m (Tc-99m) hexamethylpropyleneamine oxime (HMPAO) images show that perfusion is delayed but present, and cortical uptake is seen (C), although with a defect from the hemorrhage. (D) A follow-up study 72 hours later shows internal carotid arterial flow terminating below the head from brain death. (E) This is confirmed with absent delayed cortical uptake. Any peripheral activity is a result of external carotid flow. *ANT,* Anterior; *R LAT,* right lateral.

synthesis with F-18 fluorothymidine (FLT) can be used in aggressive, enhancing tumors, where the BBB has been broken down. However, thymidine metabolism is complex, and amino acid agents have shown potentially high specificity and sensitivity, even in lower-grade tumors and in lesions where the BBB remains intact. These agents include C-11 methionine, F-18 fluorodopa, and F-18 fluoroethyltyrosine (F-18 FET).

The SPECT agents Tc-99m HMPAO and Tc-99m ECD are generally not useful for the detection of intracranial

malignancies. Although increased uptake might be seen in tumors, slightly more commonly with Tc-99m ECD, both agents often show normal or decreased activity.

SPECT evaluation of recurrent gliomas and differentiation of intracranial lymphoma can be done with the cardiac imaging agents thallium-201 and Tc-99m sestamibi (Fig. 14.37), which have both shown accumulation in several tumor types. The potassium analog Tl-201 depends on blood flow and BBB breakdown for distribution and on metabolic activity with uptake

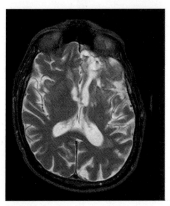 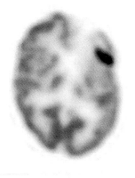

• **Fig. 14.35** Recurrent gliomas may be difficult to detect on magnetic resonance imaging (MRI). T2-weighted MRI shows posttherapy signal changes *(left)*. The recurrent tumor is seen as an intense focus on the fluorodeoxyglucose (FDG) positron emission tomography (PET) *(right)*.

through the Na+/K+ pump. Tc-99m sestamibi is transported by the endothelial cell and localizes in active mitochondria. Some accumulation of Tc-99m sestamibi occurs in the choroid plexus, which may make it less than ideal in some tumors.

The procedure for SPECT tumor imaging involves imaging approximately 20 to 30 minutes after injection of 2 to 4 mCi (74-148 MBq) of Tl-201 or 20 mCi (740 MBq) Tc-99m sestamibi. Occasionally, a 2-hour delayed Tl-201 acquisition may be helpful because the abnormal tumor tissue would be expected to wash out more slowly than normal brain or areas of BBB disruption. Visual analysis typically shows uptake equal to or greater than the scalp or the contralateral side in tumors. There is some overlap in the appearance of malignant and infectious

processes. An intracranial abscess, for example, often has increased activity. Because infections usually have lower uptake than malignancies, quantitative analysis may help improve specificity. A region of interest is drawn around the abnormal uptake and compared with the contralateral normal. Delayed images may improve sensitivity because the tumor retains activity and the background clears.

MR and CT are the main imaging modalities for visualizing issues concerning CSF leakage, ventricular CSF shunt patency, and hydrocephalus. However, for many years, dynamic radionuclide CSF studies have been employed as problem-solving tools in complex cases or when patients cannot have MR.

CSF is secreted by the ventricular choroid plexus and, to a lesser extent, from extraventricular sites. Normally, CSF drains from the lateral ventricles through the interventricular foramen of Monro into the third ventricle (Fig. 14.38). Along with the additional CSF produced by the choroid plexus of the third ventricle, it then passes through the cerebral aqueduct of Sylvius into the fourth ventricle and then leaves the ventricular system through the median foramen of Magendie and the two lateral foramina of Luschka. Subsequently, the CSF enters the subarachnoid space surrounding the brain and spinal cord. Along the base of the brain, the subarachnoid space expands into lakes called *cisterns.* The subarachnoid space extends over the surface of the brain. The CSF is absorbed through the pacchionian granulations of the pia arachnoid villi into the superior sagittal sinus. The flow of CSF can be evaluated by injecting a radiotracer intrathecally in the spine or into the port reservoir of a CSF shunt catheter.

Radiotracers that are injected into the CSF space must be produced so that they are suitable for intrathecal administration, absolutely aseptic and pyrogen-free. The use of the carrier molecule diethylenetriamine pentaacetic acid (DTPA) is highly suitable because it is not quickly metabolized, will tightly bind the radiotracer, and is nonlipophilic and so is not readily absorbed from the CSF space until it reaches the arachnoid villi. In situations where imaging will be conducted over more than a few hours, indium-111 (In-111) is the more suitable radiolabel because of its 2.8-day half-life. However, compared with Tc-99m, it has poorer imaging characteristics, with two relatively high photopeaks of 245 keV (94% abundance) and 171 keV (90%). Because of the longer half-life and higher photon energy, the amount of the radiopharmaceutical that can be administered is lower when using In-111 compared with a similar compound labeled with Tc-99m, and this differential can also affect sensitivity.

Therefore, for shorter CSF shunt studies, Tc-99m DTPA is preferred, but for cisternography, In-111 DTPA is generally used. If a study is performed to detect a CSF leak, it will be more readily visualized during imaging with Tc-99m DTPA. However, if pledgets are placed in the nose to detect leaks that are not readily seen, it may be beneficial to use In-111 so that extra time is available for the exam to deal with the more complicated procedures for assessing the pledgets for evidence of the leak.

Normal-Pressure Hydrocephalus

Hydrocephalus is an abnormal enlargement of the cerebral ventricles caused by excessive buildup of CSF that can result from

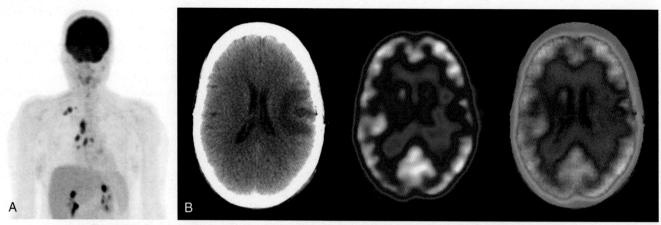

• **Fig. 14.36** F-18 fluorodeoxyglucose (FDG) images from a patient with metastatic lung cancer show (A) avid uptake in disease within the chest on the maximal-intensity projection image, but positron emission tomography (PET)/computed tomography (CT) images of the brain (B) show a left cerebral metastasis with surrounding edema on CT *(left)*, with little FDG accumulation on PET *(center)* or fused *(right)* images.

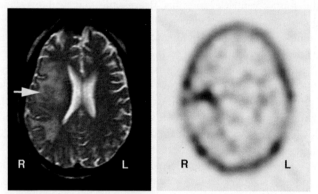

• **Fig. 14.37** Intracranial lymphoma. A mass is seen in a patient with acquired immune deficiency syndrome on the T2-weighted magnetic resonance imaging (MRI) *(left, arrow)*, with the Tl-201 single-photon emission computed tomography (SPECT) showing intense tumor uptake *(right)*.

abnormal CSF production, circulation, or absorption. This should be differentiated from hydrocephalus ex vacuo, which occurs after a stroke or traumatic brain injury causes the volume of brain tissue to shrink or atrophy because no surgical treatment will or is needed to decrease the ventricles. Hydrocephalus can present at birth from congenital causes or can be acquired later in life. The processes causing the disorder can be either noncommunicating or communicating. In *noncommunicating hydrocephalus,* flow from the ventricular system into the basal cisterns and subarachnoid space is obstructed. This is commonly the result of a mass or congenital abnormality at or above the fourth ventricle, and the diagnosis is usually made by MRI. In *communicating hydrocephalus,* CSF is free to flow from the intraventricular region into the subarachnoid space. The obstruction to CSF flow is extraventricular, in the basal cisterns, cerebral convexities, or arachnoid villi. Common causes include previous subarachnoid hemorrhage, chronic subdural hematoma, leptomeningitis, and meningeal carcinomatosis. Although an identifiable cause is often found, roughly half the cases are idiopathic, with the etiology unknown.

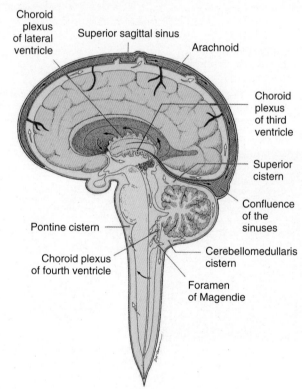

• **Fig. 14.38** Flow dynamics of cerebrospinal fluid (CSF). Originating in lateral ventricle choroid plexus, CSF flows through the third and fourth ventricles into the basal cisterns, moves over the convexities, and finally is reabsorbed in the superior sagittal sinus.

Normal-pressure hydrocephalus (NPH) is a form of communicating hydrocephalus in which the opening CSF pressure on lumbar puncture is normal. It can occur at any age but is most common in the elderly. NPH manifests clinically with progressive dementia, ataxia, and incontinence. On anatomical imaging, the ventricular system is dilated out of proportion to the prominence of cortical sulci and the basal cisterns. Shunting the CSF away through surgical placement of a drain can reduce intracranial pressure and help relieve symptoms.

BOX 14.13 Cisternography: Summary Protocol

Patient Preparation
Stop nonsteroidal medications and medications that increase bleeding risks.

Radiopharmaceutical
500 µCi (19 MBq) In-111 DTPA (pyrogen-free for intrathecal use); inject slowly into lumbar subarachnoid space using a 22-gauge needle with the bevel positioned vertically.
- The CSF opening pressure may be measured and a CSF sample may be withdrawn.
- The patient should be instructed to remain recumbent for 60 minutes after injection. Patient activity should be restricted for 24 hours.

Instrumentation
Gamma camera: Large field of view
Collimator: Medium energy
Computer setup: 256 × 256 matrix; 50,000 to 100,000 counts per image or 10 min/image
SPECT/CT (optional):
  SPECT computer setup: 128 × 128 matrix; noncircular orbit, 35 sec/stop Iterative reconstruction, 3 iterations, Butterworth filter (cutoff 0.5, order 5)
  CT: 120 kV, 50 mAs, pitch 0.813 rotation 0.75 seconds, FOV 50 cm; matrix 512 × 512

Image Acquisition
Planar: 1 hour: thoracic-lumbar spine for evaluation of injection adequacy then image the head AP.
3 hours, 24 hours, 48 hours: anterior, posterior, and both lateral views of the head
SPECT/CT if planar images equivocal at 24 hours

AP, Anteroposterior; CSF, Cerebrospinal fluid; CT, computed tomography; DTPA, diethylenetriaminepentaacetic acid; FOV, field of view; SPECT, single-photon emission computed tomography.

It is important to determine who will likely benefit from shunt placement because morbidity and mortality are high as a result of complications (approximately one-third or more of cases). In addition, not all patients will improve with shunting. Often, the patients who do not improve are subsequently found to have an underlying neurodegenerative disease that can explain the dementia. In algorithms used to assess the benefit of shunting, patients are evaluated for the presence of neurodegenerative disorders, and the MR is examined for signs that ventriculomegaly is likely the result of NPH. The opening pressure is measured at lumbar puncture, and a test removal of a large volume of CSF can be done to look for improvement. In the past, CSF patterns of flow on radionuclide cisternography were thought to be predictive of which patients would improve (with up to 88% sensitivity) from CSF shunting. However, it has since been shown that the patterns are not specific. Additionally, the lumbar puncture required for dose administration can result in complications such as headache (>25%-30%), infection, and chronic CSF fluid leak requiring intervention. Currently, cisternography is infrequently performed but may be helpful in specific cases, including patients who cannot tolerate MR.

A sample protocol for radionuclide cisternography is listed in Box 14.13. The radiotracer for intrathecal injection must be sterile and pyrogen-free. Injection may be performed by the neurologist or surgeon, and the patient should be kept supine for at least 30 to 60 minutes. Anteroposterior (AP) planar images are obtained of the spine at 1 hour, and AP and lateral images of the skull are done at 2 to 3 and 24 hours. In abnormal cases, SPECT/CT at 24 hours and planar imaging with or without SPECT/CT may be needed at 48 hours.

Cisternography Image Interpretation

Activity normally reaches the basal cisterns by 1 hour, the frontal poles and sylvian fissure area by 2 to 6 hours, the cerebral convexities by 12 hours, and the arachnoid villi in the sagittal sinus by 24 hours (Fig. 14.39). The radiotracer does not normally enter the ventricular system because physiological flow is in the opposite direction. The radiotracer is eventually absorbed and undergoes renal excretion. Early visualization of the bladder in the first couple of hours can result if the radiopharmaceutical injection is initially extravasated because it is absorbed into the bloodstream and quickly cleared into the urine.

Several patterns of flow can be observed after the introduction of the radiopharmaceutical into the intrathecal space, with the key variables being whether or not activity reaches the convexities or if reflux into the ventricles occurs (Table 14.9).

In patients with noncommunicating (obstructive) hydrocephalus, cisternography usually shows a normal pattern of flow up to the basal cisterns and over the convexities, with no ventricular reflux. However, if activity is injected into the ventricles through a ventriculostomy rather than via lumbar puncture in these patients, serial images show minimal activity in the basal cisterns.

In communicating hydrocephalus, including patients with NPH, cisternography can show a spectrum of CSF flow patterns. However, flow over the convexities of the brain will be abnormally delayed (>24 hours) or absent. Abnormal reflux of activity into the ventricles may occur transiently (pattern IIIB) or persist (pattern IV). It was previously suggested that those with NPH who were most likely to benefit from surgical shunting were those with the type IV cisternographic pattern, persistent ventricular activity and no activity over the convexities. However, false positives and false negatives occur.

Various diversionary CSF shunts (e.g., ventriculoperitoneal, ventriculoatrial, ventriculopleural, lumboperitoneal) have been used to treat obstructive hydrocephalus. Complications may include catheter blockage, infection, thromboembolism, subdural or epidural hematomas, disconnection of catheters, CSF pseudocyst, bowel obstruction, and bowel perforation.

The diagnosis of shunt patency and adequacy of CSF flow often can be made by examination of the patient and inspection of the subcutaneous CSF reservoir. When this assessment is uncertain, radionuclide studies with Tc-99m DTPA can help identify abnormal function. Familiarity with the specific shunt type and its configuration is helpful. For example, the valves may allow bidirectional or only unidirectional flow. A proximal shunt limb consists of tubing running from the ventricles into the reservoir, and the distal limb carries CSF away from the reservoir into the body.

Shunt injection should be performed with aseptic technique by a physician familiar with the type of shunt in place

4-Hour Images

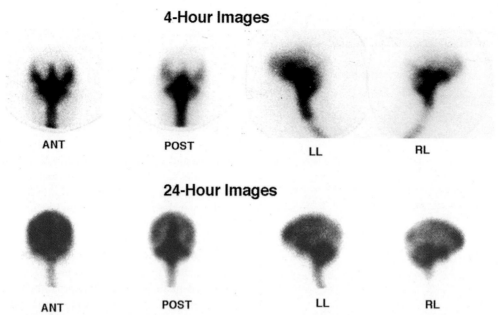

ANT   POST   LL   RL

24-Hour Images

ANT   POST   LL   RL

• **Fig. 14.39** Normal cisternogram. Anterior and lateral images 4 and 24 hours after intrathecal radiotracer injection show normal transit up over the convexities, with no ventricular reflux. *ANT,* Anterior; *LL,* left lateral; *POST,* posterior; *RL,* right lateral.

TABLE 14.9	Patterns of Flow in Cisternography for Evaluation of Hydrocephalus	

Type	Pattern	Cause
I	Tracer over convexities 24 hr	• Normal • Noncommunicating hydrocephalus
II	Delayed migration over convexities but no ventricular reflux	• Cerebral atrophy • Old age
IIIA	Transient ventricular reflux with tracer at convexities 24 hr	Indeterminate: Evolving or resolving communicating hydrocephalus
IIIB	No tracer over convexities with transient ventricular reflux	Normal-pressure hydrocephalus
IV	No tracer over convexities with persistent ventricular reflux	Normal-pressure hydrocephalus

BOX 14.14   Shunt Patency: Summary Protocol

Patient Preparation
None

Radiopharmaceutical
Technetium-99m (Tc-99m) diethylenetriaminepentaacetic acid (DTPA) 0.5 to 1 mCi (18.5-37 MBq)

Instrumentation
Gamma camera: Wide field of view; low-energy, all-purpose collimator
Computer and camera setup: 1-minute images for 30 minutes

Procedure
Using aseptic technique, clean the shaved scalp with povidone-iodine.
• Penetrate the shunt reservoir with a 25- to 35-gauge needle.
• Once the needle is in place, position the patient's head under the camera with the reservoir in the middle of the field of view.
• Inject the radiopharmaceutical.
• Take serial images for 30 minutes.
• If no flow is seen, place the patient in an upright position and continue imaging for 10 minutes.
• If still no flow is seen, obtain static images of 50k after 1 and 2 hours.
• If flow is demonstrated at any point, obtain 50k images of the shunt and tubing every 15 minutes until flow to the distal tip of the shunt tubing is identified or for 2 hours, whichever is first.
• To determine proximal patency of the reservoir, the distal catheter can be manually occluded during the procedure so that the radiotracer will reflux into the ventricular system.
• Image activity through the length of shunt and adjacent tissues at the terminal end.

(Box 14.14). The Tc-99m DTPA is generally preferred over In-111 DTPA because of the superior imaging characteristics of Tc-99m and the lack of a need to do extended delayed imaging as may be required in the assessment of hydrocephalus. The patency of the proximal shunt limb can sometimes be evaluated before checking distal patency. In patients with certain types of variable or low-pressure two-way valves, the distal catheter is initially occluded by manually pressing on the neck. The pressure may cause injected tracer to flow into the proximal limb.

Images should show prompt flow into the ventricles, followed by spontaneous distal flow through the shunt catheter (Fig. 14.40). The shunt tubing is usually seen. Catheters draining into the peritoneum show accumulation of radiotracer freely within the abdominal cavity (Fig. 14.41). In cases of obstruction, activity does not move through the distal limb on delayed images or may pool close to the tip of the catheter in a loculated collection (Fig. 14.42).

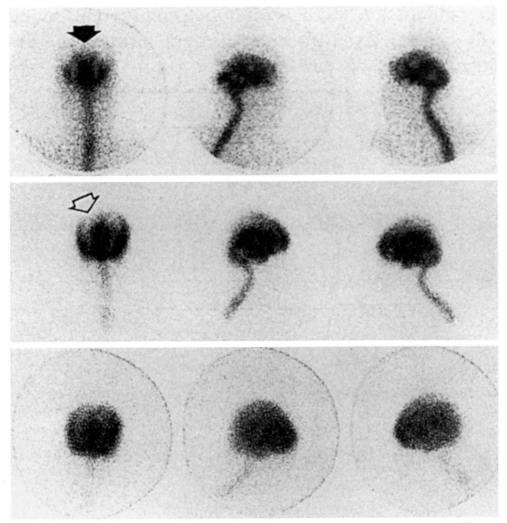

• **Fig. 14.40** Communicating normal-pressure hydrocephalus at 24 hours *(top row)*, 48 hours *(middle row)*, and 72 hours *(bottom row)* in anterior *(left)*, right lateral *(middle)*, and left lateral *(right)* projections. Ventricular reflux *(closed arrowhead)* is present, as is very delayed flow over the convexities *(open arrowhead)*. The intracerebral activity at 72 hours was caused by transependymal uptake.

Trauma and surgery (transsphenoidal and nasal) are the most common causes of CSF rhinorrhea. Nontraumatic causes include hydrocephalus and congenital defects. CSF rhinorrhea may occur at any site, from the frontal sinuses to the temporal bone (Fig. 14.43). The cribriform plate is most susceptible to fracture, which can result in rhinorrhea. Otorrhea is much less common. Accurate localization of CSF leaks can be clinically difficult.

Radionuclide studies are sensitive and accurate methods of CSF leak detection. To maximize the sensitivity of the test, nasal pledgets are placed in the anterior and posterior portion of each nasal region by an otolaryngologist and then removed and counted 4 hours later (Fig. 14.44). A ratio of nasal-to-plasma radioactivity greater than 2:1 or 3:1 is considered positive. The radiotracer is injected intrathecally via aseptic lumbar puncture (Box 14.15).

The site is most likely to be identified during a time when heavy leakage is occurring. Often, the patient position associated with the greatest leakage is reproduced during imaging. Imaging in the appropriate projection is important for identifying the site of leak; lateral and anterior imaging are used for rhinorrhea and posterior imaging for otorrhea. In cases in which no reason is known for low CSF pressure or when a leak around the lumbar region is suspected, additional views should be made of the lumbar region.

Scintigraphic studies show CSF leaks as an increasing accumulation of activity at the leak site. (Fig. 14.45). However, counting the pledgets is more sensitive than imaging for detecting CSF leaks. Pledgets are also helpful in determining the origin of the leak (anterior vs. posterior).

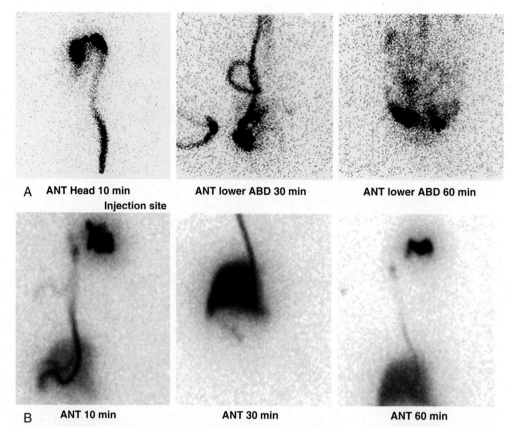

• **Fig. 14.41** Cerebrospinal shunt patency evaluation. (A) Ventriculoperitoneal shunt at 10 minutes *(left)* shows activity in the reservoir port and distal limb of the shunt moving down the neck and chest. Intraventricular activity is also seen. By 30 minutes *(middle)*, activity is in the abdomen, with free flow in the peritoneum *(right)*. (B) Ventriculopleural shunt with normal radiotracer flow through the shunt into the pleural space that decreases over time. *ANT,* Anterior.

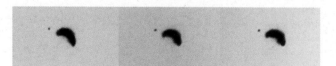

• **Fig. 14.42** Obstructed cerebrospinal shunt. After injection of technetium-99m (Tc-99m) diethylenetriaminepentaacetic acid (DTPA) into the reservoir, refluxing into the ventricles, consistent with patency of the proximal limb of the shunt, occurs. However, no distal drainage occurs over 60 minutes from obstruction.

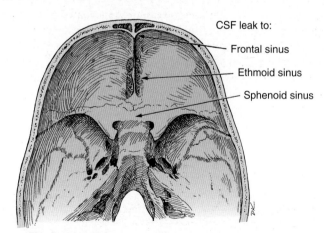

• **Fig. 14.43** Common sites of cerebrospinal fluid (CSF) leakage.

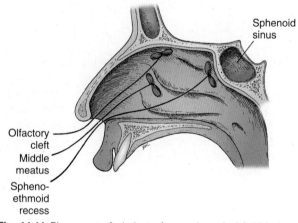

• **Fig. 14.44** Placement of pledgets for cerebrospinal fluid leak study. The labeled cotton pledgets are placed by an otolaryngologist at various levels within the anterior and posterior nares to detect leakage from the frontal, ethmoidal, and sphenoidal sinuses.

BOX 14.15 Cerebrospinal Fluid Leak Detection: Sample Protocol

Patient Preparation

No food or drink for 6 hours before lumbar puncture. Nasal pledgets are placed and labeled as to location (usually by ears, nose, and throat [ENT] physician). Pledgets should be weighed before placement. If cerebrospinal fluid (CSF) samples are taken, it should be done before radiotracer injection.

Radiopharmaceutical

In-111 diethylenetriaminepentaacetic acid (DTPA; pyrogen-free for intrathecal use) 500 μCi (19 MBq) in 5 mL dextrose 10% in water: intrathecal injection with patient adjacent to imaging table using aseptic technique. After injection, place patient in Trendelenburg position to pool the radiotracer in the basal regions until imaging begins.

Instrumentation

Gamma camera: Large field of view; medium-energy collimator
Computer setup: 256 × 256 matrix, static images 50,000 to 100,000 or 10 min/image; zoom as needed (e.g., in children)

Imaging Procedure

Positioning
- Patient is positioned supine and image activity is tracked periodically until activity reaches the basal cisterns (1-4 hours).
- Once radiotracer reaches basal cisterns, position patient in a position that increases CSF leakage:
  - Rhinorrhea: Incline patient's head forward and against camera face with the camera positioned in the lateral position.
  - Otorrhea: Obtain posterior images instead of lateral views.

Image Acquisition
- Acquire 5 minutes per frame for 1 hour in the selected view, and then acquire anterior, left lateral, right lateral, and posterior views.
- Obtain 50k images every 10 minutes for 1 hour in the original view.
- Remove pledgets and place in separate tubes. Draw a 5-mL blood sample.
- Count pledgets and 0.5-mL aliquots of plasma.
- Repeat views may be indicated at 6 and 24 hours.
- Calculate the ratio of pledgets-to-plasma activity: pledget counts/pledget capacity divided by serum counts/0.5 mL.

Interpretation

Positive for CSF leakage if the pledget-to-plasma activity ratio is greater than 2 to 3:1.

SUGGESTED READING

Chaudhry A. Pearls and pitfalls of I-123 ioflupane (DaTscan) SPECT imaging. *J Nucl Med.* 2013;54:1284.

Cummings JL, Dubois B, Molinuevo JL, Scheltens P. International work group criteria for the diagnosis of Alzheimer disease. *Med Clin N Am.* 2013;97:363–368. https://doi.org/10.1016/j.mcna.2013.01.001.

Donaghy P, McKeith I. The clinical characteristics of dementia with Lewy bodies and a consideration of the prodromal diagnosis. *Alzheimers Res Ther.* 2014;6(4):46. https://doi.org/10.1186/alzrt274. http://alzres.com/content/6/4/46.

Dubois B, Feldman HH, Jacova C, et al. Research criteria for the diagnosis of Alzheimer's disease: revising the NINCDS-ADRDA criteria. *Lancet Neurol.* 2007;6:734–746.

Frey KA. Molecular imaging of extrapyramidal movement disorders. *Semin Nucl Med.* 2017;47:18–30. https://doi.org/10.1053/j.semnuclmed.2016.09.007.

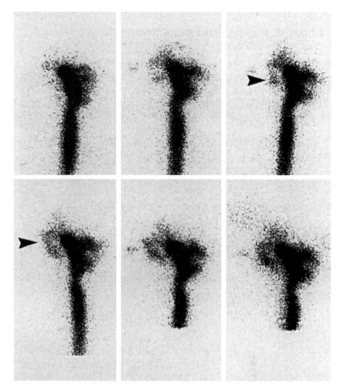

• **Fig. 14.45** Positive radionuclide cerebrospinal fluid leak study. In-111 diethylenetriaminepentaacetic acid (DTPA) left lateral views show increasing radioactivity over time originating from the nares and leaking into the nose and mouth *(arrowheads)*.

Friedman E. Epilepsy imaging in adults: getting it right. *AJR.* 2014;203:1093–1103. https://doi.org/10.2214/AJR.13.12035.

Johnson KA, Minoshima S, Bohnen NI, et al. Appropriate use criteria for amyloid PET: a report of the amyloid imaging task force, the Society of Nuclear Medicine and Molecular Imaging, and the Alzheimer's Association. *J Nucl Med.* 2013;54:476–490. https://doi.org/10.2967/jnumed.113.120618.

Johnson KA, Minoshima S, Bohnen NI, et al. Update on appropriate use criteria for amyloid PET imaging; Dementia experts, mild cognitive impairment, and education. *J Nucl Med.* 2013;54(7):1011–1013. https://doi.org/10.2967/jnumed.113.12706.

Mathis CA, Lopresti BJ, Ikonomovic MD, Klunk WE. Small-molecule PET tracers for imaging proteinopathies. *Semin Nucl Med.* 47:553–575.

McKhann GM, Knopman DS, Chertkow H, et al. The diagnosis of dementia due to Alzheimer's disease: recommendations from the National Institute on Aging-Alzheimer's Association workgroups on diagnostic guidelines for Alzheimer's disease. *Alzheimer's & Dementia.* 2011;7:263–269. https://doi.org/10.1016/j.jalz.2011.03.005.

Mountz JM, Patterson CM, Tamber MS. Pediatric epilepsy: neurology, functional imaging, and neurosurgery. *Semin Nucl Med.* 2017;47:170–187. https://doi.org/10.1053/j.semnuclmed.2016.10.003.

Nobili F, Bouwman F, Drzezga A, et al. European Association of Nuclear Medicine and European Academy of Neurology recommendations for the use of brain ^{18}F-fluorodeoxyglucose positron emission tomography in neurodegenerative cognitive impairment and dementia: Delphi consensus. *Eur J Neurol.* 2019;26(2):205–e15. https://doi.org/10.1111/ene.13818.

Rabinovici GD, Gatsonis C, Aggar C, et al. Association of amyloid positron emission tomography with subsequent change in clinical management among Medicare beneficiaries with mild cognitive impairment or dementia. *JAMA.* 2019;321(13):1286–1294. https://doi.org/10.1001/jama.2019.2000.

Shivamurthy V, Tahari A, Marcus C, Subramanian R. Brain PET and the diagnosis of dementia. *AJR*. 2015;204(1):W76–W85. https://doi.org/10.2214/AJR.13.12363.

Sperling RA, Aisen PS, Beckett LA, et al. Toward defining the preclinical stages of Alzheimer's disease: recommendations from the National Institute on Aging-Alzheimer's Association workgroups on diagnostic guidelines for Alzheimer's disease. *Alzheimer's & Dementia*. 2011;7:280–292. https://doi.org/10.1016/j.jalz.2011.03.003.

Weiner MW, Veitch DP, Aisen PS, et al. 2014 Update of the Alzheimer's disease neuroimaging initiative: a review of papers published since its inception. *Alzheimers Dement*. 2015;11(6):e1–e20. https://doi.org/10.1016/j.jalz.2014.11.001.

Zukotynski K, Kuo PH, Mikulis D, et al. PET/CT of Dementia. *AJR*. 2018;211(2):246–259. https://doi.org/10.2214/AJR.18.19822.

15

Inflammation and Infection

Infection imaging has long been an important indication for scintigraphy. Gallium-67 citrate (Ga-67) was the first infection-seeking radiopharmaceutical used clinically. It is still in use today, however, in a much more limited role than in the past. For decades now, In-111 oxine leukocytes have been the primary radiopharmaceutical used to detect infection. Tc-99m hexamethylpropyleneamine oxime (HMPAO)–labeled leukocytes have also found a role. In recent years, Fluorine-18 fluorodeoxyglucose (F-18 FDG) is increasingly being used for confirming or excluding infection (Box 15.1). Single-photon emission computed tomography with computed tomography (SPECT/CT) and positron emission tomography with computed tomography (PET/CT) have added specificity and improved localization for all of the radiopharmaceuticals.

PATHOPHYSIOLOGY OF INFLAMMATION AND INFECTION

Inflammation is a tissue response to injury attracting cells of the immune system to the site of damage. It is triggered by tissue injury (e.g., trauma, foreign particles, or neoplasm). The inflammatory response results in increased blood flow, vasodilation, increased vascular permeability, and migration of leukocytes out of blood vessels into the tissues *(chemotaxis)*. The plasma carries proteins, antibodies, and chemical mediators that modulate the inflammatory response to the site of infection (Fig. 15.1). Leukocytes are attracted to the infection site in response to chemoattractants (e.g., bacterial products). *Infection* implies the presence of microorganisms. Although infection is usually associated with inflammation, the reverse is not always true. Infection without inflammation occurs in severely immunosuppressed patients.

Leukocytes are the major cellular components of the inflammatory and immune response that protect against infection and neoplasia and assist in the repair of damaged tissue. Nucleated precursor cells differentiate into mature cells within the bone marrow. Peripheral leukocytes include granulocytes (neutrophils

60%, eosinophils 3%, basophils 1%), lymphocytes (30%), and monocytes (5%). Only 2% to 3% of neutrophils reside in the circulating blood, using it transiently when moving to sites of need. The rest are distributed in a "marginated" pool that is adherent to vascular endothelial cells in tissues, mostly in the bone marrow but also in the spleen, liver, lung, gastrointestinal tract, and oropharynx. These marginated cells can be marshaled into the circulating pool by various stimuli, including exercise, epinephrine, or bacterial endotoxins.

Neutrophils respond to an acute inflammatory stimulus by migrating toward an attractant (chemotaxis) and enter tissues between postcapillary endothelial cells (diapedesis). The neutrophils phagocytize the infectious agent or foreign body and enzymatically destroy it within cytoplasmic vacuoles. Lymphocytes, including B cells, T cells, and natural killer cells, arrive at inflammatory sites during the chronic phase. Monocytes act as tissue scavengers, phagocytosing damaged cells and bacteria and detoxifying chemicals and toxins. At sites of inflammation, they transform into tissue macrophages. Corticosteroids and ethanol inhibit the inflammatory process.

RADIOPHARMACEUTICALS

In-111-labeled leukocytes were first introduced in 1977. Indium-111 8-hydroxyquinoline (oxine) and Tc-99m hexamethylpropyleneamine oxime (HMPAO)–labeled leukocytes each have advantages and disadvantages (Table 15.1).

Indium-111 Oxine Leukocytes

The *radionuclide* Indium-111 (In-111) is cyclotron produced, decays by electron capture, emits two gamma photons (173 and 247 keV), and has a physical half-life of 67 hours (2.8 days; Table 15.2).

Adequate radiolabeling to provide good image quality usually requires 5000/mm^3 peripheral leukocytes, although sometimes the study can be performed with counts as low as 2000/mm^3. The in vitro labeling procedure requires a minimum of 2 hours. Lacking facilities and trained personnel to radiolabel the cells, imaging clinics send a patient's blood to an outside commercial radiopharmacy for radiolabeling. The time required for sending the blood to the radiopharmacy, radiolabeling the cells, returning the cells to the clinic, and reinfusing them is 3 to 4 hours.

Fifty milliliters of venous blood usually ensures sufficient leukocytes for adequate labeling; 20 to 30 mL may be acceptable for children. Radiolabeling must be performed under a laminar

---

> ### BOX 15.1 Radiopharmaceuticals for Infection Imaging
>
> Ga-67 citrate
> In-111 oxine–labeled leukocytes
> Tc-99m HMPAO–labeled leukocytes
> F-18 fluorodeoxyglucose (FDG)
> Tc-99m sulesomab (LeuTech; approved in Europe)

HMPAO, Hexamethylpropyleneamine oxime.

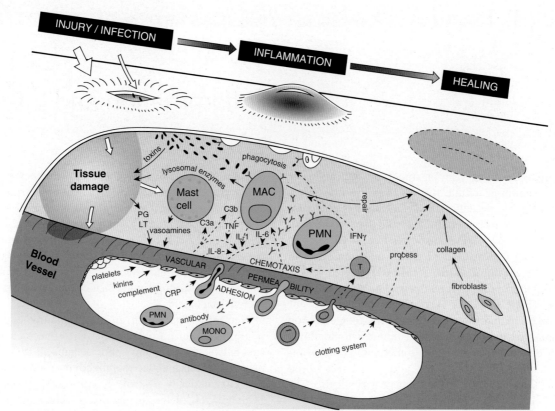

Fig. 15.1 Acute inflammation. This diagram illustrates the body's response to tissue injury and infection. The permeability of the vascular endothelium plays a central role in allowing blood cells and serum components access to the tissues. Antibodies and lymphocytes amplify or focus these primary mechanisms. If inflammation persists beyond a few days, macrophages and lymphocytes play an increasing role. *CRP,* Chronic reactive protein; *IL,* interleukin; *LT,* leukotriene; *MONO,* monocyte; *PG,* prostaglandin; *PMN,* polymorphonuclear neutrophil; *T,* T lymphocyte; *TNF,* tumor necrosis factor. (With permission, *Immunology at a Glance,* 10th edition. J.H.L. Playfair and B.M. Chain, John Wiley & Sons, Ltd. 2013.)

TABLE 15.1 Advantages and Disadvantages of In-111-Oxine Versus Tc-99m-HMPAO Leukocytes

Advantages and Disadvantages	In-111-Oxine WBCs	Tc-99m-HMPAO WBCs
Radionuclide readily available	No	Yes
Stable radiolabel, no elution from cells	Yes	No
Allows labeling in plasma	No	Yes
Radiation dosimetry	Poor	Good
Early routine imaging	No	Yes
Half-life allows for delayed imaging	Yes	No
Imaging time	Long	Short
Permits dual-isotope imaging	Yes	No
Intestinal and renal clearance	No	Yes
Image resolution	Fair	Good

HMPAO, Hexamethylpropyleneamine oxime; *WBC,* white blood cell.

TABLE 15.2 Physical Characteristics of In-111, Tc-99m, F-18, and Ga-67

Radionuclide	Half-Life	Photopeak (keV)	% Photon Abundance
In-111	67 hours	173	89
		247	94
Tc-99m	6 hours	140	89
F-18	110 minutes	511	97
Ga-67	78 hours	93	41
		185	23
		288	18
		394	4

flow hood to ensure sterility. Careful handling is required to avoid damaging cells, which could adversely affect their migration and viability. Proper labeling does not affect normal physiological function. The radiolabel remains stable in vivo for more than 24 hours.

The methodology for radiolabeling leukocytes is described in detail in Box 15.2. Radiolabeling cannot be performed in plasma, so it must be separated and retained for later resuspension with the leukocytes before reinfusion. The leukocyte pellet is suspended in saline and incubated with In-111 oxine. The lipid solubility of the In-111 oxine complex allows it to diffuse through cell membranes. Intracellularly, the complex dissociates, oxine diffuses back out of the cell, and In-111 binds to nuclear and cytoplasmic proteins. In-111 oxine binds to

BOX 15.2 Methodology for Radiolabeling of Autologous Leukocytes With Indium-111 Oxine

Preparation

1. Patient's peripheral leukocyte count should be >5000 cells/mm³.

Procedure

1. Collect autologous blood.
   Draw 30 to 50 mL into an anticoagulant citrate dextrose (ACD) anticoagulated syringe using a 19-gauge needle.
2. Isolate leukocytes:
   Separate red blood cells (RBCs) by gravity sedimentation and 6% Hetastarch, a settling agent.
   Centrifuge the leukocyte-rich plasma at 300 to 350 g for 5 minutes to remove platelets and proteins.
   A leukocyte button forms at the bottom of the tube.
   Draw off and save the leukocyte-poor plasma (LPP) for later washing and resuspension.
3. Label leukocytes:
   Suspend leukocytes (LPP) in saline.
   Incubate with In-111 oxine for 30 minutes at room temperature and gently agitate.
   Remove unbound In-111 by centrifugation. Save wash—calculate labeling efficiency.
4. Prepare injectate:
   Resuspend 500 µCi In-111-labeled leukocytes in saved plasma (LPP).
   Inject via peripheral vein within 2 to 4 hours.
5. Perform quality control:
   Microscopical examination of cells
   Calculate labeling efficiency:
   Assay the cells and wash in dose calibrator.
   Labeling efficiency = $C/([C + W] \times 100\%)$
   where C is activity associated with the cells, and W is activity associated with the wash.

TABLE 15.3 Mechanisms of Localization of Infection-Seeking Radiopharmaceuticals

Radiopharmaceutical	Mechanism
Radiolabeled leukocytes	Diapedesis and chemotaxis
F-18 fluorodeoxyglucose	Glucose metabolism
Ga-67 citrate	Iron binding to lactoferrin and bacterial siderophores

granulocytes, lymphocytes, monocytes, platelets, and erythrocytes. Pure In-111 granulocyte preparations have been radiolabeled and used clinically. However, they require density gradient centrifuge separation techniques and have not shown a clinical advantage over mixed leukocytes. They are generally not used clinically.

Standard quality-control measures (e.g., testing for sterility and pyrogenicity) cannot be performed because of the need for prompt reinfusion after labeling to ensure cell viability. However, the final radiopharmaceutical preparation should be examined for abnormal morphology, clumping, excessive red blood cell (RBC) contamination, and percent labeling efficiency, typically ranging from 75% to 90%. When labeling is less than 50%, the cells should not be administered to the patient. The final preparation contains radiolabeled granulocytes, lymphocytes, and monocytes and some platelets and erythrocytes.

After infusion of the In-111 leukocytes, no significant elution of the In-111 from the leukocytes occurs. Initial distribution is to the blood pool, lungs, liver, and spleen. Localization is the result of diapedesis and chemotaxis (Table 15.3). Lung uptake is caused by activation from in vitro cell manipulation, which may be increased by the underlying disease process. By 4 hours after

reinjection, lung and blood-pool activity markedly decrease (Fig. 15.2). By 24 hours, the greatest uptake is in the spleen, followed by the liver and bone marrow. Persistent blood pool suggests a high percentage of labeled RBCs. Genitourinary, hepatobiliary, and intestinal clearance are not normally seen. The ultimate test of the viability of leukocytes is in vivo function manifested by a normal distribution within the body and the ability to detect infection (Table 15.4). Uptake outside of expected normal uptake sites suggests infection (Figs. 15.3 and 15.4). If the infused white blood cells (WBCs) become nonviable, increased liver and lung uptake is seen.

An *imaging protocol* for In-111 oxine leukocytes is described in Box 15.3. Images are acquired on their 173- and 247-keV photopeaks (20% window) using a medium-energy collimator. Whole-body imaging is routine. High-count spot images, SPECT, and SPECT/CT are options. The spleen receives the highest radiation dose, precluding its use in pediatric patients. Dosimetry is detailed (see the Appendix). Images are routinely acquired 24 hours after reinfusion (Table 15.5). Further delayed images rarely give additional information. Early imaging (e.g., at 4 hours) is less sensitive than 24-hour imaging for detecting infection, although when the patient is quite sick, early imaging may detect the focus of infection (e.g., an abscess that requires urgent intervention). Four-hour imaging is standard for inflammatory bowel disease. Inflamed mucosal cells slough, become intraluminal, and move distally. Thus, 24-hour images can be misleading and erroneous as to the site of inflammation. Scintigraphic images reflect the distribution of leukocytes in the body. Focal or diffuse activity outside their expected normal distribution suggests inflammation or infection (see Table 15.4).

Interpretive pitfalls (i.e., potential false-positive and false-negative findings) should be kept in mind (Box 15.4). Leukocytes accumulate at sites of inflammation (e.g., intravenous catheters; nasogastric, endogastric, and drainage tubes; tracheostomies; colostomies; and ileostomies). Unless intense, this uptake should be considered normal. Uninfected postsurgical wounds show uptake for 2 to 3 weeks. If uptake is intense, persists, or extends beyond the surgical wound site, infection should be suspected (Fig. 15.5). Uptake occurs at healing bone-fracture sites, with the amount depending on the length of time since fracture, its severity, and whether it is healing properly.

A major advantage of In-111 leukocytes is the normal lack of intraabdominal activity. However, on occasion, abdominal activity may not be due to infection but rather the result of an accessory spleen, splenosis, pseudoaneurysm, or a noninfected

4 hours

24 hours

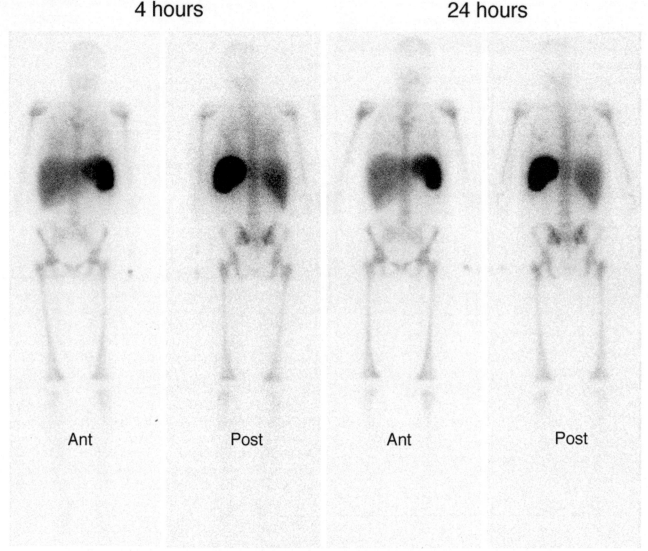

Ant   Post   Ant   Post

Fig. 15.2 Normal In-111 oxine–labeled leukocyte whole-body scan at 4 and 24 hours. Anterior *(Ant)* and posterior *(Post)* whole-body images show highest uptake in the spleen, followed by the liver, then bone marrow. The 4-hour images show mild bilateral lung uptake that has cleared by 24 hours. Image quality is superior at 24 hours due to clearance of lung background. No activity is seen in the abdomen except mild diffuse background and bone marrow.

TABLE 15.4	Normal Distribution of Infection-Seeking Radiopharmaceuticals						
Radiopharmaceutical	Liver	Spleen	Marrow	Bone	Gastrointestinal	Genitourinary	Lung
Ga-67 citrate	***	*	*	*	***	*	
In-111 oxine–labeled leukocytes	**	***	**				*
Tc-99m HMPAO–labeled leukocytes	**	***	**		**	**	*
F-18 FDG	***	**	* *		**	**	

HMPAO, Hexamethylpropyleneamine oxime.

hematoma (Figs. 15.6 and 15.7). Renal transplants normally accumulate leukocytes, probably as a result of low-grade rejection (Fig. 15.8). Intraluminal intestinal activity can result from swallowed or shedding cells that occur with pharyngitis, sinusitis, esophagitis, pneumonia, or gastrointestinal bleeding.

The sensitivity of leukocyte imaging may be reduced in conditions that alter leukocyte function (e.g., hyperglycemia, steroid therapy, and chemotherapy). Conflicting data exist regarding the sensitivity of In-111 leukocyte scintigraphy for detecting infection in patients receiving antibiotics. Investigations have not found a difference in sensitivity for detection of acute versus chronic infections. Although chronic inflammations preferentially attract lymphocytes, monocytes, plasma cells, and macrophages, they still have significant neutrophilic infiltration.

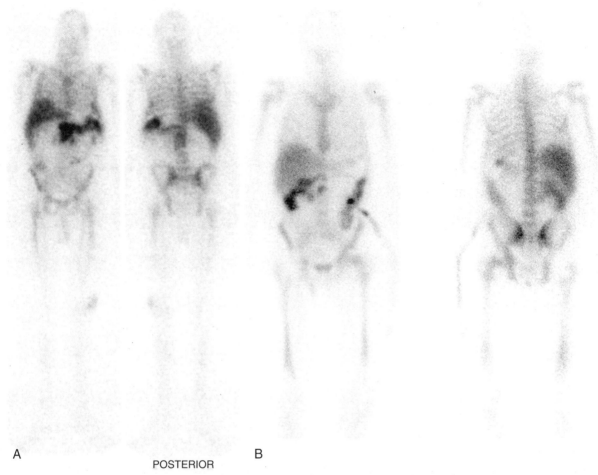

A
POSTERIOR
B

Fig. 15.3 (A) In-111 leukocyte scan in patient with postoperative lesser sac and left subphrenic infection. Note splenectomy. (B) A different patient, recently diagnosed with pancreatic cancer, has postoperative purulent infection originating from surgical bed. In-111-oxine leukocyte scan shows intraabdominal infection in the right infrahepatic and left upper quadrants and ill-defined multiloculated left paracolic gutter collection, suggestive of abscesses. Note left-sided drain with purulent drainage. See Fig. 15.4 for abdominal single-photon emission computed tomography with computed tomography (SPECT/CT) of this patient.

Tc-99m-HMPAO Leukocytes

The *radionuclide* technetium-99m (Tc-99m) is generator-produced from molybdenum-99. Tc-99m decays by isomeric transition and emits one gamma photon of 140 keV, with a 6-hour physical half-life (see Table 15.2). The *radiopharmaceutical* Tc-99m exametazime (Ceretec) is labeled to leukocytes by HMPAO. Tc-99m HMPAO was originally approved by the U.S. Food and Drug Administration (FDA) for cerebral perfusion imaging. Its lipophilicity allows it to cross cell membranes. In brain imaging, it crosses the blood–brain barrier and is taken up by cerebral cortical cells, where it changes into a hydrophilic complex and becomes trapped. This led to the use of Tc-99m HMPAO to label leukocytes. The FDA has accepted Tc-99m HMPAO–labeled leukocytes as an acceptable alternative use of Tc-99m HMPAO.

Tc-99m HMPAO–labeled leukocytes have some advantages over In-111-labeled leukocytes (see Table 15.1). The radiation dose to the patient is considerably lower (see the Appendix); thus, greater activity can be administered, resulting in higher photon yield and better image quality.

The methodology for radiolabeling leukocytes with Tc-99m HMPAO is similar to that for In-111 oxine labeling of leukocytes (see Box 15.2). The differences are that Tc-99m-HMPAO leukocyte labeling can be performed in plasma and that the resulting labeling is primarily of granulocytes. The biological half-life of Tc-99m-HMPAO leukocytes in blood is shorter than that of In-111 oxine leukocytes, 4 versus 6 hours, because of slow elution of the Tc-99m HMPAO from circulating radiolabeled cells. Tc-99m-HMPAO leukocytes distribute in the body similar to In-111-labeled cells, except that the Tc-99m leukocytes have hepatobiliary and genitourinary clearance due to elution from the leukocytes (Fig. 15.9; see also Table 15.4). In addition, a secondary labeled hydrophilic complex is excreted, also seen with Tc-99m-HMPAO brain imaging. The kidneys and bladder are normally visualized by 1 to 2 hours after injection. Biliary and bowel clearance occurs as early as 2 hours, is routinely seen by 3 to 4 hours, and increases with time (Fig. 15.10; see also Fig. 15.9).

An important advantage of Tc-99m-HMPAO leukocytes is its much lower radiation dose to the spleen, particularly in

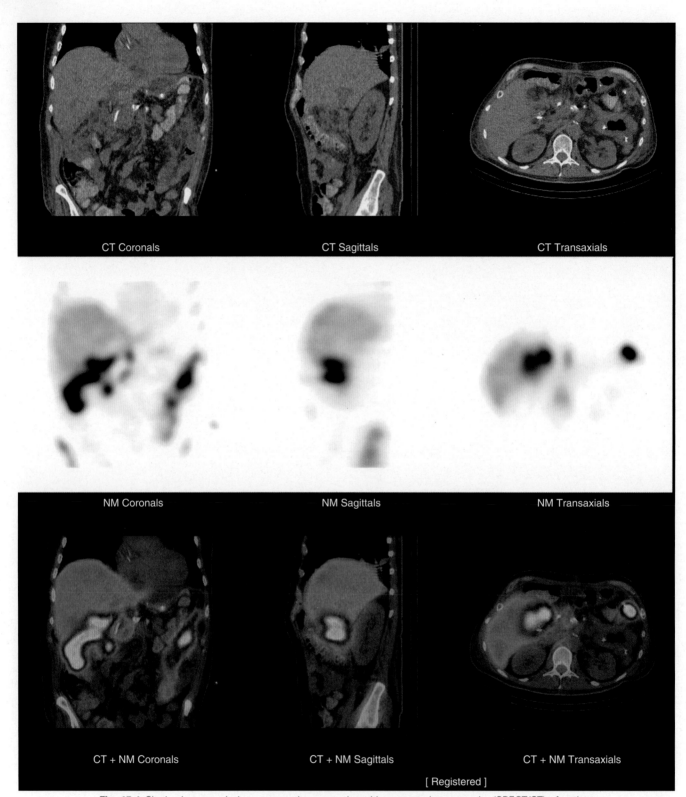

CT Coronals   CT Sagittals   CT Transaxials

NM Coronals   NM Sagittals   NM Transaxials

CT + NM Coronals   CT + NM Sagittals   CT + NM Transaxials

[Registered]

Fig. 15.4 Single-photon emission computed tomography with computed tomography (SPECT/CT) of patient with whole-body scan in Fig. 15.3B. *(Left column)* Coronal CT, SPECT, fused images; *(middle)* Sagittal images; and *(right)* Transverse images. These cross-sectional images more precisely localize infection to the right infrahepatic and left upper quadrants and left paracolic gutter infection, strongly suggesting intraabdominal abscesses.

children, <2.0 rads compared with approximately 50 rads for In-111 leukocytes (see the Appendix). Thus, Tc-99m-labeled leukocytes are not indicated for children. Because of the shorter physical half-life and hepatobiliary and urinary clearance of Tc-99m-HMPAO leukocytes, images are acquired at an earlier time point than In-111 oxine–labeled WBCs (see Table 15.5). An imaging protocol is described in Box 15.5. Abdominal imaging should be performed approximately 2 hours after reinfusion to minimize the likelihood of urinary and gastrointestinal clearance. For other body regions, such as the chest and extremities,

BOX 15.3 Indium-111-Oxine Leukocyte Scintigraphy: Protocol Summary

Radiopharmaceutical

In-111 oxine in vitro–labeled leukocytes, 500 µCi (18.5 MBq)

Instrumentation

Camera: Large field of view
Window: 20% centered over 173- and 247-keV photopeaks
Collimator: Medium energy

Patient Preparation

Draw 50 mL of blood. Radiolabel white cells (see Box 15.2).

Procedure

Inject labeled cells intravenously, preferably by direct venipuncture through a 19-gauge needle. Contact with dextrose in water solutions may cause cell damage.
Imaging at 4 hours is critical in localizing inflammatory bowel disease.
Perform routine whole-body imaging at 24 hours.
Acquire spot views as needed: anterior abdomen for 500k counts, then other images for equal time. Include anterior and posterior views of the chest, abdomen, and pelvis and spot images of specific areas of interest (e.g., feet) for a minimum of 200k counts or 20 minutes.
Perform SPECT or SPECT/CT as needed.

SPECT, Single-photon emission computed tomography; *SPECT/CT,* single-photon emission computed tomography with computed tomography.

TABLE 15.5 Optimal Imaging Time for Infection-Seeking Radiopharmaceuticals

Radiopharmaceutical	Time (hours)
Ga-67 citrate	48
In-111-oxine leukocytes	24
Tc-99m-HMPAO leukocytes	1-4
F-18 fluorodeoxyglucose	1

HMPAO, Hexamethylpropyleneamine oxime.

BOX 15.4 Interpretative Pitfalls in Leukocyte Imaging

False-Negative Results

Vertebral osteomyelitis
Chronic low-grade infection
Parasitical, mycobacterial, or fungal infections
Hyperglycemia
Corticosteroid therapy

False-Positive Results

Gastrointestinal bleeding
Healing fracture
Swallowed leukocytes; oropharyngeal, esophageal, or lung disease
Surgical wounds, stomas, or catheter sites
Hematomas
Tumors
Accessory spleens
Renal transplant
Pseudoaneurysm

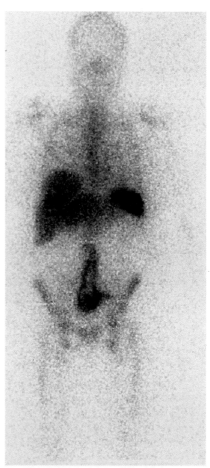

Fig. 15.5 Postoperative fever and wound infection. In-111 leukocyte whole-body scan (anterior and posterior). Dehiscence of the abdominal incision site was caused by an abscess inferior and deep to incision. Note the intense activity inferiorly. No evidence of intraabdominal infection.

later imaging at 3 to 4 hours is recommended, although further delayed imaging may at times be useful (Fig. 15.11). Blood-pool activity is commonly seen with Tc-99m leukocytes compared with In-111-labeled leukocytes because of the elution of activity from the radiolabeled cells. This can potentially complicate interpretation in the chest or major vessels. Care should be used in the interpretation of intraabdominal activity because of the normal genitourinary and hepatobiliary clearance. Potential false-positive and false-negative results are listed in Box 15.4. Delayed imaging, particularly SPECT/CT, can often improve localization.

Fluorine-18 Fluorodeoxyglucose

The radionuclide fluorine-18 (F-18) undergoes positron decay, emitting two gamma photons of 511 KeV, 180 degrees apart, with a physical half-life of 2 hours (see Table 15.2). FDG is a glucose analog. After injection, the radiopharmaceutical F-18 FDG is transported into activated granulocytes, macrophages, monocytes, giant cells, and CD4-positive T cells by upregulated glucose transporters. The degree of FDG uptake is related to the cellular metabolic rate and the number of glucose transporters. Within the cell, it is phosphorylated by hexokinase to F-18 FDG-6 phosphate but is not metabolized further and remains fixed in the cell (see Table 15.3).

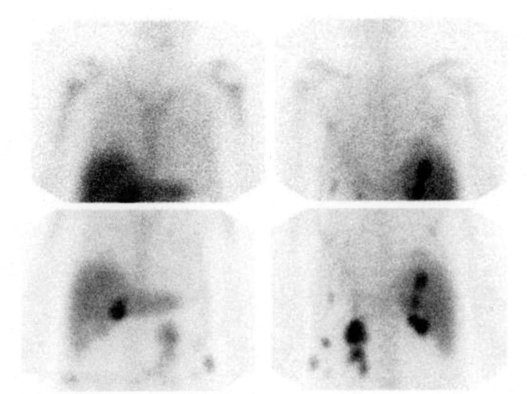

Fig. 15.6 False-positive In-111- leukocyte scan. The patient presented with recurrent fever. Planar images of the chest and abdomen (anterior and posterior). No spleen is seen because of a splenectomy in the past after trauma. Multiple very intense foci of uptake are seen in the abdominal view, all of which correlated with suspected splenules on computed tomography (CT).

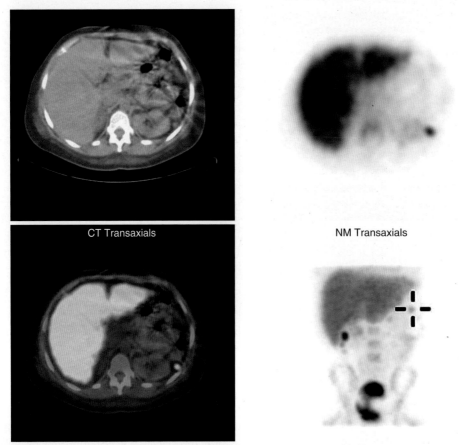

CT Transaxials   NM Transaxials

Fig. 15.7 In-111 leukocyte single-photon emission computed tomography with computed tomography (SPECT/CT) in a patient with fever and bacteremia. History of prior splenectomy. Multiple masses were seen on computed tomography (CT), suspected to be splenules. This was confirmed with SPECT/CT. The single transverse slices show one of the splenules in the left upper quadrant.

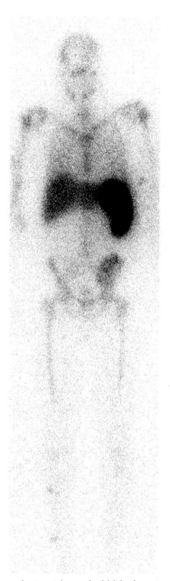

Fig. 15.8 Renal transplant uptake on In-111 leukocyte scan. Patient presented with persistent fever of uncertain etiology 4 weeks after transplantation. No definite site of infection is seen. There is moderately increased diffuse uptake in the transplant in the left pelvis, consistent with mild chronic rejection, not infection. Splenomegaly of uncertain etiology.

F-18 FDG PET has some advantages over Tc-99m and In-111 leukocytes for infection imaging. Problems associated with blood drawing, radiolabeling, and reinfusion of blood products are eliminated, and imaging is completed more rapidly. F-18 FDG PET imaging methodology is similar to oncologic imaging, beginning 1 hour after injection and completed by 2 hours (see Table 15.5). FDG PET image resolution is superior to single-photon imaging, whole-body imaging is routine, and combined PET/CT is standard. The disadvantage of FDG imaging, like Ga-67, is that uptake is not specific for infection, and it can be seen with inflammatory causes (e.g., fractures, postoperative inflammation, degenerative disease, reaction to orthopedic hardware, tumor). Infection detection in patients with poorly controlled diabetes may be poorer due to the effect of hyperglycemia on FDG uptake. Infection diagnosis in the brain and urinary tract is limited by its high cerebral uptake and urinary

excretion. Published data confirming the utility of FDG for various inflammatory and infectious indications are growing but still limited. In published studies, good data on accuracy are limited due to the lack of a gold standard and the relatively high number of patients without a final diagnosis. However, clinical utility seems to be high. Reimbursement is also an issue.

Gallium-67 (Ga-67) Citrate

The *radionuclide* Ga-67 is cyclotron-produced; decays by electron capture; emits a spectrum of gamma rays (93, 185, 288, 394 keV), all with low abundance (% likelihood of emission with each decay); and has a physical half-life of 78 hours (see Table 15.2). Image quality is limited by scatter from the lower-energy photons, and the higher-energy photons are difficult to collimate and not efficiently detected by the thin crystal (3/8 inch) of gamma cameras.

After intravenous injection, Ga-67 citrate circulates in plasma bound to transferrin, which transports it to the inflammatory site. It enters inflammatory/infectious sites as a result of locally increased blood flow and vascular permeability (see Table 15.3). The ferric ion–like properties Ga-67 permit it to bind to lactoferrin released from dying leukocytes (greater binding affinity to lactoferrin than to transferrin) and bacterial iron-containing siderophores. Ga-67 clears slowly from the blood pool. By 48 hours after injection, 10% is still bound to plasma proteins, and total body clearance is slow (25-day biological half-life), resulting in considerable image background. Sufficient uptake occurs at the site of infection by 12 to 24 hours. Excretion during the first 24 hours is primarily via the kidneys. Thereafter, the colon is the major route of excretion. Normal uptake is greatest in the liver, followed by bone marrow and spleen (Fig. 15.12; see also Table 15.4).

Inflammatory or stimulatory processes that increase lactoferrin production result in increased uptake in the salivary glands in Sjögren' syndrome, the lacrimal glands in sarcoidosis, and the breast during lactation (see Figs. 15.11 and 15.12). Normal breast uptake varies according to the menstrual cycle phase and is seen prominently postpartum. Thymic uptake is normal in children and seen in patients postchemotherapy. Postoperative sites may have increased Ga-67 uptake for 2 to 3 weeks. Uptake occurs at healing fractures (Fig. 15.13) and in sterile abscesses associated with frequent intramuscular injections. The normal distribution is altered by whole-body irradiation, multiple blood transfusions (excess ferric ions), or recent gadolinium magnetic resonance imaging (MRI). Salivary gland uptake is increased after local external-beam irradiation.

A Ga-67 *imaging protocol* is summarized in Box 15.6. Bowel preparation with laxatives/enemas is not recommended because it may cause mucosal irritation and inflammation, resulting in increased Ga-67 uptake, and is relatively ineffective. The usual administered adult dose is 5 mCi (185 MBq). A medium-energy collimator is required. The three lower photopeaks (93, 185, 300 keV) are acquired for imaging. Although 24-hour images can be diagnostic, whole-body images at 48 hours are superior and standard, due to greater background clearance and good target-to-background ratio. SPECT and SPECT/CT are most helpful for localization of uptake.

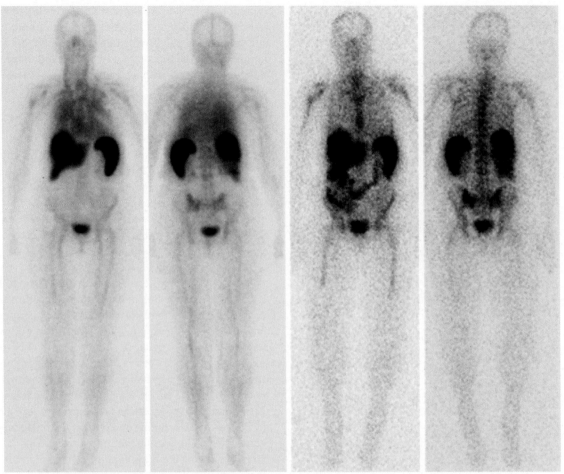

Fig. 15.9 Tc-99m HMPAO–labeled leukocyte whole-body imaging (anterior and posterior) at 4 *(left)* and 24 hours *(right)*. Considerable blood-pool activity is seen at 4 hours, but no intraabdominal activity, except for faint visualization of the renal pelvises. At 24 hours, considerable intraabdominal activity is seen, transiting the intestines and urinary tract. Image quality is inferior to that at 4 hours because of decay due to the 6-hour half-life of Tc-99m.

Radiopharmaceuticals Under Investigation or Not Approved by the Food and Drug Administration

Tc-99m fanolesomab (NeutroSpect) was approved by the FDA in the United States in 2004. It is a murine immunoglobulin (Ig) M monoclonal antibody that binds to surface CD15 antigens expressed on human neutrophils. However, approval was subsequently withdrawn because two deaths were reported. Tc-99m sulesomab (LeukoScan), a Tc-99m-labeled antigranulocyte (IgG1) murine antibody Fab' fragment, is used clinically in Europe. Fab' fragments have less immunoreactivity than whole antibodies and a better target-to-background ratio because of rapid renal clearance. Accuracy is similar to In-111 leukocytes. A number of radiopharmaceuticals under investigation are listed, and their mechanisms of uptake described, in Table 15.6.

CLINICAL APPLICATIONS FOR INFECTION SCINTIGRAPHY

Osteomyelitis

Pathophysiology

Bone infection is most commonly bacterial in origin. Microorganisms reach the bone by either hematogenous spread, extension from a contiguous site of infection, or direct introduction of organisms into bone by trauma and surgery. The terminology for acute and chronic osteomyelitis is not always consistent. *Acute* indicates hematogenous spread. *Chronic* is usually the result of an infection starting in overlying soft tissue or introduced at the time of trauma or surgery. It is an active infection and has a neutrophilic inflammatory component. Sometimes, infection initially acquired as a child or adult may recur years later as intermittent or persistent drainage from a sinus tract communicating with the involved bone, usually the femur, tibia, or humerus, or as a soft tissue infection overlying it.

Acute Hematogenous Osteomyelitis

Acute hematogenous osteomyelitis most commonly occurs in children. It typically involves the red marrow of long bones, often in the femur, due to the relatively slow blood flow in metaphyseal capillaries and sinusoidal veins in the region adjacent to the growth plate as well as a paucity of phagocytes (Figs.15.14 and 15.15). Less commonly, it occurs in the axial skeleton as discitis and then vertebral osteomyelitis (Fig. 15.16A). It is often secondary to a distant staphylococcal skin or mucosal infection. In adults, hematogenous osteomyelitis

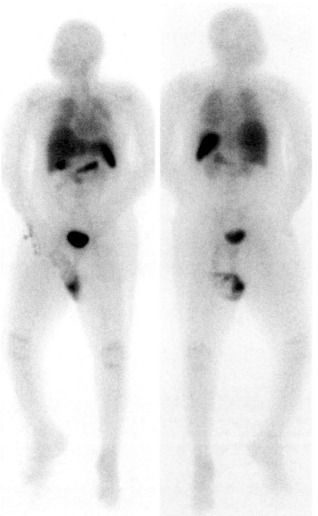

Fig. 15.10 Whole-body Tc-99m-HMPAO images at 4 hours shows radiotracer already in the gallbladder, small bowel, and urinary bladder and incidental urinary contamination in genital area.

BOX 15.5 Tc-99m-HMPAO Leukocyte Scintigraphy: Protocol Summary

Patient Preparation
Wound dressings changed before imaging

Radiopharmaceutical
Tc-99m-HMPAO in vitro–labeled WBCs, 10 mCi (370 MBq)

Instrumentation
Camera: Large field of view; two-headed camera preferable for whole-body imaging
Collimator: Low energy, high resolution
Windows: 20%, centered over 140-keV photopeaks

Patient Preparation
Draw 50 mL of blood.

Procedure
Radiolabel patient's leukocytes in vitro with Tc-99m HMPAO.
Reinject labeled cells intravenously, preferably by direct venipuncture through 19-gauge needle. Contact with dextrose in water solutions may cause cell damage.

Imaging
Imaging by 2 hours is necessary for intraabdominal imaging or to localize inflammatory bowel disease.
Imaging at 4 hours or later may be advantageous for peripheral skeleton (e.g., osteomyelitis of feet).
Whole-body imaging: Two-headed camera with whole-body acquisition for 30 minutes; 10-minute spot images for regions of special interest
SPECT or SPECT/CT in selected cases.

HMPAO, Hexamethylpropyleneamine oxime; *SPECT,* single-photon emission computed tomography; *SPECT/CT,* single-photon emission computed tomography with computed tomography; *WBC,* white blood cell.

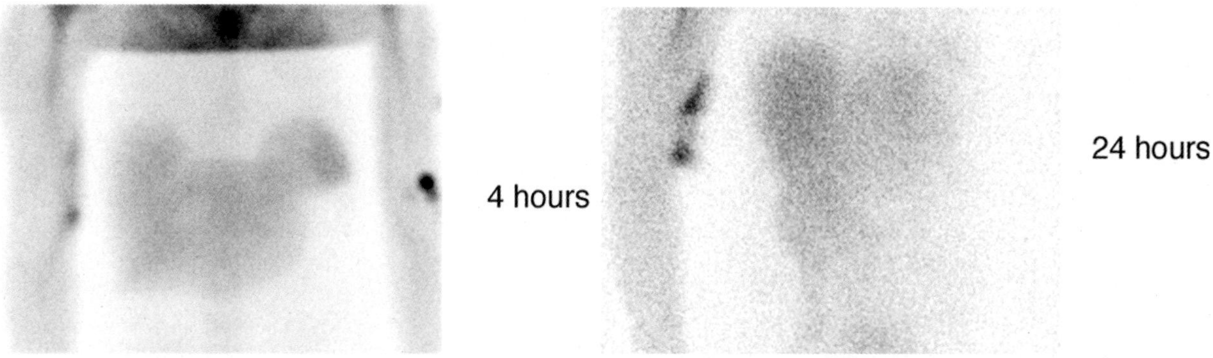

4 hours

24 hours

Fig. 15.11 Infected arteriovenous graft—Tc-99m-HMPAO white blood cells (WBCs). Image obtained at 4 hours (left) shows focal uptake within the right arm arteriovenous (AV) graft. Delayed image at 24 hours (right) shows further increase in uptake in the graft, suggestive of infection.

most commonly occurs in diabetics. The initiating event is usually septicemia from a urinary tract infection, bacterial endocarditis, or intravenous drug abuse. The infection rarely involves the long bones because adult red marrow has been replaced by yellow marrow (adipose tissue). Infection typically occurs in vertebral bodies, where the marrow is cellular, with an abundant vascular supply. It begins near the anterior longitudinal ligament and spreads to adjacent vertebrae by direct extension through the disk space or by communicating venous channels (see Fig. 15.16B). Because the adult disk does not have a vascular supply, disk-space infection is the result of osteomyelitis in an adjacent vertebra.

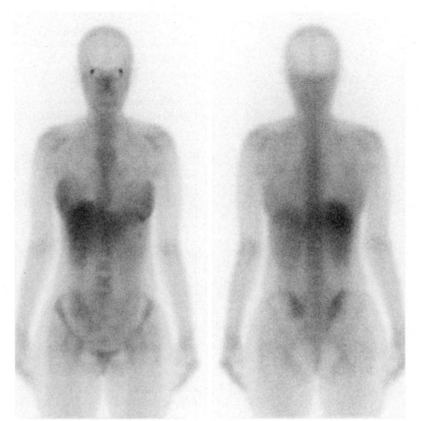

Fig. 15.12 Normal female Ga-67 citrate distribution at 48 hours. Considerable soft tissue and breast activity is seen in this thin patient. Normal lacrimal gland uptake is seen bilaterally. The highest organ uptake occurs in the liver, followed by bone and marrow. Lesser activity is seen in the spleen and nasopharyngeal region. Some large intestinal clearance is noted.

The histopathology of acute osteomyelitis includes neutrophilic inflammation, edema, and vascular congestion. Because of the bone's rigidity, intramedullary pressure increases, compromising the blood supply and causing ischemia and vascular thrombosis. The suppurative and ischemic injury may result in bone fragmentation into devitalized segments called *sequestra*. Infection may spread via Haversian and Volkmann canals to the periosteum, resulting in abscesses, soft tissue infection, and sinus tracts (see Fig. 15.15). With persistent infection, chronic inflammatory cells (e.g., lymphocytes, histiocytes, and plasma cells) join the neutrophils. Fibroblastic proliferation and new bone formation then occur. Periosteal osteogenesis may surround the inflammation to form a bony envelope, or *involucrum*. Occasionally, a dense fibrous capsule confines the infection to a localized area, or *Brodie abscess*.

Extension From a Contiguous Site of Infection

The most common cause of osteomyelitis is direct extension from overlying soft tissue infection, secondary to trauma, pressure sores, radiation therapy, or burns. In patients with diabetes and vascular insufficiency, organisms may enter soft tissues through a cutaneous ulcer, usually in the foot, producing cellulitis and then osteomyelitis.

Direct Introduction of Organisms Into Bone

Direct inoculation may occur with open fractures, open surgical reduction of closed fractures, or penetrating trauma by foreign bodies. Osteomyelitis may also arise from perioperative contamination of bone during surgery for nontraumatic orthopedic disorders (e.g., laminectomy, discectomy, or joint prosthesis placement).

Diagnosis of Osteomyelitis

Biopsy with culture is the definitive test for the diagnosis of osteomyelitis; however, it is invasive and sometimes contraindicated because noninfected bone may become contaminated by overlying soft tissue infection. There is also a risk for pathological fracture in the small bones of the hands and feet. Imaging is often required to confirm or exclude the diagnosis.

Anatomical Imaging. Plain film radiographs show the characteristic changes of soft tissue swelling, blurring of adjacent fat planes, medullary trabecular lysis, cortical destruction, and periosteal new bone formation. These findings can take 10 to 14 days to develop. The sensitivity is 50% to 75%, and the specificity is 75% to 85%. MRI can detect early marrow changes, including low signal intensity on T1-weighted images, high signal intensity on fat-suppressed T2-weighted images caused by inflammatory marrow edema, and gadolinium enhancement. Secondary changes such as sinus tracts and cortical interruption increase the diagnostic certainty. Diseases that replace marrow and result in increased tissue water may not be distinguishable from infection (e.g., healing fractures, tumors, and Charcot joints). The sensitivity and negative predictive value of MRI are high; however, the specificity is poorer.

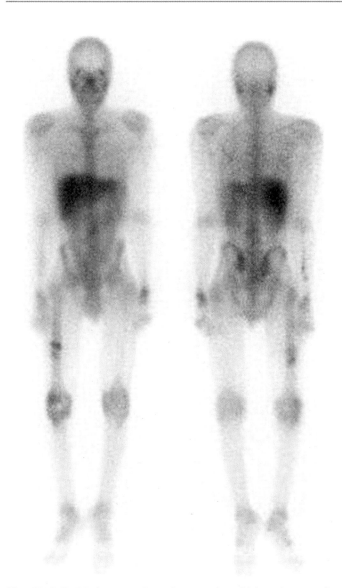

SPECT, Single-photon emission computed tomography; *SPECT/CT,* single-photon emission computed tomography with computed tomography.

TABLE 15.6 Infection Radiopharmaceuticals Under Investigation

Radiopharmaceutical	Mechanism
Tc-99m besilesomab (Scintimun)	Monoclonal antibody binds to granulocytes
Tc-99m sulesomab (LeukoScan)	Monoclonal antibody binds to leukocytes
Tc-99m interleukin 8	Cytokine binds to chemokine receptor on WBC
Tc-99m ciprofloxacin	Radiolabeled antibiotic
Tc-99m radiolabeled antimicrobial peptides	Transported by leukocytes
In-111 biotin (vitamin B_7)	Required for glucose metabolism

WBC, White blood cell.

Fig. 15.13 Ga-67 citrate uptake at fracture sites. Male patient was in an auto accident 2 weeks prior, resulting in extensive trauma. Scan requested for postoperative fever and concern for possible infection in known fractured L3 vertebral body. Images show very mild uptake, not suggestive of infection but consistent with fracture history. Moderate uptake is also seen in healing right femur fracture.

Scintigraphy—Three-Phase Bone Scan. In patients with no underlying bone pathology, such as fractures, orthopedic implants, and neuropathic joints, a three-phase bone scan should be the first scintigraphic study performed (Box 15.7). The sensitivity, specificity, and accuracy are high, greater than 95% in adults and children (Table 15.7). A negative study result excludes osteomyelitis with a high degree of certainty. However, there are reports of false-negative studies in neonates. Although the sensitivity of the bone scan remains high in patients with underlying bone disease or prior surgery, the specificity is considerably poorer (30–50%). In these cases, the first scintigraphic study should be radiolabeled leukocytes.

The positive scintigraphic findings for the *three-phase bone scan* to diagnose osteomyelitis are (1) focal hyperperfusion on the blood-flow phase, (2) focal increased activity on the immediate postflow blood-pool (extracellular-space) phase, and (3)

focal increased bone uptake on 2- to 3-hour delayed imaging (Fig. 15.17). Distinguishing soft tissue from bone uptake may be problematic with planar imaging of the lower extremities and feet because of slow soft tissue clearance due to overlying cellulitis and edema. Delayed imaging at 12 to 24 hours allows time for greater background clearance. SPECT/CT can be very helpful in separating soft tissue from bone uptake at the standard 3-hour delayed-imaging time.

Scintigraphy—Radiolabeled Leukocytes. The reported accuracy of radiolabeled leukocytes for the diagnosis of osteomyelitis has varied; however, it is clearly superior to the bone scan and Ga-67 citrate (see Table 15.7). Attempts have been made to improve its accuracy by interpreting the study in conjunction with a bone scan, and at times this can be helpful (Figs. 15.18–15.20); however, it has not significantly improved in the diabetic foot, spine, or hip and knee prostheses. SPECT/CT can improve the diagnostic accuracy in some cases (Figs. 15.21 and 15.22).

An underlying assumption of leukocyte scintigraphy interpretation for the diagnosis of osteomyelitis is that the marrow distribution is uniform and symmetrical and that an area of

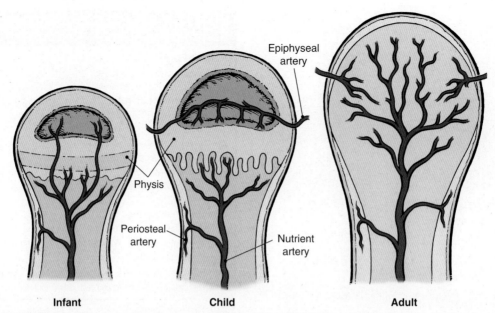

Epiphyseal
artery

Physis

Periosteal
artery

Nutrient
artery

Infant   **Child**   **Adult**

Fig. 15.14 Vascular supply of long bones in an infant, child, and adult. From infancy up to 18 months of age, small vessels perforate the physis to enter the epiphysis. After 18 months and during childhood, the perforating vessels involute. This results in the epiphysis and metaphysis having separate blood supplies. After closure of the physis, branches of the nutrient artery extend to the end of the adult bone, and the principal blood supply is again from the nutrient artery in the medullary canal. The periosteal artery supplies the outer cortex, whereas branches of the nutrient artery supply the inner cortex.

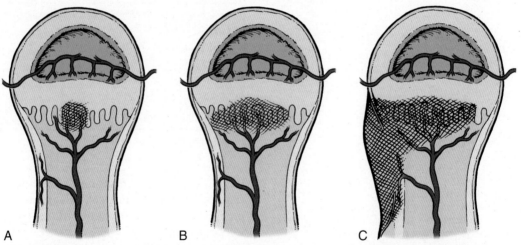

A   B   C

Fig. 15.15 Hematogenous osteomyelitis in the long bone of a child. (A) Bacterial embolization occurs via the nutrient artery, and bacteria lodge in the terminal blood supply in the metaphysis. (B) Once infection is established, it expands within the medullary canal toward the cortex and diaphysis. The physis serves as an effective barrier. (C) The infection can then extend vascular channels to the cortex to elevate and strip the periosteum from the cortex, and periosteal new bone forms. The bond between the periosteum and perichondrium at the physis prevents extension of the infection into the joint.

focally increased uptake is diagnostic of infection. However, when marrow distribution is altered by prior infection, fracture, orthopedic hardware, Charcot joint, or other factors, focal increased radiolabeled leukocyte uptake might be misinterpreted as infection. In these cases, *Tc-99m sulfur colloid* (SC) can serve as a template for the patient's bone marrow distribution. With no infection, the leukocyte and marrow scans will have a similar distribution. With infection, the radiolabeled leukocyte study will be discordant clith the marrow scan (i.e., focal increased uptake on the leukocyte study and normal or decreased uptake on marrow study; Fig. 15.23).

Different approaches have been used to combine the leukocyte and marrow studies. One is to inject and acquire the Tc-99m SC marrow scan on day 1. Blood required for In-111 WBC labeling is drawn just before the Tc-99m SC injection. Imaging of Tc-99m SC is performed 15 to 20 minutes after injection. Then the patient's radiolabeled leukocytes are infused. By 24 hours after infusion, Tc-99m activity has decayed, and In-111 WBC images are acquired.

Dual-isotope acquisition with In-111 oxine–labeled leukocytes and Tc-99m SC allows for same-day simultaneous imaging of both studies with the site of interest identically positioned.

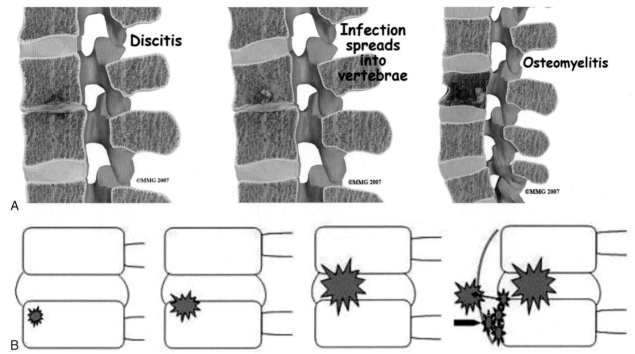

Fig. 15.16 (A) Acute hematogenous osteomyelitis in the spine of a child. The infection typically begins as discitis, then spreads to an adjacent vertebral body to become osteomyelitis. (B) In the adult, the hematogenously spread infection starts in the subchondral region of the vertebral body. As it enlarges, it may then perforate the vertebral surface, spreading to the intervertebral space. If it progresses, infection of the adjacent vertebral body can result and then spread to subligamentous and paraspinal regions.

BOX 15.7 Scintigraphic Diagnosis of Osteomyelitis by Clinical Situation

Normal radiograph: Three-phase bone scan
Neonates: Three-phase bone scan; if negative, Tc-99m-HMPAO leukocytes
Suspected vertebral osteomyelitis: Ga-67 citrate or F-18 FDG
Suspected osteomyelitis in bone marrow—containing skeleton:
  Bone marrow scan (Tc-99m SC) + leukocyte study

FDG, Fluorodeoxyglucose; *HMPAO,* hexamethylpropyleneamine oxime; *SC,* sulfur colloid.

TABLE 15.7 Diagnosis of Osteomyelitis: Accuracy of Scintigraphy and MRI

Type of Study	Sensitivity (%)	Specificity (%)
Three-phase bone scan (normal radiograph)	94	95
Three-phase bone scan (underlying bone disease)	95	33
Ga-67	81	69
In-111 oxine–labeled leukocytes	88	85
Tc-99m-HMPAO WBCs	87	81
Leukocytes (vertebral)	40	90
Leukocytes + bone marrow	95	90
MRI	95	87

HMPAO, Hexamethylpropyleneamine oxime; *MRI,* magnetic resonance imaging; *WBC,* white blood cell.

Imaging is acquired approximately 24 hours after In-111 leukocytes are reinfused and 20 minutes after Tc-99m SC. The studies are acquired simultaneously on the different radionuclide photopeaks. For Tc-99m HMPAO–labeled WBCs, imaging is usually performed on separate days, although subtraction imaging on the same day is feasible.

Scintigraphy—Gallium-67 Citrate. Gallium-67 citrate is normally taken up by both bone and bone marrow; thus, increased uptake of Ga-67 is seen at sites of increased bone turnover for whatever reason, similar to that seen on bone scans, and is nonspecific. Thus, false-positive interpretation may result in patients with underlying bone disease or orthopedic hardware. The specificity can be increased if interpreted in conjunction with a bone scan. The criteria for the diagnosis of osteomyelitis using Ga-67 scintigraphy in conjunction with a bone scan are (1) Ga-67 uptake greater than that on the bone scan or (2) Ga-67 and bone scan uptake distribution that are incongruent. The study is negative for osteomyelitis if Ga-67 uptake is less than on the bone scan (Fig. 15.24). Similar uptake on both studies is considered equivocal, and infection cannot be

excluded. The accuracy of the combined two studies is still inferior to that of radiolabeled leukocytes, except for the case of vertebral osteomyelitis. Other indications are listed in Box 15.8.

Scintigraphy—F-18 Fluorodeoxyglucose. The role of F-18 FDG for diagnosis of osteomyelitis is still evolving. The most certain indication is for suspected vertebral osteomyelitis. Limited and conflicting data have been published regarding its use for prosthesis infection and pedal osteomyelitis.

Ga-67, leukocyte scintigraphy, and F-18 FDG have all been used to monitor response to therapy (e.g., to determine whether an infection has been controlled before surgical replacement of a new prosthesis). Abnormal scintigraphic findings will revert to normal within 2 to 8 weeks of appropriate antibiotic therapy.

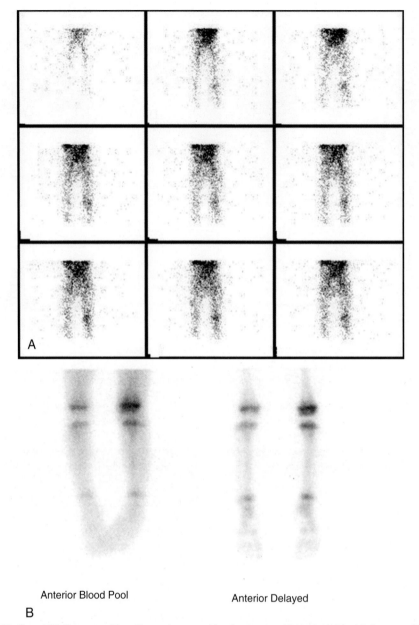

Anterior Blood Pool

Anterior Delayed

B

Fig. 15.17 (A and B) Osteomyelitis—three-phase positive bone scan. Two-year-old with fever and left knee pain. An effusion was seen on ultrasonography. The study is three-phase positive for osteomyelitis in the region of the left distal femur. (A) Increased blood flow to region of left knee. (B) Blood-pool *(left)* and delayed images *(right)* show increased uptake in the distal femur, consistent with osteomyelitis.

COMMON CLINICAL INDICATIONS

Diabetic Foot

The insensitivity of the neuropathic foot to pain often results in asymptomatic trauma, fractures, ulcers, infection, and delay in diagnosis. Overlying soft tissue infection can make the diagnosis challenging for clinicians and imagers. Radiographs and MRI may not be specific.

Interpretation of the three-phase bone scan can be complicated by the fact that the flow portion of the study may be positive due to overlying soft tissue infection, and delayed images may be positive because of fractures, Charcot joints, or degenerative disease. Although the sensitivity for the diagnosis of

osteomyelitis for the bone scan is high, the specificity is poor (see Table 15.7).

Both In-111-oxine and Tc-99m-HMPAO leukocytes can be used to diagnose osteomyelitis of the foot. The superior resolution of Tc-99m-labeled leukocytes can be an advantage because of better bone and soft tissue discrimination. However, differentiation of bone uptake from overlying soft tissue infection on planar imaging can be problematic using either agent. SPECT/CT can be valuable in separating soft tissue from bone infection (see Figs. 15.21 and 15.22).

In adults, red marrow is not normally present in the distal extremities; however, neuropathic Charcot joints form marrow and accumulate leukocytes. Fractures also stimulate marrow formation.

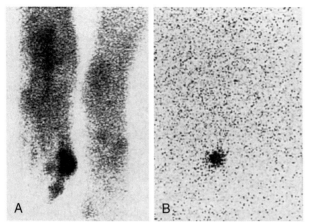

Fig. 15.18 Bone scan and In-111 leukocyte scan in diabetic patient with suspected osteomyelitis of the first metatarsal. (A) Bone scan. Three-hour delayed bone scan image of the feet shows marked increase in uptake in the region of the distal first metatarsal. Flow and blood pool (not shown) were positive. There is decreased uptake on bone scan in many digits due to severe peripheral vascular disease. (B) In-111 leukocyte scan shows intense uptake in the region of the same distal metatarsal, consistent with osteomyelitis, although there is little anatomical information to be sure this is bone and not soft tissue infection. No uptake is noted in other areas of the foot, with increased uptake on the bone scan, suggesting degenerative changes.

Bone marrow imaging with Tc-99m SC in conjunction with In-111 leukocytes can improve evaluation of the diabetic mid- and hindfoot. A mismatch strongly suggests infection (see Fig. 15.23).

Vertebral Osteomyelitis (Spondylodiscitis)

The most common route of acquisition for vertebral infection is hematogenous spread via the arterial or venous system, although postoperative infection secondary to direct implantation of microorganisms into the intervertebral disk also occurs. Tuberculous infection often affects the thoracic spine and often more than two vertebral bodies. Hematogenous pyogenic spondylodiscitis usually involves the lumbar spine. *Staphylococcus aureus* (60%) is the most common pyogenic infection, followed by *Enterobacter* (30%).

Depending on the patient age, microorganisms lodge at different sites. Below age 4, end arteries perforate the vertebral body end plates and enter the disk space to allow bacteria to cause discitis (see Fig. 15.15). In adults, the most common infection site is the subchondral (just below cartilage) region of the vertebral body, which has the richest network of nutrient arterioles, similar to the vascular tree in the childhood metaphysis. The infection is primarily spondylitis, with secondary spread into the disk space. The infection spreads from the anterior subchondral focus through the vertebral end plate into the

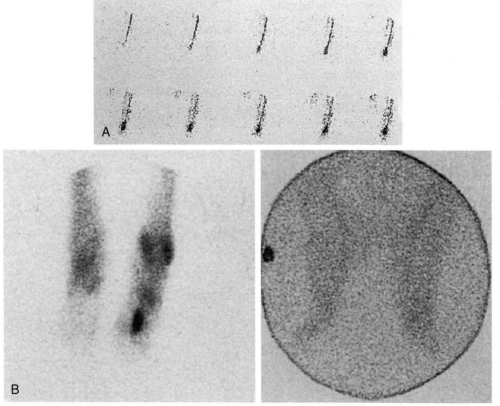

Fig. 15.19 Suspected metatarsal osteomyelitis. Positive three-phase bone scan but negative In-111-labeled leukocyte study. (A) Flow study *(top)* shows increased flow in the region of the distal left midfoot. Blood-pool images were positive (not shown). (B, *bottom left*) Three-hour delayed anterior bone scan image shows increased uptake in the third metatarsal. *(Bottom right)* In-111 leukocyte study shows no focal uptake and thus is negative for osteomyelitis. Radiograph showed a healing metatarsal fracture.

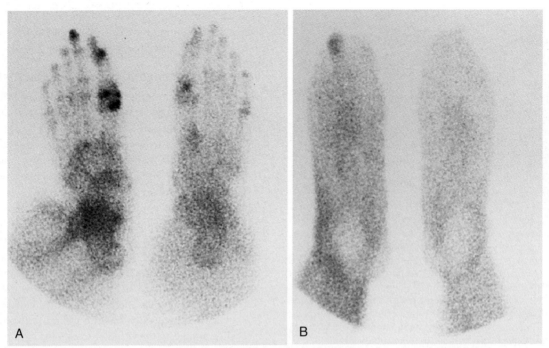

Fig. 15.20 Osteomyelitis of distal phalanx: Bone scan and Tc-99m HMPAO–labeled leukocytes. Diabetic with purulent drainage of the distal second digit of the right foot. (A) Two-hour delayed bone scan (plantar view) shows increased uptake on the distal second digit of the right. The first two phases were also positive in that area. (B) Tc-99m-HMPAO leukocyte study is positive, consistent with osteomyelitis. Other uptake on the bone scan was negative on the leukocyte study and assumed to be degenerative.

intervertebral disk. Later, it destroys the neighboring end plate, involves the opposite vertebral body, and may extend to adjacent soft tissue, resulting in epidural or paravertebral abscess.

Tc-99m methyl diphosphonate (MDP) bone scans are often used for screening for suspected infection. The usual scintigraphic pattern of discitis is increased arterial blood flow, increased blood pool, and delayed uptake at the ends of adjoining vertebral bodies. With localized osteomyelitis, the bone scan will be three-phase positive with focal bone uptake. Blood flow and pool images may be difficult to evaluate in the thoracic spine because of normal cardiac, pulmonary, and vascular structures. The bone scan has a high sensitivity and specificity in bones not affected by underlying conditions, fractures, orthopedic hardware, and similar factors.

In-111 oxine and *Tc-99m-HMPAO leukocytes* have a high false-negative rate for *vertebral osteomyelitis* (40–50%) with In-111-oxine or Tc-99m-HMPAO leukocytes. Although a positive study is diagnostic, normal or decreased uptake at the site of suspected infection is nondiagnostic (Fig. 15.25). This finding may be due to poor blood flow in bone marrow filled with pus, thrombosis, and or infarction. Infection-induced death of reticuloendothelial cells that normally take up labeled leukocytes may also be a factor. Photopenia is also seen in the spine with tumor, infarction, compression fracture, and Paget disease.

Ga-67 citrate is superior to leukocyte scintigraphy for diagnosing vertebral osteomyelitis (see Fig. 15.24). For the best accuracy, Ga-67 should be used in conjunction with a bone scan, using the criteria described (i.e., greater uptake on Ga-67 vs. bone scan). An associated disk infection or paraspinal abscess can be detected with Ga-67. SPECT and SPECT/CT can

improve localization and differentiate soft tissue from bone infection.

F-18 FDG is increasingly used as an alternative to Ga-67 for suspected vertebral osteomyelitis. The small molecule rapidly enters poorly perfused areas. Normal bone marrow uptake is low. Investigations have found it to be superior to Tc-99m MDP and Ga-67 scanning, and FDG compares favorably with MRI. A negative FDG study result is highly predictive. Orthopedic hardware and postoperative changes can complicate interpretation. After surgery or fracture, FDG uptake usually normalizes by 3 to 4 months. Focal mild to moderate increased uptake may be seen in degenerative spine disease. Foreign-body reaction around uninfected spinal implants often results in increased uptake. F-18 FDG PET/CT is superior to FDG PET alone. FDG is also valuable for monitoring treatment response (Fig. 15.26).

Prosthetic Joint Infection

The postoperative infection rate after primary hip or knee replacement is low (1–2%), as well as after revision surgery (3–5%). However, when infection occurs, morbidity can be severe. Signs and symptoms are often indolent; thus, diagnosis may be delayed. Joint aspiration with culture has poor sensitivity. Treatment of prosthetic joint infection requires excisional arthroplasty, antibiotics, and ultimately revision arthroplasty, whereas loosening is managed with only a single-stage exchange arthroplasty. Differentiating prosthesis loosening from infection can be challenging clinically and difficult for imaging. Plain radiographs lack specificity. Hardware-induced artifacts limit cross-sectional imaging.

Immediate Blood Pool

Delayed Imaging

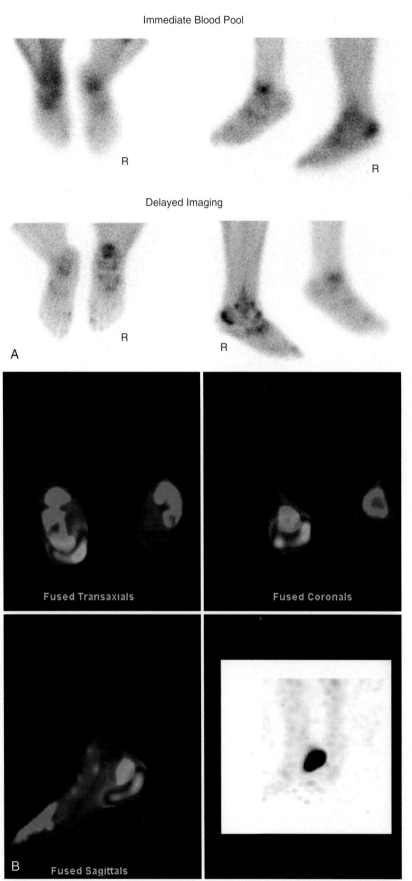

Fig. 15.21 Heel pain and single-photon emission computed tomography with computed tomography (SPECT/CT). (A, *top*) Bone scan immediate postflow blood-pool and delayed (plantar and lateral) images show abnormal increased uptake in the region of the right heel. (B) In-111 leukocyte SPECT/CT shows that the intense uptake is in soft tissue inferior to the calcaneus, consistent with soft tissue infection and not osteomyelitis.

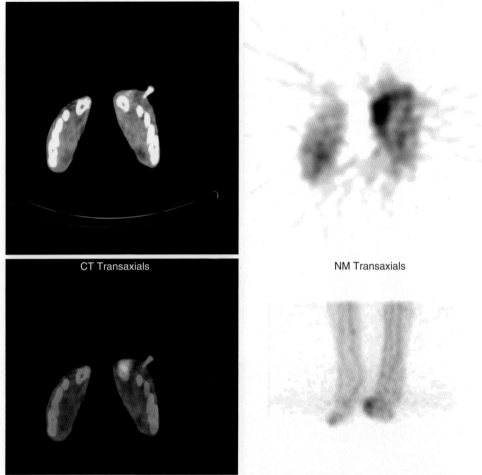

CT Transaxials

NM Transaxials

Fig. 15.22 Single-photon emission computed tomography with computed tomography (SPECT/CT) In-111 oxine–labeled leukocyte imaging of foot. Diabetic suspected of having osteomyelitis secondary to a draining infected large left toe ulcer. The maximum-intensity projection (MIP) view *(bottom right)* and the SPECT-only slice *(top right)* show diffuse uptake in the region of the distal large toe. Soft tissue cannot be differentiated from bone uptake. The fused SPECT/CT image *(bottom left)* shows that the uptake is in both soft tissue and bone, consistent with the known overlying soft tissue infection but also adjacent osteomyelitis.

Bone scan findings of increased blood flow would favor infection. Delayed uptake at the greater and lesser trochanter and prosthesis tip is suggestive of loosening, whereas diffuse uptake surrounding the femoral component is more suggestive of infection. However, the specificity of these findings is not high. Postoperative uptake usually resolves by 1 to 2 years after insertion of a cemented total hip prosthesis and up to 5 years after knee prosthesis implantation. A *cementless* or porous coated prosthesis depends on bony ingrowth for stabilization. Ongoing new bone formation is part of the fixation process, causing periprosthetic uptake in a variable pattern for a prolonged period, making interpretation difficult. Knee prostheses are also problematic for bone scintigraphy. More than half of all femoral components and three-fourths of tibial components show periprosthetic uptake more than 12 months after placement. For patients with a cementless hip or total knee replacement, bone scintigraphy is most diagnostic if the scan is normal and if serial studies are available for comparison. Even in conjunction with bone scintigraphy, *Ga-67* is only slightly more accurate for the diagnosis of an infected joint prosthesis than the bone scan alone.

Superior diagnostic accuracy results from the combined interpretation of *leukocyte and bone marrow scintigraphy*. This is because a joint prosthesis results in marrow displacement in an unpredictable manner. Discordance of uptake on leukocyte and marrow scintigraphy is diagnostic of infection (Fig. 15.27). The addition of the Tc-99m SC marrow study to WBC scintigraphy avoids the potential of a false-positive study result (e.g., interpretation of focal uptake as infection when it is merely displaced marrow). The accuracy is reported to be greater than 90%. SPECT/CT can help localize the WBC accumulation and differentiate soft tissue from bone infection. The CT component can detect joint distension, fluid-filled bursa, and intramuscular fluid collections, which suggest infection.

The reported accuracy of *F-18 FDG* for making the diagnosis of prosthetic joint infection has varied considerably. Some investigations have found high accuracy; others, not so good. Furthermore, imaging criteria have varied. One study directly compared leukocyte/marrow imaging and FDG and found WBC/marrow imaging more accurate than FDG (95% vs. 71%).

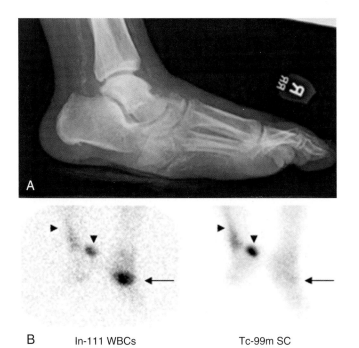

B In-111 WBCs   Tc-99m SC

Fig. 15.23 Osteomyelitis—mismatch of In-111 leukocytes and bone marrow Tc-99m sulfur colloid (SC) scan. (A) The right foot lateral radiograph shows extensive vascular calcifications and midfoot neuropathic joint. Superimposed osteomyelitis could not be excluded. Magnetic resonance imaging (MRI; not shown) was also indeterminate. (B) The In-111 leukocyte scan *(left)* shows foci of increased uptake in the right midfoot *(arrow)* and the distal left tibia and calcaneus *(arrowheads)*. On the Tc-99m *SC* bone marrow image *(right)*, no corresponding activity is seen in the right midfoot *(arrow)*, consistent with osteomyelitis. The distribution of activity in the left distal tibia and calcaneus *(arrowheads)* is virtually identical to that with In-111 leukocytes, confirming that these foci reflect marrow, not infection. Right midfoot osteomyelitis was confirmed after a below-knee amputation. (Courtesy of Christopher Palestro, MD.)

Intraabdominal Infection

Postoperative suspected intraabdominal infection is often initially evaluated with CT, which then directs further investigation, intervention, and therapy. However, in patients with nonlocalizing symptoms and negative conventional imaging, scintigraphy can be quite helpful.

In-111 oxine–labeled leukocytes are the radiopharmaceutical of choice (Figs. 15.28 and 15.29). Other than the liver and spleen uptake, there is no other normal organ uptake in the abdomen, nor is there clearance from the biliary, intestinal, or urinary tracts; thus, intraabdominal uptake is usually due to infection. The sensitivity is reported to be > 90%. Early imaging at 4 hours has a lower sensitivity for the detection of infection compared with routine 24 hours; however, in urgent situations, imaging at this time period may allow for quicker diagnosis and intervention (e.g., suspected abscess, acute appendicitis, diverticulitis). However, abnormal leukocyte uptake may be seen in a variety of noninfectious but inflammatory diseases, such as pancreatitis, acute cholecystitis, polyarteritis nodosa, rheumatoid vasculitis, ischemic colitis, pseudomembranous colitis, and bowel infarction. Delayed imaging can sometimes help confirm that early detected abnormal activity remains in a fixed pattern. A shifting pattern of activity over time implies intraluminal transit of labeled leukocytes, as seen with inflammatory or ischemic bowel disease,

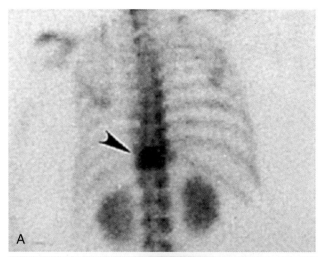

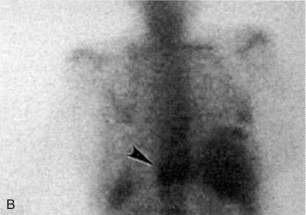

Fig. 15.24 Fever after laminectomy raised the question of osteomyelitis of the T-11 thoracic spine. (A) Tc-99m methyl diphosphonate (MDP) bone scan with *arrow* pointing to T-11. (B) Ga-67. Ga-67 uptake is less than that seen on the bone scan. The study was interpreted as negative for osteomyelitis.

BOX 15.8   Gallium-67: Clinical Indications

Severe leukopenia (<3000/m³ leukocytes)
Immunosuppressed patients
Fever of unknown origin
Malignant external otitis
Vertebral osteomyelitis
Pulmonary drug reactions (amiodarone, bleomycin)
Low-grade chronic infections
Interstitial and granulomatous pulmonary diseases

fistula, abscess in communication with bowel, or swallowed leukocytes from sinus or tracheobronchial infection (see Box 15.4).

*Tc-99m HMPAO–labeled le*ukocytes are usually preferred in children because of the high splenic radiation dose from In-111 leukocytes (see the Appendix). Early imaging is required because hepatobiliary and renal clearance may be seen by 2 to 4 hours and complicate interpretation.

Inflammatory Bowel Disease

Both ulcerative colitis and Crohn disease (granulomatous or regional enteritis) are characterized by intestinal inflammation.

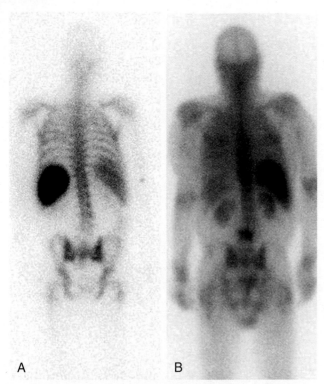

Fig. 15.25 Vertebral osteomyelitis. False-negative In-111 leukocyte scan (A) but positive Ga-67 scan (B) for spinal osteomyelitis. History of laminectomy and fusion, treated successfully for infection; now the patient has recurrent pain. Magnetic resonance imaging (MRI) was not diagnostic. Decreased In-111 uptake is seen in the lower lumbar spine. The Ga-67 scan shows intense uptake in the same region. The final diagnosis was osteomyelitis and spondylodiscitis in L4/L5.

Ulcerative colitis is typically a pattern of continuous colonic and rectal involvement, with patients at increased risk for colon cancer. Crohn disease, on the other hand, shows skip lesions and can involve any part of the gastrointestinal (GI) tract, from the mouth to the anus, classically seen in the terminal ileum, often sparing the rectum. Leukocyte scintigraphy can confirm the diagnosis, determine active disease distribution, and detect relapse (Figs. 15.30–15.32). It can aid in the evaluation of regions hard to see with endoscopy and in monitoring therapeutic effectiveness.

Tc-99m HMPAO–labeled leukocytes are reported to be superior to In-111–labeled leukocytes for the diagnosis of inflammatory bowel disease, probably because of the superior Tc-99m image resolution, enabling better disease localization. Leukocyte scintigraphy can differentiate reactivation of inflammatory bowel disease from abscess formation, a serious complication requiring surgical rather than medical therapy. Radiolabeled leukocyte uptake in an abscess is focal, whereas uptake in inflamed bowel follows the contour of the intestinal wall. Tc-99m-HMPAO imaging should be performed by 2 to 4 hours. If In-111-labeled leukocyte scintigraphy is used, images should be acquired by 4 hours rather than 24 hours because of shedding of the inflamed leukocytes into the bowel lumen from the inflammatory sites with subsequent peristalsis, potentially resulting in the incorrect assignment of disease to sites distal to the true inflammatory site.

Fever of Unknown Origin

Fever of unknown origin (FUO) has been defined as a temperature of ≥ 38.3°C (101°F) occurring on at least two occasions,

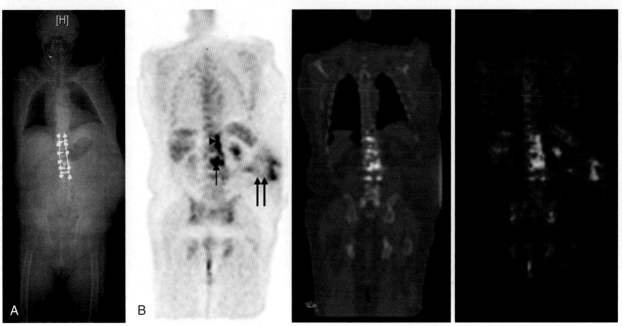

Fig. 15.26 Lumbar spine osteomyelitis and infected orthopedic hardware: Utility of fluorodeoxyglucose (FDG) positron emission tomography with computed tomography (PET/CT). (A) A 60-year-old man had spinal hardware implanted 8 years prior after a motor vehicle accident. Recent draining left flank wound, referred for suspected infected orthopedic hardware. (B) FDG PET/CT study coronal images (*left to right:* FDG, CT, fused FDG/CT) show left paraspinal hypermetabolism *(arrowhead)* along the metal rod extends from T11 to L3 (standardized uptake value [SUV] 9.3). This activity tracks to an open hypermetabolic wound in the left flank *(double arrow;* SUV 7.3). Focal hypermetabolism (SUV maximum 8.7) is seen in an upper lumbar vertebra *(arrow)* consistent with osteomyelitis. (Courtesy of Christopher Palestro, MD.)

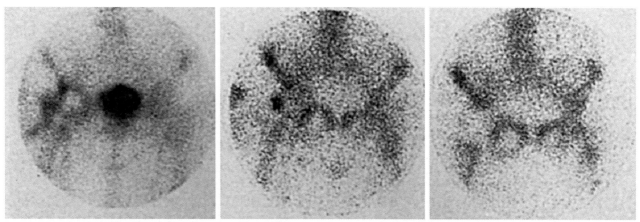

Fig. 15.27 Infected hip prosthesis. *(Left)* Tc-99m bone scan shows increased uptake in the region of the right hip prosthesis laterally, consistent with known heterotopic calcification. *(Middle)* In-111 leukocyte study shows focal intense uptake just lateral to the femoral head and more diffuse uptake within the joint space, suspicious for infection. *(Right)* Tc-99m sulfur colloid (SC) marrow study shows a normal bone marrow distribution with cold head of the femur from the prosthesis. Discordance between the bone marrow and leukocyte study is diagnostic of an infected prosthesis.

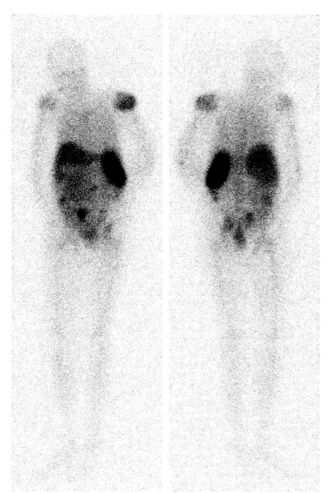

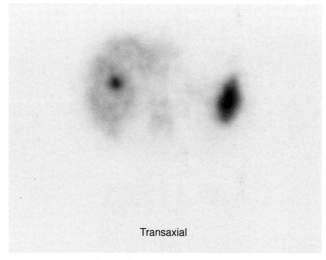

Transaxial

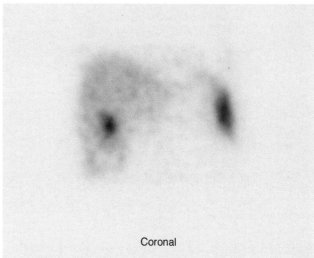

Coronal

Fig. 15.28 Peritonitis. Elderly woman with fever, sepsis, and abdominal pain. The In-111 leukocyte study shows diffuse uptake throughout the abdomen, very suggestive of peritonitis, and multiple foci of greater uptake, suggestive of abscesses. In addition, uptake in the left shoulder suggests a septic joint.

Fig. 15.29 Liver abscess diagnosed with In-111 leukocytes. Transverse *(top)* and coronal *(bottom)* cross-sectional single-photon emission computed tomography (SPECT) slices show focal uptake of leukocytes in the right lobe of the liver. An abscess was subsequently drained.

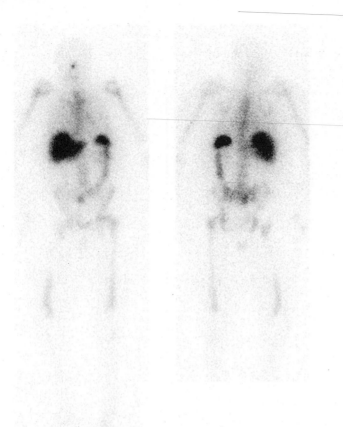

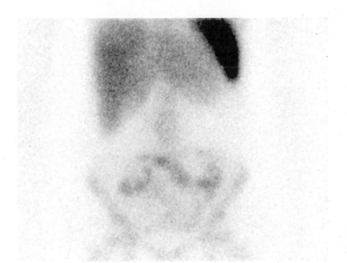

Fig. 15.30 Patient with history of ulcerative colitis and suspected recurrence, referred for confirmation of active disease and localization. In-111 leukocytes study acquired 4 hours after reinfusion shows uptake in the descending and sigmoid colon.

Fig. 15.31 Crohn disease localized with In-111 leukocytes at 4 hours after injection. Patient has several-year history of regional ileitis and 2 months of recurrent and worsening symptoms. Scintigraphy confirms active inflammation of ileum.

that remains undiagnosed for at least 3 weeks, and that results in an extensive workup during a hospital stay of at least 7 days. The source of the fever may be infection, inflammatory disease, or malignancy. Infections count for one-fifth of the cases in Western countries.

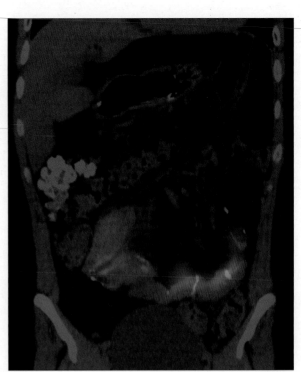

Fig. 15.32 Patient with a history of Crohn disease who had prior small bowel resections, now with suspected new obstruction. In-111 leukocyte study with single-photon emission computed tomography with computed tomography (SPECT/CT) fused coronal image shows intense uptake corresponding to a segment of thickened and collapsed small bowel at site of prior small bowel anastomosis. Consistent with active inflammation.

Ga-67 citrate has long been used to diagnose FUOs. In addition to localizing acute infection, it can detect chronic, indolent, granulomatous infections and tumor sources of fever. Ga-67 may be particularly advantageous for low-grade infections (e.g., fungal, protozoal; see Box 15.8).

Radiolabeled leukocytes have also been used because of their high sensitivity and specificity for infection, if that is the primary clinical concern. F-18 FDG-PET/CT is increasingly being used to localize the source of fever in patients with an FUO. Its advantages include the lack of a need to radiolabel the patient's leukocytes, the short duration of the study, and its ability to detect infectious and noninfectious source of infection. Like Ga-67, tumor-producing fever can also be detected. Most studies are retrospective, with varying definitions of FUO, selected patient populations, and lack of follow-up; however, nearly all have concluded that it has important clinical utility and value in 42% to 67% of patients by either identifying the etiology of the FUO or by guiding further management.

Cardiovascular Disease

Infective endocarditis has significant morbidity and mortality. The preliminary diagnosis is usually made by positive blood cultures and echocardiography. The most common infecting bacteria are staphylococci, streptococci, and enterococci; fungi are much less common. Echocardiographic findings may be difficult to interpret in patients with prosthetic valves and implantable cardiac electronic devices. The added value and higher accuracy of both radiolabeled leukocyte SPECT/CT and F-18

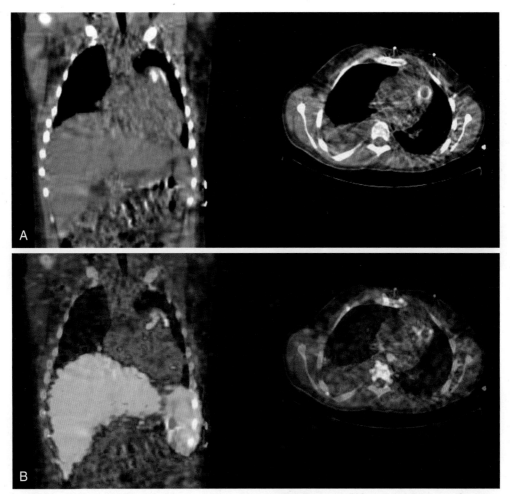

Fig. 15.33 Infected pulmonary artery conduit in a 17-year-old patient with DiGeorge syndrome, truncus arteriosus, and a right ventricular-pulmonary artery conduit. Recent chills and fever. Blood cultures were positive for *Staphylococcus aureus*. (A) Coronal and transverse computed tomography (CT) shows the pulmonary artery conduit. (B) Fused single-photon emission computed tomography with computed tomography (SPECT/CT) In-111 leukocyte images show uptake consistent with an infected pulmonary artery conduit.

FDG PET/CT over echocardiography have now been reported in a number of published investigations. Both radionuclide imaging methods have proven accurate for the diagnosis of prosthetic valve endocarditis (Fig. 15.33). They have also shown value for detecting infection of cardiac implantable devices. It is important to differentiate superficial wound infection from device infection. They are treated differently. Both leukocyte and FDG imaging are somewhat less sensitive for native valve infectious endocarditis.

F-18 FDG has advantages over radiolabeled leukocyte SPECT/CT, including its superior resolution, its short study duration, and the lack of a need for cell labeling. Another advantage of FDG PET/CT is that whole-body imaging is standard and useful for detecting unsuspected septic emboli. Early published imaging studies had reported low sensitivity attributed to high normal myocardial physiological uptake. However, much-improved accuracy has been reported by avoiding the immediate postoperative period and with patient preparation to inhibit myocardial uptake, which includes a low-carbohydrate and high-fat diet, fasting for 6 to 12 hours before the study, and, at some institutions, the use of intravenous heparin before FDG

infusion. The rationale is that heparin induces lipolysis in vivo and induces up to a 5-fold increase in blood free fatty acid (FFA) levels.

With infection of aorto-femoral or femoral-popliteal *arterial prosthetic grafts,* ultrasound, CT, and MRI may sometimes be unable to confirm the diagnosis or distinguish infection from aseptic fluid collections around the graft. In this situation, radiolabeled leukocytes can confirm a surgical prosthetic graft infection (Figs. 15.34–15.36). In-111 leukocytes have the advantage of having no blood-pool distribution, a limitation of Tc-99m HMPAO. However, early and serial imaging with Tc-99m HMPAO at 5 and 30 minutes and at 3 hours is reported to lessen this problem.

For vasculitis, FDG PET/CT can potentially make the initial diagnosis, identify an area for biopsy, evaluate the extent of disease, and determine the success or failure of therapy. A limitation is that FDG PET is only able to visualize inflammation of large to medium-sized vessels (e.g., giant-cell arteritis, Takayasu arteritis, polyarteritis nodosa, and Kawasaki disease; Fig. 15.37). Smaller-vessel arteritis imaging may result in false-negative results. Pattern recognition helps to differentiate vasculitis from

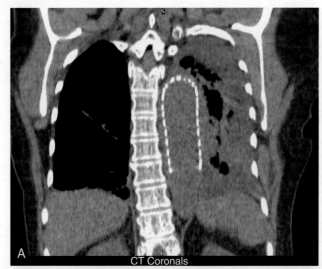

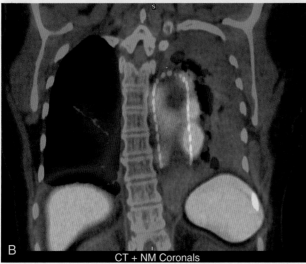

Fig. 15.34 Infected thoracic aortic-stented aneurysm in a 69-year-old female. Computed tomography (CT) showed soft tissue thickening around descending stented thoracic aortic aneurysm, suspicious for infection. The In-111 leukocyte study confirms extensive infection involving soft tissue thickening surrounding the stented aneurysm. (A) Coronal CT. (B) Fused single-photon emission computed tomography with computed tomography (SPECT/CT).

infectious etiologies and atherosclerosis. Vasculitis has homogenous diffuse uptake in the vessel wall, whereas infection shows focal intense uptake localized outside the boundaries of the vascular lumen and walls. Atherosclerosis has focal and moderate FDG uptake at the site of an inflamed plaque, with calcification seen on CT. Steroids may lead to false-negative results.

Pulmonary Infection and Inflammation

Ga-67 citrate accumulates in many types of acute and chronic pulmonary infections and inflammatory diseases (see Box 15.8) and has been used for years in the detection of sarcoidosis (Figs. 15.38–15.39), idiopathic pulmonary fibrosis, *Pneumocystis jiroveci* (formerly known as *P. carinii*; Fig. 15.40; Box 15.9), and therapeutic drug–induced pulmonary disease (Box 15.10). However, many of these indications for Ga-67 are not often requested today because other diagnostic methods have superseded them. For example, FDG PET/CT is now often preferred over Ga-67 to confirm active sarcoidosis and idiopathic

pulmonary fibrosis. Radiolabeled leukocytes are not commonly used to detect pulmonary infection. Low-grade diffuse leukocyte uptake is seen with a variety of noninfectious noninflammatory causes, including acute respiratory distress syndrome, atelectasis, and congestive heart failure, and thus is not diagnostic of infection unless it is focal and intense. Tuberculosis and fungal infections can be detected with In-111-labeled leukocytes, but the sensitivity is poorer than for Ga-67 or F-18 FDG.

Sarcoidosis

Sarcoidosis is a chronic granulomatous multisystem disease of unknown etiology characterized by the accumulation of T lymphocytes, mononuclear phagocytes, and noncaseating epithelioid granulomas, occurring in almost any organ of the body, commonly the lung, liver, and spleen. Systemic symptoms include weight loss, fatigue, weakness, malaise, and fever. Pulmonary manifestations include hilar and mediastinal adenopathy, endobronchial granuloma formation, interstitial or alveolar pulmonary infiltrates, and pulmonary fibrosis. Extrapulmonary manifestations are not rare and can involve the skin, eyes, bones, muscle, central nervous system (CNS), and heart.

The initial presentation is commonly pulmonary, with dyspnea and dry cough, although 20% of patients may be asymptomatic, with only an abnormal chest radiograph. The clinical course is variable. Spontaneous resolution occurs in 30% of patients, 40% have a smoldering or progressively worsening course, 20% develop permanent lung function loss, and 10% die of respiratory failure. Four categories of radiographic findings characterize sarcoidosis (Table 15.8). Although patients with radiographs showing type I findings tend to have a reversible form of the disease, those with types II and III usually have chronic, progressive disease.

Diagnosis is based on a combination of clinical, radiographic, and histological findings. The chest radiograph, although characteristic, is not diagnostic because bilateral hilar adenopathy may be seen with other inflammatory and malignant diseases. Biopsy evidence of a mononuclear-cell granulomatous inflammatory process is mandatory for definitive diagnosis. Bronchoalveolar lavage, Ga-67, and F-18 FDG scans have been used as indicators of disease activity. Although many patients require no specific therapy, those with more severe disease are treated with steroids that suppress the activated T cells at the disease site and the clinical manifestations.

Ga-67 citrate scintigraphy is positive in most patients with active sarcoidosis. The scan has been used to assess the magnitude of alveolitis, guide lung biopsy, choose the pulmonary segments for bronchoalveolar lavage, and distinguish active granuloma formation and alveolitis from inactive disease and fibrotic changes. Increased Ga-67 lung uptake is >90% sensitive for clinically active disease. Uptake occurs before characteristic abnormalities are present on radiographs; thus, it is more sensitive than a chest radiograph for detecting early disease. Ga-67 scans are negative in inactive cases, and these patients nearly always have a negative biopsy. Patients with a diagnosis of sarcoidosis and an abnormal chest radiograph, but inactive disease, have negative Ga-67 scans. Ga-67 is a sensitive indicator of treatment response, superior to clinical symptoms, chest radiograph, and pulmonary function tests.

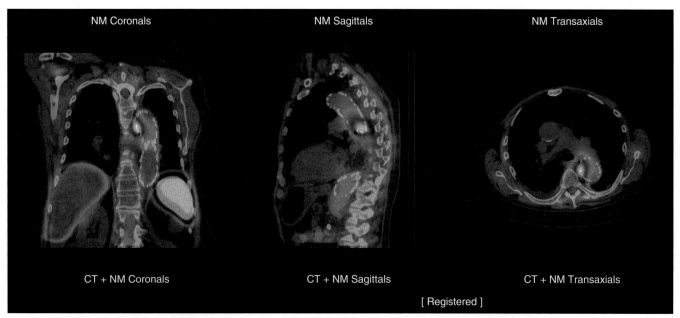

Fig. 15.35 Infected thoracic aortic graft. Patient history of thoracic aortic dissection and subsequent endovascular repair and graft. Now with fever and bacteremia. In-111 white blood cell (WBC) single-photon emission computed tomography with computed tomography (SPECT/CT) shows focal increased uptake in the midportion of the aortic graft. Fused coronal *(left)*, sagittal *(middle)*, transverse *(right)*.

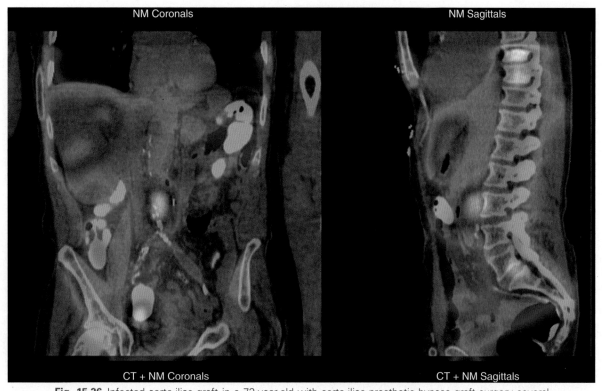

Fig. 15.36 Infected aorto-iliac graft in a 73-year-old with aorto-iliac prosthetic bypass graft surgery several years prior, now with abdominal pain and recurrent fever. Coronal *(left)* and sagittal *(right)* fused In-111 leukocyte single-photon emission computed tomography with computed tomography (SPECT/CT) study shows uptake in the graft just superior to the iliac bifurcation. Uptake in the right lower quadrant is related to inflammatory bowel disease.

F-18 FDG PET/CT is increasingly used rather than Ga-67 to confirm or exclude the diagnosis of sarcoidosis and determine its extent, distribution, and disease activity. Activated macrophages and CD4+ T lymphocytes within granulomas express high levels of glucose transporters. The extent of involvement and quantification of inflammatory activity can more accurately be assessed by FDG PET than Ga-67. FDG PET can establish the presence of previously unknown sites of active disease (e.g., bone or bone marrow involvement that is associated with a more chronic disease course), guide diagnostic biopsy, and determine the effectiveness of therapy.

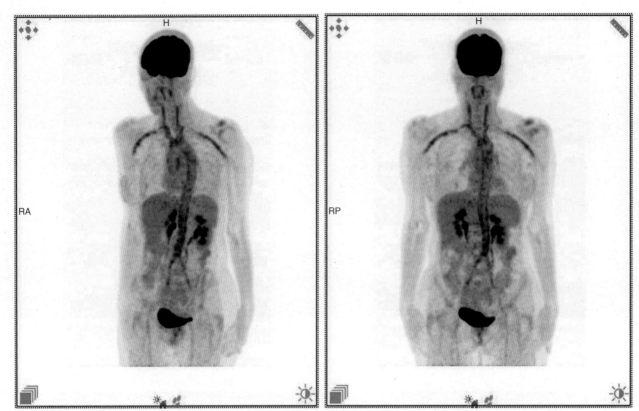

Fig. 15.37 Vasculitis. A 60-year-old female presented with fever of unknown etiology. Maximum-intensity projection (MIP) images show prominently increased fluorodeoxyglucose (FDG) uptake of the aorta, proximal iliac, left and right internal carotid up to the bifurcation, and bilateral brachiocephalic and cephalic arteries extending to the axillary arteries. Computed tomography (CT) showed diffuse circumferential wall thickening. The final diagnosis was giant-cell arteritis.

In early disease, Ga-67 and F-18 FDG typically show bilateral hilar and paratracheal uptake (*lambda sign;* see Fig. 15.38). Pulmonary parenchymal uptake may be intense and symmetrical and may or may not be associated with hilar and mediastinal involvement. Prominent Ga-67 uptake may be seen in the nasopharyngeal region and parotid, salivary, and lacrimal glands (*panda sign;* see Fig. 15.38), but this is not seen with F-18 FDG. In contrast to sarcoidosis, patients with malignant lymphoma usually have asymmetrical hilar or mediastinal uptake, often involving the anterior mediastinal and paratracheal nodes. Paraaortic, mesenteric, and retroperitoneal lymph node involvement can be seen in sarcoidosis, but this pattern of uptake is more common in lymphoma.

Idiopathic Interstitial Pulmonary Fibrosis

Idiopathic interstitial pulmonary fibrosis typically follows a progression through stages of alveolitis, with derangement of the alveolar-capillary units, leading to end-stage fibrotic disease. The cause is unknown. Ga-67 uptake is seen in approximately 70% of patients and has been used to monitor disease course and response to therapy. The degree of uptake correlates with the amount of cellular infiltration. Early data show similar findings for F-18 FDG PET/CT. Fibroblasts are thought to have a central role in the disease and are known to express glucose transporter-1. FDG uptake is a reflection of increased fibroblast metabolism.

Pulmonary Drug Reactions

Common therapeutic drugs known to cause lung injury and result in Ga-67 uptake include Cytoxan, nitrofurantoin, bleomycin, and amiodarone (see Box 15.10). Ga-67 uptake is an early indicator of drug-induced lung injury, before the radiograph becomes abnormal. F-18 FDG can be used in a similar manner.

Malignant External Otitis

Malignant external otitis is a life-threatening infection caused by *Pseudomonas.* It most commonly occurs in patients with diabetes. A bone scan can be diagnostic because of the characteristic pattern of uptake in the mastoid and temporal bone, typically three-phase positive. SPECT/CT is helpful to localize the infection (Fig. 15.41). Ga-67 and In-111 leukocytes have also been used to make the diagnosis and to evaluate response to therapy.

Renal Infection and Inflammation

Ga-67 has been used to diagnose renal parenchymal infection (e.g., pyelonephritis, diffuse interstitial nephritis, lobar nephronia [focal interstitial nephritis]) and perirenal infections. It has proven most valuable in differentiating acute tubular necrosis from acute interstitial nephritis. Acute interstitial nephritis typically has intense uptake, whereas acute tubular necrosis has faint or no uptake. Delayed 48-hour imaging is

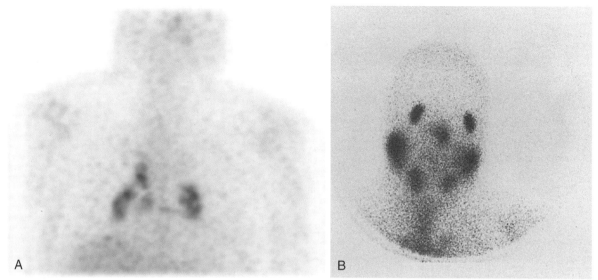

Fig. 15.38 (A) Sarcoidosis. Ga-67 scan in a 35-year-old woman with new diagnosis of sarcoidosis. Ga-67 scintigraphy demonstrates the "lambda" sign, with uptake in paratracheal and hilar adenopathy. (B) The "panda" sign in a different patient with active sarcoidosis. The prominent characteristic is increased uptake in the lacrimal, parotid, and submandibular salivary glands.

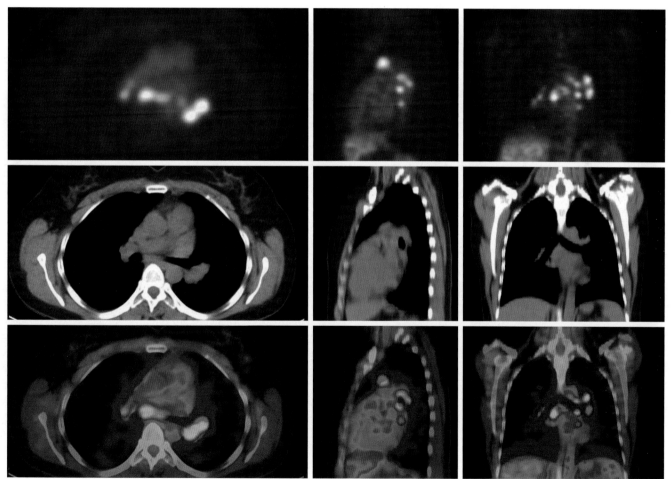

Fig. 15.39 Sarcoidosis and F-18 fluorodeoxyglucose (FDG) scan. FDG *(top)*, computed tomography (CT; *middle)*, and fused FDG/ CT images *(bottom)*. There is mediastinal and bilateral hilar adenopathy.

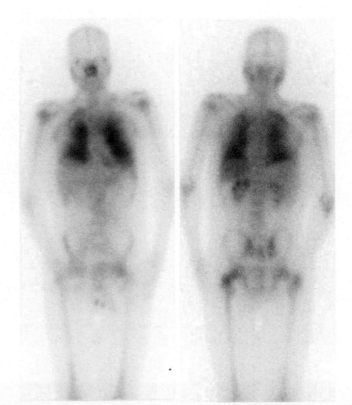

Fig. 15.40 *Pneumocystis jiroveci* (formerly *P. carinii*) infection and whole-body Ga-67 scan. A 57-year-old HIV-positive man with bilateral pulmonary pneumonitis. Diffuse bilateral Ga-67 uptake.

BOX 15.9   Ga-67 Uptake in Interstitial and Granulomatous Pulmonary Diseases

Tuberculosis
Histoplasmosis
Sarcoidosis
Idiopathic pulmonary fibrosis
Pneumocystis jiroveci
Cytomegalovirus
Pneumonoconioses (asbestosis, silicosis)
Hypersensitivity pneumonitis

TABLE 15.8   Classification of Chest Radiographic Findings in Sarcoidosis

Type	Radiographic Findings
I	Hilar and/or mediastinal node enlargement with normal lung parenchyma
II	Hilar and/or mediastinal node enlargement and diffuse interstitial pulmonary disease
III	Diffuse pulmonary disease without node involvement
IV	Pulmonary fibrosis

BOX 15.10   Therapeutic Drug Pulmonary Toxicity—Ga-67 Lung Uptake

Bleomycin
Amiodarone
Busulfan
Nitrofurantoin
Cyclophosphamide
Methotrexate
Nitrosourea

---

required because of early urinary tract clearance. Currently, most imaging involves ultrasound and CT (e.g., the characteristic striated nephrogram pattern on CT and acute perirenal stranding). Ultimately, a biopsy is required to make the diagnosis.

For pyelonephritis, Tc-99m dimercaptosuccinic acid (DMSA) has been an important scintigraphic study used most commonly in children. In adults, radiolabeled leukocyte imaging may be used (Fig. 15.42). Although radiolabeled leukocytes seem to have similar accuracy to DMSA, they are rarely used in young children because of the need for leukocyte labeling requiring 20 to 50 cc of blood and the high radiation dose to the spleen. Tc-99m HMPAO has renal clearance, limiting its use. Radiolabeled leukocytes have limited utility for the evaluation of renal transplants because all exhibit some uptake, regardless of the presence or absence of clinical infection, because of ongoing low-grade rejection (see Fig. 15.8), although focal uptake may be useful diagnostically.

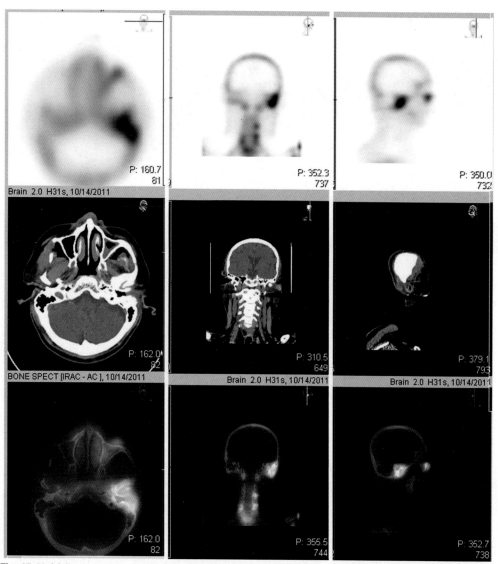

Fig. 15.41 Malignant external otitis with osteomyelitis on Tc-99 methyl diphosphonate (MDP) scan. Single-photon emission computed tomography with computed tomography (SPECT/CT) fused images localize uptake to the region of the left mastoid and temporal lobes, transverse *(left)*, coronal *(middle)*, and sagittal *(right)*.

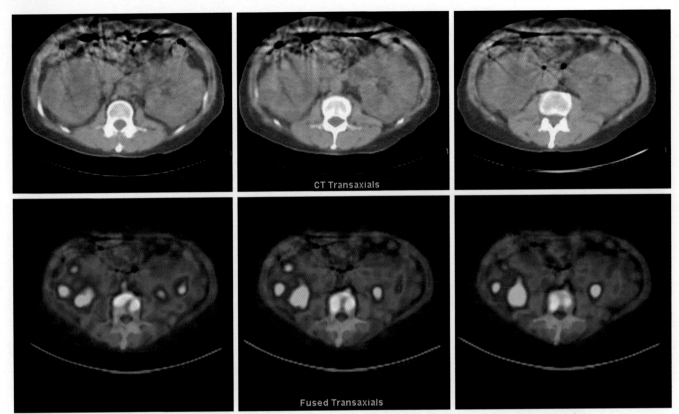

CT Transaxials

Fused Transaxials

Fig. 15.42 Infected polycystic kidneys on In-111 leukocyte scan. Renal stones, recurrent urinary tract infections (UTIs), and recent persistent fever of uncertain cause. Low-dose computed tomography (CT; *top*) demonstrates large multicystic kidneys. Fused single-photon emission computed tomography with computed tomography (SPECT/CT) images *(bottom)* show multiple areas of increased uptake *(yellow)* in the renal cysts, diagnostic of infection.

SUGGESTED READING

Adams H, Keijsers RG, Korenromp IHE, Grutters JC. FDG PET for gauging of sarcoid disease activity. *Semin Respir Crit Care Med.* 2014;35:352–361.

Andor WJM, Glaudemans MD, Israel O, Slart R. Pitfalls and limitations of radionuclide and hybrid imaging in infection and inflammation. *Semin Nucl Med.* 2015;45:500–512.

Datz FL, Taylor AT. Jr. Cell labeling: techniques and clinical utility. In: *Freeman and Johnson's Clinical Radionuclide Imaging.* 3rd ed. New York: Grune & Stratton; 1984.

Granados U, Fuster D, Pericas JM, et al. Diagnostic accuracy of 18F-FDG PET/CT infective endocarditis and implantable cardiac electronic device infection: a cross-sectional study. *J Nucl Med.* 2016;57:1726–1732.

Kouijzer IJE, Mulders-Manders M, Bleeker-Rovers CP, Oyen WJG. Fever of unknown origin: the value of FDG-PET/CT. *Semin Nucl Med.* 2017;48:100–107.

Kouranos V, Hansell DM, Sharma R, Wells TU. Advances in imaging of cardiopulmonary involvement in sarcoidosis. *Current Opinion.* 2015;21:538–545.

Lawal I, Zeevaart J, Ebenhan T, et al. Metabolic imaging of infection. *J Nucl Med.* 2017;58:1727–1732.

Matesan M, Bermo M, Cruite I, et al. Biliary leak in the post-surgical abdomen: a primer to HIDA scan interpretation. *Semin Nucl Med.* 2017;47:618–629.

Mostard RLM, Marinus JPG, Drent M. The role of the PET scan in the management of sarcoidosis. *Current Opinion.* 2013;19:538–544.

Nakahara M, Ito M, Hattori N, et al. 18F-PET/CT better localizes active spinal infection than MRI for successful minimally invasive surgery. *Acta Radiol.* 2015;56:829–836.

Palestro CJ. Radionuclide imaging of musculoskeletal infection. A review. *J Nucl Med.* 2016;57:1406–1412.

Sarrazin J-F, Philippon F, Trottier M, Tessier M. Role of radionuclide imaging for diagnosis of device and prosthetic valve infections. *World J Cardiology.* 2016;8:534–546.

Signore A, Glaudemans A, Gheysens O, et al. Nuclear medicine imaging in pediatric infection or chronic inflammatory diseases. *Semin Nucl Med.* 2017;47:286–303.

Takeuchi M, Dahabreh IJ, Nihashi T, et al. Nuclear imaging for classic fever of unknown origin: metananalysis. *J Nucl Med.* 2016;57:1913–1919.

16

Cardiovascular System

A number of noninvasive cardiac diagnostic imaging studies are available to the cardiologist, which include echocardiography, computed tomography (CT), CT angiography, and magnetic resonance imaging. The continuing value of cardiac nuclear scintigraphic studies is that they are noninvasive, contrast media is not required, and they accurately portray a wide range of physiological and metabolic parameters that predict prognosis and risk. Single-photon emission computed tomography (SPECT) and single-photon emission computed tomography with computed tomography (SPECT/CT) have become the predominant imaging modalities (Fig. 16.1). Positron emission tomography with computed tomography (PET/CT) is growing in clinical use, whereas multigated acquisition (MUGA) has an important but reduced clinical role today.

MYOCARDIAL PERFUSION SCINTIGRAPHY

The underlying physiological principles that make myocardial perfusion imaging an important diagnostic tool remain unchanged. Myocardial perfusion scintigraphy depicts the following sequential physiological events. The radiopharmaceutical must first be delivered to the myocardium. Then viable metabolically active myocardial cells must be available to extract the radiotracer. Finally, a significant amount of the radiopharmaceutical must remain within the cells to allow for imaging. The scintigraphic images are a map of regional myocardial perfusion. If a patient has reduced regional perfusion as a result of hemodynamically significant coronary artery disease (CAD) or a loss of cell viability as a result of myocardial infarction (MI), a perfusion defect or cold region is seen on the images. All diagnostic patterns in the many diverse applications follow from these observations.

SINGLE-PHOTON RADIOPHARMACEUTICALS FOR MYOCARDIAL SCINTIGRAPHY

Radiopharmaceuticals

Both Tc-99m sestamibi and Tc-99m tetrofosmin are routinely used today for cardiac perfusion imaging. They have relatively minor differences (Table 16.1). Thallium-201 was the original

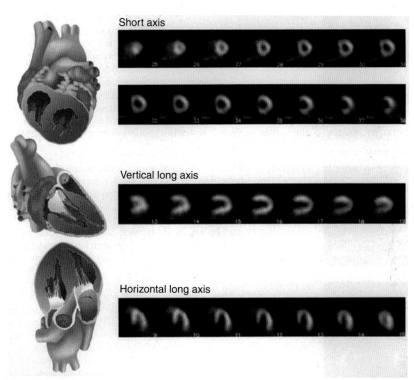

Short axis

Vertical long axis

Horizontal long axis

Fig. 16.1 Three views of the heart that correspond to the short (transaxial) and long (horizontal, vertical) axes of the heart on single-photon emission computed tomography (SPECT) myocardial perfusion images.

TABLE 16.1   Physiology and Pharmacokinetics of Thallium-201, Tc-99m Sestamibi, and Tc-99m Tetrofosmin

Physiology	Thallium-201	Tc-99m Sestamibi	Tc-99m Tetrofosmin
Chemical class/charge	Elemental cation	Isonitrile cation	Diphosphine cation
Mechanism of uptake	Active transport Na/K ATPase pump	Passive diffusion, negative electrical potential	Passive diffusion, negative electrical potential
Myocyte localization	Cytosol	Mitochondria	Mitochondria
Intracellular state	Free	Bound	Bound
Preparation	Cyclotron	Generator/kit	Generator/kit
First-pass extraction fraction	85%	60%	50%
Percent cardiac uptake	3%	1.5%	1.2%
Myocardial clearance	4-hr $T_{1/2}$	Minimal	Minimal
Body clearance	Renal	Hepatic	Hepatic
Imaging time after injection			
Stress	10 min	15–30 min	5–15 min
Rest	3–4 hr	30–90 min	30 min

perfusion agent used before the introduction of the technetium agents, but it is now reserved for special situations, as described in the following subsection.

Tc-99m Sestamibi (Cardiolite)

Tc-99m sestamibi (Cardiolite) was approved by the U.S. Food and Drug Administration (FDA) for cardiac imaging in 1990. Generic Tc-99m sestamibi became available in 2008. Sestamibi is a lipophilic cation and member of the chemical isonitrile family (Fig. 16.2A). After intravenous injection, Tc-99m sestamibi distributes in the heart in proportion to myocardial blood flow and passively diffuses into the myocardial cell because of its lipid solubility. The positively charged lipophilic molecule is attracted to the negatively charged mitochondria, where it is retained. Extraction is proportional to coronary blood flow, although it is underestimated at high flow rates and overestimated at low flow rates. This is true of all the perfusion agents (Fig. 16.3). Myocardial uptake is prompt, and the ratio of myocardium to background activity improves as the lungs clear. Blood clearance is rapid due to renal, biliary, and intestinal excretion. Radiotracer remains fixed within the myocardium, providing an imaging time window of several hours. Image acquisition begins 45 to 60 minutes after tracer administration for resting studies and as early as 30 minutes for exercise stress studies due to its more rapid background clearance.

Tc-99m Tetrofosmin (Myoview)

Tc-99m tetrofosmin (Myoview) was approved by the FDA for cardiac imaging in 1996. It is a member of the diphosphine chemical class (see Fig. 16.2B). Similar to sestamibi, tetrofosmin is a lipophilic cation that localizes near mitochondria in the myocardial cell and remains fixed there. After intravenous injection, it clears rapidly from the blood, and myocardial uptake is prompt. Extraction is proportional to blood flow, although it is underestimated at high flow rates (see Fig. 16.3). Minor differences compared with Tc-99m sestamibi are described (see Table 16.1). The heart-to-lung and heart-to-liver ratios improve with time due to

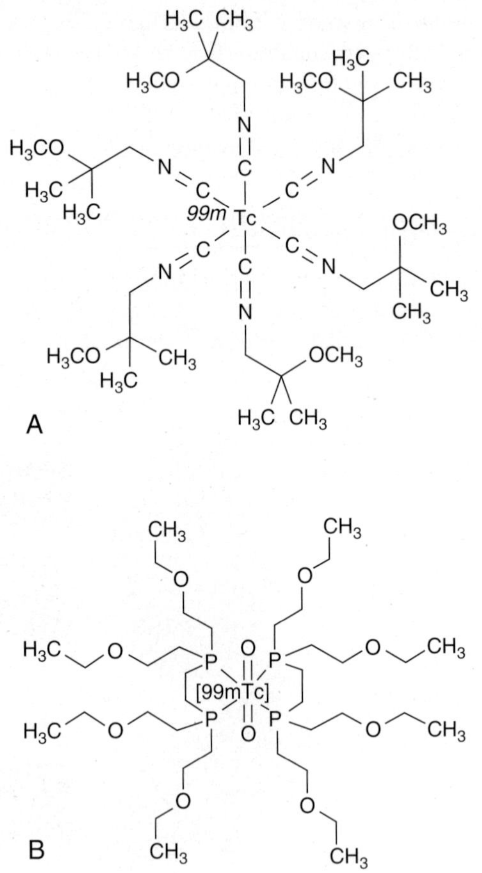

Fig. 16.2 Tc-99m sestamibi and Tc-99m tetrofosmin molecular structure. (A) Tc-99m sestamibi is composed of six isonitrile ligands (hexakis 2-methoxyisobutyl isonitrile) surrounding the Tc-99m radionuclide. (B) Tc-99m tetrofosmin has the chemical name 6,9-bis (2-ethoxyethyl)-3, 12-dioxa-6,9 diphosphatetradecane.

clearance via the liver and kidneys. The heart-to-liver ratios are higher for tetrofosmin than sestamibi because of faster hepatic clearance, allowing for earlier imaging. After exercise stress, imaging at 15 minutes is feasible; rest studies can be started at 30 minutes.

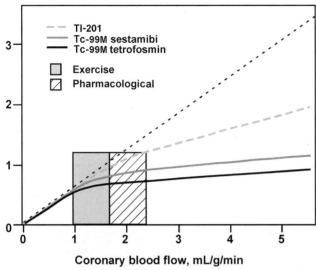

Fig. 16.3 Myocardial perfusion radiopharmaceuticals, Tl-201, Tc-99m sestamibi, and Tc-99m tetrofosmin, uptake relative to coronary blood flow. An ideal myocardial perfusion tracer would show a linear relationship to blood flow over a wide range of flow rates (straight diagonal dark dashed line). Tl-201, Tc-99m sestamibi, and Tc-99m tetrofosmin all have extraction that is proportional to blood flow but underestimate flow at high flow rates.

Thallium-201 Chloride (Tl-201)

The radionuclide Tl-201 is cyclotron-produced. It decays by electron capture to its stable mercury-201 daughter, with a physical half-life of 73 hours. The emitted photons available for imaging are mostly mercury K-characteristic x-rays ranging from 69 to 83 keV (95% abundant) and some gamma rays of 167 keV (10%) and 135 keV (3%). For imaging, a 30% camera window is set for the 69- to 83-keV x-ray emissions and a 20% window at 167 keV. After intravenous injection, Tl-201 blood clearance is rapid (Fig. 16.4). It behaves similar to K^+ and is transported across the myocardial cell membrane by the Na^+/K^+ ATPase pump. First-pass extraction and percent uptake are higher than for Tc-99m sestamibi or tetrofosmin (see Table 16.1). However, it is not ideal for gamma camera imaging, especially for large patients, because its mercury x-ray emissions have relatively low photoenergies and not a single energy photopeak, Compton scatter is high, and the administered dose (3.0 mCi) is low because of poor dosimetry (see the Appendix).

Scintigraphic images after initial uptake reflect capillary *myocardial blood flow.* Unlike the Tc-99m perfusion agents, it then undergoes *redistribution,* a process of continual dynamic exchange between myocardial cells and the vascular blood pool. Several hours after injection, the images depict an equilibrium reflecting *regional blood volume.* With normal perfusion, initial capillary blood flow and delayed regional blood-volume images are similar. Regions of decreased perfusion on early poststress images are due to either decreased blood flow (ischemia) or lack of viable cells to fix the tracer (infarction). If an initial perfusion defect persists on delayed images, it is infarcted. Defects showing "fill-in" of Tl-201 between stress and rest are viable myocardium rendered ischemic during stress. These unique pharmacokinetic characteristics of Tl-201 are the basis for "stress-redistribution"

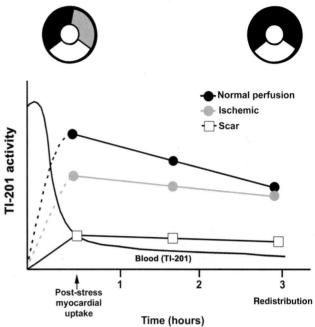

Fig. 16.4 Tl-201 pharmacokinetics: Redistribution. After intravenous injection, Tl-201 rapidly clears from the blood pool. Normal stress peak myocardial uptake occurs by 10 minutes. Redistribution begins promptly after initial uptake. There is a constant dynamic exchange of Tl-201 between the myocytes and blood pool. Normal myocardium progressively clears over 3 hours. In the presence of ischemia, uptake is delayed and reduced, and clearance is slow. With infarction, there is little uptake or change over time. The diagram relates thallium pharmacokinetics *(bottom)* to scintigraphic findings *(top).* The ischemic region, although initially hypoperfused compared with the normal region, equalizes at 3 hours.

imaging used in the past for the detection of CAD (see Fig. 16.4) but today, more commonly, for viability.

Imaging Methodologies
Planar Myocardial Perfusion Imaging

Two-dimensional (2-D) planar imaging was the standard imaging method for many years. Although three-dimensional (3-D) SPECT is now routine, 2-D planar imaging is still occasionally used for patients not able to tolerate SECT acquisition (e.g., who are too large for the SPECT camera, too heavy to lie on the camera table, or have claustrophobia). Planar images are limited by high background and overlapping structures in the standard three views (left anterior oblique, right anterior oblique, left lateral; Figs. 16.5 and 16.6). The accuracy of CAD diagnosis is generally good for planar imaging; however, localization of regional perfusion abnormalities is only moderately predictive of the coronary bed involved. This is important because scintigraphy is used for prognosis, risk stratification, and patient management.

Single-Photon Emission Computed Tomography

SPECT cross-sectional images have high-contrast resolution and are displayed in three dimensions along the short and long axes of the heart (Fig. 16.7; see also Fig. 16.1,), providing good delineation of the regional myocardial perfusion supplied by individual coronary arteries (Figs. 16.8 and 16.9). During acquisition, the gamma

ANT   LAO   LL

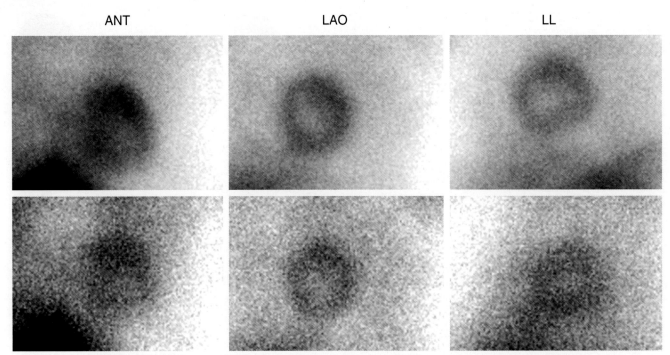

Fig. 16.5 Normal planar stress *(top row)* and rest *(bottom row)* Tc-99m sestamibi scintigraphy. The rest images *(bottom row)* are considerably noisier because of the lower administered dose (8 mCi) and count rates compared with the stress images (25 mCi). Images are acquired so that the three views are at the same angle, between stress and rest, for optimal comparison. *ANT,* Anterior; *LAO,* left anterior oblique; *LL,* left lateral.

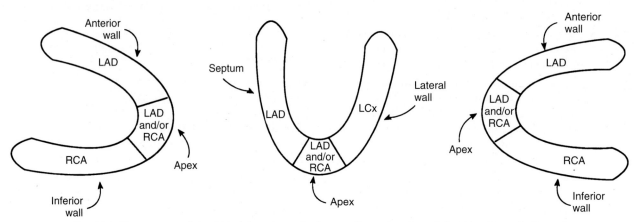

Fig. 16.6 Planar myocardial scintigraphy schematic diagram illustrating the relationship of ventricular wall segments to the coronary artery vascular supply. Anterior, left anterior oblique, and left lateral projections. *LAD,* Left anterior descending artery; *LCX,* left circumflex artery; *RCA,* right coronary artery.

camera rotates about the patient, acquiring 2-D images every few degrees of rotation. These are then processed into 3-D cross-sectional images in a manner similar to CT. Because the heart lies in the anterior lateral chest and there is considerable attenuation in the posterior projections, cardiac SPECT is acquired over a 180-degree arc from the left posterior oblique (LPO) to the right anterior oblique (RAO) projection. Using a two-headed camera with the detectors at 90 degrees maximizes sensitivity and minimizes acquisition time. High-resolution collimators take advantage of the higher counts obtained from two detectors. Image acquisition with standard SPECT systems takes 20 to 30 minutes. Some newer dedicated cardiac cameras can acquire more counts with greater image resolution in a shorter time period. Typical SPECT acquisition parameters are listed in Table 16.2.

Filtered back-projection had long been the standard method used for cross-sectional image reconstruction for both CT and SPECT; however, because of the speed of modern computers, superior *iterative reconstruction* techniques have now become routine for both. Correction for attenuation uses an attenuation map generated by the CT in SPECT/CT systems or, in older SPECT-only systems, a rotating gamma source. Software filters are chosen to optimize the trade-off between high-frequency noise and low-frequency oversmoothing.

Cardiac SPECT software reconstructs cross-sectional cardiac images along the short and long axes—transaxial (short axis), coronal (horizontal long axis), and sagittal (vertical long axis; see Figs. 16.7 and 16.9). SPECT images depict perfusion of the myocardium as it relates to the coronary artery supplying blood

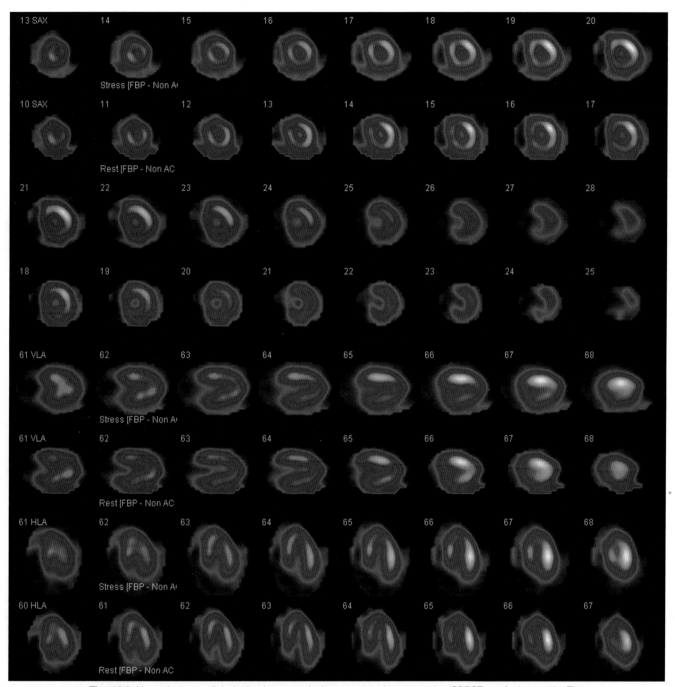

Fig. 16.7 Normal myocardial single-photon emission computed tomography (SPECT) perfusion study. The *top four rows* display the short-axis transaxial images ([*top*] stress; [*bottom*] rest), the *fifth and sixth rows* display the horizontal long-axis (sagittal) stress and rest views, and the *seventh and eighth rows* display the vertical long-axis (coronal) views.

to that region (Table 16.3) and permit estimation of the degree and extent of the perfusion abnormality.

Gated Single-Photon Emission Computed Tomography. The relatively high count rate available from 15 to 30 mCi (740–1110 MBq) of Tc-99m sestamibi or tetrofosmin and the two detector heads make electrocardiographic (ECG) gating a common practice, allowing for a cinematic 3-D display of contracting myocardial slices from summed beats over the acquisition period. Data collection is triggered by the R-wave of the electrocardiogram. Each cardiac cycle is divided into 8

frames, less than the 16 frames used for count-rich Tc-99m-labeled red blood cell (RBC) ventriculograms, because of their lower count rate. The eight frames limit only to a mild degree the temporal resolution (pinpointing end-diastole and end-systole) and accuracy of left ventricular ejection fraction (LVEF) calculation. Semiautomatic edge-detection software programs draw the endocardial surface and delineate the valve plane for LVEF calculation and wall motion (Fig. 16.10). Hybrid SPECT/CT systems are increasingly used. Low-resolution CT is used primarily for attenuation correction and

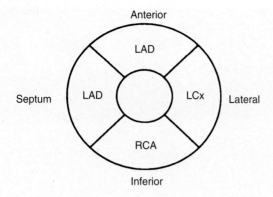

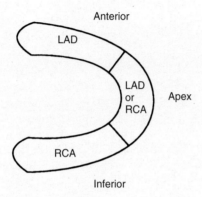

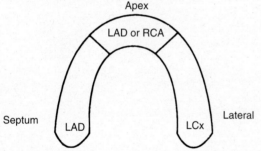

Fig. 16.8 Single-photon emission computed tomography (SPECT) myocardial scintigraphy schematic diagram illustrating the relationship of the ventricular transverse, vertical long-axis, and horizontal long-axis (coronal) segments to their coronary artery vascular supply.

TABLE 16.2 Typical Cardiac SPECT Acquisition Parameters for Dual-Headed Camera	
Matrix	128 × 128
Number of stops	64
Time per stop	28 sec
Zoom	1.46 cm
Range	90 degree/detector
Method	Step and shoot

SPECT, Single-photon emission computed tomography.

TABLE 16.3 Scintigraphic Patterns by Vascular Distribution: Stenosis and Obstruction	
Coronary Arteries	**Scintigraphic Perfusion Defects**
Left anterior descending	Septum, anterior wall, apex
Left circumflex	Lateral wall, posterior wall, posterior inferior wall, apex
Right coronary	Inferior wall, posterior inferior wall, right ventricular wall
Left main coronary	Anterior wall, septum, posterolateral wall

coronary artery calcium scoring. However, CT images should always be reviewed and may reveal incidental unknown disease (Fig. 16.11).

Diagnosis and Evaluation of Coronary Artery Disease

Ischemic perfusion abnormalities are not usually seen at rest. Although under resting conditions, high-grade stenosis (≥90%) in an epicardial coronary artery produces a downstream decline in coronary perfusion pressure to the affected vascular territory, resting blood flow is usually maintained by autoregulatory

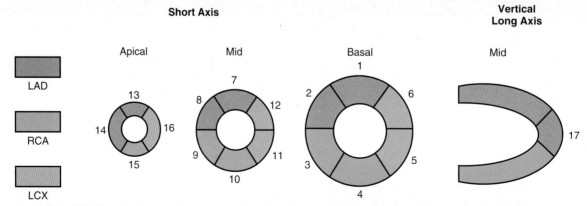

Fig. 16.9 Standardization of single-photon emission computed tomography (SPECT) myocardial segments. The left ventricular myocardium is divided into 17 regions. The diagram correlates coronary artery anatomy with regional perfusion. *LAD,* Left anterior descending artery; *LCX,* left circumflex artery; *RCA,* right coronary artery.

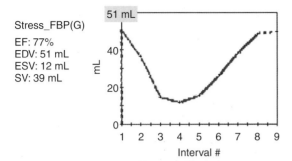

Stress_FBP(G)

EF: 77%
EDV: 51 mL
ESV: 12 mL
SV: 39 mL

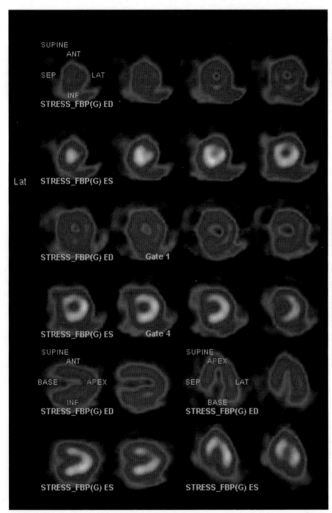

Fig. 16.10 Gated single-photon emission computed tomography (SPECT) perfusion study. End-diastolic and end-systolic images of the short-axis views (*top four rows* of images) and vertical and horizontal long-axis views *(bottom two rows)* are shown. The time–activity curve and quantification of the left ventricular ejection fraction (LVEF) is shown at the *top. ANT,* Anterior; *EDV,* end-diastolic volume; *EF,* ejection fraction; *ESV,* end-systolic volume; *FBP(G),* filtered back-projection (gated); *INF,* inferior; *Lat,* lateral; *SEP,* septal; *SV,* stroke volume.

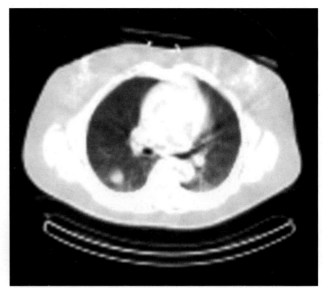

Fig. 16.11 Incidental computed tomography (CT) finding on cardiac single-photon emission computed tomography with computed tomography (SPECT/CT). Low-resolution CT scan from hybrid SPECT/CT system shows previously unknown nodule in the left posterior lung.

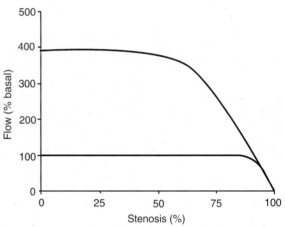

Fig. 16.12 Relationship between blood flow and severity of coronary stenosis. At rest, myocardial blood flow is not reduced until a coronary stenosis approaches 90%. It then begins to drop off. However, with increased coronary blood flow produced by exercise or pharmacological stress, less severe stenoses (50–75%) result in reduced coronary flow.

dilation of the coronary arterioles (Fig. 16.12). Exercise increases cardiac work and the demand for oxygen and blood flow. In the absence of CAD, maximum exercise increases coronary flow by 3 to 5 times. *Coronary flow reserve* (maximum increase in blood flow above normal resting flow) across a fixed mechanical stenosis is limited because most of the coronary arteriolar vasodilator reserve has already been used to maintain resting flow. However, with exercise, myocardium in the watershed of a coronary artery with a hemodynamically significant stenosis becomes ischemic, resulting in less delivery and localization of the radiopharmaceutical. Hypoperfusion on scintigraphy is seen as a perfusion defect ("photopenic" or cold) surrounded by normal blood flow in the adjacent nonischemic cardiac regions (Fig. 16.13). Coronary artery stenoses of more than 70% are considered clinically significant based on the usually rapid fall-off in flow reserve augmentation above this level (see Fig. 16.12). Myocardial perfusion scintigraphy is often used to evaluate the clinical significance of a known stenosis, particularly in the range of 50% of 70%.

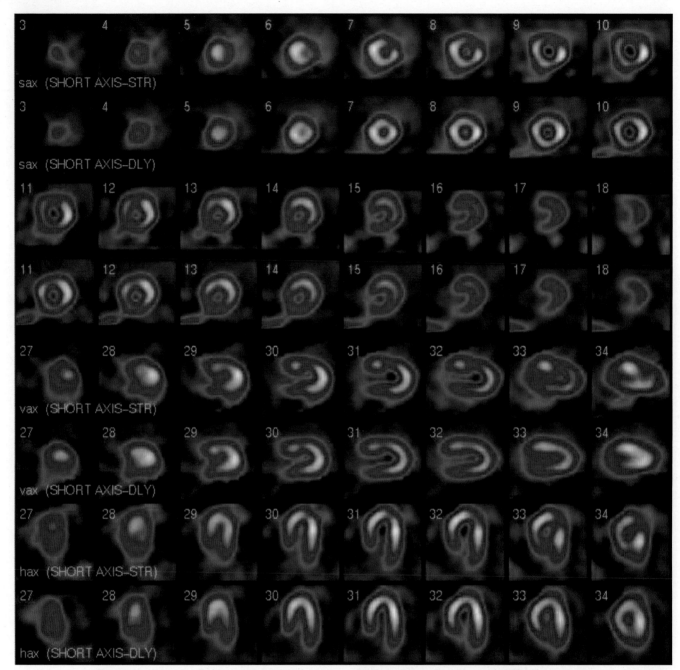

Fig. 16.13 Ischemia—Tc-99m sestamibi single-photon emission computed tomography (SPECT) myocardial perfusion scintigraphy. Reduced perfusion (cold, photopenic) at stress in the anterior lateral left ventricle; near normal perfusion at rest. *DLY*, Delay; *hax*, horizontal long axis; *sax*, short axis; *STR*, stress; *vax*, vertical long axis.

Cardiac Stress

Exercise Stress. Graded treadmill exercise with ECG monitoring has long been the standard method to diagnose ischemic CAD (Fig. 16.14). Exercise increases cardiac workload and oxygen demand. The degree of stress must be sufficient to unmask underlying ischemia (Box 16.1). The treadmill study allows for an assessment of the patient's functional cardiac status by monitoring exercise tolerance, heart rate, blood pressure, and ECG response to graded exercise. Contraindications to cardiac stress testing are listed (Box 16.2).

Exercise-induced myocardial ischemia produces characteristic ECG ST-T segment depression (Fig. 16.15). The adequacy of exercise is critical for interpretation. Patients achieving more than 85% of the age-predicted maximum heart rate (220 − age) are considered to have achieved adequate exercise stress. The product of heart rate × blood pressure, metabolic equivalents (METS), and exercise time (minutes) are also used to judge the adequacy of exercise. Failure to achieve adequate exercise is the most common reason for a false-negative stress test result (Box 16.3).

The accuracy of the cardiac treadmill exercise test for the diagnosis of CAD is modest, approximately 75%, with many false-negative and false-positive results. The specificity is particularly poor in women, in patients with resting ECG ST-T abnormalities, left

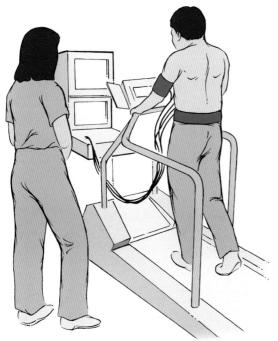

Fig. 16.14 Treadmill graded patient exercise with electrocardiographic, blood pressure, heart rate, and symptom monitoring.

BOX 16.1 Exercise Testing: Rationale and Endpoint Measures

Physiological Rationale
Physical exercise increases cardiac work.
Increased work increases myocardial oxygen demand.
Normal coronary arteries dilate, and flow increases.
Stenotic vessels cannot dilate, and flow reserve is limited.
Myocardial ischemia is induced.

Manifestations of Myocardial Ischemia
Electrocardiogram: Ion flux across cell membrane is impaired, producing ST-segment depression.
Perfusion scintigraphy: Decrease in regional flow produces cold defect on scintigraphy.
Radionuclide ventriculography: Regional wall-motion abnormality or fall in left ventricular ejection fraction with stress

ventricular hypertrophy, or bundle branch block, and for those on digoxin. These patients often require myocardial perfusion scintigraphy to confirm or exclude the diagnosis of CAD.

Methodology for Exercise Stress. The patient must fast for 4 to 6 hours before the test to prevent gastric symptoms and minimize splanchnic blood distribution. Cardiac medications may be held depending on the indication for the stress test (e.g., whether for diagnosis or to determine the effectiveness of therapy; Table 16.4). Beta-blockers may prevent achievement of maximum heart rate, and nitrates and calcium channel blockers may block or prevent cardiac ischemia, limiting the test's diagnostic value. In addition to a standard 12-lead electrocardiogram, an intravenous line is kept open. Graded treadmill exercise is usually performed according to the Bruce protocol (Table 16.5). When the patient has achieved maximal exercise or peak patient tolerance, the radiotracer is injected. Exercise is continued for another minute to ensure adequate myocardial uptake. Early discontinuation of exercise may result in uptake reflecting perfusion at submaximal exercise levels. Indications for terminating exercise are listed in Box 16.4. Many are manifestations of ischemia; others are due to underlying medical, cardiac, or pulmonary conditions.

Pharmacological Stress. Patients receive pharmacological stress with coronary vasodilators rather than exercise stress when it is anticipated that they will not be able to achieve adequate exercise due to concurrent medical problems (e.g., pulmonary disease or lower extremity musculoskeletal problems). The disadvantage of this approach is the lack of functional cardiac information provided by exercise.

BOX 16.2 Contraindications for Stress Testing

Acute myocardial infarction
Unstable angina
Severe tachyarrhythmias or bradyarrhythmias
Uncontrolled symptomatic heart failure
Critical aortic stenosis
Acute aortic dissection
Pulmonary embolism
Poorly controlled hypertension

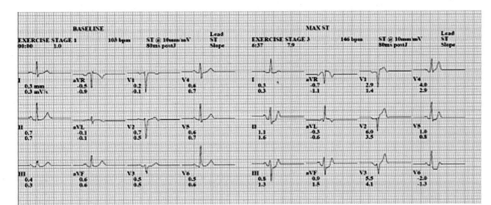

Fig. 16.15 Treadmill electrocardiographic ischemia. Baseline *(left)* and maximal stress *(right)* 12-lead electrocardiogram demonstrates ST-T wave depression in II, III, aV_F, and V_6, consistent with stress-induced ischemia.

BOX 16.3 Reasons for Failing to Achieve Adequate Exercise

Poor general conditioning, low exercise tolerance
Poor motivation
Arthritis, other musculoskeletal problems
Lung disease
Peripheral vascular disease
Medications (beta-blockers)
Angina
Arrhythmia
Cardiac insufficiency

BOX 16.4 Indications for Terminating a Stress Test

Patient request
Inability to continue because of fatigue, dyspnea, or faintness
Moderate to severe chest pain
Dizziness, near syncope
Pallor, diaphoresis
Ataxia
Claudication
Ventricular tachycardia
Atrial tachycardia or fibrillation
Onset of second- or third-degree heart block
ST-segment depression greater than 3 mm
Decrease in systolic blood pressure from baseline
Increase in systolic blood pressure above 240 mm Hg or diastolic above 120 mm Hg

TABLE 16.4 Drugs That Interfere With Stress Testing: Recommended Withdrawal Interval

Drugs	Withdrawal Interval
Exercise	
Beta-blockers	48–96 hr
Calcium channel blockers	48–72 hr
Nitrates (long acting)	12 hr
Pharmacological	
Theophylline derivatives	48 hr
Caffeine	24 hr

TABLE 16.5 Drugs That Interfere With Stress Testing: Recommended Withdrawal Interval

Stage (min)	Total Time (min)	Speed (mile/hr)	Grade (%)
Standard Bruce Protocol			
1 (3)	3	1.7	10
2 (3)	6	2.5	12
3 (3)	9	3.4	14
4 (3)	12	4.2	16
5 (3)	15	5.0	18
6 (3)	18	6.0	20
Modified Bruce Protocol			
1 (3)	3	1.7	0
2 (3)	6	1.7	5
3 (3)	9	1.7	10
4 (3)	12	2.5	12
5 (3)	15	3.4	14
6 (3)	18	4.2	16
7 (3)	21	5.0	18

The modified Bruce starts with the same speed as the standard Bruce, but with no slope, followed by a slight increase in slope and then in speed. This protocol is suited for elderly patients or when one anticipates difficulties with physical performance.

Dipyridamole (Persantine) and adenosine (Adenoscan) have long been used for pharmacological stress myocardial perfusion imaging. Regadenoson (Lexiscan) was approved by the FDA in 2009 and is the most recently FDA-approved drug.

Coronary vasodilators increase coronary blood flow by 3 to 5 times in normal vessels. Because coronary arteries with significant stenoses cannot increase blood flow to the same degree, vasodilator stress results in vascular regions of relative hypoperfusion on myocardial perfusion scintigraphy, similar to that seen with exercise-induced ischemia. This is really not a test of ischemia because cardiac work is not involved but, rather, a test of coronary flow reserve. However, comparative studies have shown similar scintigraphic patterns and diagnostic accuracy for exercise and pharmacological stress.

Endogenous adenosine is normally physiologically released from the coronary endothelial cells and activates four coronary receptor subtypes, A1, A2A, A2B, and A3. Only A2A activation produces coronary vasodilation. Activation of the other receptors is responsible for side effects. The adenosine analog (Adenoscan) used for stress testing has a similar effect. It is short acting, and discontinuation of infusion promptly resolves any adverse symptoms. Dipyridamole exerts its pharmacological effect by blocking the reuptake of adenosine and thus raising endogenous adenosine blood levels. Regadenoson is a selective A2A receptor.

Methodology. Because vasodilators are counteracted by drugs and food containing methylxanthines (e.g., theophylline and caffeine), they should be held for 12 to 24 hours before the study (see Table 16.4). The technical details for dipyridamole, adenosine, and regadenoson infusion protocols vary somewhat (Fig. 16.16) due to their different pharmacokinetics (Table 16.6). Unlike adenosine and dipyridamole, which are given as constant infusions based on weight, regadenoson is given in a fixed dose as an intravenous bolus. A mild to moderate increase in heart rate and a reduction in blood pressure confirm the drugs' pharmacological effect.

Not uncommon side effects of these drugs include dizziness, headache, and flushing. Infrequently, patients experience chest pain; however, it is not usually caused by ischemia. A coronary steal syndrome may sometimes produce true ischemia, manifested by ECG ST-T depression during the infusion, suggesting significant CAD. Dyspnea and atrioventricular (AV) conduction blocks occur predominantly with adenosine.

Although dipyridamole was the first agent approved, it is less often used today because of its long physiological effect, often

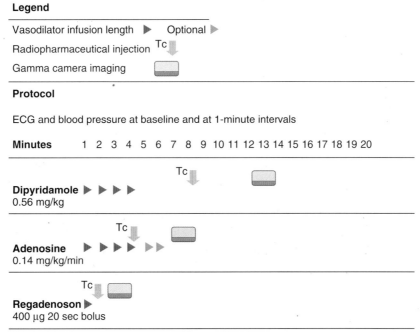

Legend

Vasodilator infusion length ▶   Optional ▶

Radiopharmaceutical injection ^{Tc}⬇

Gamma camera imaging 🔲

Protocol

ECG and blood pressure at baseline and at 1-minute intervals

Minutes   1 2 3 4 5 6 7 8 9 10 11 12 13 14 15 16 17 18 19 20

Dipyridamole ▶ ▶ ▶ ▶
0.56 mg/kg

Adenosine   ▶ ▶ ▶ ▶ ▶ ▶
0.14 mg/kg/min

Regadenoson ▶
400 µg 20 sec bolus

Fig. 16.16 Coronary vasodilator stress protocols compared for dipyridamole, adenosine, and regadenoson.

TABLE 16.6 Adenosine, Dipyridamole, and Regadenoson Pharmacokinetics

Pharmacokinetics	Dipyridamole	Adenosine	Regadenoson
Administration	Intravenous infusion	Intravenous infusion	Intravenous bolus
Dose	0.56 mg/kg	140 µgm/kg/min	400 µg
Mode of action	Blocks reuptake of adenosine, raising endogenous adenosine blood levels	Nonselective	Selective A2A agonist
Duration of infusion	4–8 min	4–6 min	10-sec bolus
Time to peak	6.5 min	30 sec	33 sec
Duration of action	12 min	6 sec after infusion stopped	2.3 min
Elimination	Liver	Cellular uptake/metabolism	Renal (57%)

causing adverse symptoms and requiring reversal with aminophylline. Both adenosine and dipyridamole may cause bronchospasm in patients with asthma and chronic obstructive pulmonary disease. Regadenoson is somewhat safer in patients with mild to moderate reactive airway disease and may have fewer side effects overall.

Because of adenosine's short half-life (<10 seconds), side effects resolve promptly when the infusion is stopped. Because the effect of dipyridamole and regadenoson is prolonged after stopping the infusion, intravenous aminophylline may be required to reverse the side effects.

Dobutamine. For patients unable to exercise and with contraindications to vasodilator therapy (e.g., symptomatic asthma), dobutamine can be used as an alternative. It is a synthetic catecholamine that acts on alpha- and beta-adrenergic receptors, producing inotropic and chronotropic effects that increase cardiac work. In normal coronary arteries, increased blood flow results. With significant stenosis, regional flow does not increase, producing scintigraphic patterns similar to those seen with exercise and pharmacological stress.

Methodology. The initial dopamine infusion rate is 5 µg/kg/min over 3 minutes, then increased to 10 µg/kg/min for another 3 minutes and increased further by the same amount every 10

TABLE 16.7 Protocols for Stress Myocardial Perfusion Scintigraphy

Method	Radiopharmaceutical	Rationale
2 day	Tc-99m sestamibi/tetrofosmin	Obesity, image quality
1 day	Tc-99m sestamibi/tetrofosmin	Image quality, efficiency
1 day	Tl-201	Viability
Dual isotope	Tl-201 and Tc-99m sestamibi/tetrofosmin	Image quality, viability, logistics

minutes until a maximum of 40 µg/kg/min is achieved. The radiopharmaceutical is injected 1 minute after the maximal tolerable dose. Dobutamine infusion is continued for 1 minute.

The accuracy of dobutamine perfusion imaging is similar to that of exercise or pharmacological stress. However, it is limited by the frequent occurrence of side effects, including chest pain, arrhythmias, and the inability of patients to tolerate the maximum dose. The main adverse effects are hypotension and arrhythmias, which are dose related and require cessation of infusion.

Imaging Protocols. The specific stress/rest perfusion imaging protocol used depends on the radiopharmaceutical chosen, physician preference, and clinic logistics (Table 16.7; Box 16.5).

BOX 16.5 Tc-99m Sestamibi and Tetrofosmin SPECT Myocardial Perfusion Imaging: Summary Protocol

Patient Preparation
Patient should fast for 4 hours before the study.

Radiopharmaceutical
10 to 30 mCi (370–1110 MBq) intravenously (see the following individual protocols)

SPECT Imaging Protocol
1-Day rest–stress imaging
Rest: 10 mCi (370 MBq); imaging at 30 to 90 minutes
Stress: 30 mCi (1110 MBq); imaging at 15 to 30 minutes
2-Day rest–stress or stress–rest imaging: 30 mCi (1110 MBq)

SPECT Acquisition Parameters
Patient position: supine, left arm raised (180-degree arc)
Rotation: counterclockwise
Matrix: 128 × 128 word mode
Image/arc: 64 views (180-degree and 45-degree right anterior oblique; 135-degree left posterior oblique)

SPECT Reconstruction Parameters[a]
Ramp filter
Convolution filter: Butterworth
Attenuation correction: Review images with and without correction.
Oblique-angle reformatting: Short axis, vertical long axis, and horizontal long axis
Gated SPECT
Electrocardiogram synchronized data collection: R-wave trigger, 8 frames/cardiac cycle

Planar Imaging Protocol
Collimator: High resolution
Window: 20% centered at 140 keV
For 1-day rest and stress studies, give 10 mCi (370 MBq) at rest and image at 30 to 60 minutes.
Rest studies: Begin imaging at 60 to 90 minutes after tracer injection.
Obtain anterior, 45-degree left anterior oblique and left lateral images.
Obtain 750,000 to 1 million counts per view.
Wait 4 hours and give 30 mCi (1110 MBq) with repeat imaging at 15 to 30 minutes.
Stress studies: Begin imaging at 15 to 30 minutes after tracer injection.
Obtain stress and rest images in identical projection.

[a]Choice of SPECT acquisition and reconstruction parameters is influenced by the equipment used.
SPECT, Single-photon emission computed tomography.

Tc-99m Sestamibi and Tc-99m Tetrofosmin

Single-Day Protocol. Separate injections are required for the rest and stress studies. The patient receives a lower administered dose of the radiopharmaceutical for the initial study (8–10 mCi [266–370 MBq]) and a several-fold-higher dose (25–30 mCi [925–1110 MBq]) for the second study, so that the first study will be only in background. The most common approach is to perform the rest study first, followed by the stress study with the administered dose approximately 3 times higher. Some centers are doing the stress study first with the lower dose. If normal, no rest study is performed. If abnormal, the rest study

is acquired after administering the larger dose. This approach can improve patient throughput and reduce patient radiation. The downside is that the stress test has fewer counts, and the image quality is sometimes suboptimal.

Two-Day Protocol. Tissue attenuation can be quite marked in large patients and result in poor image quality and interpretative problems, particularly for the lower-dose rest study. A 2-day approach allows administration of the maximum dose (25–30 mCi) for both studies.

Thallium-201 Chloride. Only one injection of radiopharmaceutical is required. After peak stress injection, initial stress images are acquired at 10 to 15 minutes and delayed rest images at 3 hours (Fig. 16.17).

Dual-Isotope Protocol With Tc-99m Sestamibi and Thallium-201 Chloride. The dual-isotope approach is used at some centers because the entire study can be completed more rapidly than with Tc-99m protocols. Imaging begins earlier, immediately after the rest study (Tl-201) and 10 minutes after the stress study (Tc-99m sestamibi). It takes advantage of the different photopeaks of Tc-99m (140 keV) and Tl-201 (69–83 keV). The Tl-201 rest study is performed first with 3 to 3.5 mCi (110–130 MBq), followed by the stress study, using 20 to 30 mCi (740–1110 MBq) of the Tc-99m radiopharmaceutical. The downside is the poorer resolution of Tl-201.

Quality Control and Image Quality. Gamma camera quality control is required to routinely obtain high-quality images and is described in detail in Part I, Radiation Detection and Instrumentation. Image quality may be poor because of insufficient myocardial counts due to a low administered dose, inadvertent subcutaneous injection, or soft tissue attenuation. Patient motion and scatter from radioactivity in the liver or bowel can degrade image quality. Review of the acquisition raw data for patient movement and significant attenuation should be routine. The 2-D unprocessed planar images acquired every few degrees for 180 degrees from each camera head can be displayed in a cinematic loop to look for motion. Another method for confirming movement is to review the "sinogram." Each projection image is stacked vertically and compressed, with maintenance of the count density distribution in the x-axis but minimization in the y-axis. Because the heart is not in the center of the camera radius of rotation, the position of the left ventricle in the stacked frames varies sinusoidally. Motion is seen as a break in the sinogram (Fig. 16.18). With significant motion, the study should ideally be reacquired. If this is not possible due to poor patient cooperation or logistical issues, software motion-correction programs are available with most camera computer systems. However, these programs usually correct only in the vertical axis, and patients often move in multiple dimensions.

Image quality can sometimes be limited by activity below the diaphragm from the liver or bowel activity scattering into the heart, causing artifacts and sometimes interpretative problems. When serious, further delayed imaging can be performed, allowing time for clearance.

Image Interpretation

Although the anatomy of the coronary circulation varies in detail, the distribution of the major vessels is reasonably

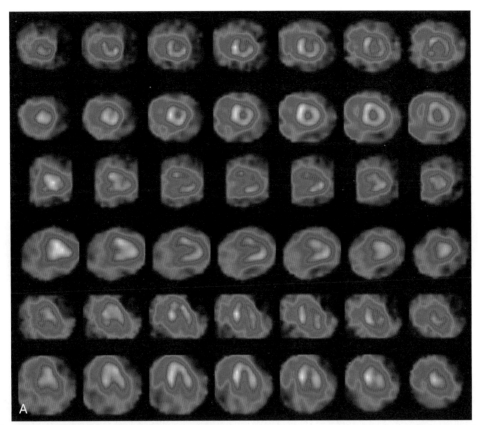

Fig. 16.17 TI-201 1-day protocol shows hypoperfusion in the anterior apical wall 10 minutes after stress *(top)* and complete redistribution *(bottom)* 3 hours later.

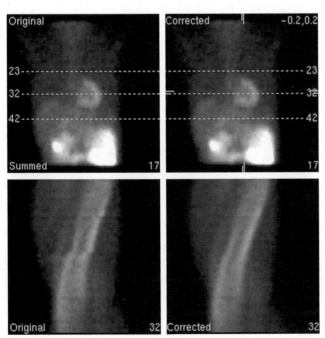

Fig. 16.18 Sinogram—detection of patient motion. The projection images are stacked vertically. Because the heart is not in the center of the camera radius of rotation, the position of the left ventricle in the stacked frames varies sinusoidally. Any significant motion is seen as a break in the sinogram. There is a horizontal break in the midsinogram *(left)*. The repeat acquisition shows no break and thus no significant motion *(right)*.

predictable (Fig. 16.19; see also Table 16.3). The left anterior descending (LAD) coronary artery serves most of the septum and the anterior wall of the left ventricle. Its diagonal branches course over the anterior lateral wall, and septal perforators penetrate into the septum. The left circumflex coronary artery (LCX) and its marginal branches serve the lateral wall and the inferior segment of the lateral wall. The right coronary artery (RCA) and its branches serve the right ventricle, the inferior portion of the septum, and the inferior wall of the left ventricle.

Planar Images. The cardiac scintigraphic configuration depends on patient habitus and the orientation of the heart in the chest, but it is usually circular or ellipsoid in different views (see Figs. 16.5 and 16.6). The right ventricle has much less uptake than the left. The anterior view best shows the anterior wall and apex. The inferior wall and septum overlap in this view. The LAO view best demonstrates the lateral wall and septum, but the apex and inferior wall may overlap depending on the orientation of the heart. The left lateral view best demonstrates the inferior wall and apex. Stress and rest images should be acquired at the same angle.

Single-Photon Emission Computed Tomography Images. The cinematic rotating 2-D raw (unprocessed) data should be reviewed for the presence of attenuation and motion. Regions of reduced myocardial activity from breast or soft tissue and subdiaphragmatic attenuation could potentially be misinterpreted as myocardial infarction. If attenuation is noted on the cine display, this could help explain a finding on cross-sectional images. If the breasts are in different positions during

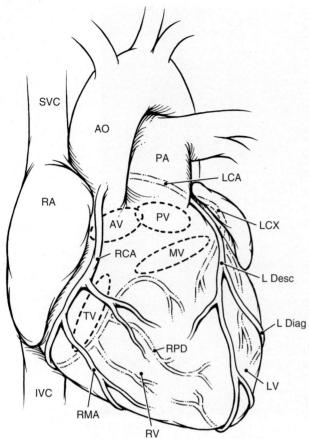

Fig. 16.19 Normal coronary anatomy and cardiac perfusion beds. The left main coronary artery is only 0 to 15 mm in length before dividing into the left anterior descending and left circumflex arteries. Major branches of the left anterior descending artery are the diagonal and septal branches. The left circumflex artery *(LCX)* has obtuse marginal branches. The right coronary artery (RCA) originates separately and has important branches that include the posterior right ventricular branches and the posterior descending artery. "Dominance" refers to which coronary artery (RCA or LCX) supplies the diaphragmatic surface of the left ventricle and posterior septum by giving rise to the posterior descending and posterior left ventricular branches. Right posterior descending *(RPD)*, right marginal branch artery (RMA). The apex may be perfused by branches from any of the three main vessels. *AO,* Aorta; *AV,* aortic valve; *IVC,* inferior vena cava; *LCA,* left coronary artery; *LCX,* left circumflex; *L Desc,* left anterior descending; *L Diag,* left diagonal; *LV,* left ventricle; *MV,* mitral valve; *PA,* pulmonary artery; *PV,* pulmonary valve; *RA,* right atrium; *RMA,* right mesenteric artery; *RV,* right ventricle; *SVC,* superior vena cava; *TV,* tricuspid valve.

the two studies, this could be misinterpreted as ischemia if not noted on the rotating raw data views.

With normal myocardial perfusion there is relatively uniform uptake throughout the left ventricle (LV) myocardium (see Fig. 16.7). On short-axis SPECT views, the LV has a doughnut appearance. The lateral wall usually has more uptake than the anterior or inferior wall. Near the base of the heart, there is less or no uptake in the septum because of the membranous septum and valve planes, giving the heart a horseshoe- or U-shaped appearance on vertical and horizontal long-axis SPECT slices. Reduced uptake in the apex (apical thinning) is a normal finding. The right ventricle (RV) has less uptake than the left ventricle due to its lesser myocardial muscle mass. RV hypertrophy

results in increased uptake (Fig. 16.20). Atria are not visualized. Although some normal lung uptake is seen, increased uptake on rest most commonly occurs in heavy smokers and patients with underlying lung disease or heart failure.

Stress images after exercise or pharmacological stress are not strikingly different in distribution from those at rest, although there are some differences. The stress image cardiac-to-background ratio is higher because of the increased myocardial blood flow and thus radiotracer uptake. RV uptake is often increased but is still considerably less than the LV. With good treadmill exercise, reduced liver activity is seen because of the diversion of blood flow from the splanchnic bed to the leg muscles. Vasodilator pharmacological stress results in increased liver activity.

Soft tissue attenuation is seen on most SPECT images and is marked in large patients. Males typically have decreased activity in the inferior wall (Fig. 16.21). This is referred to as *diaphragmatic attenuation,* specifically attenuation due to subdiaphragmatic organs interpositioned between the heart and gamma camera. The amount of attenuation effect is dependent on patient size, shape, and internal anatomy. Women often have reduced activity in the anterior, apex, or anterior lateral wall due to *breast attenuation,* the extent depending on the size and position of the breasts (Fig. 16.22). Anterior and lateral wall attenuation may be seen in males with excessive adipose tissue or muscle hypertrophy and is marked in patients not able to elevate their arms during imaging.

Attenuation correction improves the specificity (Fig. 16.23; see also Fig. 16.21). There are two methods. An older method used a rotating gadolinium-153 gamma source attached to the camera head to produce an attenuation map. Hybrid SPECT/CT systems use the CT transmission data for this purpose. SPECT and CT images are usually acquired during tidal volume breathing as the heads rotate around the patient. Thus, some misregistration is not unusual. Fused images should be checked for significant misregistration because this could result in incorrect attenuation correction.

Gated SPECT has become routine at most centers (see Fig. 16.10), obtained immediately after stress. In addition to analyzing global and regional myocardial wall motion and calculating an LVEF, it can be helpful for differentiating the decreased activity from attenuation artifact from myocardial infarction. Good wall motion and myocardial thickening suggest that the decreased counts are due to attenuation and not infarction.

Extracardiac uptake is always present because the radiopharmaceuticals are normally taken up in all metabolically active tissues in the body except for the brain. Structures accumulating the cardiac radiopharmaceuticals often in the field of view are the thyroid, salivary glands, skeletal muscle, and kidneys. Gallbladder, biliary, and intestinal activity are also routinely seen. Uptake may be seen in many benign and malignant tumors.

Activity emanating from the liver and bowel adjacent to the heart may cause *scatter* of counts into the inferior wall and adjacent walls of the heart, increasing apparent uptake and causing artifacts, which can complicate interpretation. The activity scattering into the inferior wall may cause focal hot spots. Intense subdiaphragmatic radioactivity adjacent to the heart may also

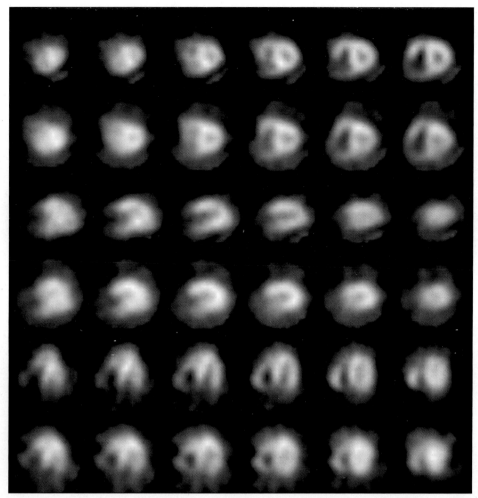

Fig. 16.20 Right ventricular hypertrophy. Patient has severe pulmonary hypertension secondary to interstitial pulmonary fibrosis. Stress and rest Tc-99 sestamibi show prominent uptake in the hypertrophied right ventricle.

produce cold defects due to reconstruction artifacts. Both may cause interpretive problems.

Diagnostic Patterns in Coronary Artery Disease. Terms used to characterize the status of the myocardium, such as *ischemia, infarction, hibernating,* and *stunning,* are defined in Table 16.8.

Ischemia and Infarction. Diagnostic interpretation makes use of the difference in the appearance of the scans at stress and rest (Table 16.9). The stress study is initially assessed for the presence or absence of perfusion defects, noting the location, size, severity, and likely vascular distribution of visualized abnormalities. The rest study is then compared with stress, looking for stress-induced perfusion deficits not present at rest. Computer quantitative methods are routinely used in conjunction with image analysis to enhance interpretation (Fig. 16.24). Perfusion defects caused by CAD are most commonly distal in the vascular bed, rather than limited to the base of the heart. A true perfusion defect is seen on more than one cross-sectional slice. Certainty increases with lesion size and the degree or severity of the photon deficiency.

Left Bundle Branch Block. Exercise-induced reversible hypoperfusion of the septum can be seen in patients with left bundle branch block (LBBB) in the absence of coronary disease. The apex and anterior wall are not involved, as would be expected with left anterior descending CAD. The stress-induced decreased septal blood flow is thought due to asynchronous relaxation of the septum, which is out of phase with diastolic filling of the remainder of the ventricle when coronary perfusion is maximal. This is not seen with pharmacological stress.

Multiple Perfusion Defects. Perfusion defects in more than one coronary artery distribution indicate multiple-vessel CAD. The prognosis worsens with increasing number and size of perfusion defects (Fig. 16.25). Not all significant coronary artery stenoses are seen on stress perfusion scans. Stress-induced ischemia of the most severe stenotic lesion may limit further exercise, and thus other stenoses may not be seen, and multiple-vessel disease may be underestimated. Three-vessel balanced disease may not be apparent at all.

Transient Ischemic Dilation. The normal cardiac response is to dilate during stress and return to normal size promptly with cessation of exercise. Poststress ventricular dilation is abnormal and suggests multivessel disease. There are two possible explanations for the finding, widespread subendocardial ischemia or myocardial stunning during stress.

Stunned Myocardium. After a transient period of severe ischemia followed by reperfusion, there may be delayed recovery of regional left ventricular function (*stunned*

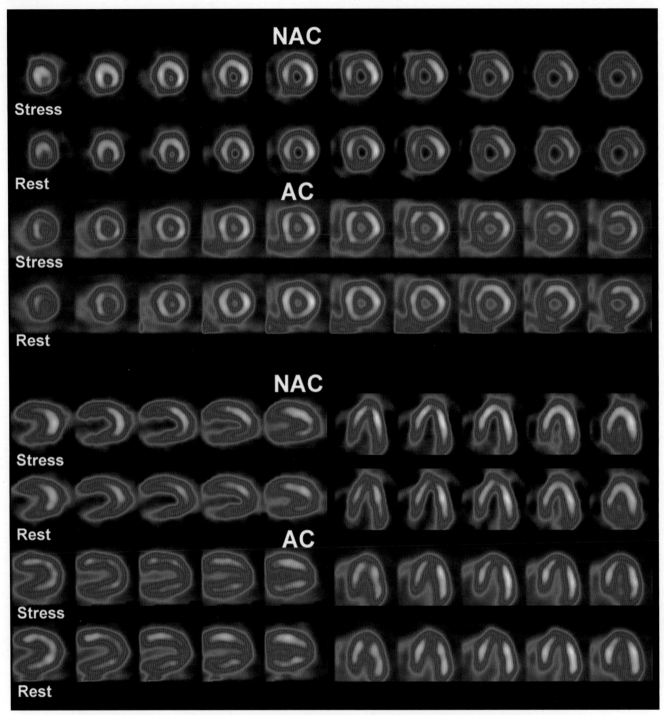

Fig. 16.21 Inferior wall attenuation correction. Dipyridamole (Persantine) stress and rest Tc-99m sestamibi single-photon emission computed tomography with computed tomography (SPECT/CT) study. Non–attenuation corrected *(NAC)* stress and rest images and the attenuation-corrected images *(AC)*. Note the improvement in inferior wall perfusion with attenuation correction. The study was interpreted as normal.

myocardium; Fig. 16.26). The ischemic episode may be a single event, multiple, brief, or prolonged but is not severe enough to cause necrosis. It is most commonly seen after thrombolysis or angioplasty in patients who have had acute coronary occlusion. Tissue in the affected perfusion watershed is viable and accumulates the radiopharmaceutical immediately after reperfusion. However, the myocardial segment is akinetic. If it is only stunned and not infarcted, wall motion will improve with time. Stress-induced transient ischemic dilation and gated

poststress SPECT ventricular dysfunction are manifestations of stunned myocardium.

Myocardial Viability (Hibernating Myocardium). Although the scintigraphic findings of regional hypoperfusion at stress and rest along with myocardial dysfunction are usually due to myocardial infarction, some of these patients do not have infarction but, rather, severe chronic ischemia or *hibernating myocardium* (see Fig. 16.26). Although severely underperfused, the myocytes have preserved cell membrane integrity and

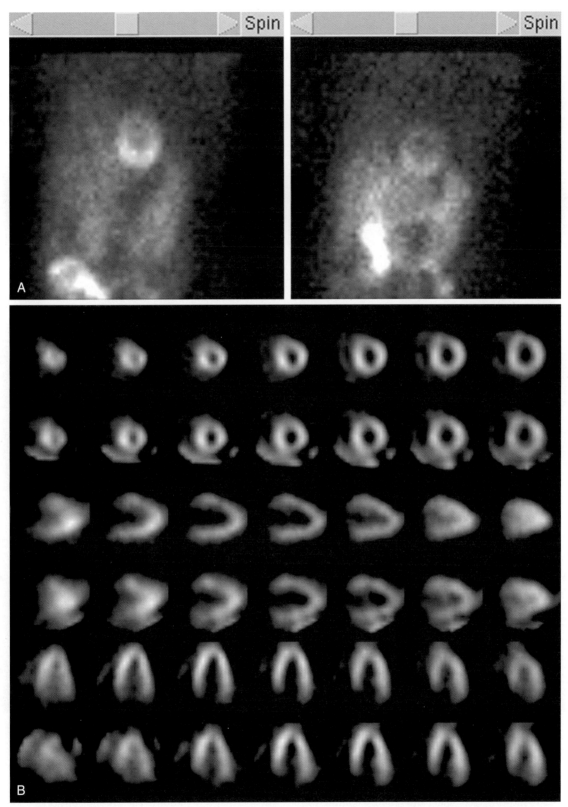

Fig. 16.22 Breast attenuation. (A) Single-projection images from a cinematic display at stress *(left)* and rest *(right)* illustrate breast attenuation seen as decreased activity in the superior portion of the heart. (B) The patient's single-photon emission computed tomography (SPECT) cross-sectional slices show mild to moderate reduced activity in the anterior wall, best seen in the short-axis and sagittal views.

sufficient metabolic activity to maintain cellular viability but not contractility and thus will have reduced myocardial contraction. These segments are "hibernating" in a functional and metabolic sense. Patients with viable but hypoperfused myocardium benefit from coronary revascularization, with resulting improvement in cardiac function and reduction in mortality. Patients with hibernating myocardium usually have known CAD, prior myocardial infarction, and ventricular dysfunction.

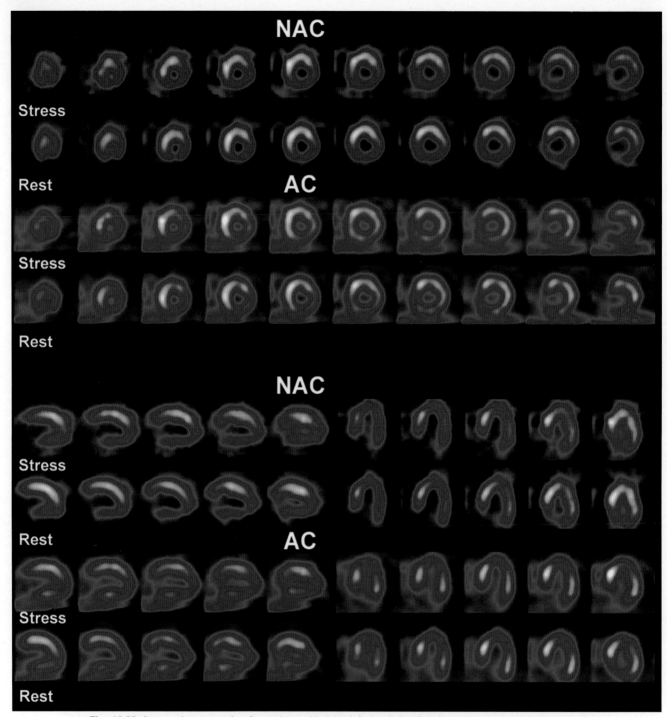

Fig. 16.23 Attenuation correction for patient with prior inferior wall infarction. Uncorrected images show much-reduced activity in the inferior wall. Corrected images continue to show reduced uptake but to a much lesser extent. A fixed apical perfusion defect is also seen. *AC,* Attenuation-corrected images; *NAC,* noncorrected images.

A perfusion study shows a fixed defect and reduced contraction. Infarction must be differentiated from hibernating myocardium. In patients being considered for bypass surgery, the surgeon wants to know whether sufficient viable myocardium exists to justify revascularization.

Tl-201 has been used to evaluate for viability/hibernating myocardium. Uptake is an energy-dependent process requiring intact cell-membrane integrity; thus, uptake implies preserved myocardial cell viability. The amount of uptake correlates with the extent of tissue viability. Various protocols have been used to diagnose viability based on Tl-201 pharmacokinetics. Two methods use a stress–rest Tl-201 study. If this shows a fixed perfusion defect, further delayed images are acquired 8 to 24 hours later or, alternatively, reinjecting Tl-201 at the time of redistribution and repeat imaging 20 minutes later (Fig. 16.27). With both methods, viability is confirmed with Tl-201 uptake. A

TABLE 16.8 Definitions Describing Myocardial Status

Term	Definition and Scan Appearance
Myocardial ischemia	Oxygen supply below metabolic requirements because of inadequate blood circulation caused by coronary stenosis
	Hypoperfusion (cold defect) on stress perfusion scintigrams and normal at rest
Myocardial infarction	Necrosis of myocardial tissue as a result of coronary occlusion
	Hypoperfusion on both rest–stress perfusion and decreased uptake with metabolic imaging
Transmural infarction	Necrosis involves all layers, from endocardium to epicardium
	High sensitivity for detection by perfusion imaging
Subendocardial infarction	Necrosis involves only muscle adjacent to endocardium
	Lower sensitivity for detection on perfusion imaging
Myocardial scar	Late result of infarction; hypoperfusion on scintigraphy
Hibernating myocardium	Chronic ischemia with decreased blood flow and down-regulation of contractility; reversible with restoration of blood flow
	No perfusion on rest imaging, poor ventricular contraction
	Improved perfusion given a long recovery between rest–rest imaging or delayed reinjection Tl-201
	Increased uptake by FDG metabolic imaging mismatched to reduced uptake on perfusion scan
Stunned myocardium	Myocardium with persistent contractile dysfunction despite restoration of perfusion after a period of ischemia; usually improves with time
	Normal perfusion imaging, poor ventricular contraction
	Uptake by FDG metabolic imaging

FDG, fluorodeoxyglucose.

TABLE 16.9 Diagnostic Patterns: Stress Myocardial Perfusion

Stress	Rest	Diagnosis
Normal	Normal	Normal
Defect	Normal	Ischemia
Defect	Defect (unchanged)	Infarction
Defect	Some normalization with areas of persistent defect	Ischemia and scar
Normal	Defect	Reverse redistribution[a]

[a]The term *reverse redistribution* was first described with Tl-201, and thus the reason for the terminology. It signifies a larger defect at rest than stress but has no real clinical significance.

third approach can be used, a *rest–rest study*. After Tl-201 injection at rest, images are obtained at 15 minutes and 3 to 4 hours later or the next day. Uptake reflects viability and the likely benefit from revascularization (Fig. 16.28). *F-18 fluorodeoxyglucose (FDG)* PET/CT is now most commonly used for viability and is discussed with cardiac PET.

Quantitative Analysis

Relative regional perfusion is often illustrated on a 2-D polar map or bull's-eye display generated with circumferential slice count profiles obtained from the SPECT study, with the apex at the center of the display and the base of the ventricle at the periphery (see Figs. 16.25B and 16.26B). Three-dimensional displays are also available. Stress–rest difference polar maps are commonly used to analyze for reversible ischemia. Gated SPECT analysis of wall motion and thickening is standard (see Fig. 16.24C). Calculation of an LVEF is obtained by measuring the change in the size of the ventricular cavity during the cardiac cycle using edge-detection algorithms.

Clinical Scenarios

Although diagnosis continues to be an important indication for SPECT myocardial perfusion imaging, risk stratification and prognosis have become its primary role.

Acute Ischemic Syndromes

Emergency Room Chest Pain. Clinical decision making requires triage of patients into risk categories based on the probability of infarction or unstable angina and risk assessment. SPECT perfusion imaging can provide information critical to this decision-making process. The accuracy of diagnosis is highest when the radiopharmaceutical is injected during pain, although good accuracy is obtainable for several hours thereafter.

Tc-99m sestamibi or tetrofosmin can be injected in the emergency room and the patient transferred for imaging when initial evaluation and stabilization is complete. Because the radiopharmaceutical is fixed and does not redistribute, this delayed imaging still reflects blood flow at the time of injection. Negative SPECT studies are highly predictive of a good prognosis. Cardiac events occur in less than 1.5% of patients compared with a 70% incidence in those with a positive study. SPECT perfusion scintigraphy has a high sensitivity (>90%) for the detection of transmural infarction immediately after the event. The sensitivity decreases with time as the edema and ischemia resolve. By 24 hours, small infarctions may not be detectable, and the overall sensitivity for larger ones decreases. The sensitivity is lower for nontransmural infarctions.

Acute Myocardial Infarction With ST Elevation. Infarct size, LVEF, and residual myocardium at risk provide important prognostic management information. Submaximal exercise (achieving less than target heart rate) SPECT perfusion scintigraphy after infarction can be used to detect the presence and extent of stress-induced residual ischemia. However, pharmacological stress can be safely done earlier than submaximal exercise, 2 to 5 days after infarction. Evidence for ischemia warrants aggressive management, coronary angiography, or revascularization. If negative, the patient can be treated conservatively.

Unstable Angina and Non–ST Elevation Myocardial Infarction. Early invasive interventional therapy is recommended for patients with high-risk indicators such as positive myocardial perfusion scintigraphy. SPECT can be used for predischarge risk stratification of patients with unstable angina. Ischemia is seen in a high percentage (90%) of patients who develop subsequent cardiac events compared with those without evidence of ischemia (20%).

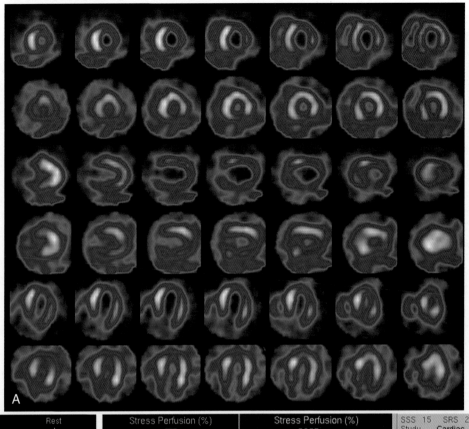

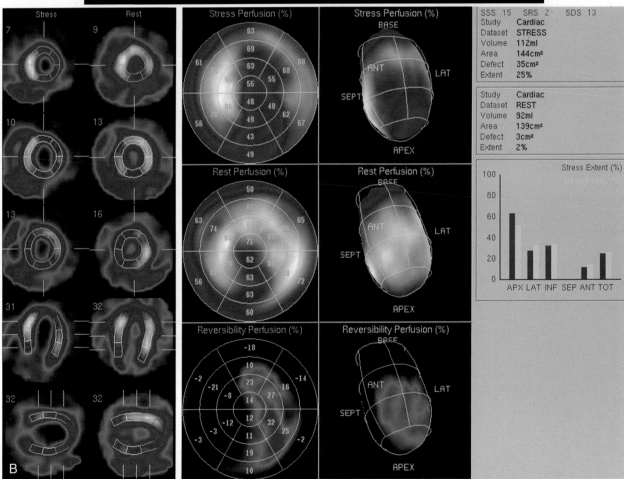

Fig. 16.24 Anterior lateral and inferior lateral wall ischemia—dipyridamole stress and rest study. (A) Stress images *(top)* show hypoperfusion of the apical-anterior lateral wall and no perfusion to the inferior lateral wall. Rest images *(bottom)* show markedly improved perfusion to the anterior lateral wall but still incomplete perfusion of the inferior wall. (B) Polar map display in two dimensions and three dimensions confirms definite ischemia. The reversibility percentage is as high as 23% to 32% in the anterior lateral and inferior lateral walls.

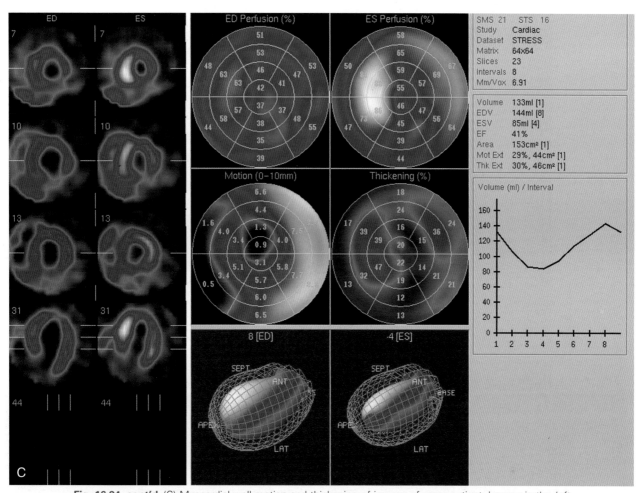

Fig. 16.24, cont'd (C) Myocardial wall motion and thickening of images of same patient. Images in the *left* column show septal wall thickening (manifested by brightening) and, to a lesser degree, lateral wall thickening. Reduced thickening is seen in the inferior wall. The cardiac time–volume curve and calculated left ventricular ejection fraction (LVEF; 41%) show diffuse hypokinesis. *ANT,* Anterior; *LAT,* lateral; *SEPT,* septal.

Chronic Ischemic Syndromes, Patient Management. Identification of patients at high risk but minimal symptoms can reduce mortality with coronary artery bypass grafting (CABG) or angioplasty. High risk and low risk are defined as >3% and <1% cardiac mortality rate per year, respectively. Factors assessed by SPECT that determine patient prognosis include the extent of infarcted myocardium, amount of jeopardized myocardium supplied by vessels with hemodynamically significant stenosis, and severity of ischemia. A normal stress SPECT perfusion study predicts a good prognosis, with <1% annual risk for cardiac death or infarct. An abnormal study is associated with an increased risk for cardiac death or infarction. Multivessel disease is associated with high risk. Reduced LVEF is a strong negative prognostic predictor.

Assessment of Coronary Bypass Surgery and Angioplasty. Because 40% to 60% of angiographically detected stenotic lesions of 50% to 75% are of uncertain significance, myocardial perfusion scintigraphy can help stratify risk and assess which patients require revascularization. Those with no ischemia have a low risk for cardiac events, even with left main or three-vessel disease on angiography. Those with ischemia will be helped by successful intervention.

After Percutaneous Coronary Intervention. Symptom status and exercise electrocardiography are not reliable indicators of restenosis. Of patients with recurrent chest pain within a month of intervention, 30% have restenosis. Stress perfusion imaging can identify recurrent ischemia.

After Coronary Bypass Surgery. Abnormal perfusion suggests bypass graft disease in the native coronary arteries beyond the distal anastomosis, nonrevascularized coronaries or side branches, or new disease. SPECT can determine the location and severity of ischemia and has prognostic value early and late after coronary bypass surgery. Ischemia occurring less than 12 months after surgery is usually caused by perianastomotic graft stenosis. Ischemia developing after 1 year postoperatively is usually caused by new stenoses in graft conduits or native vessels.

Heart Failure, Assessment for Coronary Artery Disease. Heart failure in the adult can be due to various causes, including hypertrophic cardiomyopathy, hypertensive or valvular heart disease, and ischemic and idiopathic cardiomyopathy. Determining whether left ventricular dysfunction is due to the consequences of CAD or other causes is critical for patient management. If it is the result of coronary disease, revascularization can reverse the dysfunction.

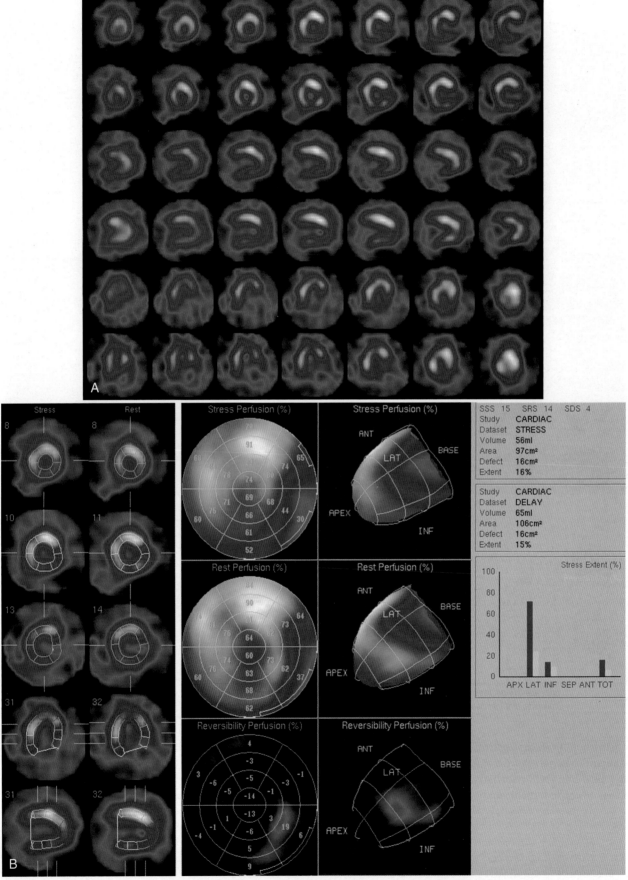

Fig. 16.25 Multivessel disease. (A) Lateral wall infarction and inferior lateral wall ischemia. Dipyridamole stress images show no perfusion of the lateral wall and reduced perfusion to the inferior wall. Rest images show no improvement in the lateral wall but improved perfusion to the inferior wall. (B) Polar map and quantitative volume display from this patient. The reversibility percentage on the polar map shows one inferior wall region with 19%. The graph in the right column shows the discrepancy between the stress extent and the reversibility extent, representing the infracted lateral wall. *ANT,* Anterior; *INF,* inferior; *SEPT,* septal.

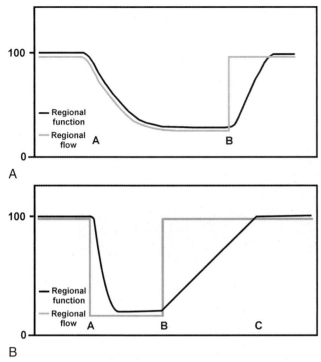

A

B

Fig. 16.26 Hibernating versus stunned myocardium. (A) Hibernating myocardium (chronic ischemia) develops over time as a result of chronic hypoperfusion, causing regional wall-motion dysfunction. When perfusion is reestablished by surgical intervention, myocardial function gradually returns. (B) Stunned myocardium is often due to an acute ischemic episode, such as thrombosis, which, when relieved (e.g., with angioplasty), results in prompt reperfusion. Functional recovery is considerably delayed. (Modified with permission from Dilsizian V, Narula J. *Atlas of nuclear cardiology.* 2nd ed. Philadelphia: Current Medicine LLC; 2006.)

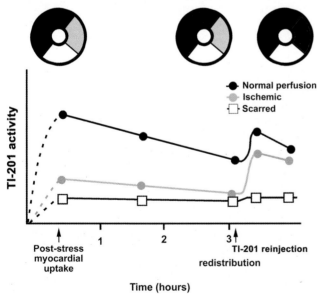

Fig. 16.27 Pharmacokinetics of the Tl-201 reinjection method for diagnosing hibernating myocardium for viability. During routine Tl-201 imaging, delayed images may show a persistent fixed perfusion defect in a region of severe or chronic ischemia. Low blood levels of Tl-201 do not allow for adequate redistribution of Tl-201 to the myocardium. Augmenting the Tl-201 blood levels permits greater myocardial uptake and scintigraphic evidence for redistribution and thus viable myocardium. (Modified with permission from Dilsizian V, Narula J. *Atlas of nuclear cardiology.* 2nd ed. Philadelphia: Current Medicine LLC; 2006.)

Left ventricular dysfunction resulting from ischemic cardiomyopathy is the result of either large or multiple prior myocardial infarctions with subsequent remodeling or moderate infarction associated with considerable inducible ischemia or hibernation. SPECT sensitivity is high for the detection of CAD in patients with cardiomyopathy, although the specificity is lower. False-positive study findings are due to perfusion abnormalities seen in many patients with nonischemic cardiomyopathy. Some have regions of fibrosis and decreased coronary blood-flow reserve, resulting in both fixed and reversible defects. More extensive and severe perfusion defects are likely to be due to CAD, whereas smaller and milder defects are likely to occur in patients with coronary microvascular disease or nonischemic cardiomyopathy.

Coronary Artery Calcium Screening. Calcium scoring has become routine at many centers. It is a simple add-on procedure for SPECT/CT and PET/CT. The risk for cardiac events is low with coronary calcium scores of ≤ 100. Stress SPECT myocardial perfusion is positive in <1% of these patients. With scores of 101 to 399, the risk for future cardiac events is moderate, with 12% having abnormal stress SPECT perfusion. Scores >400 identify patients at high risk, with 50% having abnormal SPECT.

MYOCARDIAL INFARCTION IMAGING

Tc-99m bone scan radiopharmaceuticals are taken up by the heart in the region of a recent myocardial infarction. Tc-99m pyrophosphate has been used for this purpose because it has higher soft tissue uptake than other Tc-99m diphosphonates. This imaging test is no longer requested by cardiologists to confirm the diagnosis of infarction. However, diffusely increased uptake may also be seen with myocarditis, postradiation injury, doxorubicin cardiotoxicity, and one form of amyloidosis, as discussed in the following subsection. After cell death, an influx of calcium occurs. Calcium phosphate complexes are formed, and these microcrystalline deposits act as sites for bone tracer uptake. Binding also occurs on denatured macromolecules.

CARDIAC AMYLOIDOSIS

Cardiac amyloidosis presents as heart failure. There are two types of amyloidosis, light-chain (AL) and transthyretin (TTR) cardiac amyloid. AL-type disease is a secondary manifestation of a systemic disease of plasma cells, and cardiac involvement is a poor prognostic factor. TTR-type amyloidosis has a relatively milder disease course. Tc-99m pyrophosphate can confirm the TTR type because there is cardiac uptake (Fig. 16.29). The AL type has no uptake and cannot be confirmed. Tc-99m methylene diphosphonate (MDP) and F-18 NaF have also been reported to be uptake-positive for TTR-type amyloidosis but negative for AL-type amyloidosis. C-11 PiB (Pittsburg Compound B) and F-18 florbetaben and florbetapir have demonstrated uptake with cardiac AL-type amyloidosis.

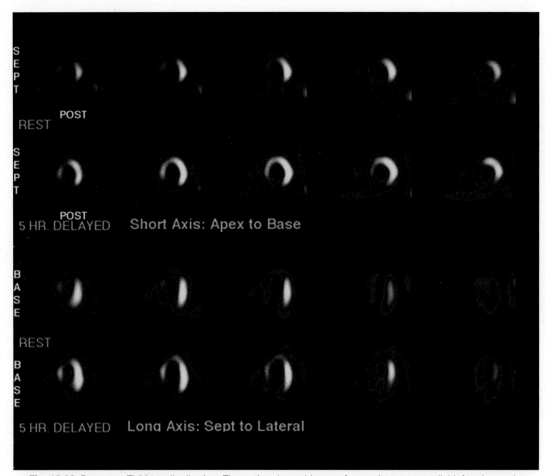

Fig. 16.28 Rest–rest Tl-201 redistribution. The patient has a history of a previous myocardial infarction and a low left ventricular ejection fraction (LVEF) and is being considered for revascularization. The initial rest study shows hypoperfusion of the inferior and anterior septal wall at rest; however, 5-hour delayed images show evidence of viability in the septum and adjacent anterior and apical wall. *POST,* Posterior.

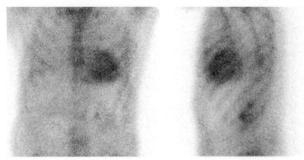

Fig. 16.29 Cardiac amyloidosis in a 62-year-old male with chronic congestive heart failure. Echocardiography was suggestive of an infiltrative cardiomyopathy. Tc-99m pyrophosphate was administered intravenously. Diffuse uptake greater than bone is seen in the myocardium. This is consistent with transthyretin-related amyloidosis of the left ventricle.

CARDIAC SYMPATHETIC HYPERACTIVITY—I-123 METAIODO-BENZYL-GUANIDINE

Heart failure is growing in incidence and has a high 1-year mortality rate. Implantable cardiac devices (ICDs; e.g., cardiac defibrillators) and resynchronization therapy can improve survival. Selecting appropriate patients is important but uncertain. Many ICDs are not really needed, whereas other patients have operative complications or malfunction after placement.

Cardiac sympathetic hyperactivity is associated with fatal arrhythmias. I-123 metaiodo-benzyl-guanidine (mIBG) can help identify patients who will most benefit from ICD implantation. I-123 mIBG was approved by the FDA for this purpose in 2013. I-123 mIBG is a norepinephrine analog that has the same presynaptic uptake, storage, and release mechanism as norepinephrine. Because it is not metabolized, its accumulation over several hours is a measure of myocardial neuronal sympathetic integrity. Parameters of I-123 mIBG myocardial uptake and washout have been shown to be of clinical value, particularly for assessment of prognosis.

Planar scintigraphy has been best validated. After administration of 5 mCi (185 MBq) I-123 mIBG, 10-minute images are acquired at 15 minutes and 4 hours. Regions of interest (ROIs) for the heart and mediastinum are drawn. Early and late heart/mediastinal (H/M) ratios and cardiac washout (WO) rates are calculated. The early H/M ratio reflects the integrity of the sympathetic nerve terminals. The late H/M ratio provides information about neuronal function resulting from uptake, storage, and release. WO reflects the neuronal integrity of sympathetic tone. Cardiac sympathetic hyperactivity is reflected by a decreased I-123 mIBG late H/M ratio and increased WO. Both are associated with increased fatal arrhythmia and cardiac mortality.

CARDIAC POSITRON EMISSION TOMOGRAPHY

Positron Emission Tomography Perfusion Scintigraphy

PET cardiac perfusion imaging is growing in use due to the increased availability of PET/CT cameras, the availability of Rb-82 generators, its superior spatial resolution and image quality, and the ability to better perform attenuation correction compared with SPECT. All of this contributes to improved accuracy. Its use is particularly advantageous in obese patients.

Radiopharmaceuticals

Nitrogen-13 (N-13) ammonia is the preferred PET myocardial perfusion agent because of its superior imaging characteristics. However, it has a very short physical half-life of 10 minutes, requiring on-site cyclotron production. It decays 100% by positron ($\beta+$) emission (Table 16.10). At physiological pH, the major form of ammonia is NH_4^+. When injected intravenously, it clears rapidly from the circulation, with 85% leaving the blood in the first minute and only 0.4% remaining after 3.3 minutes. It diffuses across the myocardial cell capillary membrane, is converted by glutamine synthetase to N-13 glutamine, and is subsequently trapped within tissues by incorporation in the cellular pool of amino acids.

Myocardial N-13 ammonia uptake is proportional to coronary blood flow. It has a 70% to 80% extraction rate by myocardial cells at normal coronary flow rates (see Table 16.10). As with other perfusion tracers, its extraction efficiency drops at higher flow rates. The N-13 label remains within the myocardium with a relatively long biological residence time, although

its physical half-life is short. Its range of 5.4 mm in tissue contributes to its good imaging characteristics.

N-13 ammonia, 10 to 20 mCi (370–740 MBq), is administered intravenously. Imaging begins 4 minutes after injection, allowing time for pulmonary background clearance. In the diagnosis of CAD, a second study is performed after pharmacological stress with protocols similar to those described for SPECT myocardial perfusion scintigraphy (Fig. 16.30).

Rubidium-82 Chloride

The commercial availability of strontium-82 (Sr-82)/Rb-82 generator systems is a relatively inexpensive alternative to having an on-site cyclotron for N-13 ammonia. The half-life of the Sr-82 parent is 25 days (see Table 16.10); thus, facilities using Rb-82 require one new generator system each month. This is still expensive, and thus a sufficient volume of cardiac studies, four per day, is needed to make it financially feasible. Some regional radiopharmacies now deliver Rb-82 from a single generator to multiple sites on specified days, reducing the cost for low-volume centers.

Rb-82 is a monovalent cation and true analog of potassium. Like Tl-201, Rb-82 is taken up by the myocardium via active transport through the Na^+/K ATPase pump. Its extraction is lower than that of N-13 ammonia (60%). The relative myocardial extraction and localization of Rb-82 are proportional to blood flow. The short 70-second half-life of Rb-82 (see Table 16.10) allows sequential myocardial perfusion studies before and after pharmacological interventions (Fig. 16.31). Rb-82 decays by positron emission (95%) and electron capture (5%). In addition to 511-keV annihilation photons, it emits a 776-keV gamma (15% abundance) and 1395-keV gamma (0.5% abundance). It has a range of 13 to 15 mm in soft tissue before undergoing annihilation, resulting in inferior resolution and image quality compared with N-13. However, the image quality is superior to that of SPECT, and there is less attenuation effect and subdiaphragmatic scatter.

Rb-82 (40–60 mCi [1480–2220 MBq]) is infused intravenously over 30 to 60 seconds. Imaging is delayed for about 90 seconds in individuals with normal left ventricular function or 120 seconds in patients with low LVEF (e.g., <30%) to allow time for blood-pool clearance. The study is completed 8 minutes after injection. Imaging time is short because of rapid decay and the need to minimize reconstruction artifacts. About 80% of the useful counts are acquired in the first 3 minutes and 95% in the first 5 minutes. Sequential studies can be performed within 10 minutes.

TABLE 16.10 Cardiac Positron Radiopharmaceuticals

Mechanism	Radionuclide	Pharmaceutical	Half-Life	Extraction	Energy (MeV)	Range in Soft Tissue	Production Method
Perfusion	N-13	Ammonia	10 min	70–80%	1.09	5.4 mm	Cyclotron
	Rb-82	Rubidium chloride	1.3 min	60%	3.15	15.0 mm	Generator
	O-15	Oxygen	2.0 min	95%	1.73	7.3 mm	Cyclotron
Glucose metabolism	F-18	Fluorodeoxyglucose	110 min		0.635	2.4 mm	Cyclotron

Oxygen-15 (O-15) Water

Because it is a freely diffusible perfusion tracer with 95% extraction by the myocardium (see Table 16.10) and not affected by metabolic factors, O-15 water is an excellent radiotracer for quantitative regional myocardial flow measurements (mL/min/gram). Unlike other perfusion agents, extraction remains linear at very high flow rates; therefore, the myocardial distribution reflects regional perfusion. However, the image quality is far inferior to that of other PET myocardial perfusion agents. Tracer circulating in the blood pool remains within the

ventricular chamber and must be subtracted to visualize the myocardium. Its 2-minute half-life requires that on-site cyclotron production occur in an adjacent facility. Its use is primarily reserved for research.

Future Cardiac Positron Emission Tomography Radiopharmaceuticals

N-13 ammonia and Rb-82 are currently the only FDA-approved myocardial perfusion PET tracers for the evaluation of CAD. Limits to their widespread use include the high cost of both the

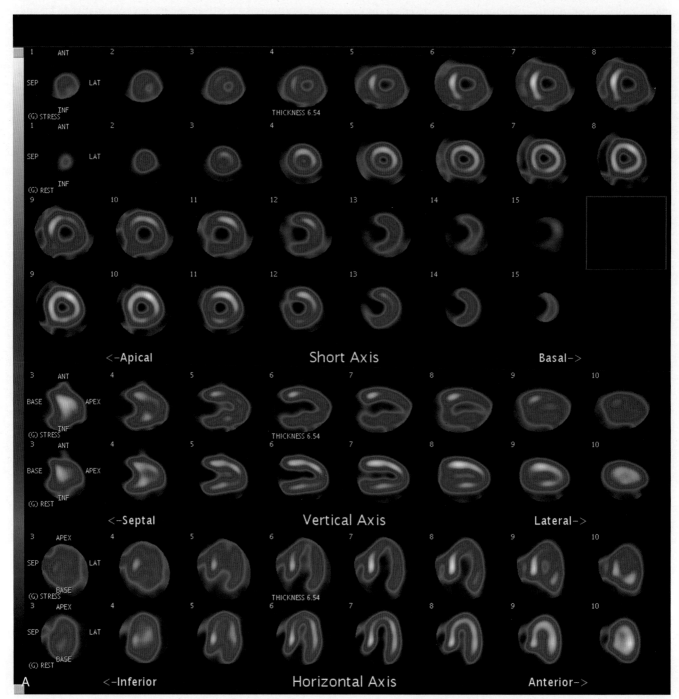

Fig. 16.30 N-13 ammonia myocardial perfusion scintigraphy in severe multivessel ischemia. (A) The stress study shows extensive hypoperfusion of the anterior lateral, lateral, inferior-lateral, and inferior wall. The rest study shows normal perfusion. Stress images suggest dilatation compared with rest (transient ischemic dilation).

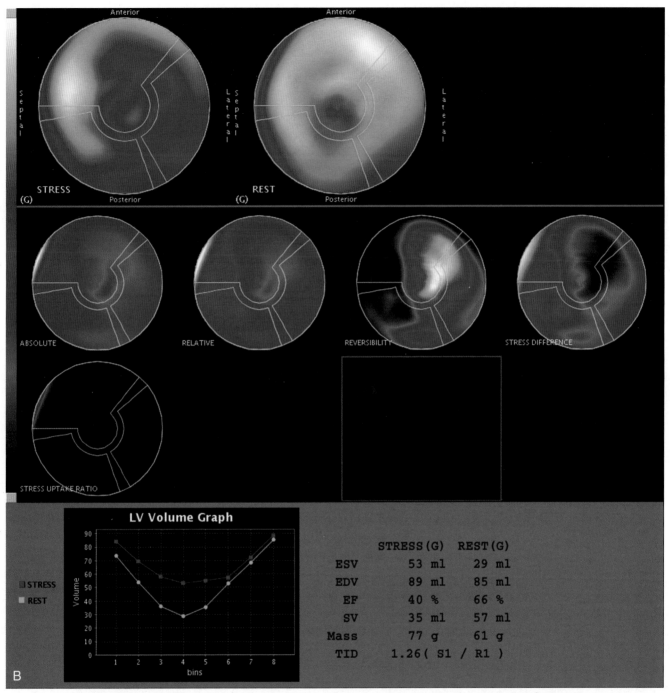

Fig. 16.30, cont'd (B) Bull's-eye display showing significant reperfusion of multiple segments. Stress and rest left ventricular ejection fraction (LVEF) are also calculated and shown. *ANT*, Anterior; *EDV*, end-diastolic volume; *EF*, ejection fraction; *ESV*, end-systolic volume; *LAT*, lateral; *LV*, left ventricle; *SEPT*, septal; *SV*, stroke volume; *TID*, transient ischemic dilatation.

on-site cyclotrons required for N-13 ammonia and the generators for Rb-82 and their short half-lives, which impose logistical difficulties.

These issues may be overcome in the near future with the development of cyclotron-produced fluorinated perfusion tracers. F-18 flurpiridaz is presently under active investigation. It complexes to a mitochondrial protein in myocardial cells. The long half-life (110 minutes) will allow it to be shipped from off-site cyclotron facilities, similar to F-18 FDG. It will also make

possible exercise stress protocols. F-18 has the highest resolution of clinically used positron emitters, approximately 2 mm, because emitted positrons travel only 1.2 mm before annihilation.

Diagnosis of Coronary Artery Disease

Present-day cardiac PET stress tests use pharmacological rather than exercise stress because of the short half-life of the radiopharmaceuticals and because, unlike SPECT, images are

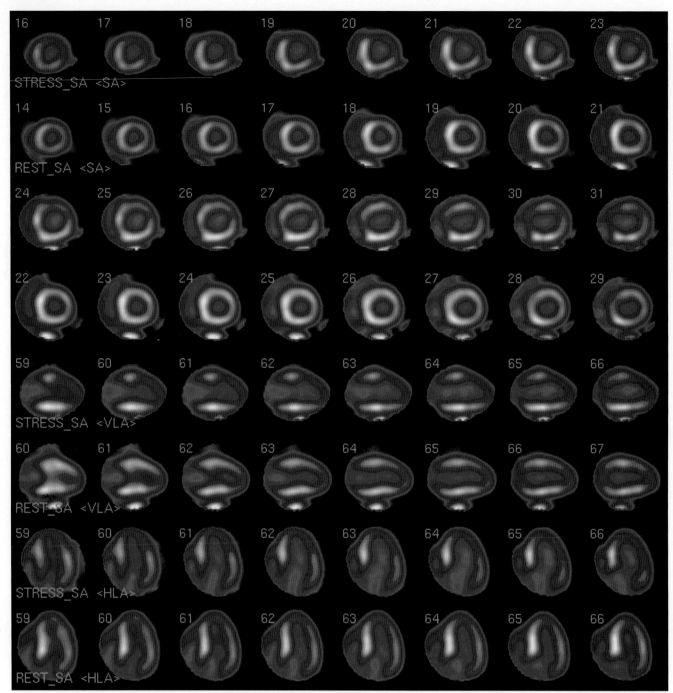

Fig. 16.31 Rb-82 stress myocardial perfusion study. Reversible ischemia is seen in the anterior lateral and apical myocardium. *HLA*, horizontal long axis; *SA*, short axis; *VLA*, vertical long axis.

acquired during stress testing. After a resting baseline study, pharmacological stress is used to challenge coronary flow reserve, similar to single-photon protocols. The scintigraphic appearance of the heart and the diagnostic criteria for Rb-82 and N-13 ammonia studies are the same as for SPECT perfusion scans (see Table 16.9).

Accuracy of PET Versus SPECT

PET myocardial perfusion tracers have superior pharmacokinetic properties because of their greater myocardial net uptake rates at higher coronary flow than their SPECT counterparts,

translating into better PET sensitivity for the diagnosis of single-vessel or multivessel CAD. PET instrumentation provides superior spatial resolution than SPECT (5–7 mm vs. >15 mm); better temporal resolution, allowing for data acquisition in dynamic sequences to delineate radiotracer kinetics for quantification of absolute myocardial blood flow; increased ability to detect tissue radiotracer concentration; and improved correction methods for photon scatter, random events, and photon attenuation. This translates into higher image quality, interpretive certainty, and diagnostic accuracy compared with SPECT, particularly for obese patients and females. The sensitivity and specificity of PET to detect coronary luminal stenotic lesions of ≥50% is 92% and 85%, respectively, versus 87% and 80%, respectively, for SPECT.

Absolute Myocardial Blood Flow Quantification

PET makes possible in vivo dynamic quantitative measurement of radiotracer in the heart so that estimation of absolute myocardial blood flow at baseline and during vasodilator-induced peak hyperemia is possible.

Coronary Flow Reserve

Low coronary flow reserve is thought to be an independent predictor of adverse cardiovascular events, even in the presence of normal regional myocardial perfusion imaging. Patients with severe triple-vessel coronary disease may on occasion demonstrate no perfusion abnormalities on rest–stress PET imaging because of balanced three-vessel ischemia; however, coronary flow reserve measured by PET will be decreased in these patients, enabling diagnosis of this high-risk population missed by standard myocardial perfusion imaging. It can also suggest multiple-vessel disease when standard perfusion imaging demonstrates only one ischemic coronary bed, and in other patients, it can confirm small-vessel disease.

Myocardial Viability/Hibernating Myocardium

Hibernating myocardium refers to a state of persistent left ventricular dysfunction secondary to chronically compromised resting myocardial blood flow in patients with CAD, in whom a revascularization procedure can result in partial or complete recovery of cardiac function. The combination of perfusion imaging and metabolic imaging with F-18 FDG can diagnose the presence of hibernating myocardium and assess the potential utility of revascularization (see Table 16.8). Under normal conditions, the energy needs of the heart are met through fatty acid metabolism. The rationale for using F-18 FDG is that severely ischemic, dysfunctional, but viable myocardium switches from fatty acid metabolism to glucose metabolism. Thus, FDG uptake is increased in severely hypoperfused hypokinetic or akinetic myocardial segments compared with the remainder of the heart. This is referred to as metabolic–perfusion mismatch, diagnostic of hibernating myocardium (Fig. 16.32). The combination of matched perfusion and FDG uptake is indicative of scar formation (Fig. 16.33).

Fluorine-18 Fluorodeoxyglucose

F-18 FDG is a marker of myocardial glucose metabolism. The radionuclide F-18 has a physical half-life of 110 minutes (see Table 16.10). Only 1% to 4% of the injected F-18 FDG radiopharmaceutical is trapped in the myocardium. The target-to-background ratio is high. Blood clearance of FDG takes considerably longer than perfusion agents. Imaging begins 45 to 60 minutes after tracer injection (10–15 mCi [370–555 MBq]), allowing for maximal myocardial uptake and blood and soft tissue background clearance.

For the evaluation of myocardial viability with F-18 FDG, high serum glucose and insulin levels and low free fatty acids promote uptake (Fig. 16.34). Thus, patient preparation requires glucose loading after a fasting period of at least 6 hours to induce an endogenous insulin response. The temporary increase in plasma glucose levels stimulates insulin production, which in turn reduces fatty acid levels. A common method of glucose loading is to give an oral load of 25 to 100 g, although intravenous loading can also be used. The intravenous route avoids potential problems due to variable gastrointestinal absorption times or the inability to tolerate oral administration. However, most clinics use the simpler oral glucose-loading approach, with supplemental insulin administered as needed. Diabetic patients pose a challenge, either because they have limited ability to produce endogenous insulin or because their cells are less able to respond to insulin stimulation. Thus, the fasting/oral glucose-loading method is often not effective. Use of insulin infusion along with close monitoring of blood glucose can yield satisfactory results (Box 16.6).

An FDG metabolic–perfusion mismatch is accurate in predicting improvement of regional wall motion and global LVEF after revascularization. The sensitivity and specificity for predicting improvement of regional function after revascularization are reported to be approximately 95% and 80%, respectively. The positive predictive value of preserved F-18 FDG uptake in predicting functional recovery has been reported to be 85%, and the negative predictive value has been reported as 92%. FDG uptake is the most important independent predictor of future cardiac events.

Cardiac Sarcoidosis

Cardiac sarcoidosis is being increasingly recognized in patients with sarcoidosis and is associated with a poor prognosis. Although it is frequently associated with pulmonary sarcoidosis, this is not always the case. It manifests as dysrhythmias, conduction defects, heart failure, and sudden death. It is difficult to diagnose clinically because its manifestations are nonspecific, and the diagnostic modalities are of limited value. Endomyocardial biopsy can confirm sarcoidosis; however, the sensitivity is poor (25%) due to its heterogeneity and thus sampling error. Any region of the heart can become the site of granuloma deposition, including the myocardium, endocardium, and pericardium. The most frequently involved areas are the ventricular septum (32%) followed by the inferior wall, anterior left ventricle, right ventricle, and lateral left ventricle. SPECT or PET perfusion scintigraphy may detect fixed defects in the right and the left ventricle in some patients; however, no abnormalities are seen in others. Ga-67 was used in the past; however, FDG PET is clearly superior. Cardiac magnetic resonance (MR) can detect the active inflammatory phase of the disease and the chronic scarring and fibrosis phase.

With inflammation, there is increased glucose metabolism. The inflammation can be visualized using the glucose analog F-18 FDG. In healthy subjects as well as oncologic patients, uptake is sometimes inhomogeneous throughout the left ventricle, particularly the lateral and basal walls. This must not be confused with myocardial inflammation. Normal myocardial uptake must be suppressed for the study. Patient preparation varies between institutions, but the general consensus is that it

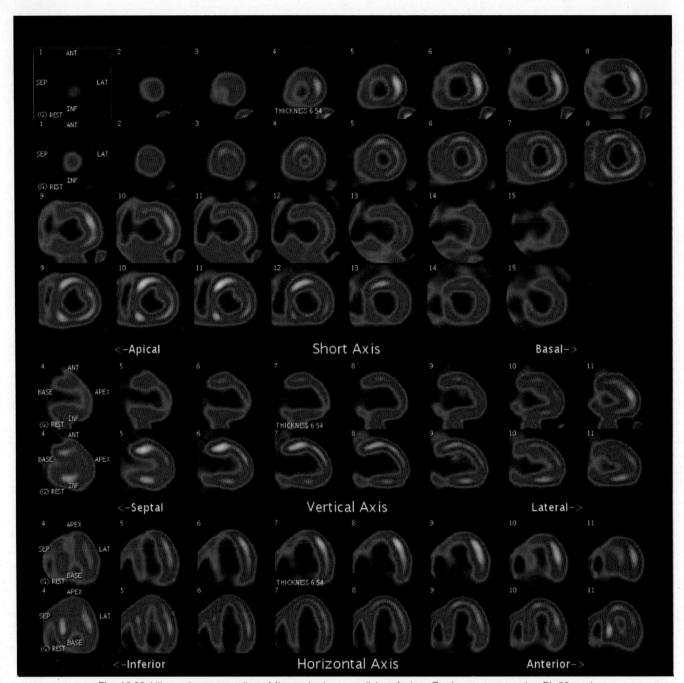

Fig. 16.32 Hibernating myocardium. Mismatched myocardial perfusion. *Top* images are resting Rb-82, and *bottom* images are F-18 fluorodeoxyglucose (FDG). There is a perfusion–metabolic mismatch in the anterior, septal, and apical walls. *ANT,* Anterior; *INF,* inferior; *LAT,* lateral; *SEP,* septal.

requires a low-carbohydrate, high-fat diet the evening before the study, then prolonged fasting (12–18 hours) and, in some clinics, also heparin loading. Heparin increases plasma free fatty acid levels and thus suppresses glucose metabolism.

A patchy, focal FDG pattern of uptake is suggestive of cardiac sarcoid (Figs. 16.35 and 16.36). More diffuse uptake suggests that myocardial suppression has been insufficient. The FDG study is usually preceded by or combined with a perfusion study. Normal perfusion but abnormal FDG suggests early disease, whereas abnormal perfusion and increased FDG is likely due to advanced disease. Late-stage scarring may result in abnormal perfusion without FDG uptake. Uptake resolves with

successful therapy, usually corticosteroids. On cardiac MR, delayed enhancement represents cardiac damage. There is only mild to moderate correlation between FDG and MR. Cardiac MR is reported to have higher specificity but lower sensitivity than FDG.

RADIONUCLIDE VENTRICULOGRAPHY

Tc-99m RBC radionuclide ventriculography (RVG), or the multigated acquisition (MUGA) study, has been used clinically since the 1970s to analyze global and regional ventricular function. A major advantage of the radionuclide method versus

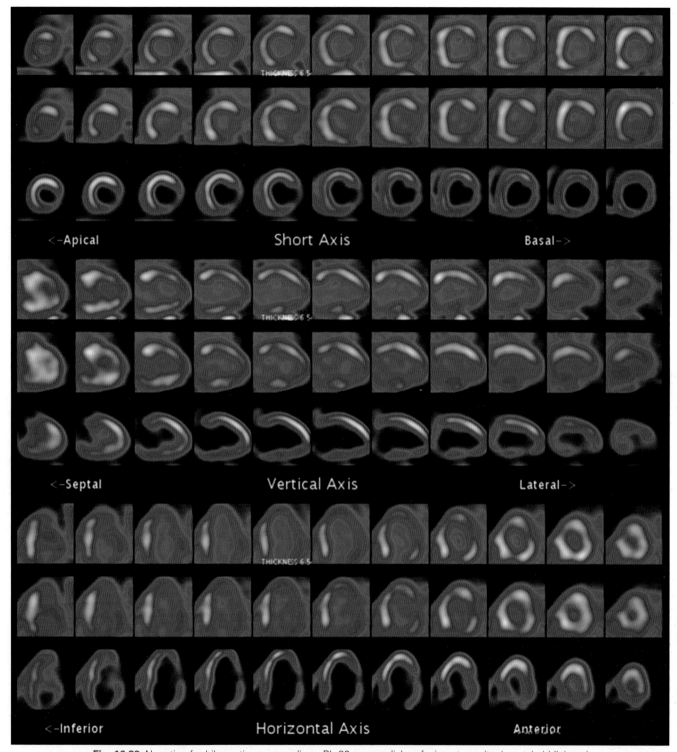

Fig. 16.33 Negative for hibernating myocardium. Rb-82 myocardial perfusion stress *(top)*, rest *(middle)*, and F-18 fluorodeoxyglucose (FDG; *bottom*) with matching defects consistent with myocardial infarction and nonviable myocardium.

echocardiography or other anatomical methods is that calculation of LVEF is not dependent on mathematical assumptions of ventricular shape. LV emitted counts are proportional to its volume, making possible accurate LVEF quantification. Two approaches have been used: the *first-pass method,* in which all data collection occurs during the initial transit of a tracer bolus through the central circulation; and the *equilibrium method,* in which data are collected over many cardiac cycles using ECG gating and a tracer that remains in the blood pool. The latter has become the standard method at most centers.

Equilibrium Blood-Pool Method

Radiolabeling RBCs is most commonly done using either the modified in vivo method or the in vitro method (Ultra-Tag), as

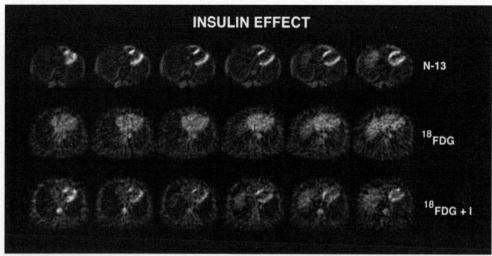

Fig. 16.34 Importance of glucose loading for fluorodeoxyglucose (FDG) cardiac imaging. N-13 ammonia images *(top row)* and two sets of F-18 FDG images of a patient with diabetes. The N-13 ammonia images show a large perfusion defect at the cardiac apex. The initial F-18 FDG images show uptake in the blood pool but essentially no myocardial uptake *(middle row)*. After insulin (I) administration *(bottom row)*, FDG accumulates in the myocardium and reveals a matched defect at the apex.

BOX 16.6   Fluorine-18 Fluorodeoxyglucose Positron Emission Tomography Cardiac Viability: Summary Protocol

Patient Preparation
Patient should fast after midnight.
Obtain rest myocardial perfusion scan.
Obtain serum fasting blood sugar (BS).

Nondiabetic
If BS ≤150 mg/dL: 50 g oral glucose solution + regular insulin 3 units intravenously
If BS 151 to 300 mg/dL: 25 g oral glucose solution + regular insulin 3 units intravenously
If BS 301 to 400 mg/dL: 25 g oral glucose solution + regular insulin 5 units intravenously
If BS >400 mg/dL: 25 g oral glucose solution + regular insulin 7 units intravenously
Inject F-18 FDG at least 45 minutes after glucose loading and when BS <150 mg/dL

Diabetic
If BS <150 mg/dL: 25 g oral glucose solution
If BS 151 to 200 mg/dL: Regular insulin 3 units intravenously
If BS 201 to 300 mg/dL: Regular insulin 5 units intravenously
If BS 301 to 400 mg/dL: Regular insulin 7 units intravenously
If BS ≥ 401 mg/dL: Regular insulin 10 units intravenously
    Obtain BS every 15 mins for 60 minutes. If BS elevated, administer additional insulin per scale. At least 45 minutes after glucose loading and when BS ≤150 mg/dL, inject F-18 FDG.

Radiopharmaceutical
F-18 FDG 0.22 mCi/kg (100 μCi/lb)

Time of Imaging
After 60-minute uptake phase

Procedure
PET acquisition: Cardiac field of view

Processing
Reconstruct along the short and long axis of the heart similar to the perfusion study

FDG, Fluorodeoxyglucose; *PET,* positron emission tomography.

---

described in the gastrointestinal chapter (Box 10.10). The in vitro kit method has the highest labeling efficiency, >97% versus 85% for the modified in vivo method. Poor RBC labeling is uncommon using the in vitro method.

ECG leads are placed on the patient, and a gating signal triggered by the R wave of the ECG tracing is sent to the computer. The R wave occurs at the beginning of systole. The cardiac cycle is divided into 16 frames (bins) by computer processing software (Fig. 16.37A). Sufficient frames are needed to catch the peaks and valleys of the cardiac cycle (temporal sampling). During each heartbeat, data are acquired sequentially into the 16 bins spanning the cardiac cycle. With imaging of 100 to 300 cardiac cycles, sufficient counting statistics are obtained for valid quantitative analysis and reasonable spatial resolution. Approximately 250,000 counts per frame are acquired. An equilibrium gated MUGA protocol is described in Box 16.7.

An underlying assumption of R-wave gating and 16 bins is that the patient has a normal sinus rhythm so that data can be added together from corresponding segments of each cardiac cycle over the entire study period. Arrhythmia results in misplacement of data into bins, thus reducing the accuracy of quantitative analysis. Significant quantitative error can result with >10% premature ventricular contractions. A rhythm strip should be obtained before injection of the radiotracer to ensure a regular rhythm (Fig. 16.38). Review of the beat (phase) histogram display (time between beats) is also helpful for analyzing the cardiac rhythm (see Fig. 16.37). A widened histogram suggests rhythm variability. Potential gating problems include spurious signals from skeletal muscle activity, giant T waves triggering the gating device, and pacemaker artifacts.

The standard computer software method that attempts to correct for premature beats is to exclude the subsequent beat that also has an abnormal R-to-R wavelength due to a compensatory pause. The premature beat has already been accepted. So one beat is premature, and the following one is excluded. If this

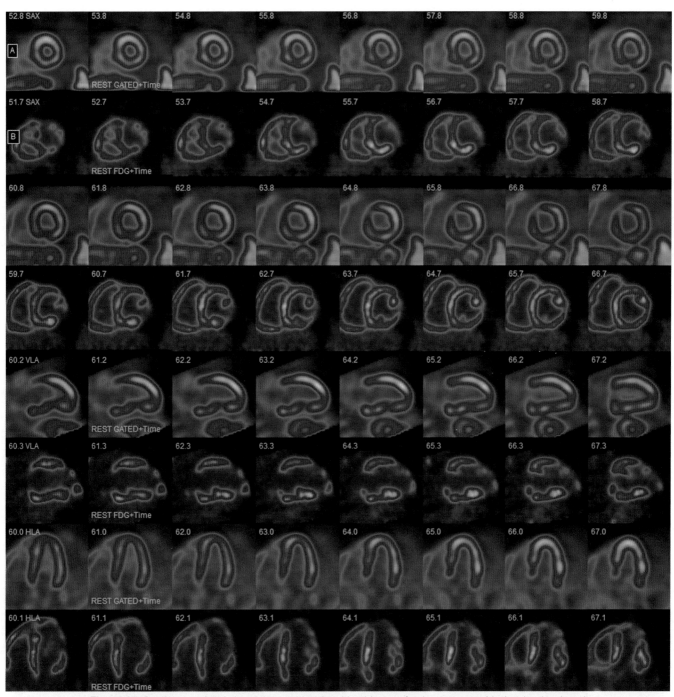

Fig. 16.35 Cardiac sarcoidosis in a 35-year-old male with a history of pulmonary sarcoidosis who developed an atrial-ventricular conduction block. Echocardiography showed a reduced left ventricular ejection fraction (LVEF) of 45%, and magnetic resonance imaging (MRI) showed biventricular enlargement and patchy fibrosis of the left ventricle and septum. The rest N-13 ammonia images *(top)* show hypoperfusion of the inferior, inferoseptal wall, and basal septum. The fluorodeoxyglucose (FDG) images show a mismatch with uptake in the regions of hypoperfusion, as well as patchy uptake in the right ventricle.

happens frequently, data are reduced, image quality suffers, and quantification becomes less accurate.

For studies at rest, multiple views (anterior, left anterior oblique, left lateral) are obtained to evaluate regional ventricular wall motion. The exact camera angle for the left anterior oblique view, the one used to calculate the LVEF, is determined by moving the gamma camera head to find the view that best separates the left and right ventricles, usually 35% to 45% left anterior oblique.

Data Analysis and Multigated Acquisition Study Interpretation
Qualitative Analysis

Comprehensive analysis and interpretation of MUGA studies require both qualitative and quantitative assessments. Wall motion is analyzed by viewing a repetitive cinematic closed-loop display. Ventricular contraction is evaluated by noting a reduction in the size of the ventricular cavity from diastole to systole and evidence of normal wall motion. Septal contraction is usually less than other walls. The complete absence of wall motion is termed *akinesis,* diminished contraction is termed *hypokinetic,* and paradoxical wall motion (outward bulge during systole) is dyskinetic. In normal subjects, all wall segments should contract, with the greatest incursion seen in the left ventricular free wall and apex. Areas of ventricular scar are typically akinetic or dyskinetic.

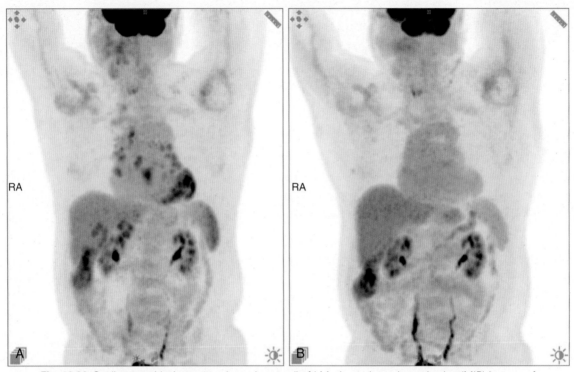

Fig. 16.36 Cardiac sarcoidosis—pre- and posttherapy. *(Left)* Maximum-intensity projection (MIP) images of a 40-year-old patient with cardiomegaly, multiple areas of focal fluorodeoxyglucose (FDG) uptake in the right and left ventricle, consistent with clinically suspected cardiac sarcoidosis. *(Right)* After therapy, there has been complete resolution of cardiac involvement.

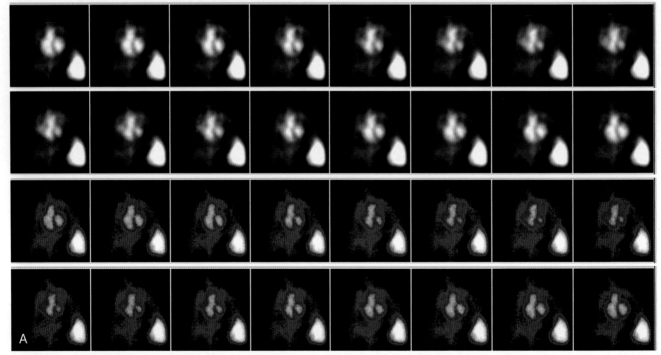

Fig. 16.37 (A) Normal multigated acquisition (MUGA) study. Sixteen sequential frames of R-wave gated MUGA study acquired in the left anterior oblique (LAO) view. Displayed in grayscale and a color scale. Note the change in size and count density of the cardiac chambers during the cardiac cycle. End-diastole is the *first* image, and end-systole is the *seventh* frame. The grayscale and four-color images are from the same date.

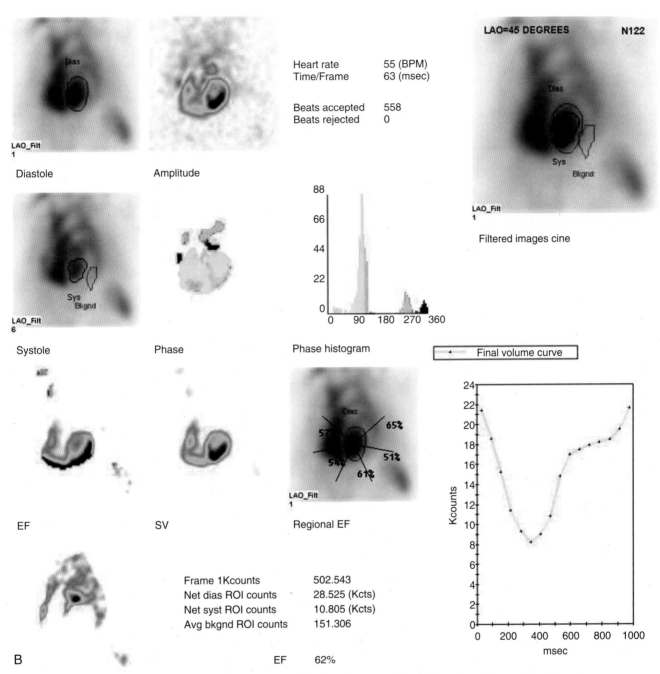

Fig. 16.37, cont'd (B) Computer-processed display shows end-diastolic, end-systolic, and background regions of interest. The normal left ventricular time–activity curve (TAC) is shown with the atrial kick during the later phase. Phase and functional images are shown and the rate histogram. Left ventricular ejection fraction (LVEF) is 62%. *Avg,* Average; *bkgnd,* background; *EF,* ejection fraction; *filt,* filter; *Kcts,* kilocounts; *ROI,* region of interest; *SV,* stroke volume.

Cardiac muscle contraction is inferred from noting brightening with systole. Complete qualitative or visual analysis includes assessment of cardiac chamber size, overall biventricular function and regional wall motion, and any extracardiac abnormalities (e.g., aortic aneurysm or pericardial effusions).

Quantitative Data Analysis

The LVEF is defined as the fraction of the left ventricular volume expelled during each contraction. Ventricular counts are determined by placing an ROI around the left ventricle for end-diastole and end-systole and a background region, a crescent adjacent to the left ventricular apex (see Fig. 16.37B). End-diastole is the frame demonstrating the highest counts, and end-systole is the frame with the fewest counts. A background-corrected ventricular time–activity curve (TAC) is generated.

The LVEF is calculated as follows, with count corrected for background:

$$\text{Ejection fraction} = \frac{\text{End diastolic counts} - \text{End systolic counts}}{\text{End diastolic counts}}$$

The normal ejection fraction is 50% to 75%.

The time–activity (cardiac volume) curve should be inspected as a quality-control measure. The count values at the beginning and end of the curve should be identical. The trailing frames in late diastole may have fewer counts, owing to variations in cardiac

cycle length, even in patients with normal sinus rhythm. In patients with frequent premature ventricular contractions (PVCs) and rapid atrial fibrillation with an irregular ventricular response, the fall-off in counts at the end of the curve is much greater.

Calculation of a right ventricular ejection fraction (RVEF) from equilibrium data can be performed similarly, although the ROIs are more difficult to draw because of overlap of the right ventricle with the right atrium and RV outflow tract. Thus, the results are subject to some error. The RVEF is normally lower than the LVEF. The stroke volume is the same for both, but the right ventricular volume is larger than the left ventricular volume.

Clinical Applications
Coronary Artery Disease

In the past, stress MUGA studies were performed to detect regional myocardial ischemia and infarction, showing wall motion abnormalities and a decrease of LVEF with exercise. MUGA studies are not used for this purpose today but, rather, sometimes to quantify the LVEF when echocardiography is unsuccessful or, most commonly, to detect cardiac toxicity.

Assessment of Cardiac Toxicity

Anthracycline drugs (e.g., doxorubicin [Adriamycin]), commonly used in the treatment of breast cancer and malignant lymphoma, produce a cumulative dose-dependent depression of left ventricular function (Fig. 16.39). Cardiac toxicity leads to

---

BOX 16.7 Equilibrium Gated Blood-Pool Ventriculography: Summary Protocol

Patient Preparation

Rhythm strip to confirm normal sinus rhythm (<10% premature ventricular contractions)

Radiopharmaceutical

Tc-99m red blood cells 20 mCi (740 MBq) intravenously

Instrumentation

Collimator: low-energy general-purpose or high-resolution collimator

Window: 15% to 20% centered at 140 keV

Imaging: Anterior, left anterior oblique (LAO; best septal view), and left lateral views.

Gamma camera persistence scope to determine optimal LAO view for separating left and right ventricular activity

Sixteen frames per cardiac with frame duration of 50 msec or less

250k counts per frame for studies performed at rest

100k counts per frame in the optimum LAO view for studies obtained during an intervention

---

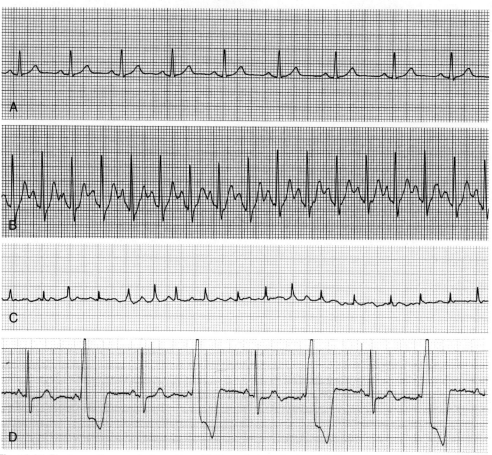

Fig. 16.38 Electrocardiogram rhythm strips. (A) Normal sinus rhythm. (B) Sinus tachycardia. (C) Atrial fibrillation with irregular ventricular response. (D) Premature vascular contractions with bigeminy.

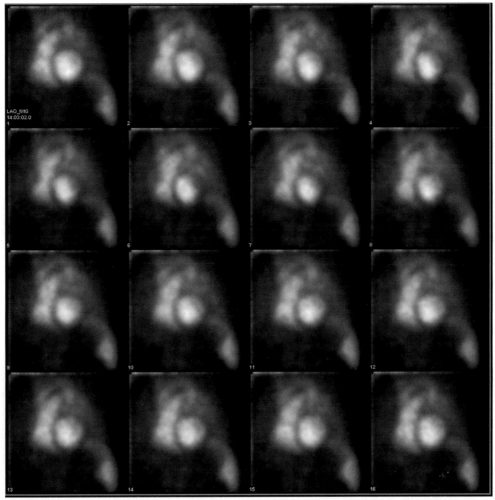

Fig. 16.39 Abnormal multigated acquisition (MUGA) scan. Sixteen sequential frames show diffuse hypokinesis of both the right and left ventricle. Left ventricular ejection fraction (LVEF) was 25%. *LAO,* Left anterior oblique.

progressive left ventricular dysfunction and heart failure. Trastuzumab (Herceptin), used for the treatment of breast cancer, is also cardiotoxic. However, the dose is not cumulative, and there is a high likelihood of reversal of new dysfunction within 2 to 4 months if the medication is discontinued.

Doxorubicin doses of more than 450 to 500 mg/m² can result in cardiotoxicity and heart failure. Overt failure is preceded by a progressive fall in the LVEF. Serial monitoring can detect a change in cardiac function, and the drug can be stopped or reduced when a reduction in the LVEF is observed. Complete recovery may occur if therapy is discontinued at an early stage.

In patients with a normal baseline LVEF (>50%), moderate toxicity is defined as a decline of >10% in the absolute LVEF, with a final LVEF of <50% (Box 16.8). In patients with abnormal baseline (>30% and <50%), a study is performed before each dose. Doxorubicin is discontinued with an absolute decrease in the LVEF of ≥10% or a final LVEF of ≤30%. Trastuzumab should be discontinued at least temporarily if the LVEF falls by >10% to a level of <50%.

Pulmonary Disease

Right ventricular enlargement can be seen with the MUGA study. In patients with a new onset of dyspnea, it can help differentiate left ventricular from pulmonary dysfunction. Normal wall motion, LVEF, and chamber size strongly suggest a pulmonary cause.

BOX 16.8   Guidelines for Monitoring Doxorubicin Cardiotoxicity

Baseline evaluation: Before the start of therapy or at least before 100 mg/m² has been given
Subsequent evaluations: 3 weeks after the last dose at recommended intervals
Patients with normal baseline LVEF (>50%):
   Obtain second study after 250 to 300 mg/m².
   Obtain a repeat study after 400 mg/m² in patients with heart disease, hypertension, radiation exposure, abnormal electrocardiogram, cyclophosphamide therapy or after 450 mg/m² in the absence of risk factors.
   Obtain sequential studies thereafter before each dose. Discontinue therapy if >10% decrease in LVEF to <50%.
Patients with abnormal baseline LVEF (<50%):
   With baseline LVEF <30%, do not start therapy.
   With baseline LVEF >30% and <50%, perform a study before each dose.
Discontinue drug in patients with an absolute decrease in LVEF ≥30% or final LVEF ≤30%.

LVEF, Left ventricular ejection fraction.

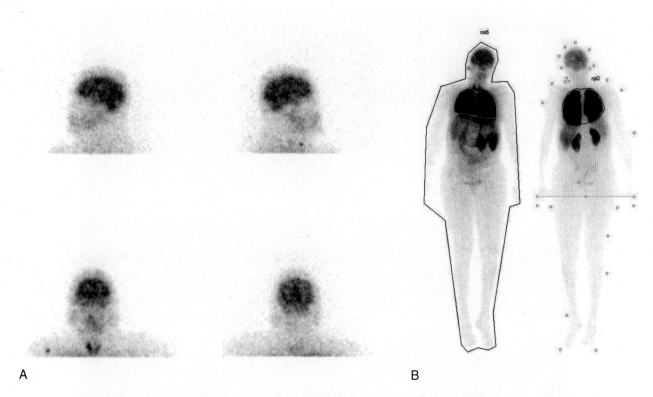

A   B

Fig. 16.40 Right-to-left shunt. (A) Brain cortical uptake is seen. (B) Whole-body quantification of right-to-left shunt. Regions of interest are drawn for the whole body and lungs. Quantification found the percent shunt to be 15%.

Congenital Heart Disease—Right-to-Left Shunts

Right-to-left shunts result from a variety of congenital cardiac diseases. The shunts can be confirmed and quantified with Tc-99m macroaggregated albumin (MAA). With shunting, images show uptake in other organs of the body (Fig. 16.40A). Cerebral cortex uptake is easiest to see and is diagnostic. If not seen, there is no significant shunt. Different methods of quantification have been used. One method uses whole-body imaging. ROIs are drawn for the lungs and total body (see Fig. 16.40B). A caution, however, is that the % shunt calculation does not accurately quantify the actual % shunt but does correlate with its severity. A calculated shunt >10% is usually abnormal. Right-to-left shunts have been considered a relative contraindication to the use of Tc-99m MAA because of the theoretical risk for embolizing the capillary bed of the brain. In practice, this is not a clinical problem, although it is still recommended that the number of particles be reduced.

SUGGESTED READING

Al Jaroudi WA, Iskandrian AE. Regadenoson: a new myocardial stress agent. *J Am Coll Cardiol*. 2009;54:1123–1130.

Arumugam P, Tout D, Tonge C. Myocardial perfusion scintigraphy using rubidium-82 positron emission tomography. *Br Med Bull*. 2013;107:87–100.

Cerqueira MD, Weissman NJ, Dilsizian V, et al. Standardized myocardial segmentation and nomenclature for tomographic imaging of the heart. *Circulation*. 2002;105:539–549.

Chareonthaitawee P, Beanlands RS, Chen W, et al. Joint SNMMI–ASNC Expert consensus document on the role of 18F-FDG PET/CT in cardiac sarcoid detection and therapy monitoring. *J Nucl Med*. 2017;58:1341–1353.

De Jong MC, Genders TS, van Geuns RJ, Moelker A, Hunink MG. Diagnostic performance of stress myocardial perfusion imaging for coronary artery disease: a systematic review and meta-analysis. *Eur Radiol*. 2012;66:477–492.

Di Carli MF, Asgarzadie F, Schelbert HR, et al. Quantitative relation between myocardial viability and improvement in heart failure symptoms after revascularization in patients with ischemic cardiomyopathy. *Circulation*. 1995;92:3436–3444.

Dilsizian V, Bacharach SL, Beanlands RS, et al. ASNC imaging guidelines/SNMMI procedure standard for positron emission tomography (PET) nuclear cardiology procedures. *J Nucl Cardiol*. 2016;23:1187–1226.

Dilsizian V, Narula J, Braunwald E. *Atlas of Nuclear Cardiology*. 3rd ed. Philadelphia: Current Medicine; 2013.

Eitzman D, Al-Aouar Z, Kanter HL, et al. Clinical outcome of patients with advanced coronary artery disease after viability studies with positron emission tomography. *J Am Coll Cardiol*. 1992;20:559–565.

Henzlova MJ, Duvall Wl, Einstein AJ, et al. ASNC imaging guidelines for SPECT nuclear cardiology procedures: Stress, protocols, and tracers. *J Nucl Cardiol*. 2016;23:606–639.

Lim SP, McArdle BA, Beanlands RS, Hessian RC. Myocardial viability: it is still alive. *Semin Nucl Med*. 2014;44:358–374.

Murthy VL, Bateman TM, Beanlands RS, et al. Clinical quantification of myocardial blood flow using PET: Joint position paper of the SNMMI Cardiovascular Council and the ASNC. *J Nucl Cardiol*. 2018;25:269–27.

Nandalur KR, Dwamena BA, Choudhri AF, et al. Diagnostic performance of positron emission tomography in the detection of coronary artery disease: a meta-analysis. *Acad Radiol.* 2008;15:444–451.

Rischpler C, Nekolla SG, Kunze KP, Schwaiger M. PET/MRI of the heart. *Semin Nucl Med.* 2015;45:234–247.

Sampson UK, Dorbala S, Limaye A, et al. Diagnostic accuracy of rubidium-82 myocardial perfusion imaging with hybrid positron emission tomography/computed tomography in the detection of coronary artery disease. *J Am Coll Cardiol.* 2007;49:1052–1058.

Schatka I, Bengel FM. Advanced imaging of cardiac sarcoidosis. *J Nucl Med.* 2014;55:99–106.

Zaret BL, Beller GA. *Clinical Nuclear Cardiology: State of the Art and Future Directions.* 4th ed. Philadelphia: Elsevier; 2010.

17

Pearls, Pitfalls, and Frequently Asked Questions

This chapter reinforces concepts presented in this textbook. Students of medicine gather pearls of wisdom from their mentors that may not fit well into a didactic treatment of a subject but are valuable in day-to-day practice. We all learn to avoid pitfalls that arise that have escaped our formal education. Interpretive questions require assembling multiple bits of information for a correct answer, and these questions are not necessarily asked in quite the same way that subject material was presented didactically. This chapter is neither comprehensive nor necessarily weighted toward the relative importance of the topics.

RADIOPHARMACEUTICALS

> **PEARL:** *Radiopharmaceuticals are radioactive molecules comprised of a radionuclide that permits external detection and a biologically active molecule or drug that acts as a carrier that determines localization and biodistribution. Exceptions are radioiodine, gallium, thallium, and oxygen-15, in which the radioactive atoms themselves confer the localization properties.*

Q: What is the relationship between the half-lives of a parent radionuclide and a daughter radionuclide in a generator system?

A: A longer-lived parent decays to a shorter-lived daughter in all clinical generator systems. The parent radionuclide must have a long enough half-life to permit the formulation and distribution of the generator. The daughter half-life must be long enough for the clinical application.

Q: How are parent and daughter radionuclides separated in generator systems?

A: Because the parent and daughter are different elements, they can be chemically separated (e.g., molybdenum-99 and technetium-99m).

> **PEARL:** *The most common radionuclide contaminant in the generator eluate is the parent radionuclide, Mo-99. Tc-99, the daughter product of the isomeric transition of Tc-99m, is also present but is not considered an impurity or contaminant, although significant Tc-99 can be a problem from a radiolabeling standpoint.*

Q: What quality-assurance procedure is used to detect radionuclide impurities?

A: Thin-layer chromatography.

> **PEARL:** *If 5% of a Tc-99m-labeled radiopharmaceutical activity remains as free pertechnetate in a radiolabeling procedure, the radiochemical purity is reported as 95%.*

Q: What is the legal limit for Mo-99 in Tc-99m-containing radiopharmaceuticals?

A: The Nuclear Regulatory Commission (NRC) limit is 0.15 microcurie of Mo-99 activity per 1 mCi of Tc-99m activity in the administered dose.

Q: How does the ratio of Mo-99 to Tc-99m change with time?

A: In any preparation in which the radionuclidic contaminants have longer half-lives than the desired radionuclide label, the relative activity of the contaminant increases with time.

Q: What is the purpose of stannous ion in Tc-99m-labeling procedures?

A: Stannous ion is used to reduce technetium pertechnetate from a +7 valence state to lower valence states necessary to allow for labeling a wide range of agents.

Q: What constitutes a medical event, formerly known as a misadministration of a radiopharmaceutical?

A: Previously, a misadministration was defined by the NRC as a radiopharmaceutical given to the wrong patient, receiving the ordered radiopharmaceutical by the wrong route of administration, or the administered dose differing from the prescribed dose by greater than an allowable standard. Although these are all of concern and need reporting within a department and institution, as well as a record of the event, the NRC now requires reporting them only when they are medical events, defined as an event where the effective dose equivalent to the patient exceeds 5 rem to the whole body or 50 rem to an individual organ.

Q: Describe the general response to the spill of radioactive material.

A: The person who recognizes that a spill has occurred should notify all persons in the vicinity, and the area should be restricted. If possible, the spill should be covered. For minor spills, cleanup using appropriate disposable and protective clothing can be accomplished until background or near-background radiation levels are observed. For major spills, the source of the radioactivity should be shielded. For both major and minor spills, all personnel potentially exposed in the area should be surveyed, with appropriate removal of contaminated clothing and decontamination of skin. The radiation safety officer should be notified of all spills and has the primary responsibility for supervising cleanup for major spills and determining what reports must be made to regulatory agencies.

NUCLEAR MEDICINE PHYSICS

> **PEARL:** *Positrons are positive electrons, and thus they are particles. With radioactive decay, an emitted positron travels 2 to 10 mm in tissue (depending on the radionuclide) before losing its kinetic energy, then interacts with an electron. The two particles annihilate each other and emit two 511-keV gamma photons at approximately 180-degree angles from each other. The gamma photons can be detected by positron emission tomography (PET) coincidence detectors. This conversion of mass to energy is predicted by Einstein's well-known formula:* $E = mc^2$.

Q: What is the difference between x-rays and gamma rays?

A: Both x-rays and gamma rays are ionizing radiation. X-rays originate outside the atomic nucleus; gamma rays originate inside the atomic nucleus. The respective energy spectra for x-rays and gamma rays substantially overlap at the high-energy end of the spectrum for all forms of electromagnetic radiation.

Q: What is the energy equivalent of the rest mass of an electron?

A: The energy equivalent is 511 keV. This is also the energy equivalent of a positron (positive electron).

Q: What is the difference between the rad, roentgen, and rem?

A: These terms are frequently confused with each other but have important distinctions.

The *roentgen* is defined as radiation exposure, specifically the quantity of x-radiation or gamma radiation that produces 1 electrostatic unit of charge per cubic centimeter of air at standard temperature and pressure. In the International System of Units (SI), radiation exposure is expressed in terms of coulombs per kilogram (C/kg). One roentgen is equal to 2.58×10^{-4} C/kg air.

A *rad,* or the radiation absorbed dose, is the traditional unit of absorbed dose equal to the absorption of 100 ergs of energy per gram of absorbing material. The gray (Gy) is the unit of absorbed dose in the SI system; 1 Gy = 100 rads.

The unit *rem* is an acronym for *roentgen* equivalent *man.* The rem is calculated by multiplying the absorbed dose in rads by a factor to correct for the *relative biological effectiveness* (RBE) of the type of radiation in question. In the SI system, 1 *sievert* (Sv) = 100 rem.

Q: Which is more penetrating in soft tissues—alpha or beta particles of the same kinetic energy?

A: Alpha particles have very low penetration in soft tissue because of their rapid loss of kinetic energy through the interaction of their electrical charge with electrons in the tissues. Beta particles of the same respective kinetic energy of alpha particles have higher velocity, lower mass, and a single negative charge. They demonstrate considerably greater penetration in soft tissues, although penetration still is typically measured in millimeters.

Q: Define the two systems for expressing radioactive decay.

A: The traditional unit of radioactive decay is the curie (Ci). One curie is equal to 3.7×10^{10} disintegrations per second (dps). This number was derived from the decay rate of 1 g of radium. (Modern measurements indicate that the actual decay rate for 1 g of radium is 3.6×10^{10} dps.) In the SI system, decay is expressed in becquerels (Bcq). One becquerel equals 1 disintegration per second; 1 mCi = 37 MBq.

Q: How are the half-life and the decay constant related?

A: The physical half-life ($T_{1/2}$) of a radionuclide is defined as the time for half the atoms in a sample to decay. The $T_{1/2}$ is expressed in units of time, typically seconds, minutes, hours, days, or years. The decay constant indicates the fraction of the sample decaying in a unit of time. The units of the decay constant are "per unit time" (per second, per hour). Mathematically, the $T_{1/2}$ and the decay constant (λ) are related by the following equation: $\dfrac{T_1}{2} = \dfrac{\ln 2}{\lambda}$

Q: After a photon has undergone Compton scattering, how does the energy of the scattered photon compare to the original photon energy?

A: In Compton scattering, the photon gives up energy to a recoil or Compton electron. The "scattered" photon has correspondingly lower energy. The amount of energy lost increases as the angle of scattering increases.

Q: What factors speed up or slow down radioactive decay?

A: Unlike chemical reactions, radioactive decay is a physical constant that cannot be sped up or slowed down by heating or cooling or by applying other physical or chemical influences.

Q: What special term is used to designate the electrons in the outermost shell of an atom?

A: They are called valence electrons and are responsible for many of the chemical characteristics of the element.

Q: What is the binding energy of an electron?

A: Binding energy refers to the amount of energy required to remove that electron from the atom. Electrons in shells close to the nucleus have higher binding energy than electrons farther from the nucleus. This energy is typically expressed in terms of electron volts (eV). The binding energy for each electron shell and subshell is characteristic for the respective element; the higher the atomic number of the element, the greater is the binding energy for each shell and subshell.

RADIATION DETECTION AND INSTRUMENTATION

Q: What are examples of the uses of ionization chambers in nuclear medicine?

A: Ionization chambers are used for radiation survey meters and some pocket dosimeters. The radionuclide dose calibrator incorporates an ionization chamber.

Q: What is the purpose of the thallium impurity added to sodium iodide crystals in gamma detectors?

A: The thallium is used to "activate" the sodium iodide crystal. The thallium impurity provides "easier" pathways for the return of electrons from the conduction band of the crystal to the valence bands of atoms.

Q: What is the relationship between photon energy and detection efficiency in a sodium iodide crystal?

A: For a given crystal size, detection efficiency decreases with increasing photon energy.

Q: Why do photopeaks appear as bell-shaped curves in pulse height spectra rather than as discrete spikes corresponding to the energy of the gamma ray?

A: Although gamma rays have discrete energies, the detection process is subject to statistical factors at each step of the process. The bell-shaped curve corresponding to the gamma-ray photopeak reflects these statistical variations, which results in different events being measured as having slightly different energies. The better the "energy resolution" of a pulse height analyzer, the narrower the bell-shaped curve.

Q: In using a gamma scintillation camera, what does it mean to "set" the energy window?

A: Gamma cameras are equipped with pulse-height analyzers that allow the operator to select a range of observed energies for accepting photons to be used in making the scintigraphic image. The window is usually described by giving the photopeak energy of interest and a percentage range that defines the limits of acceptance above and below the photopeak energy. A typical window for the 140-keV photon of Tc-99m is 20%, or ±14 keV.

Q: What are the causes of inhomogeneous flood field images in gamma camera quality control?

A: Causes include improper photomultiplier tube voltage adjustment, off-peak camera pulse-height analyzer setting, crystal imperfections or damage, poor coupling of the crystal and the photomultiplier tubes, and inadequate mixing of radiotracer in the flood phantom.

Q: What effects do Compton-scattered photons have on scintigraphic image quality?

A: Compton-scattered photons are the enemy! Scattered photons that fall within the acceptance limits of the energy window are included in the image. They represent false data because they are recorded in a different spatial location than the origin of the primary photon. Thus, Compton scattering reduces image contrast and spatial resolution. Compton-scattered photons falling outside the energy window still must be processed by the gamma camera pulse-height-analyzer circuitry. These rejected events contribute to dead time and reduce the count-rate capability of gamma cameras.

Q: What photons are desired in the scintigraphic image?

A: Primary (unscattered) photons that arise in the organ of interest in the body and travel parallel to the axis of the gamma camera collimator field of view are the photons desired in the image. Intuitively, one may think of these as "good" photons. All other photons are "bad" photons. The good photons include (unscattered) photons that arise in the object or organ of interest but travel "off axis," primary photons that arise in front of or behind the organ of interest (background photons), and all scattered photons.

Q: What is the purpose of the collimator?

A: The collimator defines the geometrical field of view of the gamma camera crystal. Off-axis photons, whether they are primary photons or scattered photons, are absorbed in the septa of the collimator and do not get to the crystal.

PEARL: Pinhole collimators allow resolution of objects below the spatial resolution of the gamma camera through geometrical magnification.

Q: What is the construction difference between a low-energy, all-purpose collimator and a low-energy, high-resolution collimator?

A: A high-resolution collimator has more holes that are smaller and deeper.

Q: How does poor energy resolution degrade spatial resolution?

A: Gamma cameras with poor energy resolution have reduced ability to reject scattered photons on the basis of pulse-height analysis, as well as reduced ability for accurate determination of *x*- and *y*-coordinates for spatial localization of events.

SINGLE-PHOTON EMISSION COMPUTED TOMOGRAPHY AND POSITRON EMISSION TOMOGRAPHY

PEARL: *Most nuclear medicine imaging clinics use 180-degree single-photon emission computed tomography (SPECT) acquisition for cardiac studies and 360 degrees for imaging most other organs, including the brain.*

PEARL: *For SPECT imaging, the highest-resolution collimator that provides sufficient count rate should be selected, usually the high-resolution parallel-hole collimator.*

PITFALL: *In addition to equipment factors, patient motion is the most important cause of image degradation in SPECT and positron emission tomography (PET) studies.*

Q: What special importance does the biological half-life of a radiotracer have in SPECT imaging?

A: In SPECT imaging, two-dimensional data are acquired from sequential sampling angles. If significant biological change in the distribution of a radiopharmaceutical takes place between the start of data acquisition and completion, the reconstruction of tomographic images can be significantly distorted.

Q: What is a filter?

A: Filters are special mathematical functions applied to SPECT and PET data that enhance desired characteristics in the image, such as background subtraction, edge enhancement, and suppression of statistical noise. A ramp filter is designed to eliminate or reduce the star artifact during reconstruction.

PEARL: *With SPECT and PET, flexible reformatting of image data can be performed in multiple image planes, typically transverse, coronal, and sagittal. For cardiac imaging, short-axis, vertical long-axis, and horizontal long-axis views of the heart are typically obtained.*

PEARL: *Two quick ways of assessing patient motion during SPECT imaging are to view the projection images as a cinematic closed-loop display or to create slice sinograms. In the cinematic display, patient motion is seen as a change in position from one projection image to another. It best shows vertical motion. On sinograms, patient motion is seen as a discontinuity in the stacked projection profiles.*

PITFALL: *SPECT is subject to various artifacts. Field flood nonuniformity can result in ring artifacts. Center-of-rotation misalignment results in loss of image resolution and, if severe, also ring artifacts.*

PEARL: *The spatial resolution of PET is twice or greater than that of SPECT.*

PITFALL: *Spatial resolution in PET is limited by positron travel distance in soft tissue before annihilation and photon emission.*

PEARL: *PET imaging with transmission attenuation correction and detector sensitivity calibration allows for absolute quantitative uptake determinations.*

PEARL: *Positron emitters, such as carbon, nitrogen, oxygen, and fluorine (as a replacement for hydrogen), make possible the potential radiolabeling of any biological compound. However, the chemistry for developing and radiolabeling single-photon radiopharmaceuticals can be complex.*

ENDOCRINE

Q: What is the origin of lingual and sublingual thyroid tissue?

A: The main thyroid anlage begins as a down-growth from the foramen cecum. Thyroid tissue may be seen anywhere along the tract of the thyroglossal duct from the foramen cecum to the usual location of the gland. However, with lingual thyroid tissue, usually a failure of normal development occurs, with no tissue in the normal location of the thyroid.

Q: What is the difference in mechanism of thyroid uptake between Tc-99m pertechnetate and radioiodine?

A: Radioiodine is taken up or extracted (trapped) by the thyroid follicular cell and organified, binding to tyrosine residues on thyroglobulin, and stored in the colloid of the follicle. Tc-99m pertechnetate is trapped but not organified.

Q: What has happened to the range for normal percent thyroid uptake of radioiodine in the United States over the last 50 or more years?

A: The normal range has dropped significantly as a result of iodination of salt and the use of iodine in foods. The normal 24-hour range was 20% to 45% in the 1960s but is now 10% to 30%.

PEARL: *Radioiodine is administered orally. Tc-99m pertechnetate is administered intravenously.*

PITFALL: *A potentially serious pitfall is to confuse microcuries with millicuries.*

PEARL: *The following are the approximate adult doses of iodine-123 and iodine-131 used for uptakes, scans, and therapy. Serious consequences can result from confusing these doses, particularly if a therapeutic dose is administered instead of a diagnostic dose.*

I-123 uptake (50–100 microcuries [µCi])
I-123 scan (200–400 µCi)
I-131 uptake (10 µCi)
I-131 scan substernal goiter (50 µCi)—however, I-123 has replaced I-131 for this indication
I-131 therapy for Graves disease (7–15 millicuries [mCi])
I-131 therapy for thyroid cancer (30–200 mCi)

Q: What is the normal distribution of radioiodine and Tc-99m pertechnetate?

A: Radioiodine is taken up by the thyroid, salivary glands, and stomach and excreted by the kidneys. Tc-99m pertechnetate has identical uptake and clearance, except that because it is not organified, it remains in the thyroid and salivary glands for a much shorter time.

PEARL: *After injection of the radiopharmaceutical, Tc-99m pertechnetate scans are acquired at 15 to 20 minutes. Routine I-123 thyroid scans after oral ingestion are acquired at 4 hours. The delayed imaging for I-123 is to allow background clearance. Tc-99m is not organified like I-123; thus, it must be imaged earlier because of the rapid thyroid washout.*

Q: What are common causes of falsely low thyroid uptakes?

A: Patients taking thyroid hormones, iodine-containing drugs, organification blockers such as propylthiouracil or methimazole, and recent administration of intravenous iodine-containing radiographic contrast are common causes.

PEARL: *A thyroid scan should not be performed within 6 to 8 weeks of the patient receiving a CT scan with intravenous iodine contrast.*

Q: How does the methodology differ for a thyroid scan and thyroid uptake?

A: A thyroid uptake is a nonimaging study using a gamma-detector counting probe, whereas a thyroid scan results from gamma camera imaging.

PEARL: *Swallowed activity from salivary secretions on Tc-99m pertechnetate or radioiodine scans occasionally remains in the esophagus and can confuse interpretation. The nature of the activity can be determined by having the patient drink water, followed by reimaging of the neck.*

Q: How can a thyroid uptake test differentiate the two most common causes of thyrotoxicosis, Graves disease, and subacute thyroiditis? Why?

A: In the initial phase of subacute thyroiditis, thyroid hormones are released from the inflamed gland, causing thyrotoxicosis. Both radioiodine and Tc-99m uptake require thyroid-stimulating hormone (TSH) stimulation for uptake. As a result of pituitary feedback of elevated serum thyroid hormones,

TSH is suppressed. Thus, the uptake of radioiodine or Tc-99m pertechnetate is suppressed. With Graves disease, although TSH is suppressed, the gland is autonomous, and the uptake is high.

Q: What is the mechanism of action of antithyroid drugs propylthiouracil (PTU) and methimazole (Tapazole)?

A: Both are thiourea antithyroid drugs that block the organification of iodine.

Q: What medical conditions are associated with an increased incidence of pheochromocytomas and paragangliomas?

A: Both forms of multiple endocrine neoplasia type II are associated with pheochromocytoma, as are von Hippel–Lindau disease and neurofibromatosis.

> **PITFALL:** *Autonomous nodules are not synonymous with toxic nodules. Patients with small autonomous nodules (<2.5 cm in diameter) are often euthyroid. They do not produce enough thyroid hormone to suppress TSH.*

> **PEARL:** *The incidence of thyroid cancer in a patient with a single cold nodule is approximately 15%; a hot nodule, less than 1%.*

Q: Which radiopharmaceutical is used most commonly to localize a clinically diagnosed parathyroid adenoma? Describe its characteristic and diagnostic pharmacokinetics.

A: Tc-99m sestamibi is taken up by both thyroid and hyperfunctioning parathyroid tissue; however, it typically clears faster from the thyroid, thus the rationale for early (15 minutes) and delayed (2 hour) imaging. At early imaging, uptake in the thyroid is dominant and hyperfunctioning parathyroid may or may not be apparent as focal hot uptake. On delayed imaging, thyroid uptake has usually mostly washed out, leaving residual uptake in a hyperfunctioning parathyroid.

> **PEARL:** *The most common false positive for parathyroid scanning is a thyroid adenoma. Benign and malignant tumors are other potential causes for false-positive scintigraphy.*

BONE

Q: What percentage of Tc-99m-labeled bone radiopharmaceuticals is retained in the skeleton at the usual time of imaging?

A: In normal adult subjects, 40% to 60% of the injected dose is in the skeleton 2 to 3 hours after tracer administration.

> **PITFALL:** *The greatest pitfall in interpreting a bone scan is a failure to appreciate its nonspecificity. The bone scan is very sensitive; however, specificity is considerably lower. The most common pitfalls are diagnosing areas of arthritis or prior trauma as metastases, or vice versa. Correlative anatomical imaging is advisable.*

Q: Which factors favor osteoarthritis versus metastatic disease as the cause of increased activity?

A: Osteoarthritis has characteristic locations in the extremities. Because metastatic lesions are relatively rare below the proximal femurs or beyond the proximal humeri, osteoarthritis

should be considered first in the elbows, wrists, hands, knees, and feet of older patients. The involvement of both sides of a joint is common in arthritis but unusual in metastatic disease. The lower lumbar spine is the most problematic area because both arthritis and metastases are common there. Degenerative disease is often more posterior and lateral, compared with metastases. Anatomical imaging is advised to help differentiate.

Q: What is the distribution of metastatic deposits from epithelial primary malignancies in the skeleton?

A: A rule of thumb is that 80% of metastases are found in the axial skeleton (spine, pelvis, ribs, and sternum). The remaining metastases are distributed equally between the skull (10%) and the long bones (10%). A single rib with uptake has a low likelihood of being a metastasis. A sternal lesion in a patient with breast cancer has a high likelihood of being a metastasis.

> **PEARL:** *The majority of epithelial tumor metastases localize first in the red marrow. The skeletal tracers do not localize in the tumor tissue but, rather, in the reactive bone around the metastatic deposits.*

> **PITFALL:** *A small amount of activity is frequently seen at the injection site; this should not be confused with pathology. Extravasation at the injection site may result in proximal nodal uptake. Variable degrees of urinary contamination on the skin may be superimposed on skeletal structures and could be confused with activity caused by metastatic disease. Multiple views can be helpful to make the distinction.*

> **PEARL:** *In many diseases, the bone scan has a very high sensitivity for the detection of bone metastases. Sensitivity is lower in tumors with a lytic rather than blastic response, such as multiple myeloma, thyroid cancer, and renal-cell carcinoma. The bone scan is also less sensitive for tumors that preferentially go to bone marrow, such as lymphoma.*

Q: How can the radiation dose to the bladder, ovaries, and testes be reduced?

A: The radiation dose to these structures is largely caused by radioactivity in the bladder. Frequent voiding reduces the patient's radiation dose.

> **PEARL:** *Faint or absent visualization of the kidneys should alert the observer to the possibility of a superscan. This may be misinterpreted as indicating lack of excretion of tracer through the kidneys. In cases of superscan resulting from metastatic or metabolic disease, visualization of the kidneys is faint (1) because the skeleton accumulates more tracer than usual, leaving less available for renal excretion, and (2) because of the increased skeletal tracer uptake, the renal activity may actually fall below the grayscale threshold. The presence of renal activity is readily established by adjusting the intensity-setting window.*

Q: What factors distinguish a superscan resulting from metastatic disease from a superscan resulting from metabolic disease?

A: In the usual superscan caused by metastatic disease, the increased uptake is usually restricted to the axial skeleton and the proximal parts of the femurs and humeri, the red marrow–bearing areas. Usually there is some focality to it as well. In metabolic bone disease, the entire skeleton is typically affected, with increased uptake seen in the extremities and axial skeleton.

Q: What is the mechanism of the "flare" phenomenon?

A: In some patients treated with chemotherapy for metastatic disease, regression of the tumor burden is associated with increased osteoblastic activity, caused by skeletal healing in response to chemotherapy. This can appear on bone scans as a paradoxical increase or apparent worsening of the abnormal tracer. This may last for up to 6 months after therapy.

Q: What is the postmastectomy appearance of the thorax?

A: With a radical mastectomy, the majority of the soft tissue is removed from the corresponding anterior thorax. The ribs appear "hotter" than on the contralateral side. This is caused by less attenuation of rib activity by soft tissue. Alternatively, if the patient is imaged with a breast prosthesis in place, the rib activity may be attenuated.

Q: What factors contribute to prolonged fracture positivity on scintigrams?

A: Displaced and comminuted fractures and fractures involving joints tend to have prolonged positivity scintigraphically. Elderly patients have delayed healing.

Q: What factors favor shin splints versus stress fracture scintigraphically in the tibia?

A: Stress fractures are classically focal or fusiform. The uptake can involve the entire width of the bone but more commonly extend partially across the shaft of the bone. Shin splints are classically located along the posterior medial tibial cortex and involve a third or more of the length of the bone. In pure shin splints, a focal component is not present, and superficial linear activity runs parallel to the long axis of the bone.

Q: The three-phase bone scan is used to diagnose osteomyelitis. What are other causes of a positive three-phase scan?

A: Recent fracture, tumor, Charcot's joint, and soft-tissue infection overlying chronic noninfectious bone disease are other causes.

> **PITFALL:** *False-negative scintigrams may sometimes be seen in neonates with osteomyelitis. Sometimes the lesions appear photopenic.*

HEPATOBILIARY

Q: What are the two Tc-99m hepatobiliary iminodiacetic acid (HIDA) analog radiopharmaceuticals approved by the U.S. Food and Drug Administration (FDA) in clinical use, and how are they different?

A: Tc-99m DISIDA (disofenin) and Tc-99m mebrofenin (Choletec) are the approved agents. Mebrofenin has greater hepatic extraction, 98% versus 88%, and less renal excretion, 1% versus 9%. The higher extraction of mebrofenin is particularly preferable in patients with hepatic insufficiency and young children.

> **PEARL:** *Tc-99m HIDA is extracted by the same cellular mechanism as bilirubin, but it is not conjugated. The radiopharmaceutical then follows the path of bile through the biliary system into the bowel.*

> **PEARL:** *The alternative route of excretion for Tc-99m HIDA radiopharmaceuticals is via the kidneys. The amount of excretion is usually small but increases with hepatic dysfunction.*

Q: What is the most important question to ask a patient before starting cholescintigraphy for suspected acute cholecystitis, and why?

A: When did the patient last eat? If the patient has eaten in the last 4 hours, the gallbladder may be contracted secondary to endogenous stimulation of cholecystokinin, and therefore radiotracer cannot gain entry into the gallbladder. If the patient has not eaten for more than 24 hours, the gallbladder may not have had the stimulus to contract and may contain thick, concentrated bile, which can prevent tracer entry. Sincalide (of an analog cholecystokinin [CCK]) is indicated to empty the gallbladder.

> **PEARL:** *If the patient receives sincalide before the study to empty the gallbladder, the HIDA radiopharmaceutical should not be administered until at least 30 minutes later to allow time for the gallbladder to relax.*

Q: What are other common indications for sincalide infusion than mentioned previously?

A: Common indications are (1) to differentiate common duct obstruction from functional causes, as an alternative to delayed imaging, (2) to exclude acute acalculous cholecystitis if the gallbladder fills in a patient strongly suspected of having the disease (a diseased gallbladder will not contract from either acute or chronic disease), and (3) to confirm or exclude chronic acalculous gallbladder disease (gallbladder dyskinesia).

Q: Cholescintigraphy is a very sensitive and specific test for acute cholecystitis. In what clinical settings can an increased number of false-positive study findings for acute cholecystitis be seen?

A: False positives may be seen in patients who have fasted less than 4 hours or more than 24 hours, those receiving hyperalimentation, and patients who have chronic cholecystitis, hepatic dysfunction, or a concurrent serious illness.

Q: What is the rim sign seen during cholescintigraphy, and what is its significance?

A: The rim sign is increased activity in the liver parenchyma adjacent to the gallbladder fossa. This finding has been associated with severe acute cholecystitis and an increased incidence of the complications of perforation and gangrene.

Q: At what time after Tc-99m HIDA injection is nonfilling of the gallbladder diagnostic of acute cholecystitis?

A: One hour is abnormal. However, the diagnosis of acute cholecystitis cannot be made unless the gallbladder does not fill by 3 to 4 hours after radiopharmaceutical injection or 30 minutes after morphine administration.

Q: What is the mechanism of morphine-augmented cholescintigraphy?

A: Morphine increases tone at the sphincter of Oddi, producing increased intraductal pressure. This results in bile flow preferentially through the cystic duct, if patent.

Q: What is acute acalculous cholecystitis?

A: Acute acalculous cholecystitis occurs in sick hospitalized patients who have sustained trauma, burns, or sepsis or have other serious illness. It is associated with high morbidity and mortality. The cystic duct may be obstructed by debris or inflammatory changes. In some cases, the acute cholecystitis is caused by direct inflammation of the gallbladder wall as a result of infection, ischemia, or toxemia, without cystic duct obstruction.

Q: The diagnosis of common duct obstruction is often made by sonographic detection of a dilated common duct. In what clinical situations would cholescintigraphy be diagnostically helpful?

A: It is helpful in early acute obstruction before the duct has had time to dilate (24–72 hours) and in patients with previous obstruction who have chronically dilated ducts.

Q: What are the cholescintigraphic findings of high-grade common duct obstruction?

A: The findings include prompt hepatic uptake but a persistent hepatogram without clearance into biliary ducts. This is caused by high backpressure from the obstruction.

Q: What are the cholescintigraphic findings of partial common duct obstruction?

A: The findings include good hepatic uptake, delayed biliary-to-bowel clearance, and poor ductal clearance on delayed imaging or after sincalide.

Q: What ancillary maneuver increases the sensitivity of cholescintigraphy for detection of biliary atresia?

A: The administration of phenobarbital for 5 days before the HIDA study activates liver enzymes and increases biliary excretion. A serum phenobarbital level should be in the therapeutic range at the time of imaging.

Q: How is the diagnosis of biliary atresia made with cholescintigraphy?

A: No clearance of Tc-99m HIDA tracer is seen by 24 hours. The many causes of neonatal hepatitis usually have clearance by that time, although not always.

Q: What is the postcholecystectomy syndrome, and what are common causes for it?

A: In patients who have had a cholecystectomy, some develop recurrent biliary, colic-like pain. Causes include a retained or recurrent stone, inflammatory stricture, sphincter of Oddi dysfunction, or, very rarely, an inflamed or obstructed cystic duct remnant.

GENITOURINARY

Q: What percentage of renal plasma flow is filtered through the glomerulus, and what percentage is secreted by the tubules?

A: Twenty percent of renal plasma flow is cleared by glomerular filtration and 80% by tubular secretion.

Q: What are the mechanisms of renal uptake for Tc-99m diethylenetriaminepentaacetic acid (DTPA), Tc-99m mercaptylacetyltriglycine (MAG3), and Tc-99m dimercaptosuccinic acid (DMSA)?

A: Tc-99m DTPA, glomerular filtration; Tc-99m MAG3, tubular secretion; Tc-99m DMSA, cortical proximal tubular binding

Q: What is the percent cortical binding of Tc-99m DMSA?

A: The percent cortical binding is 40% to 45%.

Q: What time interval is used to calculate a differential renal function for dynamic renal scintigraphy?

A: Because cortical uptake of the renal radiopharmaceutical is the interest, the optimal interval is after the initial flow but before the collecting system activity appears, usually 1 to 3 minutes. With good function, activity may be seen before 3 minutes, especially in children. Thus, the 1- to 2-minute interval may be optimal overall.

Q: What are the general methods for calculating absolute glomerular filtration rate (GFR)?

A: Blood sampling, blood sampling and urine collection, and camera-based methods can be used to calculate the absolute GFR.

Q: What is the proper renal region-of-interest (ROI) selection for diuresis renography?

A: The ROI should include the dilated collecting system and mostly exclude the cortex.

Q: What factors can affect the accuracy of diuresis renography?

A: The state of hydration, renal function, diuretic dose, choice of radiopharmaceutical, and bladder capacity can affect the accuracy. Adequate hydration is required for good urine flow and adequate response to the diuretic. A full bladder may cause a functional delay in clearance. Urinary catheterization is strongly suggested in children and in adults who cannot void. Because of its high extraction efficiency and good image resolution, Tc-99m MAG3 is the radiopharmaceutical of choice. Tc-99m DTPA works well in patients with good renal function. Poor renal function is a limitation to diuresis renography. The kidney must be able to respond to the diuretic challenge. Therefore, the dose of diuretic must be increased in renal insufficiency, but the exact dose required is only an educated estimate.

Q: What is the most sensitive technique for diagnosing scarring secondary to reflux?

A: Tc-99m DMSA cortical imaging is the most sensitive. CT is good but results in a considerably higher radiation dose to a child. Ultrasonography has lower sensitivity.

Q: How can radionuclide imaging differentiate upper from lower urinary tract infection, and why is this differentiation important?

A: With upper tract infection or pyelonephritis, Tc-99m DMSA shows tubular dysfunction, manifested by decreased uptake. This is a reversible process. With appropriate therapy, tubular function will return in 3 to 6 months. Upper tract infection may lead to subsequent renal scarring, hypertension, and renal failure.

Q: What is the advantage of radionuclide versus contrast cystography?

A: The radionuclide test is more sensitive for the detection of reflux than contrast-enhanced voiding cystourethrography and results in much less radiation exposure, by a factor of 50- to 200-fold. However, in the first evaluation of a male child, the better resolution of the contrast study can permit the diagnosis of an anatomical abnormality such as posterior urethral valves.

ONCOLOGY: POSITRON EMISSION TOMOGRAPHY

Q: What is the difference in uptake mechanism between glucose and F-18 fluorodeoxyglucose (FDG)?

A: After initial cellular uptake via glucose transporters, both are phosphorylated by hexokinase. Unlike glucose-6-phosphate, F-18 FDG-6-phosphate does not undergo further metabolism and is trapped within cells. Also unlike glucose, F-18 FDG is cleared by the kidneys.

Q: The sensitivity of FDG PET is high for detection of many malignancies. For which tumors is the sensitivity of FDG PET often not as high?

A: FDG PET has poor sensitivity for primary hepatocellular carcinoma, renal carcinoma, and prostate cancer. This is less true of metastatic disease than primary tumors.

> **PEARL:** *For thyroid cancer imaging, I-131 or I-123 is more sensitive than F-18 FDG for the detection of well-differentiated papillary or follicular thyroid carcinoma. In patients who have been treated with I-131 and have a negative I-131 whole-body scan on follow-up evaluation but have an elevated serum thyroglobulin value, F-18 FDG PET has good sensitivity for the detection of malignancy. The reason is that the tumor has dedifferentiated into a higher-grade malignancy.*

> **PEARL:** *With positron emission tomography with computed tomography (PET/CT), misregistration caused by patient or respiratory motion or organ movement (bowel) can introduce potential false-positive interpretations. PET/CT is usually acquired during tidal volume breathing. Still, there may be artifacts resulting from errors in anatomical registration and attenuation correction.*

Q: What are some limitations of FDG PET in tumor staging?

A: PET imaging does not detect microscopical metastases, tumor involvement in local lymph nodes may be obscured by activity in an adjacent tumor, concurrent infection/inflammatory processes may cause false-positive results, and the sensitivity for intracranial metastases is low.

Q: What are limitations of tumor restaging by FDG PET?

A: Posttherapy inflammatory effects of surgery, chemotherapy, and especially radiation therapy may cause increased F-18 FDG uptake, which can be confused with tumor uptake. Even patients scheduled for imaging after an appropriate delay after therapy may require further follow-up imaging. If activity is diminishing, this helps confirm a benign process.

> **PEARL:** *The usual recommended FDG PET/CT imaging time to evaluate response to therapy is 3 weeks after chemotherapy, but for radiation therapy, at least 2 and preferably 3 months. It is not always possible from a clinical standpoint to follow these guidelines, but an awareness of the potential problem is critical for interpretation.*

> **PEARL:** *FDG PET/CT can help direct biopsy to the most metabolically active area of a mass to help avoid sampling areas of necrosis.*

Q: Which is the most accurate method for the detection of osseous metastases?

A: It depends. Magnetic resonance imaging (MRI) is highly sensitive and often detects lesions not seen on bone scan because it can visualize changes in the bone marrow and does not depend on secondary reactive cortical bone changes to develop. Bone scintigraphy has the advantage that it routinely images the whole body. It is particularly helpful for sclerotic (blastic) metastases. FDG PET scanning is more sensitive than bone scan for detection of lytic tumors. At times, the modalities complement each other by detecting different lesions in the same patient. F-18 sodium fluoride PET is a very sensitive bone scan agent but at the expense of specificity. PET/CT improves the specificity.

Q: What are some differences between nonattenuation-corrected and attenuation-corrected FDG PET images?

A: The noncorrected image has an appearance quite different from that of the corrected image. Without attenuation, structures near the surface appear more intense because fewer photons are attenuated before hitting the detector. This explains why the skin looks like it is outlined with a charcoal pencil. The air-filled lungs are also intense. Because fewer counts are seen in central areas, lesions may be missed. However, this is a preferable way to detect skin lesions. For accurate quantification (standard uptake value [SUV]), attenuation corrected images must be used.

ONCOLOGY: BEYOND FLUORODEOXYGLUCOSE

Q: Which of the following are true statements regarding indium-111 OctreoScan (pentetreotide)?

a. It is a somatostatin receptor imaging agent.
b. The sensitivity for all neuroendocrine tumors is very high.
c. The highest uptake is seen in the spleen and kidneys.
d. Only neuroendocrine tumors have somatostatin receptors.

A: a, c. Although the sensitivity for the detection of many neuroendocrine tumors is high (e.g., carcinoid), it has a poorer sensitivity for others (e.g., insulinomas and medullary carcinoma of the thyroid). Somatostatin receptors are found on a variety of nonneuroendocrine tumors, including astrocytomas, meningiomas, malignant lymphoma, and breast and lung cancer.

PEARL: Ga-68 dotatate PET/CT is now FDA approved for somatostatin imaging of neuroendocrine tumors. It has superior image quality and higher sensitivity for tumor detection than In-111 pentetreotide. As with other PET studies, it is completed by 2 hours after injection, compared with 24-hour imaging for In-111 pentetreotide.

PEARL: The sentinel node is the first lymph node draining a malignant tumor site and the most likely one to have a metastatic tumor. Radionuclide lymphoscintigraphy is commonly used to detect the sentinel node. Surgeons sometimes use blue dye as well at the time of surgery.

Q: Which patients with malignant melanoma require sentinel node lymphoscintigraphy?

A: Lymphoscintigraphy is indicated for patients with primary lesions >1 mm and <4 mm thickness. Patients with a primary lesion <1 mm in thickness are at low risk for recurrence and have a good prognosis. Patients with a primary lesion thickness >4 mm are at high risk for metastatic regional and distant metastases.

Q: What information does sentinel node lymphoscintigraphy provide?

A: Lymphoscintigraphy can localize the sentinel node for the surgeon, who can then detect it at surgery with a gamma probe. After immunohistochemical staining of tissue from this lymph node, the presence of metastases can be determined. The results will determine whether the patient requires further dissection of the nodal bed. If the sentinel node is negative, no further surgery is necessary.

Q: In what other malignant disease is sentinel node lymphoscintigraphy commonly performed? What is the method of injection?

A: Sentinel node lymphoscintigraphy is commonly performed in breast cancer. The method of radiopharmaceutical injection varies. At some hospitals, it is injected intratumorally. Others inject it subdermally, whereas still others inject in the periareolar region. The rationale for the latter is that all lymphatics drain to the areolar region before further drainage to the axillary region.

PEARL: In patients with acquired immunodeficiency syndrome (AIDS) and an intracerebral mass, thallium-201 can differentiate malignancy, usually lymphoma, from inflammatory causes, commonly toxoplasmosis. Tl-201 is rarely taken up in inflammation but is taken up by many malignant tumors. The predictive value is greater than 85%. F-18 FDG performs similarly.

PEARL: In-111 ProstaScint is no longer commonly used for imaging metastatic prostate cancer. F-18 fluciclovine (Axumin) PET, an amino acid analog, has been approved for imaging of metastatic prostate cancer. Ga-68 prostate-specific membrane antigen (PSMA) and F-18 PSMA-targeted radiopharmaceuticals are both PET tracers under active investigation for imaging metastatic prostate cancer, and at least one is likely to be approved in the near future. The target of these small-molecule radiopharmaceuticals is the enzyme site in the extracellular domain. It is then internalized by endocytosis. Image quality is clearly superior to ProstaScint and very likely better than F-18 fluciclovine.

GASTROINTESTINAL

PEARL: The radionuclide gastrointestinal reflux study ("milk study") is a sensitive method for the detection of reflux because of its rapid acquisition rate (5–10 sec/frame). However, it is not particularly sensitive for aspiration (<25%). A salivagram, essentially an esophageal transit scintigraphic study where a small amount of activity is placed in the child's mouth, is much more sensitive for the detection of aspiration.

Q: What are the different functional roles of the proximal and distal stomach?

A: The proximal stomach (fundus) undergoes receptive relaxation and accommodation after ingestion of a meal and is responsible for liquid emptying. The distal stomach (antrum) grinds and sieves solid food and is responsible for solid emptying.

Q: Describe the difference in emptying patterns between solids and liquids.

A: Liquids empty in an exponential pattern. Solid emptying is biphasic, with an initial lag phase before linear emptying begins. The lag phase is due to the time required for food to be broken down into small enough pieces to allow passage through the pylorus.

Q: Which of these factors will affect the rate of gastric emptying: meal content, time of day, position (standing, sitting, lying), stress, exercise?

A: All. The gastric-emptying study should be standardized for the size and contents of the meal, time of day, patient position, acquisition method, processing, and normal values. A standardized meal has been recommended, with normal values based on that method.

Q: What is the published recommendation for a standardized solid gastric-emptying study?

A: The published consensus for a standardized gastric-emptying study involves the ingestion of specific amounts of an egg-white sandwich, jam, and water. Images are acquired immediately after ingestion and at 1, 2, and 4 hours in the anterior and posterior view. Attenuation correction is performed. Normal values are established for percent emptying: >10% at 1 hour, >40% at 2 hours, and >90% at 4 hours.

> **PEARLS:** *Gastric emptying may be underestimated when an anterior acquisition alone is obtained. The geometrical mean method is considered the standard method for attenuation correction.*

Q: What is the red blood cell labeling efficiency of these three methods: in vivo, in vitro, and in vivtro labeling methods?

A: The efficiency is 75% for in vivo, 85% for modified in vivo (in vivtro), and >97% for the in vitro method.

> **PEARL:** *An in vitro commercial kit method (Ultra-Tag) for labeling Tc-99m erythrocytes is the method of choice today because of its high labeling efficiency.*

Q: What are the essential criteria needed to confidently diagnose the site of active bleeding on a radionuclide gastrointestinal bleeding study?

A: A radiotracer "hot spot" appears where there was none, transit is in a pattern conforming to bowel anatomy, the activity increases over time, and it moves antegrade and or retrograde.

> **PITFALL:** *A poor label (free Tc-99m pertechnetate) for a gastrointestinal (GI) bleeding study can result in activity that might be construed as GI bleeding.*

> **PEARL:** *Look for thyroid and salivary gland uptake when in doubt about the presence of free Tc-99m pertechnetate. If the patient has recently had a contrast CT scan, the thyroid may not be visualized.*

> **PEARL:** *A lateral view or left anterior oblique (LAO) view of the pelvis at the end of a GI bleeding study acquisition can help to differentiate bladder, rectal bleeding, and penile activity.*

> **PITFALL:** *Focal activity seen on a Tc-99m red blood cell (RBC) GI bleeding study that does not move but remains fixed in position may be due to an accessory spleen, hemangioma, varices, or aneurysm.*

> **PEARL:** *The RBC gastrointestinal bleeding study can detect bleeding rates of approximately 0.1 mL/min versus 1 mL/min for contrast angiography.*

> **PEARL:** *This most common congenital anomaly of the gastrointestinal tract is a Meckel diverticulum, which results from failure of closure of the omphalomesenteric duct of the embryo, which connects the yolk sac to the primitive foregut via the umbilical cord.*

> **PEARL:** *The Meckel diverticulum is a true diverticulum that occurs on the antimesenteric side of the bowel, usually 80 to 90 cm proximal to the ileocecal valve, although it can occur elsewhere.*

> **PEARL:** *Gastric mucosa is present in 10% to 30% of all Meckel diverticula, in 60% of symptomatic patients, and in 98% of those with bleeding.*

> **PITFALL:** *False-positive study results reported for Meckel scans include those of urinary tract origin (e.g., horseshoe kidney, ectopic kidney), those resulting from inflammation (e.g., inflammatory bowel disease, neoplasms), bowel obstruction (seen most often with intussusception and volvulus), and other areas of ectopic gastric mucosa (e.g., gastrointestinal duplication cyst).*

INFECTION AND INFLAMMATION

Q: Which photopeaks are used for In-111-leukocyte imaging, and what is their abundance?

A: 173 keV (89%) and 247 keV (94%)

Q: Which collimator should be used for In-111 leukocyte imaging?

A: Medium-energy collimator

> **PEARL:** *Characteristic scintigraphic patterns of uptake with sarcoidosis on Ga-67 imaging are (1) the "panda" sign, due to uptake in the salivary glands, parotids, and nasopharyngeal region, and (2) the "lambda" sign, which results from paratracheal and hilar lymph node uptake. The lambda sign is also seen with FDG PET; however, the panda sign is not.*

Q: Which leukocytes are labeled with In-111 oxine and Tc-99m hexamethylpropyleneamine oxime (HMPAO)?

A: In-111 oxine binds to neutrophils, lymphocytes, monocytes, erythrocytes, and platelets. Tc-99m HMPAO binds only to neutrophils.

Q: Which of the following statements is true regarding In-111 oxine leukocytes?

a. They are useful for evaluating inflammatory lung disease.

b. They have a high sensitivity for detecting osteomyelitis of the spine.

c. They should not be used when the peripheral leukocyte count is less than 3000/mm³.

d. They are the radiopharmaceutical of choice for intraabdominal infection.

A: c and d are true, with explanations as follows:

a. False. Ga-67 or F-18 FDG is a better choice for inflammatory disease of the lung.

b. The sensitivity for vertebral osteomyelitis is poor, with a 40% false-negative rate. Ga-67 or FDG would be preferable.

c. Fewer than 3000/mm³ leukocytes is inadequate for radiolabeled leukocyte studies.

d. The lack of intraabdominal hepatobiliary and genitourinary clearance makes In-111 leukocytes ideal for detecting intraabdominal infection and superior to Tc-99m HMPAO, which is cleared by both of these routes.

> **PEARL:** *Tc-99m HMPAO is the preferred agent for localizing infection in children because In-111 leukocytes result in a high radiation dose to the spleen of 30 to 50 rads (15–20 rads in adults). Tc-99m HMPAO results in less than 2.2 rads to the spleen.*

Q: What is the optimal imaging time for In-111 and Tc-99m-HMPAO leukocytes?

A: In-111 leukocytes are usually imaged at 24 hours. Imaging at 4 to 6 hours is less sensitive for detection of infection. Tc-99m-HMPAO leukocytes should be imaged by 2 hours for intraabdominal infection before biliary and renal clearance occurs. Extraabdominal infection can be imaged later, usually at 4 hours, allowing time for background clearance.

> **PEARL:** *An exception to 24-hour imaging for In-111 leukocytes is for inflammatory bowel disease, in which imaging should be done at 4 hours because intraluminal shedding of inflamed cells may result in inaccurate localization at 24 hours.*

> **PITFALL:** *Leukocytes may accumulate at the site of inflammation without infection (e.g., intravenous catheters; nasogastric, endogastric, and drainage tubes; tracheostomies; and colostomies). Leukocytes may accumulate at postoperative surgical sites for 2 to 3 weeks, and low-grade uptake may be seen at healing fracture sites. Accessory spleens could be misinterpreted as infection, and renal transplants always accumulate leukocytes.*

> **PITFALL:** *In a radiolabeled leukocyte study, intraluminal intestinal radioactivity can result from swallowed or shedding cells from pharyngitis, sinusitis, pneumonia, herpes esophagitis, or GI bleeding.*

> **PITFALL:** *A radiolabeled leukocyte study for suspected osteomyelitis of the extremities may have a false-positive result because of displaced bone marrow. The addition of a bone marrow study (Tc-99m sulfur colloid) can confirm or exclude the diagnosis. Osteomyelitis will show increased uptake on the leukocyte study and normal or decreased uptake on the bone marrow study. A similar distribution of the two radiopharmaceuticals is negative for infection.*

CENTRAL NERVOUS SYSTEM

Q: How is the diagnosis of brain death made?

A: Brain death is a clinical diagnosis, usually made in a patient in a deep coma with a total absence of brainstem reflexes and spontaneous respiration. Reversible causes must be excluded (e.g., drugs, hypothermia), the cause of the dysfunction must be diagnosed (e.g., trauma, stroke), and the clinical findings of brain death must be present for a defined period of observation (6–24 hours). Confirmatory tests such as electroencephalography (EEG) and radionuclide brain perfusion imaging are used to increase diagnostic certainty.

Q: Which radiopharmaceutical(s) are indicated to evaluate for brain death?

A: Tc-99m HMPAO or Tc-99m ethyl cysteinate dimer (ECD) is indicated. A flow study is optional. Delayed images at 15 to 20 minutes are diagnostic.

> **PEARL:** *A "hot nose" may be seen on the flow-phase images and delayed images of a brain death study as a result of shunting of blood from the internal to the external carotid system supplying the face and nose.*

Q: How can SPECT brain perfusion or FDG PET imaging be useful in the differential diagnosis of dementia?

A: Such imaging is useful by noting the distribution pattern. Multiinfarct dementia is characterized by multiple areas of past infarcts, recognized as areas of decreased uptake that correspond to vascular distribution, as well as changes in the deep structures, such as the basal ganglia and thalamus. Alzheimer disease exhibits a characteristic pattern of bitemporal and parietal hypoperfusion and hypometabolism. Pick disease or frontal temporal dementia has decreased frontal lobe and temporal lobe uptake.

> **PEARL:** *Although Alzheimer disease has a characteristic bitemporal-parietal pattern on perfusion imaging, it is often not symmetrical. Decreased frontal lobe uptake may be seen in late-stage disease. Decreased uptake is also characteristically seen in the posterior cingulate and precuneus regions of the brain.*

> **PEARL:** *F-18 florbetapir (Amyvid) was approved to estimate β-amyloid neuritic plaque density in patients with cognitive impairment. A negative study rules out Alzheimer' disease as the cause. A study that is positive for amyloid plaques is not diagnostic of Alzheimer' disease because this may be seen in normal individuals without dementia.*

Q: What is the purpose of cerebral perfusion imaging in patients with seizures? What is the expected PET or SPECT pattern?

A: Interictal studies performed with F-18 FDG PET and Tc-99m HMPAO or ECD SPECT show decreased metabolism on FDG PET and decreased perfusion on SPECT. Increased activity is seen during a seizure (ictal). The SPECT tracer must be injected during the seizure. Imaging can be delayed because the tracer is fixed. The logistics of FDG PET make detection of a seizure focus unlikely.

CARDIAC

> **PEARL:** *Myocardial perfusion scintigraphy, whether performed with SPECT or PET, is a "map" of relative blood flow to viable myocardium. That is, for activity to be recorded in the image, it must be delivered (blood flow) and taken up by a myocardial cell (viable myocardium).*

Q: What percentage of Tc-99m sestamibi and Tc-99m tetrofosmin localizes in the heart?

A: Tc-99 sestamibi, 1.5%; tetrofosmin, 1.2%

Q: What quality control should be routinely performed to detect patient motion?

A: Review raw data in cinematic display. Review of the sinogram can also confirm motion.

> **PEARL:** *The best method for correcting the problem of patient motion is to repeat the study. If this is not possible, software motion-correction programs can be used. However, the software usually corrects for motion only in one axis, vertical. Motion typically occurs in multiple dimensions.*

> **PITFALL:** *Attenuation of photons by soft tissue can result in decreased activity seen in the myocardium, which might suggest myocardial infarction if seen on both rest and stress or as ischemia if only apparent on the stress study. With females, breast attenuation results in decreased activity of the anterior, septal, or lateral wall, depending on their size, shape, and position. Males characteristically have attenuation of the inferior wall, so-called diaphragmatic attenuation.*

Q: In what ways can the image interpreter determine whether fixed myocardial decreased activity is pathological (i.e., infarction) or merely caused by attenuation?

A: Review the raw data in the cinematic display to look for soft tissue attenuation. Review of the gated SPECT can help determine whether ventricular wall motion and thickening are present, which would indicate that it is not an infarction but, rather, the result of attenuation. Attenuation-correction programs can be helpful in differentiating attenuation from infarction.

> **PEARL:** *To correct for cardiac attenuation, a transmission map must be acquired. This can be done by acquiring transmission counts from a gamma source (e.g., gadolinium-153). Today, most commonly the CT portion of the SPECT/CT examination is used for attenuation correction.*

Q: What is the significance of exercise-induced dilation on SPECT perfusion studies?

A: The normal heart dilates during exercise stress, but gated SPECT images are acquired after stress, when normal hearts should have returned to baseline size. Poststress dilation suggests cardiac decompensation and three-vessel disease.

> **PEARL:** *Patients with left bundle branch block (LBBB) may have exercise-stress-inducible reversible hypoperfusion of the septum. Patients with true ischemia do not typically have isolated septal involvement but also have apical and anterior wall ischemia. This can be avoided by performing pharmacological stress in patients with LBBB.*

> **PEARL:** *The primary cause of a false-negative exercise study that results in the diagnosis of coronary artery disease is a failure to achieve an adequate exercise level.*

> **PEARL:** *After exercise stress, significant uptake in the liver usually indicates a poor exercise level was achieved. At peak exercise, blood flow is diverted from the splanchnic circulation.*

Q: What is the mechanism of action of dipyridamole and regadenoson?

A: Dipyridamole inhibits the reuptake of adenosine deaminase and thus augments the effects of endogenous adenosine. Regadenoson is a selective A2A coronary receptor.

Q: What effect can a cup of coffee have on pharmacological stress?

A: The types of caffeine in coffee, tea, soft drinks, or foods such as chocolate are chemically related and can block the effect of pharmacological stress testing.

Q: What percentage of stenosis at rest is necessary in the coronary arteries for resting blood flow to be affected?

A: Coronary artery stenosis greater than 85% to 90% is required before flow is diminished at rest. Not all stenoses are created equal. Long, irregular stenotic segments have more effect than discrete, short-segment stenoses.

Q: Why is imaging delayed for 30 to 60 minutes after administration of Tc-99m sestamibi or Tc-99m tetrofosmin?

A: Although myocardial uptake is rapid with both Tc-99m sestamibi and Tc-99m tetrofosmin, the lungs and liver also have high uptake. The lungs and liver clear with time, and the target-to-background ratio improves. The liver clears somewhat more rapidly with Tc-99m tetrofosmin.

Q: What are the considerations for selecting the number of frames in a gated blood-pool study?

A: Selecting the number of frames to divide the cardiac cycle is a balance between having enough frames to capture the peaks and valleys of the ventricular time–activity curve versus the need to acquire a statistically valid number of counts in each frame. Too many frames will increase the imaging time required for a given number of counts per frame. For gated ventriculography (multiple gated acquisition [MUGA]), using 16 frames achieves this compromise. For gated SPECT myocardial perfusion imaging, the usual compromise is 8 frames because of lesser counts. Too few frames will "average out" the peaks and valleys.

> **PEARL:** *Variations in the length of the cardiac cycle can be recognized on gated perfusion or blood-pool studies if the time–activity curve (ventricular volume curve) trails off or fails to approximate the height of the initial part of the curve.*

PULMONARY

Q: What are the two most commonly used radiopharmaceuticals for ventilation imaging? What are their advantages and disadvantages?

A: Xenon-133 and Tc-99m DTPA aerosol are commonly used. Xe-133 demonstrates the physiology of respiration and is very sensitive to the detection of obstructive airway disease, as manifested by delayed washout. The disadvantage is the normally rapid washout, limiting the views obtainable (with two-headed cameras, two views), and its suboptimal image quality that is due to the low photopeak (81 keV) and poor-count-rate images. Tc-99m DTPA aerosol results in high-count images in all projections; however, the images are similar to those with Xe-133 only in the inspiratory phase. With obstructive airway disease, particles become impacted in the proximal bronchi, and fewer get to the periphery of the lung, potentially causing interpretation difficulties.

> **PEARL:** *Xe-133 is fat soluble and will be taken up and cleared slowly from livers with fatty metamorphosis. This should not be confused with delayed pulmonary washout.*

Q: What is the minimum number of particles recommended for pulmonary perfusion imaging?

A: At least 100,000 particles are required for a statistically reliable image in normal adults; 300,000 to 400,000 particles are generally administered.

Q: What is the size range of macroaggregated albumin (MAA) particles?

A: In commercial preparations, the majority of particles are 20 to 40 μm (range, 10–90 μm).

> **PITFALL:** *Withdrawing blood into a syringe with Tc-99m MAA particles may result in a small radioactive embolus that shows up as a hot spot or hot spots on subsequent images. Failure to resuspend the Tc-99m MAA particles with gentle agitation before administration may result in clumping of particles together and the presence of hot spots on subsequent imaging.*

> **PEARL:** *Tc-99m MAA is used to confirm a right-to-left shunt. Uptake in the cerebral cortex is confirmatory. If no brain uptake is seen, no significant right-to-left shunt exists. Free Tc-99m pertechnetate does not localize in the brain cortex but, rather, in the thyroid, salivary glands, and stomach.*

Q: What is the preferred patient position during administration of Tc-99m MAA?

A: Administering Tc-99m MAA with the patient supine results in a more homogeneous distribution of particles in the lung than when the patient is sitting or standing. Gravitational effects result in more basilar distribution than when the injection is accomplished with the patient upright.

> **PITFALL:** *In the analysis of perfusion scintigrams, failure to recognize the significance of decreased versus absent activity is a potential pitfall. Not every clot is 100% occlusive of the circulation. Diminished activity needs to be recognized as one of the patterns caused by pulmonary emboli.*

> **PITFALL:** *The pulmonary hili on lung scans are relatively photon-deficient structures caused by the displacement of lung parenchyma by large vascular and bronchial structures. Failure to remember this might result in false-positive interpretations, especially for defects seen on posterior oblique images.*

> **PITFALL:** *If the patient is placed supine for ventilation–perfusion imaging but the chest radiograph was obtained with the patient upright, it can make correlation of the findings difficult. For example, free fluid may collect in a subpulmonic location or obscure the lung base in the upright position. With the patient supine, the fluid may layer out posteriorly or collect in the fissures. Also, the apparent height of the lungs may be different, as may the heart size. Ideally, imaging studies should be performed with the patient in the same position for all examinations. On the other hand, if significant pleural fluid is present, it may be desirable to image the patient in more than one position to prove that a defect is caused by mobile fluid.*

Q: What is the "stripe" sign?

A: The stripe sign refers to linear activity seen at the pleural surface of a proximal perfusion defect. Because pulmonary emboli are typically pleura based, the stripe sign suggests another diagnosis, often emphysema. Rarely, in the resolution of pulmonary emboli, a stripe sign can be seen as circulation is restored.

Q: What is the physiological basis for perfusion defects in areas of poor ventilation?

A: The classic response to hypoxia at the alveolar level is vasoconstriction. Shunting of blood away from the hypoxic lung zone maintains oxygen saturation.

Q: What is the classic appearance of multiple pulmonary emboli on lung ventilation–perfusion scintigraphy?

A: The classic appearance is multiple pleura-based, wedge-shaped areas of significantly diminished or absent perfusion. The size of the defects may vary from subsegmental to segmental or may even involve an entire lobe or lung. Ventilation is mismatched. The chest radiograph is clear, without infiltrates, atelectasis, or effusions in regions of perfusion–ventilation mismatches.

Dosimetry

Radiopharmaceutical	ADULT ADMINISTERED DOSE		Organ Receiving Highest Dose	DOSE TO TARGET ORGAN		TOTAL EFFECTIVE DOSE EQUIVALENT	
	mCi	MBq		rem	mg ray	rem	mSV
Iodine-123 (25% uptake)	0.200	7.5	Thyroid	2.4	24.0	0.008	0.1
Iodine-131 (25% uptake)	0.010	3.7	Thyroid	13.00	130.0	0.410	4.1
Tc-99m pertechnetate	5	185	Large intestine	1.150	11.5	0.24	2.4
Tc-99m MDP	20	0.74	Bone cortex	0.7	7.0	0.130	1.3
Tc-99m sestamibi	30	1110	Gallbladder	2.7	27.0	0.700	7.0
Tc99m tetrofosmin	40	1480	Gallbladder	4.4	44.0	1.000	10.0
Thallium-201	3	111	Kidneys	5.1	51.0	2.55	25
Tc-99m red blood cells	20	740	Heart	1.7	17.0	0.62	62
Tc-99m mebrofenin	5	185	Gallbladder	2.1	21.0	0.32	3.2
Tc-99m disofenin	5	185	Gallbladder	2.1	21.0	0.32	3.2
Tc-99m SC liver/marrow?	5	185	Liver	1.7	17.0	0.17	1.7
Tc-99m SC/egg white	2	74	Large intestine	0.66	6.6	0.14	1.4
Tc-99m DTPA liquid meal	1	37	Large intestine	0.48	4.5	0.08	0.8
In-111 DTPA liquid meal	0.2	7.4	Large intestine	1.8	18.0	0.2	2.0
Tc-99m DTPA aerosol	1	37	Bladder wall	0.17	1.7	0.023	0.23
Tc-99m DTPA renal	20	740	Bladder wall	5.4	54.0	0.12	1.2
Tc-99m MAG3	10	370	Bladder wall	0.33	3.3	0.065	0.65
Tc-99m DMSA	5	185	Renal cortex	5	51.0	0.09	0.9
Tc-99m MAA	4	148	Lungs	8.8	88.0	0.06	0.6
Xenon-133	20	750	Lungs	0.41	4.1	0.0026	0.03
Tc-99m Technegas	0.8	30	Lungs	0.41	4.1	0.555	5.55
Radionuclide cystography Tc-99m DTPA	1	37	Bladder	0.03	0.3	0.002	0.02
F-18 FDG	10	370	Bladder	5.9	59.0	0.703	7.03
Gallium 67 citrate	5	185	Colon	4.5	45.0	1.9	18.5
Tc-99m ECD	20	740	Bladder	2.5	25.0	0.82	8.2
Tc-99m HMPAO	20	740	Kidneys	3.5	35.0	1.28	12.8
Tc-99m HMPAO white blood cells	10	370	Spleen	5.6	56.0	0.63	6.3
In-111 leukocytes	0.5	185	Spleen	20	200.0	0.70	7.0
I-123 MIBG	10	370	Liver	0.1	1.0	0.50	5.0
In-111 OctreoScan	6	222	Bladder	6.1	60.5	2.61	26.1
In-111 DatScan	5	185	Bladder	1	12.0	0.39	3.9
Gallium-68 dotatate	5	185	Spleen	1.95	19.5	0.373	3.73
F-18 florbetapir (Amyvid)	10	370	Gallbladder	1.43	14.3	0.73	7.3

Continued

Radiopharmaceutical	ADULT ADMINISTERED DOSE		Organ Receiving Highest Dose	DOSE TO TARGET ORGAN		TOTAL EFFECTIVE DOSE EQUIVALENT	
	mCi	MBq		rem	mg ray	rem	mSV
F-18 flutemetamol (Vizamyl)	5	185	Gallbladder	5.3	53.0	0.59	5.9
F-18 florbetaben (Neuraceq)	8	296	Large intestine	1.15	11.5	0.56	5.6
F-18 fluorodeoxyglucose	10	370	Bladder	2.7	27.0	0.703	7.0
Ga-68 PMSA	4	148	Testes	0.95	9.5	0.3	3.0
F-18 PMSA	10	370	Kidneys	3.5	35.0	0.6	6
Rubidium 82	50	1850	Kidneys	3.3	33.0	0.37	3.7
Ammonia NH_3	20	740	Bladder	0.34	4.3	0.2	2.0
F-18 fluciclovine	10	370	Pancreas	3.8	38.0	0.8	8.0
Tc-99m tilmanocept (Lymphoseek)	0.5	18.5	Kidneys	0.03	0.3	0.03	0.3
F-18 sodium fluoride	10	370	Bladder	0.18	1.8	0.19	1.9
DEXA bone density						0.0001	0.001
CT scan—chest or abdomen						0.8	8

CT, Computed tomography; *DEXA,* dual-energy x-ray absorptiometry.

The Periodic Table of the Elements

Periodic Table of the Elements

1 IA 1A																	18 VIIIA 8A
1 H Hydrogen 1.008	2 IIA 2A											13 IIIA 3A	14 IVA 4A	15 VA 5A	16 VIA 6A	17 VIIA 7A	**2 He** Helium 4.003
3 Li Lithium 6.941	**4 Be** Beryllium 9.012											**5 B** Boron 10.811	**6 C** Carbon 12.011	**7 N** Nitrogen 14.007	**8 O** Oxygen 15.999	**9 F** Fluorine 18.998	**10 Ne** Neon 20.180
11 Na Sodium 22.990	**12 Mg** Magnesium 24.305	3 IIIB 3B	4 IVB 4B	5 VB 5B	6 VIB 6B	7 VIIB 7B	8 VIII 8	9 VIII 8	10 VIII 8	11 IB 1B	12 IIB 2B	**13 Al** Aluminum 26.982	**14 Si** Silicon 28.086	**15 P** Phosphorus 30.974	**16 S** Sulfur 32.066	**17 Cl** Chlorine 35.453	**18 Ar** Argon 39.948
19 K Potassium 39.098	**20 Ca** Calcium 40.078	**21 Sc** Scandium 44.956	**22 Ti** Titanium 47.867	**23 V** Vanadium 50.942	**24 Cr** Chromium 51.996	**25 Mn** Manganese 54.938	**26 Fe** Iron 55.845	**27 Co** Cobalt 58.933	**28 Ni** Nickel 58.693	**29 Cu** Copper 63.546	**30 Zn** Zinc 65.38	**31 Ga** Gallium 69.723	**32 Ge** Germanium 72.631	**33 As** Arsenic 74.922	**34 Se** Selenium 78.972	**35 Br** Bromine 79.904	**36 Kr** Krypton 83.798
37 Rb Rubidium 85.468	**38 Sr** Strontium 87.62	**39 Y** Yttrium 88.906	**40 Zr** Zirconium 91.224	**41 Nb** Niobium 92.906	**42 Mo** Molybdenum 95.95	**43 Tc** Technetium 98.907	**44 Ru** Ruthenium 101.07	**45 Rh** Rhodium 102.906	**46 Pd** Palladium 106.42	**47 Ag** Silver 107.868	**48 Cd** Cadmium 112.411	**49 In** Indium 114.818	**50 Sn** Tin 118.711	**51 Sb** Antimony 121.760	**52 Te** Tellurium 127.6	**53 I** Iodine 126.904	**54 Xe** Xenon 131.294
55 Cs Cesium 132.905	**56 Ba** Barium 137.328	57-71	**72 Hf** Hafnium 178.49	**73 Ta** Tantalum 180.948	**74 W** Tungsten 183.84	**75 Re** Rhenium 186.207	**76 Os** Osmium 190.23	**77 Ir** Iridium 192.217	**78 Pt** Platinum 195.085	**79 Au** Gold 196.967	**80 Hg** Mercury 200.592	**81 Tl** Thallium 204.383	**82 Pb** Lead 207.2	**83 Bi** Bismuth 208.980	**84 Po** Polonium [208.982]	**85 At** Astatine 209.987	**86 Rn** Radon 222.018
87 Fr Francium 223.020	**88 Ra** Radium 226.025	89-103	**104 Rf** Rutherfordium [261]	**105 Db** Dubnium [262]	**106 Sg** Seaborgium [266]	**107 Bh** Bohrium [264]	**108 Hs** Hassium [269]	**109 Mt** Meitnerium [278]	**110 Ds** Darmstadtium [281]	**111 Rg** Roentgenium [280]	**112 Cn** Copernicium [285]	**113 Nh** Nihonium [286]	**114 Fl** Flerovium [289]	**115 Mc** Moscovium [289]	**116 Lv** Livermorium [293]	**117 Ts** Tennessine [294]	**118 Og** Oganesson [294]

Symbol key:
- Atomic Number
- **Symbol**
- Name
- Atomic Mass

Lanthanide Series

57 La Lanthanum 138.905	**58 Ce** Cerium 140.116	**59 Pr** Praseodymium 140.908	**60 Nd** Neodymium 144.242	**61 Pm** Promethium 144.913	**62 Sm** Samarium 150.36	**63 Eu** Europium 151.964	**64 Gd** Gadolinium 157.25	**65 Tb** Terbium 158.925	**66 Dy** Dysprosium 162.500	**67 Ho** Holmium 164.930	**68 Er** Erbium 167.259	**69 Tm** Thulium 168.934	**70 Yb** Ytterbium 173.055	**71 Lu** Lutetium 174.967

Actinide Series

89 Ac Actinium 227.028	**90 Th** Thorium 232.038	**91 Pa** Protactinium 231.036	**92 U** Uranium 238.029	**93 Np** Neptunium 237.048	**94 Pu** Plutonium 244.064	**95 Am** Americium 243.061	**96 Cm** Curium 247.070	**97 Bk** Berkelium 247.070	**98 Cf** Californium 251.080	**99 Es** Einsteinium [254]	**100 Fm** Fermium 257.095	**101 Md** Mendelevium 258.1	**102 No** Nobelium 259.101	**103 Lr** Lawrencium [262]

Legend:
- Alkali Metal
- Alkaline Earth
- Transition Metal
- Basic Metal
- Semimetal
- Nonmetal
- Halogen
- Noble Gas
- Lanthanide
- Actinide

INDEX

Note: Page numbers followed by *f* refer to figures, by *t* to tables, and by *b* to boxes.